LIBRARY

College of Physicians and Surgeons
of British Columbia

Myeloma: Pathology, Diagnosis, and Treatment

Myeloma: Pathology, Diagnosis, and Treatment

Edited by

Stephen A. Schey
Professor of Plasma Cell Dyscrasias, King's College London;
Consultant Haematologist,
King's College Hospital NHS Foundation Trust, London, UK

Kwee L. Yong
Professor of Haematology, University College London;
Consultant Haematologist,
University College London Hospitals, London, UK

Robert Marcus
Consultant Haematologist,
King's College Hospital NHS Foundation Trust, London, UK

Kenneth C. Anderson
Kraft Family Professor of Medicine, Harvard Medical School;
Medical Director, Kraft Family Blood Donor Center,
Dana-Faber Cancer Institute, Boston, MA, USA

CAMBRIDGE
UNIVERSITY PRESS

2014

CAMBRIDGE
UNIVERSITY PRESS

University Printing House, Cambridge CB2 8BS, United Kingdom

Published in the United States of America by Cambridge University Press, NewYork

Cambridge University Press is part of the University of Cambridge.

It furthers the University's mission by disseminating knowledge in the pursuit of education, learning and research at the highest international levels of excellence.

www.cambridge.org
Information on this title: www.cambridge.org/9781107010574

© Cambridge University Press 2014

First published 2014

Printed in Spain by Grafos SA, Arte sobre papel

A catalog record for this publication is available from the British Library

Library of Congress Cataloging-in-Publication data
Myeloma (2013)
Myeloma : pathology, diagnosis, and treatment / edited by Stephen A. Schey, Kwee L. Yong, Robert Marcus, Kenneth C. Anderson.
p. ; cm.
Includes bibliographical references and index.
ISBN 978-1-107 01057-4 (Hardback)
I. Schey, Stephen A., editor of compilation.   II. Yong, Kwee L., editor of compilation.   III. Marcus, Robert, 1940– editor of compilation.
IV. Anderson, Kenneth C., editor of compilation.   V. Title.
[DNLM: 1. Multiple Myeloma. WH 540]
RC280.M37
616.99′418–dc23   2013027999

ISBN 978-1-107-01057-4 Hardback

....

Contents

Contents

Contributors

Pooja Advani
Department of Internal Medicine, State University
of New York at Buffalo, Buffalo, NY, USA

Kenneth C. Anderson
Harvard Medical School, and Kraft Family Blood
Donor Center, Dana-Faber Cancer Institute,
Boston, MA, USA

Nabeel Aslam
Department of Nephrology and Hypertension,
Mayo Clinic, Jacksonville, FL, USA

Kevin D. Boyd
Haemato-oncology Research Unit, Division of
Molecular Pathology, The Institute of Cancer
Research, Sutton, Surrey, UK

A. Broyl
Department of Hematology, University Hospital
Rotterdam, Rotterdam, Netherlands

Asher Alban Chanan-Khan
Department of Hematology and Oncology,
Mayo Clinic, Jacksonville, FL, USA

Andrew Chantry
Department of Oncology, Medical School,
The University of Sheffield, Sheffield, UK

Raymond L. Comenzo, MD
Blood Bank and Neely Cell Processing and Collection
Center; Division of Hematology-Oncology,
Department of Medicine, Tufts Medical Center;
and Tufts University School of Medicine, Boston,
MA, USA

Christopher P. Conlon
Nuffield Department of Medicine, John Radcliffe
Hospital, Oxford, UK

Shirley D'Sa
Department of Haematology, University College
London Hospital, London, UK

Meletios A. Dimopoulos
Department of Clinical Therapeutics, University
of Athens School of Medicine, Athens, Greece

Angela Dispenzieri
Division of Hematology, Mayo Clinic College
of Medicine, Rochester, MN, USA

Simon W. Dubrey
Department of Cardiology, Hillingdon and
Mount Vernon Hospitals NHS Trust, Middlesex;
Department of Cardiology, Royal Brompton and
Harefield NHS Trust, London; and Imperial College
School of Medicine, London, UK

Eve Gallop-Evans
Department of Clinical Oncology, Velindre Cancer
Centre, Cardiff, UK

Charise Gleason
Department of Hematology and Medical Oncology,
Winship Cancer Institute of Emory University,
Atlanta, GA, USA

T. Guglielmelli
Unit of Hematology, "S. Luigi Gonzaga" Hospital,
Orbassano, Torino, Italy

Suzanne R. Hayman
Division of Hematology, Mayo Clinic College of
Medicine, Rochester, MN, USA

Martin F. Kaiser
Haemato-oncology Research Unit, Division of
Molecular Pathology, The Institute of Cancer
Research, Sutton, Surrey, UK

Efstathios Kastritis
Department of Clinical Therapeutics, University of Athens School of Medicine, Athens, Greece

Asim Khwaja
Department of Haematology, University College London, and University College London Hospitals NHS Trust, London, UK

Jacob Laubach
Hematologic Malignancies Center, Dana-Faber Cancer Institute, Boston, MA, USA

Sagar Lonial
Department of Hematology and Medical Oncology, Winship Cancer Institute of Emory University, Atlanta, GA, USA

Robert Marcus
King's College Hospital NHS Foundation Trust, London, UK

Giampaolo Merlini
Department of Biochemistry, University of Pavia, and Biotechnology Research Laboratories, University Hospital Policlinico San Matteo, Pavia, Italy

Gareth J. Morgan
Haemato-oncology Research Unit, Division of Molecular Pathology, The Institute of Cancer Research, Sutton, Surrey, UK

Paul Moss
School of Cancer Sciences, University of Birmingham, Edgbaston, Birmingham, UK

Nicola Mulholland
Department of Nuclear Medicine, King's College Hospital, London, UK

Roger Owen
HMDS Laboratory, St James' University Hospital, Leeds, UK

Antonio Palumbo
Myeloma Unit, Division of Hematology, University of Torino, Torino, Italy

Aneel Paulus
Department of Hematology and Oncology, Mayo Clinic, Jacksonville, FL, USA

Guy Pratt
Department of Haematology, School of Cancer Sciences, University of Birmingham, Edgbaston, Birmingham, UK

John Quinn
Department of Haematology, RCSI/Beaumont Hospital, Dublin, Ireland

Neil Rabin
Department of Haematology, University College London Hospitals NHS Trust, London, UK

Karthik Ramasamy
Department of Haematology, Oxford University Hospitals NHS Trust and Royal Berkshire NHS Foundation Trust, UK

Paul Richardson
Hematologic Malignancies Center, Dana-Faber Cancer Institute, Boston, MA, USA

Eve Roman
Department of Health Sciences and Hull York Medical School, University of York, York, UK

Stephen A. Schey
Department of Haematology, King's College London, and King's College Hospital NHS Foundation Trust, London, UK

Alexandra G. Smith
Department of Health Sciences and Hull York Medical School, University of York, York, UK

P. Sonneveld
Department of Hematology, University Hospital Rotterdam, Rotterdam, Netherlands

Matthew J. Streetly
Department of Haematology, Guy's and St Thomas' NHS Foundation Trust, London, UK

Yu-Tzu Tai
Department of Medical Oncology, Dana-Farber Cancer Institute, Harvard Medical School, Boston, MA, USA

Steven P. Treon
Bing Center for Waldenstrom's Macroglobulinemia, Dana Farber Cancer Institute, Harvard Medical School, Boston, MA, USA

Ming Young Simon Wan
Department of Radiology, King's College Hospital, London, UK

Melanie Watson
Department of Hematology and Medical Oncology, Winship Cancer Institute of Emory University, Atlanta, GA, USA

Ashutosh D. Wechalekar
National Amyloidosis Centre, University College London Medical School, London, UK

Kwee L. Yong
UCL Cancer Institute, University College London, London, UK

Epidemiology of myeloma

Eve Roman and Alexandra G. Smith

Introduction

Epidemiology is the basic quantitative science of public health; and as such is concerned with the distribution, determinants, treatment, management and potential control of disease. Concentrating on the first two of these, this chapter reviews the epidemiology of myeloma, which accounts for around 1%–2% of all newly diagnosed cancers, and 10%–15% of all newly diagnosed hematological malignancies [1,2].

Descriptive epidemiology

The accurate description of underlying disease patterns and trends provides the foundation for etiological research [3], hence before considering the epidemiology of myeloma in any depth issues relating to disease ascertainment and classification are briefly discussed below.

Cancer ascertainment and classification

Whilst cancer registration has a long history in many countries, particularly those in the more affluent regions of the world, nearly 80% of the global population is not covered by such systems [1]. Furthermore, for hematological cancers, information gathering and dissemination has long been acknowledged to be a major problem even in countries that have adequate collations processes. These concerns were summarized in EUROCARE 4 in their 2009 statement that *"the evolving classification and poor standardization of data collection on haematological malignancies vitiate the comparison of disease incidence and survival over time and across regions"* [4]. The main issue here is that, unlike many other cancers, the majority of hematological neoplasms are diagnosed by using multiple parameters, including a combination of histology, cytology, immunophenotyping, cytogenetics, imaging

and clinical information. This range and depth of data is difficult for cancer registries and other researchers to access routinely, forming a barrier both to complete ascertainment and to the collection of diagnostic data at the level of detail required to systematically implement the latest disease classifications. Hence although WHO's 2001 consensus classification of hematological malignancies [5,6] and its successor [2] were adopted into clinical practice almost uniformly around the world, their publication had no immediate effect on population-based cancer registration systems, where data on hematological malignancies continue to be largely presented using the four broad ICD-10 [7] groupings of multiple myeloma, leukemia, non-Hodgkin lymphoma and Hodgkin lymphoma [8–10].

Whilst continued use of ICD-10 may not be as challenging for the myelomas as it is for lymphomas and leukemias, the appropriateness of this topographic classification (which includes, for example, historical entities such as plasma cell leukemia) undoubtedly impacts on the accuracy of the cancer registration process. Misdiagnosis and undernumeration are particularly problematic for multiple myeloma since, in contrast to many other non-hematological cancers, diagnosis and need for treatment are based on a combination of laboratory tests and clinical findings [2,11,12]. Patients with symptomatic multiple myeloma often present at older ages (see variations with age and sex below) with intermittent and nonspecific symptoms such as bone pain in the back or chest, as well as general fatigue. Such symptoms are relatively common in the general population, particularly in older people, and patients may present late and referral to appropriate specialists may be delayed.

In addition to symptomatic disease, in countries with well-developed health care systems, around one in five myelomas are diagnosed in patients who have no obvious symptoms; such asymptomatic "smoldering" myelomas often being detected through routine blood tests taken for other purposes [12,13]. Furthermore, in addition to smoldering myeloma, pre-malignant monoclonal plasma cell proliferation is estimated to occur in around 3%–4% of those over 50 years in populations of European descent, resulting in the asymptomatic disorder Monoclonal Gammopathy of Undetermined Significance (MGUS) [14]. MGUS, which like asymptomatic myeloma is usually diagnosed incidentally, is poorly captured by most cancer registries since it is grouped in ICD-10 with other neoplasms of uncertain or unknown behavior (D47). Accordingly, most information about the epidemiology of MGUS is derived from specialist patient cohorts [14–19]. With respect to pathogenic process, both MGUS and smoldering myeloma are associated with increased risks of multiple myeloma, the estimated progression rates being around 1% and 10% per year respectively [2,13].

Variations in incidence with age and sex

With a median age of diagnosis of around 73 years, and hardly any cases recorded before 40 years of age, myeloma is predominantly a disease of older people [8,18,20,21]. The strong relationship with older age, together with the fact that the disease is around 40%–50% more common in men than women, is clearly evident in Figure 1.1 which shows the average number of cases and age-specific rates recorded in the

UK 2006–08. The trends with age and sex are similar to those reported by other population-based registers: the incidence rising steeply with age and the sex-specific curves diverging as age increases. In affluent regions of the world such as the UK, the fact that more diagnoses occur in women in the oldest age group reflects the fact that more women than men survive to reach old age.

Evidence from specialist registers in Sweden, the USA and the UK suggest that the age and sex distributions of patients diagnosed with MGUS are broadly similar to those of patients diagnosed with myeloma [14,19,22]. This is illustrated in Figure 1.2 where data on myeloma (ICD-03, M9731/3-9732/3) and MGUS (ICD-O3, M9765/1) diagnosed over the six years 2004–10 in the UK's specialist population-based Haematological Malignancy Research Network (www.HMRN.org) are shown. This register collects information on all hematological malignancies and pre-malignancies diagnosed within two UK Cancer Networks (population 3.6 million); and for comparability purposes (Figure 1.2), the numbers of cases are scaled-up to the UK as a whole [18,22]. The similarity between the two distributions is striking: the median ages at diagnosis and age-standardized sex-rate ratios respectively being 73.0 years and 1.4 for myeloma and 72.2 years and 1.4 for MGUS.

Changes over time

Monitoring disease trends over time is a fundamental activity of descriptive epidemiology, with such analyses often yielding important etiological clues.

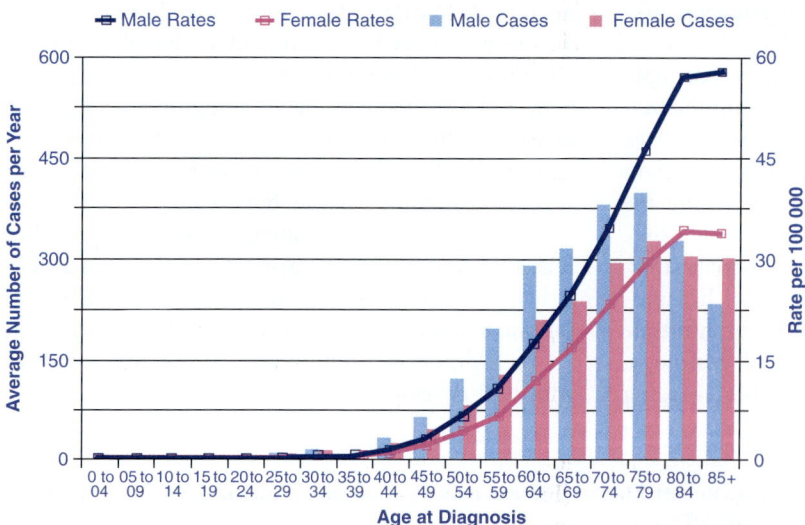

Figure 1.1 Age-specific incidence of myeloma (ICD-10, C90); UK 2006–2008.

(a)

(b)

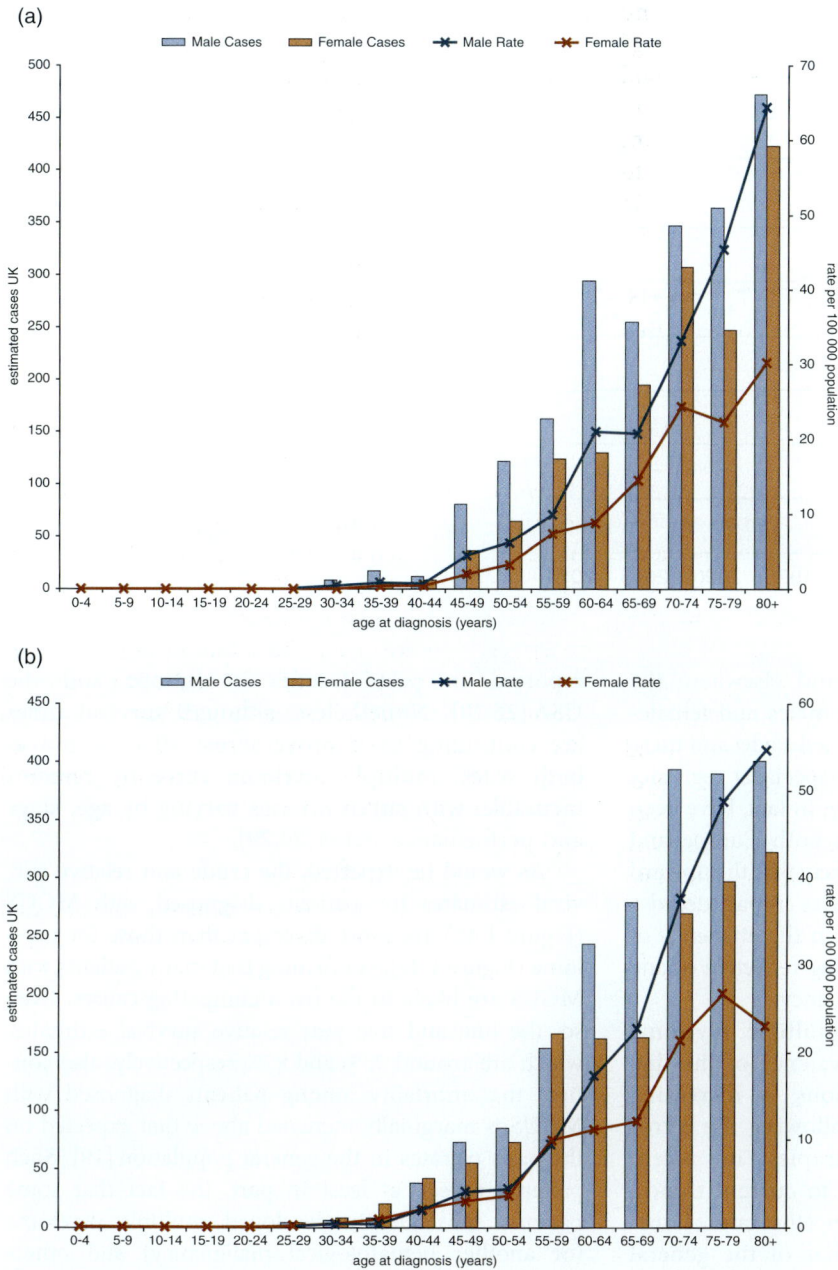

Figure 1.2 Age-specific incidence of (a) myeloma and (b) MGUS (ICD-O3, M9732/3 + 9731/3 and 9765/1 respectively); HMRN 2004–10.

Indeed, there are many examples in the field of cancer epidemiology where this has been the case, particularly in relation to the identification of hazardous occupational and environmental exposures. In this context, the temporal changes reported for myeloma in earlier decades are marked, as can be seen from Figure 1.3, which shows the estimated age-adjusted incidence rates from the Surveillance, Epidemiology and End Results (SEER) Program in the United States (www.seer.cancer.gov).

The increase in the estimated incidence of myeloma seen in the SEER registries in the 1970s and 1980s (Figure 1.3) was mirrored in England and Wales, as well as several other European populations [20,23].

3

• Male Rate — Male Modeled Rate ♦ Female Rate — Female Modeled Rate

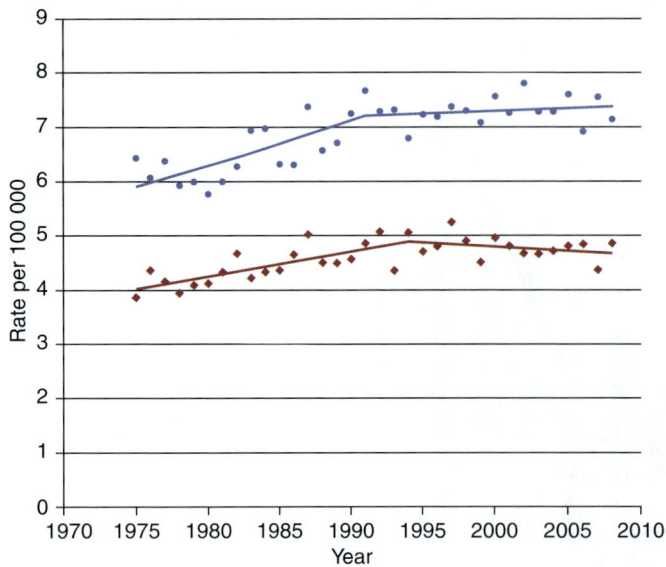

Figure 1.3 Age-adjusted incidence rates by sex; SEER 9 areas (San Francisco, Connecticut, Detroit, Hawaii, Iowa, New Mexico, Seattle, Utah and Atlanta), 1975–2008.

However, in the SEER regions and elsewhere the estimated rates of disease in both males and females have been stable now for more than a decade; and there is evidence from several long-term specialist registries that the age-adjusted incidence may, in fact, have been stable in the 1960s and 1970s in both Europe and America [20,24]. Indeed, it seems likely that the upward trend seen in many national registries in past decades may have been due to an increase in the efficiency of case ascertainment, rather than being reflective of any underlying increase in disease frequency.

Although the incidence of multiple myeloma may be relatively stable, the prevalence of the disease in more affluent populations is increasing markedly as survival improves following the introduction of several novel therapies in recent decades [11,25–29]. With respect to current trends, crude and relative survival curves (the rate of survival of patients compared to that of the general population) of patients newly diagnosed with myeloma (ICD-03, M9731/3 -9732/3; N = 1226) and/or MGUS (ICD-O3, M9765/1; N = 1134) in the UK's HMRN region 2004–9 (followed through to December 2011) are shown in Figure 1.4. The one and five year relative survival estimates for multiple myeloma diagnosed at any age were around 72% (85% < 60 years; 68% ≥ 60 years) and 41% (64% < 60 years; 34% ≥ 60 years) respectively. These population-based estimates are roughly twice those

reported in past decades in Europe and the USA [26,29]. Nonetheless, although survival times are continuing to improve across all ages and in both sexes, multiple myeloma currently remains incurable, with survival times varying by age, stage and performance status [26,29].

As would be expected, the crude and relative survival estimates for patients diagnosed with MGUS (Figure 1.4b) are more divergent than those for myeloma (Figure 1.4a); confirming that many patients with MGUS are likely to die from competing causes. Even so, the one and five year relative survival estimates, which are around 93% and 87% respectively, also confirm that mortality among patients diagnosed with MGUS is marginally increased above that expected on the basis of rates in the general population [19]. Such patterns reflect, at least in part, the fact that some patients subsequently developed multiple myeloma (or another hematological malignancy) and others had MGUS detected as part of routine testing for another more serious disease. The potential contribution that MGUS itself may play is currently unknown.

International incidence variations and ethnicity

Incidence rates from IARC's most recent series of estimates are shown in Figures 1.5 and 1.6. Of the

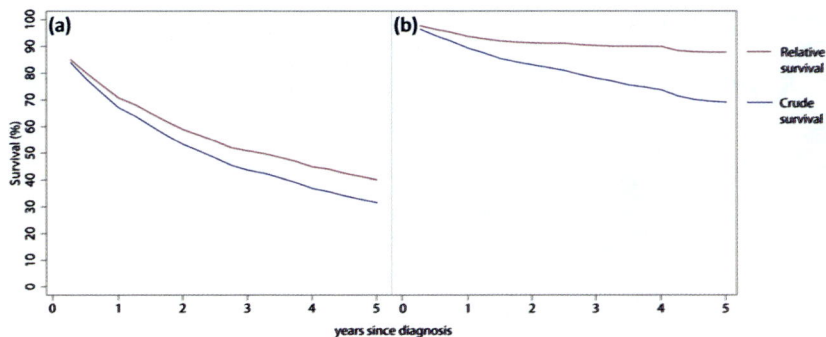

Figure 1.4 Crude and relative survival of (a) myeloma and (b) MGUS (ICD-O3 = M9732/3 + 9731/3 and 9765/1 respectively); HMRN diagnoses 2004–2009, followed-up to end of 2011.

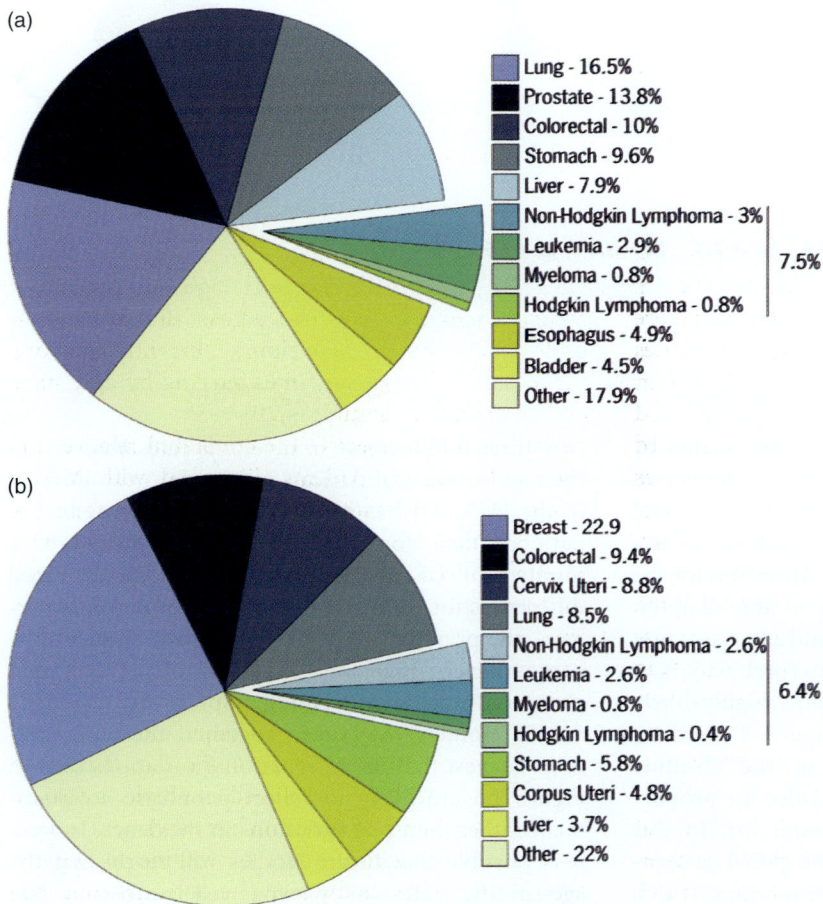

Figure 1.5 Estimated global cancer frequency for (a) males and (b) females; GLOBOCAN.

12.67 million new cancers estimated to have occurred around the world in 2008, 6.62 million were in men and 6.05 million were in women (Figure 1.5). Combined, hematological malignancies were estimated to comprise around 7.5% of cancers in males and 6.4% in females, with myelomas accounting for around 12% of hematological malignancies in both men and women (www.globocan.iarc.fr/).

The age-standardized incidence rates for both sexes combined are globally distributed in Figure 1.6.

5

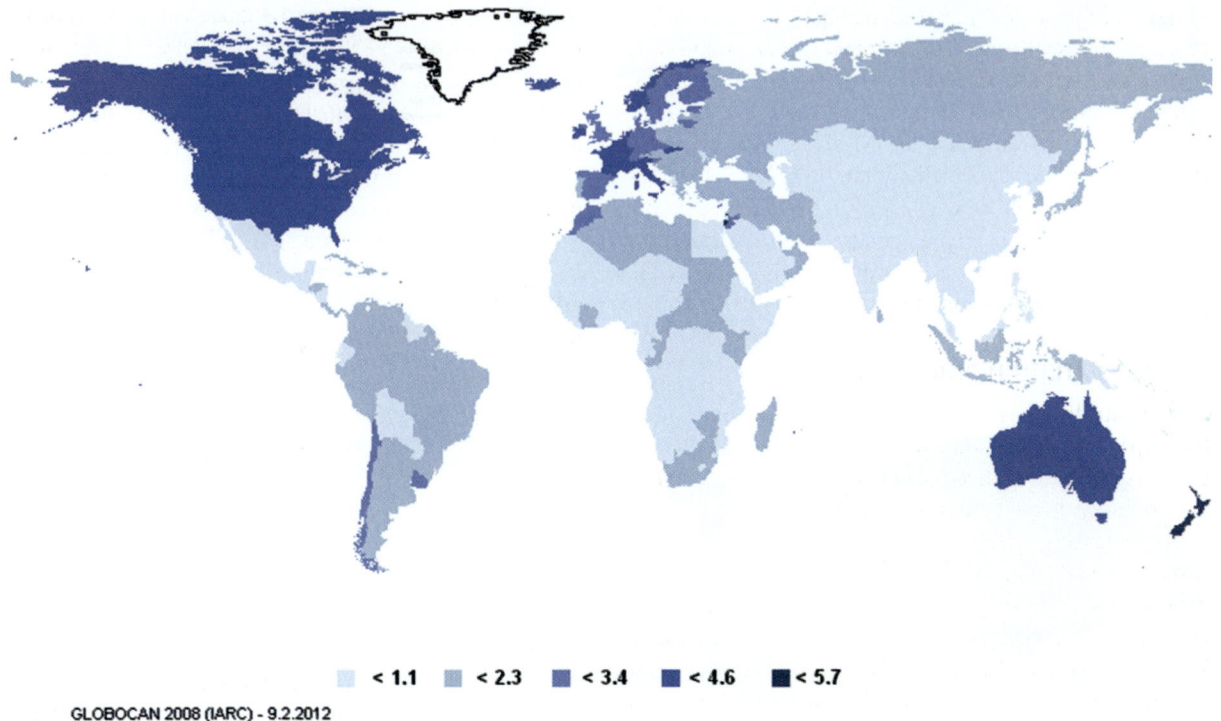

Figure 1.6 Estimated numbers and age-standardized (world population) incidence rates by region for myeloma, both sexes combined; GLOBOCAN.

In general, the geographical pattern is dominated by the high rates in the more economically developed regions of the world: the estimated rates being several fold higher in North America, Europe and Australasia than in large parts of Africa and Asia. However, for the reasons stated in previous sections of this chapter, problems with disease classification and ascertainment make these patterns difficult to interpret with any degree of confidence. Indeed, it seems highly likely that the global estimates shown in Figures 1.3 and 1.4 are conservative, both in terms of the absolute numbers of myelomas occurring and also the proportion of total cancers that they account for. In this regard it is interesting to note that the global patterning of other cancers, including the lymphomas which share many of the same ascertainment problems as myeloma, are broadly similar to that shown in Figure 1.6 [10,30].

Significantly, there is also accumulating evidence that, compared with persons of European descent, both myeloma and MGUS are, in fact, at least twice as common in persons of African descent and lower in those of Asian descent [9,16,17,31–34]. Indeed, the two–three fold increase in myeloma rates observed in men and women of African descent for over 40 years in the USA [34] has recently been confirmed in UK national data for 2003–2006 [9]. Furthermore, a number of US studies have shown similar racial differences for MGUS [14,31]. More importantly perhaps, the prevalence of MGUS has been shown to be comparatively high in Ghanaian men [17,35] and comparatively low in Japanese populations, especially among women [16]. Taken together, these observations suggest that the international variations seen in Figure 1.6 are likely to reflect poor case ascertainment rather than real variations in incidence. Indeed, it is possible that future studies will reveal that the age-specific rates of plasma cell neoplasms are highest in Africa and lowest in Asia.

Etiology

As with most cancers, the causal pathway leading to the development of myeloma is likely to involve the interaction of several individual genetic and environmental components. Examination of descriptive epidemiological patterns and trends (see above) has revealed associations with increasing age, male sex, and ethnicity; the prevalence of MGUS displaying broadly similar associations [15–18,35], although interestingly no increase in MGUS with age was found in the survey of Ghanaian men [17]. In addition, MGUS itself is a precursor to multiple myeloma, but the frequency of progression is quite low, seemingly occurring at a constant rate of around 1% per year in all populations that have been studied [31].

Genetic variation and family history

Several studies have reported that first-degree relatives (parent, sibling or child) of myeloma or MGUS patients are two to three times more likely to develop myeloma or MGUS themselves, in comparison with people without a close family history of these conditions [36–39]. This, coupled with the distributional differences with ethnicity and sex, has resulted in considerable speculation and wide-ranging research in the area of genetic susceptibility [40–42].

Neither myeloma nor MGUS are single disease entities [13,44], and it seems likely that genetic variation in several pathways could contribute to their pathogenesis. Genes of interest obviously include those involved in normal plasma cell development, as well as inflammation and immune response. In addition, genes involved in key metabolic pathways such as DNA repair, the metabolism of folate and the metabolism of various xenobiotics have received much attention [43,45]. Thus far, however, few consistent genetic findings have emerged; although results from a recent genome-wide association study (GWAS) in a European population led investigators to conclude that genetically determined dysregulation of *MYC* could be a common mechanism underlying several mature B-cell malignancies [40].

Infections and immunity

As with other mature B-cell malignancies, associations with infection and factors potentially causing immune dysregulation have been the focus of much of the etiological research on plasma cell malignancies conducted to date. In general, for broad categories of autoimmune, infectious and inflammatory conditions relative risks ranging between 1.1 and 1.5 have been reported for both subsequent myeloma and MGUS development – such risks being similar to, but weaker than, those seen for many of the lymphomas [46,47].

In general, reported relationships have tended to be non-specific, one of the most consistent associations being that seen for pernicious anemia, although the underpinning mechanism remains to be elucidated [46,47]. In addition, as might be expected, the risks of both myeloma and MGUS have been observed to be increased in immunocompromised individuals, such as transplant recipients and those infected with HIV, although again the magnitudes are generally smaller than those seen for many of the non-Hodgkin lymphomas [14,48].

Diet and obesity

As well as infectious agents and comorbidities associated with the immune system, several recent studies have reported on the relationship between anthropometric characteristics and myeloma and/or MGUS [49–52]. Increased risks ranging from around 1.1 to 2.0 have been reported for obesity, measured as having a body mass indexes (BMI kg/m^2) of 30 or more; and studies that have used other anthropometric measures, such as waist-to-hip ratio, have found similar results [49–52]. Importantly, as with the associations for autoimmunity these relationships are similar to those reported for other B-cell malignancies – and indeed for several other cancers [49,53]. The important public health message here being that, if such associations are real, then disease could be prevented by maintaining a healthy body weight. However, whilst a wide - range of biological mechanisms have been suggested as possible explanations for the association between excess body weight and plasma cell myeloma, including the effects on growth factor signaling and various inflammatory processes, the underpinning mechanisms remain to be clarified (49–53).

Environmental exposures

A number of studies have examined the relation between myeloma and various physical and chemical exposures, notably ionizing radiation in the case of the former and various organic compounds in the case of the latter. Ionizing radiation is mutagenic, but debate surrounds the potentially hazardous effects of exposure at the low-levels encountered in some workplaces (such as nuclear plants) and certain medical procedures (such as X-rays). With respect to myeloma, the available evidence does not support an association with levels of exposure [54,55]. Likewise, evidence that myeloma is associated with exposure to organic pesticides and/or solvents is weak and inconsistent [56,57].

Conclusion

Multiple myeloma is currently incurable, accounting for around 10% of all hematological malignancies in Western populations. It is a heterogeneous disease with respect to presentation, biological characteristics and response to treatment; its etiology is poorly understood. Currently, the main identified risk factors are old age, male sex, personal history of MGUS, family history of plasma cell disease, and African ethnicity; and the underpinning reasons for these associations are the subject of current research. Within populations, disease incidence is comparatively stable but, following the introduction of new therapies, disease prevalence is rising markedly.

References

1. Ferlay, J., Shin, H.-R., Bray, F., et al. Estimates of worldwide burden of cancer in 2008: GLOBOCAN 2008. Int. J. Cancer 2010;**127**(12):2893–917.

2. Swerdlow, S. WHO classification of tumours of haematopoietic and lymphoid tissues, 4th edn. Lyon France: International Agency for Research on Cancer; 2008.

3. Boyle, P. World cancer report 2008. Lyon: IARC Press; 2008.

4. Sant, M., Allemani, C., Santaquilani, M., et al. EUROCARE-4. Survival of cancer patients diagnosed in 1995–1999. Results and commentary. Eur. J. Cancer. 2009;**45**(6):931–91.

5. Jaffe, E., World Health Organization. Pathology and genetics of tumours of haematopoietic and lymphoid tissues. Lyon; Oxford: IARC Press; Oxford University Press (distributor); 2001.

6. Fritz, A. International classification of diseases for oncology: ICD-O. 3rd edn. Geneva: World Health Organization; 2000.

7. International statistical classification of diseases and related health problems, ICD-10. Vol. 3, Alphabetical index. Geneva: World Health Organization; 1994.

8. Siegel, R., Naishadham, D., Jemal, A. Cancer statistics, 2012. CA Cancer J. Clin. 2012;**62**(1):10–29.

9. National Cancer Intelligence Network. Cancer incidence and survival by major ethnic group, England, 2002–2006 [Internet]. 2009; Available from: http://www.ncin.org.uk/publications/reports/default.aspx

10. Ferlay, J., Shin, H.-R., Bray, F., et al. Estimates of worldwide burden of cancer in 2008: GLOBOCAN 2008. Int. J. Cancer [Internet]. 2010 Jun 17 [cited 2010 Aug 26]; Available from: http://www.ncbi.nlm.nih.gov/pubmed/20560135

11. Rajkumar, S. V., Gahrton, G., Bergsagel, P. L. Approach to the treatment of multiple myeloma: a clash of philosophies. Blood 2011;**118**(12):3205–11.

12. Bird, J. M., Owen, R. G., D'Sa, S., et al. Guidelines for the diagnosis and management of multiple myeloma 2011. Br. J. Haematol. 2011;**154**(1):32–75.

13. Landgren, O. Monoclonal gammopathy of undetermined significance and smoldering myeloma: new insights into pathophysiology and epidemiology. ASH Education Program Book. 2010 December **4**(1):295–302.

14. Wadhera, R. K., Rajkumar, S. V. Prevalence of monoclonal gammopathy of undetermined significance: a systematic review. Mayo Clin. Proc. 2010;**85**(10):933–42.

15. Kyle, R. A., Therneau, T. M., Rajkumar, S. V., et al. Prevalence of monoclonal gammopathy of undetermined significance. N. Engl. J. Med. 2006;**354**(13):1362–9.

16. Iwanaga, M., Tagawa, M., Tsukasaki, K., Kamihira, S., Tomonaga, M. Prevalence of monoclonal gammopathy of undetermined significance: study of 52,802 persons in Nagasaki City, Japan. Mayo Clin. Proc. 2007;**82**(12):1474–9.

17. Landgren, O., Katzmann, J. A., Hsing, A. W., et al. Prevalence of monoclonal gammopathy of undetermined significance among men in Ghana. Mayo Clin. Proc. 2007;**82**(12):1468–73.

18. Smith, A., Howell, D., Patmore, R., Jack, A., Roman, E. Incidence of haematological malignancy by sub-type: a report from the Haematological Malignancy Research Network. Br. J. Cancer 2011;**105**(11):1684–92.

19. Kristinsson, S. Y., Björkholm, M., Andersson, T. M.-L., et al. Patterns of survival and causes of death following a diagnosis of monoclonal gammopathy of undetermined significance: a population-based study. Haematologica 2009;**94**(12):1714–20.

20. Turesson, I., Velez, R., Kristinsson, S. Y., Landgren, O. Patterns of multiple myeloma during the past 5 decades: stable incidence rates for all age groups in the population but rapidly changing age distribution in the clinic. Mayo Clin. Proc. 2010;**85**(3):225–30.

21. Phekoo, K. J., Schey, S. A., Richards, M. A., *et al.* A population study to define the incidence and survival of multiple myeloma in a National Health Service Region in UK. *Br. J. Haematol.* 2004;**127**(3):299–304.

22. Smith, A., Roman, E., Howell, D., *et al.* The Haematological Malignancy Research Network (HMRN): a new information strategy for population based epidemiology and health service research. *Br. J. Haematol.* 2010;**148**(5):739–53.

23. Levi, F., Lucchini, F., Negri, E., Boyle, P., La Vecchia, C. Cancer mortality in Europe, 1995–1999, and an overview of trends since 1960. *Int. J. Cancer* 2004;**110**(2): 155–69.

24. Kyle, R. A., Therneau, T. M., Rajkumar, S. V., *et al.* Incidence of multiple myeloma in Olmsted County, Minnesota: trend over 6 decades. *Cancer* 2004;**101**(11): 2667–74.

25. Kaya, H., Peressini, B., Jawed, I., *et al.* Impact of age, race and decade of treatment on overall survival in a critical population analysis of 40,000 multiple myeloma patients. *Int. J. Hematol.* 2012;**95**(1):64–70.

26. Pulte, D., Gondos, A., Brenner, H. Improvement in survival of older adults with multiple myeloma: results of an updated period analysis of SEER data. *The Oncologist* 2011; **16**(11):1600–3.

27. Kumar, S. K., Rajkumar, S. V., Dispenzieri, A., *et al.* Improved survival in multiple myeloma and the impact of novel therapies. *Blood* 2008;**111**(5):2516–20.

28. Raab, M. S., Podar, K., Breitkreutz, I., Richardson, P. G., Anderson, K. C. Multiple myeloma. *Lancet* 2009;**374** (9686):324–39.

29. Renshaw, C., Ketley, N., Møller, H., Davies, E. A. Trends in the incidence and survival of multiple myeloma in South East England 1985–2004. *BMC Cancer* 2010;**10**:74.

30. Roman, E., Smith, A. G. Epidemiology of lymphomas. *Histopathology* 2011;**58**(1):4–14.

31. Greenberg, A. J., Vachon, C. M., Rajkumar, S. V. *Disparities in the prevalence, pathogenesis and progression of monoclonal gammopathy of undetermined significance and multiple myeloma between blacks and whites.* *Leukemia* [Internet]. 2011 Dec 23 [cited 2012 Feb 9]; Available from: http://www.ncbi.nlm.nih.gov/ pubmed/22193966

32. Waxman, A. J., Mink, P. J., Devesa, S. S., *et al.* Racial disparities in incidence and outcome in multiple myeloma: a population-based study. *Blood* 2010;**116**(25):5501–6.

33. Jemal, A., Siegel, R., Xu, J., Ward, E. Cancer statistics, 2010. *CA Cancer J. Clin.* 2010;**60**(5): 277–300.

34. Howlader, N., Noone, A. M., Krapcho, M., *et al. SEER Cancer Statistics Review* 1975–2008 [Internet]. [cited 2012 Feb 19]; Available from: http://seer.cancer. gov/csr/1975_2008/

35. Landgren, O, Weiss, B. M. Patterns of monoclonal gammopathy of undetermined significance and multiple myeloma in various ethnic/racial groups: support for genetic factors in pathogenesis. *Leukemia* 2009;**23**(10):1691–7.

36. Landgren, O., Kristinsson, S. Y., Goldin, L. R., *et al.* Risk of plasma cell and lymphoproliferative disorders among 14621 first-degree relatives of 4458 patients with monoclonal gammopathy of undetermined significance in Sweden. *Blood* 2009;**114**(4): 791–5.

37. Kristinsson, S. Y., Björkholm, M., Goldin, L. R., *et al.* Patterns of hematologic malignancies and solid tumors among 37,838 first-degree relatives of 13,896 patients with multiple myeloma in Sweden. *Int. J. Cancer* 2009; **125**(9):2147–50.

38. Vachon, C. M., Kyle, R. A., Therneau, T. M., *et al.* Increased risk of monoclonal gammopathy in first-degree relatives of patients with multiple myeloma or monoclonal gammopathy of undetermined significance. *Blood* 2009;**114** (4):785–90.

39. Greenberg, A. J., Rajkumar, S. V., Vachon, C. M. Familial monoclonal gammopathy of undetermined significance and multiple myeloma: epidemiology, risk factors and biological characteristics. *Blood* 2012;**119** (23):5359–66.

40. Broderick, P., Chubb, D., Johnson, D. C., *et al.* Common variation at 3p22.1 and 7p15.3 influences multiple myeloma risk. *Nat. Genet.* 2012;**44**(1): 58–61.

41. Boyd, K. D., Ross, F. M., Chiecchio, L., *et al.* Gender disparities in the tumor genetics and clinical outcome of multiple myeloma. *Cancer Epidemiol. Biomarkers Prevention* 2011; **20**(8):1703–7.

42. Purdue, M. P., Lan, Q., Menashe, I., *et al.* Variation in innate immunity genes and risk of multiple myeloma. *Hematol. Oncol.* 2011;**29**(1):42–6.

43. Vangsted, A., Klausen, T. W., Vogel, U. Genetic variations in multiple myeloma I: effect on risk of multiple myeloma. *Eur. J. Haematol.* 2012;**88**(1): 8–30.

44. Hervé, A.-L., Florence, M., Philippe, M., *et al.* Molecular heterogeneity of multiple myeloma: pathogenesis, prognosis, and therapeutic implications. *J. Clin. Oncol.* 2011;**29**(14):1893–7.

9

Clonality assessment using kappa and lambda can also be incorporated into these assays but it is not essential as previous extensive evaluation has conclusively proven that aberrant phenotype plasma cells are monotypic [10,11].

It is now widely accepted that, in addition to the morphological assessment of bone marrow aspirate smears and trephine biopsy sections, a diagnosis of myeloma should be confirmed by demonstrating monoclonality and/or an aberrant plasma cell phenotype. Flow cytometry should not be used to formally assess the extent of infiltration as it systematically underscores the extent of disease typically due to the fact that first-pull aspirates are used for morphology and second-pull specimens for additional assessments such as flow cytometry, cytogenetics and FISH [10,14]. Flow enumeration is, however, more reproducible than morphology and appears to be a better predictor of outcome in patients with symptomatic myeloma with a cut-off value of 15% being most informative [14].

One of the principal advantages of the flow cytometry assays is the ability to identify and enumerate both normal and neoplastic plasma cells when they are present within the same sample. This is useful in the routine diagnostic setting as the majority of patients with myeloma have exclusively aberrant plasma cells while the majority of patients with MGUS have some residual normal plasma cells [14–18]. It is essential, however, that final diagnoses are not made solely on the basis of these immunophenotypic patterns as ultimately diagnoses depend on the overall level of marrow infiltration and the associated clinical features [1]. It has also been established that the plasma cell populations in lymphoproliferative disorders such marginal zone lymphoma (MZL) and Waldenstrom macroglobulinemia (WM) also differ considerably from that seen in MM [19–22]. This is very useful in the definitive diagnosis of IgM myeloma and extramedullary plasmacytoma (EMP) (see below). The assessment of BMPC is also a highly informative technique in patients with primary AL amyloidosis and solitary plasmacytoma of bone (see relevant chapters) [23,24].

Plasma cell phenotyping may also be achieved by using immunohistochemistry on bone marrow trephine biopsies and other tissue specimens. In this regard the most useful antibodies to identify plasma cells are CD138 and MUM1/IRF4 whose expression at least in the context of bone marrow pathology appears to be confined to plasma cells. It is useful to use both CD138 and MUM1/IRF4 as the former is widely expressed in non-hemopoietic tumours. Other less specific antibodies include CD38, VS38c (p63) and COX2. Aberrant phenotypes may again be demonstrated using antibodies to CD19, CD20, CD56, CD27 and CD117. One additional advantage of immunohistochemical techniques is the ability to demonstrate the aberrant expression of both PAX5 and cyclin D1 which is not readily achieved with flow cytometry. The latter is aberrantly expressed in approximately 50% of myeloma but this is not confined to cases with the t (11;14) as it may also be seen in cases with hyperdiploidy and indeed expression appears to correlate with CCND1 copy number [25,26].

Prognostic assessment

Plasma cell phenotyping particularly by flow cytometry can also provide useful prognostic data. For instance, in patients with symptomatic myeloma phenotypically aberrant plasma cells comprise the great majority (>95%) of total BMPC. This relative proportion of normal and neoplastic plasma cells appears to have prognostic significance. In patients with asymptomatic MM and MGUS the presence of >95% aberrant phenotype plasma cells defines a greater risk of progression whilst the presence of ≥5% normal phenotype plasma cells in patients with symptomatic myeloma appears to be associated with favorable clinical features, a lower incidence of adverse cytogenetic abnormalities and an improved overall clinical outcome at least in the context of conventional chemotherapy treatment [16–18]. Flow cytometric evaluation of BMPC is also useful in the evaluation of patients with solitary plasmacytoma of bone and AL amyloidosis [23,24] and also in the assessment of so-called minimal residual disease (MRD, see below) (Table 2.1).

It has become clear with more detailed immunophenotypic studies that strong phenotypic–genotypic correlations exist in some hematological malignancies. For example, in acute myeloid leukemia the balanced translocations t(15;17), t(8;21) and inversion 16 are each characterized by a highly specific immunophenotypic profile. Such strong correlations have not however been demonstrated in myeloma. In a detailed assessment of 915 cases Mateo and colleagues were able to demonstrate some statistically significant associations [27]. It was noted that non-hyperdiploid myeloma was associated with a higher frequency of

Table 2.1 Applications of plasma cell immunophenotyping by flow cytometry

Differential diagnosis of myeloma, MGUS, amyloidosis and reactive plasmacytoses
Prognostic factor
• symptomatic myeloma
• asymptomatic myeloma and MGUS
• solitary plasmacytoma of bone
• AL amyloidosis
Minimal residual disease (MRD)
Identification of potential therapeutic targets

CD28 and CD20 expression but a lower frequency of CD56 and CD117 expression. The t(11;14) was also strongly associated with CD20 expression but absence of CD56 and CD117 while cases with alternative *IGH* translocations were typically CD20- and CD117-. These associations, although statistically significant, are not absolute and hence the underlying genotype cannot for individual patients be inferred from their immunophenotypic profile [27]. Immunophenotyping cannot therefore act as a surrogate for formal cytogenetic assessment. Similarly the prognostic impact of specific immunophenotypic determinants has been assessed by the same group. They demonstrated that the expression of CD19 and CD28 and the absence of CD117 were all associated with an inferior outcome and a prognostic stratification model incorporating CD28 and CD117 was proposed [28]. The clinical utility of this stratification model is, however, debatable given that there is a significant association with known adverse cytogenetic factors such as the t(4;14), t(14;16) and del (17p). Smaller studies have also suggested that a CD27- immunophenotype is also associated with adverse clinical features and overall outcome [29,30].

Minimal residual disease

The assessment of therapeutic response in MM has relied heavily upon demonstrating sequential changes in the concentration of paraprotein and/or free light chains along with an improvement in clinical parameters such as anemia and renal function. Repeat BM assessment has previously been largely used for the confirmation of complete response (CR) or the assessment of patients with non-secretory disease in whom no serum or urine monoclonal protein is available for sequential quantitative assessment.

It has however become clear that the assessment of so-called minimal residual disease (MRD) in the BM is highly informative and of significant prognostic relevance [31–35]. The flow cytometric assays employed in the routine diagnostic setting can similarly be applied in the assessment of post-treatment samples as they allow the discrimination between aberrant phenotype and normal phenotype plasma cells [10,11]. The latter become readily demonstrable in the post-treatment setting particularly in those patients with high quality responses and compromise the value of disease assessments that rely upon the demonstration of monoclonality such as immunohistochemistry and consensus primer polymerase chain reaction (PCR) for *IGH* rearrangements. Indeed immunohistochemical staining for kappa and lambda on trephine biopsy sections has been shown to be a relatively insensitive technique that provides limited added value over standard assessment with immunofixation [36]. Flow cytometry is currently regarded as the method of choice for assessing MRD in MM as it is applicable to the vast majority of patients (>90%) and has a reproducible sensitivity of 0.01% and allows for the provision of results in real-time for clinical decision making [37,38]. Allele-specific PCR based techniques may also be used and have the advantage of an increased potential sensitivity of 0.001%. Sensitivity, however, will vary from patient to patient and fewer patients will have an informative marker [32,38,39]. Similarly they are currently more labor intensive and less applicable to routine laboratory practice. Molecular techniques may, however, eventually supersede flow cytometry given the continued improvement and cost effectiveness of sequencing technologies as well as continued therapeutic advances that are resulting in further improvements in depth of response [39].

The prognostic relevance of MRD has traditionally been evaluated in patients treated with stem cell transplantation. A number of groups have demonstrated (by flow cytometry) that approximately 40% of patients have no demonstrable bone marrow disease at the traditional day 100 assessment following autologous transplantation and that this appears to predict for a significant improvement in both progression free and overall survival [31,33,35]. Patients with no demonstrable BM disease at the end of induction chemotherapy as well as following high-dose therapy appear to have particularly favorable outcome. It has also become clear that MRD is demonstrable in approximately 1/3 of patients who achieve an immunofixation negative CR and in this context the presence of MRD again predicts for an inferior outcome [31,33,35]. The prognostic value of MRD assessment has also been demonstrated in patients with standard risk and adverse cytogenetics although the magnitude of benefit appears greatest in those with standard risk features [35].

Recent studies have shown that MRD-negative responses are also demonstrable in a significant proportion of patients following treatment with novel agent combinations particularly those containing bortezomib [34,35,39,40]. Although the overall proportion of patients achieving MRD negativity with these combinations is lower than that demonstrable following high-dose therapy, recent studies have again demonstrated a highly significant prognostic advantage of achieving MRD-negativity in these non-transplant cohorts [34,35].

Scheduled BM assessments within clinical trials can also provide important information regarding the efficacy of individual components of sequential multi-agent therapy including stem cell transplantation. For instance, post-induction assessments may allow for a more detailed comparison of induction regimens as conventional paraprotein assessments may underestimate the CR rate in this setting because of the slow rate of decline of some paraproteins particularly those of IgG Isotype [41,42]. Similarly MRD assessment can also provide useful insights into the efficacy of maintenance/consolidation strategies following stem cell transplantation as demonstrating changes in categorical paraprotein responses in this setting is frequently not possible [35].

Identification of therapeutic targets

Monoclonal antibodies such as rituximab and alemtuzumab are widely used in the treatment of B-cell lymphoproliferative disorders but have been less widely applied in the treatment of MM and related disorders. Immunophenotypic studies have generally shown that CD20 is variably expressed in a subset of myeloma patients while clinical studies have suggested that rituximab has limited single agent activity even in cases expressing the antigen [43]. It has also been argued that rituximab may have a role in depleting clonogenic B-cells that may be responsible for relapse but this is a controversial area. Similarly CD52, the alemtuzumab target, is expressed at low levels in MM plasma cells and below that typically

associated with depletion with the therapeutic antibody. Indeed clinical studies in WM have shown that while alemtuzumab effectively depletes B-cells there is apparent sparing of the plasma cell component of the disease [44,45].

There are, however, now a number of new monoclonal antibodies at various stages of clinical application that have been developed specifically for the treatment of myeloma. These include elotuzumab which targets the CS1 antigen (CD319) which appears to be extensively expressed in both normal and neoplastic plasma cells [46]. A number of other antibodies targeting antigens such as CD38, CD138 and CD56 are in development but clearly further progress in this area will require extensive immunophenotypic studies given the variability in expression of some antigens in both normal and neoplastic plasma cell populations.

Specific syndromes
Plasma cell leukemia

Plasma cell leukemia (PCL) is conventionally defined by the presence of $\geq 20\%$ circulating plasma cells and/or an absolute level of $>2 \times 10^9/l$ and is typically associated with a poor outcome [1]. This can occur as the primary presenting feature or as a secondary progression event in patients with established MM. Circulating plasma cells are, however, demonstrable, by using sensitive PCR or flow cytometric based techniques, in the majority of patients with active myeloma and hence the value of defining PCL as a distinct entity by using such arbitrary cut-offs is debatable [47]. There are, however, a number of clinicopathological correlates that are consistently reported in PCL. Most studies have demonstrated a lower incidence of CD56 expression and indeed where analysis of peripheral blood and bone marrow has been performed in the same patients CD56 expression appears lower in the circulating PC than in BMPC [47–49]. A number of reports have also highlighted aberrant expression of CD23 [50]. Similarly cytogenetic studies have also highlighted a higher incidence of the t(11;14), t(14;16) along with deregulation of *TP53* and *MYC* [51,52].

Detailed morphological and immunophenotypic studies are essential in the diagnosis of PCL. The diagnosis can be mistaken for other hematological malignancies and indeed, in rare instances of high circulating levels of polyclonal plasma cells, have been described in diverse clinical situations such as angioimmunoblastic T cell lymphoma and autoimmune disorders [53–55].

t(11;14) myeloma

The t(11;14) which deregulates *CYCLIN D1* as a consequence of its juxtaposition to the *IGH* locus is the commonest of the immunoglobulin translocations in MM, occurring in approximately 20% of patients [56,57]. Whilst the majority of studies have failed to demonstrate a significant impact on outcome it remains distinctive from a clinicopathological perspective and worthy of specific discussion with this in mind. The majority of studies have demonstrated "small cell" or "lymphoplasmacytoid" cytology and expression of CD20 which can lead to an erroneous diagnosis of lymphoma [25–27,58–60]. The expression of CD20 has been documented in up to 2/3 of patients with the t(11;14) and is associated with strong uniform nuclear expression of cyclin D1 protein in tissue sections but also aberrant expression of PAX5 protein and CD23 in a significant proportion of cases [25,26,60,61]. Similarly there appears to be a lower incidence of CD56 and CD117 expression [27]. It should, however, be noted that cyclin D1 protein expression is not confined to t(11;14) MM as it is also demonstrable in hyperdiploid MM presumably as a consequence of extra copies of *CCND1*[25,26]. Cyclin D1 immunohistochemistry cannot therefore be used in the routine laboratory as a definitive marker of the t(11;14) as is routinely done in the diagnosis of mantle cell lymphoma. SOX11 protein, which has recently been identified as a useful immunohistochemical marker in mantle cell lymphoma, does not appear to be expressed in MM [62,63].

The t(11;14) is also associated with specific clinical correlates including paraprotein concentrations of less than 10 g/l, AL amyloidosis, plasma cell leukemia and IgM MM [51,52,56,64–69].

IgM myeloma

Myeloma is typically a disorder of class-switched immunoglobulin secreting plasma cells but rare cases of IgM secreting myeloma have been described. These account for approximately 0.3% of all cases of myeloma and have, at least in the context of conventional chemotherapy and stem cell transplantation, an inferior survival compared to standard myeloma [70]. The main differential diagnosis is Waldenstrom macroglobulinemia (WM) but it is possible with the use of detailed morphological and immunophenotypic assessment to make a definitive distinction between IgM myeloma and WM. The latter is defined by bone marrow infiltration by lymphoplasmacytic lymphoma and as such it should be possible to demonstrate both monotypic B cells and monotypic plasma cells by flow cytometry and/or immunohistochemistry even in those cases where plasma cells are the predominant cell type [19,20,22]. Monotypic B cells are not demonstrable in IgM myeloma and the infiltrate is composed entirely of cytoplasmic IgM containing plasma cells which have an aberrant phenotype [69]. The immunophenotypic profile seen in IgM myeloma may differ somewhat from standard myeloma as the recorded incidence of CD56 expression appears to be lower but should allow a distinction from the PC of WM which typically show normal expression of CD19, CD45 and CD56 [19,20,22]. Similarly, in contrast to WM, there is a high incidence of immunoglobulin translocations and in particular the t(11;14) in IgM myeloma [68,69,71–73].

References

1. International Myeloma Working Group. Criteria for the classification of monoclonal gammopathies, multiple myeloma and related disorders: a report of the International Myeloma Working Group. *Br. J. Haematol.* 2003;**121**:749–57.

2. Bird, J. M., Owen, R. G., D'sa, S. *et al.* Guidelines for the diagnosis and management of multiple myeloma 2011. *Brit. J. Haematol.* 2011;**154**: 32–75.

3. Rajkumar, S. V., Fonseca, R., Dispenzieri, A. *et al.* Methods of estimation of bone marrow plasma cell involvement in myeloma: predictive value for response and survival in patients undergoing autologous stem cell transplantation. *Am. J. Hematol.* 2001;**68**:269–75.

4. Ng, A. P., Wei, A., Bhurani, D. *et al.* The sensitivity of CD138 immunostaining of bone marrow trephine specimens for quantifying marrow involvement in MGUS and myeloma, including samples with a low percentage of plasma cells. *Haematologica* 2006;**91**:972–5.

5. Al-Quran, S. Z., Yang, L., Magill, J. M. *et al.* Assessment of bone marrow plasma cell infiltrates in multiple myeloma: the added

value of CD138 immunohistochemistry. *Hum. Pathol.* 2007;**38**:1779–87.

6. Joshi, R., Horncastle, D., Elderfield, K. *et al.* Bone marrow trephine combined with immunohistochemistry is superior to bone marrow aspirate in follow up of myeloma patients. *J. Clin. Pathol.* 2008;**61**: 213–16.

7. Greipp, P. R., Raymond, N. M., Kyle, R. A. *et al.* Multiple myeloma: significance of plasmablastic subtype in morphological classification. *Blood* 1985;**65**:305–10.

8. Bartl, R., Frisch, B., Fateh-Moghadam, A. *et al.* Histologic classification and staging of multiple myeloma. A retrospective and prospective study of 674 cases. *Am. J. Clin. Pathol.* 1987;**87**:342–55.

9. Greipp, P. R., Leong, T., Bennett, J. M. *et al.* Plasmablastic morphology – an independent prognostic factor with clinical and laboratory correlates: Eastern Cooperative Oncology Group (ECOG) Myeloma Trial E9486 report by the ECOG Myeloma Laboratory Group. *Blood* 1998;**91**:2501–7.

10. Rawstron, A. C., Orfao, A., Beksac, M. *et al.* Report of the European Myeloma Network on multiparametric flow cytometry in multiple myeloma and related disorders. *Haematologica* 2008;**93**:431–8.

11. Paiva, B., Almeida, J., Perez-Andres, M. *et al.* Utility of flow cytometry immunophenotyping in multiple myeloma and other clonal plasma cell-related disorders. *Cytometry Part B (Clinical Cytometry)* 2010;**78B**:239–52.

12. Morice, W. G., Hanson, C. A., Kumar, S. *et al.* Novel multi-parameter flow cytometry sensitively detects phenotypically distinct plasma cell subsets in plasma cell proliferative disorders. *Leukemia* 2007;**21**:2043–6.

13. de Tute, R. M., Jack, A. S., Child, J. A. *et al.* A single-tube six-colour flow cytometry screening assay for the detection of minimal residual disease in myeloma. *Leukemia* 2007;**21**:2046–9.

14. Paiva, B., Vidriales, M. B., Perez, J. J. *et al.* Multiparameter flow cytometry quantification of bone marrow plasma cells at diagnosis provides more prognostic information than morphological assessment in myeloma patients. *Haematologica* 2009;**94**: 1599–602.

15. Ocqueteau, M., Orfao, A., Almeida, J. *et al.* Immunophenotypic characterization of plasma cells from monoclonal gammopathy of undetermined significance patients. Implications for the differential diagnosis between MGUS and multiple myeloma. *Am. J. Pathol.* 1998;**152**:1655–65.

16. Perez-Persona, E., Vidriales, M. B., Mateo, G. *et al.* New criteria to identify risk of progression in monoclonal gammopathy of uncertain significance and smoldering multiple myeloma based on multiparameter flow cytometry analysis of bone marrow plasma cells. *Blood* 2007;**110**:2586–92.

17. Paiva, B., Vidriales, M. B., Mateo, G. *et al.* The persistence of immunophenotypically normal residual bone marrow plasma cells at diagnosis identifies a good prognostic subgroup of symptomatic multiple myeloma patients. *Blood* 2009;**114**:4369–72.

18. Perez-Persona, E., Mateo, G., Garcia-Sanz, R. *et al.* Risk of progression in smouldering myeloma and monoclonal gammopathies of unknown significance: comparative analysis of the evolution of monoclonal component and multiparameter flow cytometry of bone marrow plasma cells. *Br. J. Haematol.* 2010;**148**:110–14.

19. San Miguel, J. F., Vidriales, M. B., Ocio, E. *et al.* Immunophenotypic analysis of Waldenstrom's macroglobulinemia. *Semin. Oncol.* 2003;**30**:187–95.

20. Ocio, E., Hernandez, J. M., Mateo, G. *et al.* Immunophenotypic and cytogenetic comparison of Waldenstrom's macroglobulinemia with splenic marginal zone lymphoma. *Clin. Lymphoma* 2005;**5**:241–5.

21. Seegmiller, A. C., Xu, Y., McKenna, R. W. *et al.* Immunophenotypic differentiation between neoplastic plasma cells in mature B-cell lymphoma vs plasma cell myeloma. *Am. J. Clin. Pathol.* 2007;**127**:176–81.

22. Morice, W. G., Chen, D., Kurtin, P. J. *et al.* Novel immunophenotypic features of marrow lymphoplasmacytic lymphoma and correlation with Waldenstrom's macroglobulinemia. *Mod. Pathol.* 2009;**22**:807–16.

23. Paiva, B., Vidriales, M. B., Perez, J. J. *et al.* The clinical utility and prognostic value of multiparameter flow cytometry immunophenotyping in light-chain amyloidosis. *Blood* 2011;**117**:3613–16.

24. Hill, Q., Rawstron, A., de Tute, R. *et al.* Outcome prediction in solitary plasmacytoma of bone (SPB): Development of a risk stratification model utilising bone marrow flow cytometry and light chain analysis. *Haematologica* 2011;**96(s1)**:158.

25. Cook, J. R., Hsi, E. D., Worley, S. *et al.* Immunohistochemical analysis identifies two cyclin D1 +subsets of plasma cell myeloma, each associated with favourable survival. *Am. J. Clin. Pathol.* 2006;**125**:615–24.

26. Owen, R. G., Ross, F., O'Connor, S. J. M. *et al.* Cyclin D1, CD20 and

PAX5 expression in myeloma: correlation with karyotype. *Haematologica* 2007;**92(s2)**:101–2.

27. Mateo, G., Castellanos, M., Rasillo, A. *et al.* Genetic abnormalities and patterns of antigenic expression in multiple myeloma. *Clin. Cancer Res.* 2005;**11**:3661–7.

28. Mateo, G., Montalban, M. A., Vidriales, M. *et al.* Prognostic value of immunophenotyping in multiple myeloma: a study by the PETHEMA/GEM Cooperative Study Groups on patients uniformly treated with high-dose therapy. *J. Clin. Oncol.* 2008;**26**:2737–44.

29. Moreau, P., Robillard, N., Jego, G. *et al.* Lack of CD27 in myeloma delineates different presentation and outcome. *Br. J. Haematol.* 2006;**132**:168–70.

30. Guikema, J. E., Hovenga, S., Vellenga, E. *et al.* CD27 is heterogeneously expressed in multiple myeloma: low CD27 expression in patients with high-risk disease. *Br. J. Haematol.* 2003;**121**:36–43.

31. Rawstron, A. C., Davies, F. E., DasGupta, R. *et al.* Flow cytometric disease monitoring in multiple myeloma: the relationship between normal and neoplastic plasma cells predicts outcome after transplantation. *Blood* 2002;**100**:3095–100.

32. Bakkus, M. H., Bouko, Y., Samson, D. *et al.* Post-transplantation tumour load in bone marrow, as assessed by quantitative ASO-PCR, is a prognostic parameter in multiple myeloma. *Br. J. Haematol.* 2004;**126**:665–74.

33. Paiva, B., Vidriales, M. B., Cervero, J. *et al.* Multiparameter flow cytometric remission is the most relevant prognostic factor for multiple myeloma patients who undergo autologous stem cell transplantation. *Blood* 2008;**112**:4017–23.

34. Paiva, B., Matinez-Lopez, J., Vidriales, M. B. *et al.* Comparison of immunofixation, serum free light chain, and immunophenotyping for response evaluation and prognostication in multiple myeloma. *J. Clin. Oncol.* 2011;**29**:1627–33.

35. Rawstron, A., de Tute, R., Child, A. *et al.* Minimal residual disease (MRD) assessment using multiparameter flow cytometry (MFC) predicts outcome in both intensively and non-intensively treated patients: results from the MRC Myeloma IX trial. *Haematologica* 2011;**96(s1)**:30–1.

36. Tatsas, A. D., Jagasia, M. H., Chen, H. *et al.* Monitoring residual myeloma: high-resolution serum/urine electrophoresis or marrow biopsy with immunohistochemical analysis. *Am. J. Clin. Pathol.* 2010;**134**:139–44.

37. Owen, R. G., Rawstron, A. C. Minimal residual disease monitoring in multiple myeloma: flow cytometry is the method of choice. *Br. J. Haematol.* 2004;**126**:665–74.

38. Sarasquete, M. E., Garcia-Sanz, R., Gonzalez, D. *et al.* Minimal residual disease monitoring in multiple myeloma: a comparison between allelic-specific oligonucleotide real-time quantitative polymerase chain reaction and flow cytometry. *Haematologica* 2005;**90**:1365–72.

39. Ladetto, M., Pagliano, G., Ferrero, S. *et al.* Major tumor shrinking and persistent molecular remissions after consolidation with bortezomib, thalidomide, and dexamethasone in patients with autografted myeloma. *J. Clin. Oncol.* 2010;**28**:2077–84.

40. Paiva, B., Vidriales, M. B., Montalban, M. A. *et al.* Analysis of immunophenotypic response (IR) by multiparameter flow cytometry in 516 myeloma patients included in three consecutive Spanish trials. *Blood* 2010;**116**:1910.

41. Davies, F. E., Forsyth, P. D., Rawstron, A. C. *et al.* The impact of attaining a minimal disease state after high-dose melphalan and autologous transplantation for multiple myeloma. *Br. J. Haematol.* 2001;**112**: 814–19.

42. Drayson, M. T., Morgan, G. J., Jackson, G. H. *et al.* Prospective study of serum FLC and other M-protein assays: when and how to measure response? *Clin. Lymphoma Myeloma* 2009;**9s1**:51.

43. Kapoor, P., Greipp, P. T., Morice, W. G. *et al.* Anti-CD20 monoclonal antibody therapy in multiple myeloma. *Brit. J. Haematol.* 2008;**141**:135–48.

44. Rawstron, A. C., Laycock-Brown, G., Hale, G. *et al.* CD52 expression patterns in myeloma and the applicability of alemtuzumab therapy. *Haematologica* 2006;**91**:1577–8.

45. Owen, R. G., Hillmen, P., Rawstron, A. C. CD52 expression in Waldenstrom's macroglobulinemia: implications for alemtuzumab therapy and response assessment. *Clin. Lymphoma* 2005;**5**: 278–81.

46. Hsi, E. D., Steinle, R., Balasa, B. *et al.* CS1, a potential new therapeutic antibody target for the treatment of multiple myeloma. *Clin. Cancer. Res.* 2008;**14**:2775–84.

47. Rawstron, A. C., Owen, R. G., Davies, F. E. *et al.* Circulating plasma cells in multiple myeloma: characterization and correlation with disease stage. *Br. J. Haematol.* 1997;**97**:46–55.

48. Garcia-Sanz, R., Orfao, A., Gonzalez, M. *et al.* Primary plasma cell leukemia: clinical, immunophenotypic, DNA ploidy, and cytogenetic

17

characteristics. *Blood* 1999;**93**:1032–7.

49. Kraj, M., Kopec-Szlezak, J., Poglod, R. *et al.* Flow cytometric immunophenotypic characteristics of 36 cases of plasma cell leukemia. *Leuk. Res.* 2011;**35**:169–76.

50. Walters, M., Olteanu, H., Van Tuinen, P. *et al.* CD23 expression in plasma cell myeloma is specific for abnormalities of chromosome 11, and is associated with primary plasma cell leukaemia in this cytogenetic subgroup. *Br. J. Haematol.* 2010;**149**: 292–3.

51. Tiedemann, R. E., Gonzalez-Paz, N., Kyle, R. A. *et al.* Genetic aberrations and survival in plasma cell leukemia. *Leukemia* 2008;**22**:1044–52.

52. Chiecchio, L., Dagrada, G. P., White, H. E. *et al.* Frequent upregulation of MYC in plasma cell leukemia. *Genes Chromosomes Cancer* 2009;**48**:624–36.

53. van Veen, J. J., Reilly, J. T., Richards, S. J. *et al.* Diagnosis of plasma cell leukaemia: findings of the UK NEQAS for Leucocyte Immunophenotyping Scheme. *Clin. Lab. Haematol.* 2004;**26**: 37–42.

54. Touzeau, C., Pellat-Deceunynck, C., Gastinne, T. *et al.* Reactive plasmacytoses can mimic plasma cell leukemia: therapeutical implications. *Leuk. Lymphoma* 2007;**48**:207–8.

55. Ahsanuddin, A. N., Brynes, R. K., Li, S. Peripheral blood plasmacytosis mimicking plasma cell leukemia in patients with angioimmunoblastic T-cell lymphoma: report of 3 cases and review of the literature. *Int. J. Clin. Exp. Pathol.* 2011;**4**:416–20.

56. Fonseca, R., Blood, E. A., Oken, M. M. *et al.* Myeloma and the t(11;14)(q13;q32): evidence for a biologically defined unique subset of patients. *Blood* 2002;**99**: 3735–41.

57. Avet-Loiseau, H., Attal, M., Moreau, P. *et al.* Genetic abnormalities and survival in multiple myeloma: the experience of the Intergroupe Francophone du Myelome. *Blood* 2007;**109**:3489–95.

58. Garand, R., Avet-Loiseau, H., Accard, F. *et al.* t(11;14) and t(4;14) translocation correlated with mature lymphoplasmacytoid and immature morphology, respectively, in multiple myeloma. *Leukemia* 2003;**17**:2032–5.

59. Robillard, N., Avet-Loiseau, H., Garand, R. *et al.* CD20 is associated with a small mature plasma cell morphology and t(11;14) in multiple myeloma. *Blood* 2003;**102**:1070–1.

60. Lin, P., Mahdavy, M., Zhan, F. *et al.* Expression of PAX5 in CD20-positive multiple myeloma assessed by immunohistochemistry and oligonucleotide microarray. *Mod. Pathol.* 2004;**17**:1217–22.

61. Buonaccorsi, J. N., Kroft, S. H., Harrington, A. M. *et al.* Clinicopathologic analysis of the impact of CD23 expression in plasma cell myeloma with t(11;14)(q13;q32). *Ann. Diagn. Pathol.* 2011;**15**(6):385–8.

62. Mozos, A., Royo, C., Hartmann, E. *et al.* SOX11 protein expression is highly specific for mantle cell lymphoma and identifies the cyclin D1-negative subtype. *Haematologica* 2009;**94**:1555–62.

63. Diktor, M., Ek, S., Sundberg, M. *et al.* Strong lymphoid nuclear expression of SOX11 transcription factor defines lymphoblastic neoplasms, mantle cell lymphoma and Burkitt's lymphoma. *Haematologica* 2009;**94**:1563–8.

64. Fonseca, R., Ahmann, G. J., Jalal, S. M. *et al.* Chromosomal abnormalities in systemic amyloidosis. *Br. J. Haematol.* 1998;**103**:704–10.

65. Hayman, S. R., Bailey, R. J., Jalal, S. M. *et al.* Translocations involving the immunoglobulin heavy-chain locus are possible early genetic events in patients with primary systemic amyloidosis. *Blood* 2001;**98**: 2266–8.

66. Harrison, C. J., Mazzullo, H., Ross, F. M. *et al.* Translocations of 14q32 and deletions of 13q14 are common chromosomal abnormalities in systemic amyloidosis. *Br. J. Haematol.* 2002;**117**:427–35.

67. Bryce, A. H., Ketterling, R. P., Gertz, M. A. *et al.* Translocation t(11;14) and survival of patients with light chain (AL) amyloidosis. *Haematologica* 2009;**94**:380–6.

68. Avet-Loiseau, H., Garand, R., Lode, L. *et al.* Translocation t(11;14)(q13;q32) is the hallmark of IgM, IgE, and nonsecretory multiple myeloma variants. *Blood* 2003;**101**:1570–1.

69. Feyler, S., O'Connor, S. J. M, Rawstron, A. C. *et al.* IgM myeloma: a rare entity characterized by a CD20-CD56-CD117- immunophenotype and the t(11;14). *Br. J. Haematol.* 2007;**140**:547–51.

70. Morris, C., Drake, M., Apperley, J. *et al.* Efficacy and outcome of autologous transplantation in rare myelomas. *Haematologica* 2010;**95**:2126–33.

71. Ackroyd, S., O'Connor, S. J., Rawstron, A. C. *et al.* IgM myeloma with t(4;14)(p16; q32). *Cancer Genet. Cytogenet.* 2005;**162**:183–4.

72. Schuster, S. R., Rajkumar, S. V., Dispenzieri, A. *et al.* IgM multiple myeloma: Disease definition, prognosis, and differentiation from Waldenstrom's macroglobulinemia. *Am. J. Hematol.* 2010;**85**:853–5.

73. Owen, R. G., O'Connor, S. J. M., Bond, L. R. *et al.* Translocation t(14;16) in IgM multiple myeloma. *Br. J. Haematol.* 2011;**155**:402–3.

Monoclonal gammopathy of undetermined significance (MGUS)

Monoclonal gammopathy of undetermined significance (MGUS) has traditionally been considered as a single entity but it is crucial to consider the heavy chain isotype of the monoclonal protein. It is important that IgG and IgA MGUS be distinguished from IgM MGUS as the latter is considered the precursor of Waldenstrom macroglobulinemia and other lymphoproliferative disorders rather than myeloma. IgM MGUS is discussed in more detail elsewhere in this book.

The value of bone marrow assessment in asymptomatic individuals with IgG and IgA (and light-chain only) monoclonal gammopathy is somewhat controversial but the majority of international guidelines recommend it in patients with intermediate/high-risk features such as a paraprotein concentration of >15 g/l, IgA paraproteins and/or an abnormal serum free light chain ratio or any patients with suspicious clinical features or suspected amyloidosis [1,2]. When marrow assessment is performed it is recommended that both a bone marrow aspirate and a trephine biopsy are obtained as the latter provides for a better assessment of the extent of marrow infiltration and also ensures that a diagnosis can be made when the bone marrow aspirate specimen is of poor quality. It is well recognized that bone marrow aspirate plasma cell counts consistently underestimate the overall level of infiltration [3–6]. MGUS is by definition characterized by <10% BMPC and absence of confluent areas of infiltration on the trephine but it should be recognized that this 10% cut-off is somewhat arbitrary and that MGUS and myeloma form part of a continuous spectrum and therefore definitive diagnoses should only be made following detailed correlation with other clinical and laboratory features. The extent of infiltration can most accurately be determined by using CD138 immunohistochemical staining of trephine biopsy sections [3–6].

There is, however, some rationale for considering detailed marrow assessment in the majority of patients with suspected MGUS as flow cytometry can provide useful prognostic information. Plasma cells with an aberrant phenotype are demonstrable in the majority of patients with MGUS and the antigenic profiles are very similar to that demonstrable in myeloma. They comprise a median of approximately 60%–70% of BMPC and are monotypic but in contrast to patients with symptomatic myeloma residual normal phenotype plasma cells are also frequently demonstrable [7–9]. This may be useful additional information in the differential diagnosis of MGUS and myeloma but more importantly it appears to be an independent prognostic factor for progression to symptomatic myeloma. Studies have demonstrated that MGUS patients in whom aberrant phenotype plasma cells comprise >95% of total BMPC have a significantly greater risk of progression. Such a pattern is demonstrable in approximately 20% of MGUS patients and is associated with a median time to progression of 107 months and cumulative risk of progression at 5 years of 25% versus not reached and 5% respectively for those patients in which aberrant phenotype plasma cells comprise ≤95% of BMPC [8]. This flow cytometric profile also appears to be predictive of progression in patients with conventionally determined low risk disease [8] as well as those patients with both stable and evolving paraproteins [9]. Defining risk of progression in this way could be used to identify patients suitable for therapeutic intervention in future clinical trials.

References

1. Bird, J., Behrens, J., Westin, J. et al. UK Myeloma Forum (UKMF) and Nordic Myeloma Study Group (NMSG): guidelines for the investigation of newly detected M-proteins and the management of monoclonal gammopathy of undetermined significance (MGUS). Br. J. Haematol. 2009;147:22–42.

2. Kyle, R. A., Durie, B. G., Rajkumar, S. V. et al. Monoclonal gammopathy of undetermined significance (MGUS) and smoldering (asymptomatic) multiple myeloma: IMWG consensus perspectives risk factors for progression and guidelines for monitoring and management. Leukemia 2010;24:1121–7.

3. Rajkumar, S. V., Fonseca, R., Dispenzieri, A. et al. Methods of estimation of bone marrow plasma cell involvement in myeloma: predictive value for response and survival in patients undergoing autologous stem cell transplantation. Am. J. Hematol. 2001;68:269–75.

4. Ng, A. P., Wei, A., Bhurani, D. et al. The sensitivity of CD138 immunostaining of bone marrow trephine specimens for quantifying marrow involvement in MGUS and myeloma, including samples with a low percentage of plasma cells. Haematologica 2006;91:972–5.

5. Al-Quran, S. Z., Yang, L., Magill, J. M. *et al.* Assessment of bone marrow plasma cell infiltrates in multiple myeloma: the added value of CD138 immunohistochemistry. *Hum. Pathol.* 2007;**38**:1779–87.

6. Joshi, R., Horncastle, D., Elderfield, K. *et al.* Bone marrow trephine combined with immunohistochemistry is superior to bone marrow aspirate in follow up of myeloma patients. *J. Clin. Pathol.* 2008;**61**:213–16.

7. Ocqueteau, M., Orfao, A., Almeida, J. *et al.*

Immunophenotypic characterization of plasma cells from monoclonal gammopathy of undetermined significance patients. Implications for the differential diagnosis between MGUS and multiple myeloma. *Am. J. Pathol.* 1998;**152**:1655–65.

8. Perez-Persona, E., Vidriales, M. B., Mateo, G. *et al.* New criteria to identify risk of progression in monoclonal gammopathy of uncertain significance and smoldering multiple myeloma based on multiparameter flow

cytometry analysis of bone marrow plasma cells. *Blood* 2007;**110**:2586–92.

9. Perez-Persona, E., Mateo, G., Garcia-Sanz, R. *et al.* Risk of progression in smouldering myeloma and monoclonal gammopathies of unknown significance: comparative analysis of the evolution of monoclonal component and multiparameter flow cytometry of bone marrow plasma cells. *Br. J. Haematol.* 2010;**148**: 110–14.

Solitary plasmacytoma of bone

Solitary plasmacytoma of bone (SPB) are localized plasma cell tumors with evidence of local bone destruction but no features to suggest underlying myeloma. SPB typically arise in the axial skeleton with vertebral location most commonly reported whilst presentation in the distal appendicular skeleton is very unusual. It is recommended that a formal tissue biopsy is obtained for the diagnosis of SPB as fine needle aspiration cytology is of limited value [1]. Similarly formal biopsy is encouraged in all patients with destructive bone lesions as a diagnosis of SPB cannot be inferred by the presence of a paraprotein in the serum given the prevalence of the latter in older individuals. SPB are typically characterized by a monomorphic plasma cell infiltrate with little or no inflammatory background. CD138 and MUM1/IRF4 are the most useful markers although CD38 and VS38c (p63) may also be used. In confirming the nature of the infiltrate it should also be noted that CD138 is extensively expressed in non-hemopoietic tumors and CD45 is frequently not expressed in neoplastic plasma cells. There is very limited specific immunophenotypic data in SPB but it is generally considered that the plasma cells will have an aberrant immunophenotype and in tissue sections CD19,

CD56, CD117, CD27 and cyclin D1 are the most useful markers [1,2]. There is no specific data on cytogenetics in SPB.

Despite the apparently localized nature of SPB 30%–70% of patients will progress (typically to myeloma) at a median of 18–24 months [3–11]. Given that local control rates following involved field irradiation typically exceed 90% it is assumed that this progression occurs as a result of occult marrow disease not detected by standard investigations at the time of diagnosis. By utilizing multi-parameter flow cytometry it is possible to demonstrate aberrant phenotype plasma cells, indicative of occult marrow disease, in the staging bone marrows of approximately 2/3 of patients with SPB. When present they comprise 70% of bone marrow plasma cells and a median of 0.5% of bone marrow leucocytes. A recent study has demonstrated that the presence of occult marrow disease is highly predictive of outcome as progression occurred in 72% of patients with occult marrow disease compared to 12.5% of patients without (median time to progression 26 months versus not reached) [11]. A prognostic stratification model incorporating bone marrow flow cytometry and urinary light chain assessment has also been proposed [11].

References

1. Hughes, M., Soutar, R., Lucraft, H. *et al. Guidelines on the diagnosis and management of solitary plasmacytoma of bone, extramedullary plasmacytoma and multiple solitary plasmacytomas:*

2009 update. http://www.bcshguidelines.com/documents/solitary_plasmacytoma_bcsh_FINAL_190109.pdf

2. Zuo, Z., Liu, W. P., Tang, Y. *et al.* Solitary plasmacytoma of bone: a clinicopathologic,

immunohistochemical and immunoglobulin gene rearrangement study. *Zhonghua Bing Li Xue Za Zhi* 2010;**39**: 177–82.

3. Dimopoulos, M. A., Goldstein, J., Fuller, L. *et al.* Curability of

solitary bone plasmacytoma. *J. Clin. Oncol.* 1992;**10**:587–90.

4. Dingli, D., Kyle, R. A., Rajkumar, S. V. *et al.* Immunoglobulin free light chains and solitary plasmacytoma of bone. *Blood* 2006;**108**:1979–83.

5. Knobel, D., Zouhair, A., Tsang, R. W. *et al.* Prognostic factors in solitary plasmacytoma of bone: a multicenter Rare Cancer Network study. *BMC Cancer* 2006;**6**:118.

6. Ozsahin, M., Tsang, R. W., Poortmans, P. *et al.* Outcomes and patterns of failure in solitary plasmacytoma: a multicenter Rare

Cancer Network study of 258 patients. *Int. J. Radiat. Oncol. Biol. Phys.* 2006;**64**:210–17.

7. Kilciksiz, S., Celik, O. K., Pak, Y. *et al.* Clinical and prognostic features of plasmacytomas: a multicenter study of Turkish Oncology Group-Sarcoma Working Party. *Am. J. Hematol.* 2008;**83**:702–7.

8. Dagan, R., Morris, C. G., Kirwan, J. *et al.* Solitary plasmacytoma. *Am. J. Clin. Oncol.* 2009;**32**:612–17.

9. Jawad, M. U., Scully, S. P. Skeletal plasmacytoma: progression of disease and impact of local treatment; an analysis of SEER

database. *J. Hematol. Oncol.* 2009;**2**:41–9.

10. Reed, V., Shah, J., Medeiros, L. J. *et al.* Solitary plasmacytomas: outcome and prognostic factors after definitive radiation therapy. *Cancer* 2011;**117**: 4468–74.

11. Hill, Q., Rawstron, A., de Tute, R. *et al.* Outcome prediction in solitary plasmacytoma of bone (SPB): Development of a risk stratification model utilising bone marrow flow cytometry and light chain analysis. *Haematologica* 2011; **96(s1)**:158.

Extramedullary plasmacytoma

Extramedullary plasmacytoma (EMP) are rare tumors that typically present as solitary lesions at soft tissue sites without evidence of local bone destruction or signs of multiple myeloma. They frequently arise in the upper aerodigestive tract but have been described in numerous other anatomical locations including lymph nodes, gastrointestinal tract and skin. Owing to their sites of presentation, excellent response to local therapy and low rate of progression to myeloma it has been considered by some that EMP do not form part of the spectrum of plasma cell disorders but may represent a form of extranodal marginal zone lymphoma (ENMZL) exhibiting marked plasma cell differentiation [1]. Recent data have, however, demonstrated that EMP are in fact characterized by a similar range of immunophenotypic and genotypic abnormalities to those encountered in standard myeloma [2–7]. It is clear the plasma cells of EMP have an aberrant immunophenotype in >90% of cases and this is extremely useful in the differential diagnosis of EMP and ENMZL. Aberrant expression of CD19, CD56, CD117, CD27, CD20 and cyclin D1 has been demonstrated by a number of investigators although the incidence of CD56 and cyclin D1 protein expression may be lower than that typically seen in myeloma [3,5,7].

Similarly recent cytogenetic data have demonstrated a high incidence of deletion 13, hyperdiploidy and immunoglobulin heavy chain rearrangements including both the t(11;14)(q13;q32) and the t(4;14)(p16;q32) with no evidence of rearrangements of *MALT1*, *PAX5*, *FOXP1* or *BCL6* [2,4,6,7].

It is essential that a diagnosis of EMP is made following formal assessment of surgical biopsy material as fine needle cytology is inadequate in this setting [8]. In histological sections CD138 and MUM1/IRF4 are the most useful antibodies to confirm the nature of the plasma cell infiltrate although CD38 and VS38c may also be used. EMP are characterized by a monomorphic infiltrate of monotypic plasma cells but additional steps are required to definitively exclude ENMZL. In the latter it is possible in virtually all cases even in the presence of extensive plasma cell differentiation to show the presence of a concomitant small B-cell component. This may be highlighted by CD20 staining although PAX5 protein may also be needed if the plasma cells show aberrant expression of CD20. Similarly the aberrant of expression of CD19, CD56, CD117, CD27, CD20 and cyclin D1 is confined to EMP [7–9]. Local amyloid deposition may also be seen in EMP and in some instances may account for the bulk of the tumor.

References

1. Hussong, J. W., Perkins, S. L., Schnitzer, B. *et al.* Extramedullary plasmacytoma. A form of marginal zone cell lymphoma? *Am.* *J. Clin. Pathol.* 1999;**111**: 111–16.

2. Y. Aalto, S. Nordling, A. H. Kivioja, et al. Among numerous DNA copy number changes, losses of chromosome 13 are highly recurrent in plasmacytoma. *Genes Chromosomes Cancer* 1999;**25**:104–7.

seen on giemsa stained sections or highlighted with CD117 or mast cell tryptase immunohistochemistry) and intranuclear and cytoplasmic immunoglobulin inclusions, termed Dutcher and Russell bodies respectively.

The overall extent of plasma cell differentiation varies considerably from patient to patient and it appears that this is the major determinant of paraprotein concentration rather than the overall extent of marrow infiltration [6]. In a significant minority (20%) of cases the degree plasma cell differentiation may be such that plasma cells are the predominant cell type and IgM myeloma becomes part of the differential diagnosis [7].

Immunophenotypic studies are necessary for a definitive diagnosis of WM [1] and this may be achieved using either flow cytometry or immunohistochemistry although the former allows for a more extensive assessment of antigenic determinants. In WM it is generally possible to demonstrate both monotypic B cells and monotypic plasma cells but extended phenotyping is usually only performed on the B cell component [5,7–9]. This component of the disease shows almost universal expression of the pan B cell antigens CD19, CD20 and CD79 while CD5 and CD23 are expressed in a minority of cases only. Distinguishing WM from CLL is not usually difficult but mantle cell lymphoma may require specific exclusion in those cases showing strong CD5 expression and this is readily done by cyclin D1 immunostaining or FISH studies for the t(11;14). The germinal center associated antigens CD10 and BCL6 are not demonstrable but most cases show expression of the memory B cell marker CD27 as well as CD52. Distinguishing WM form marginal zone lymphoma can however be difficult although the expression patterns of CD22, CD25 and CD103 may be helpful as WM may show a CD25+ CD22 weak CD103− pattern whilst MZL may be CD22+ CD25− and CD103+. Clinical correlation is, however, essential for definitive diagnosis [5,7–10].

There are limited data on plasma cell immunophenotyping in WM but the published data would suggest that the antigenic patterns seen in myeloma plasma cells (CD19− CD45− CD56+) are not seen in WM plasma cells [7–9]. This can be useful in those cases of WM in which plasma cells predominate and plasma cell phenotyping should allow a definitive distinction between WM and the very rare entity of IgM myeloma [11].

It is also recognized that a proportion of patients with LPL have IgG or IgA rather than an IgM paraprotein but the clinicopathological features of such cases are poorly characterized at this time and their relationship to WM is unclear.

Cytogenetics. Conventional karyotyping has limited applicability in WM as it is difficult to obtain tumor metaphases because of the low rate of cell proliferation. There are no disease defining cytogenetic abnormalities but translocations involving the immunoglobulin heavy chain (*IGH*) locus at 14q32 are characteristically rare [12–14]. This is of course in contrast to IgM myeloma, which is characterized by a high incidence of *IGH* translocations and the t(11;14) in particular [11,13,15–18]. Deletion of chromosome 6q appears to be the commonest cytogenetic abnormality in WM occurring in up to 50% of patients and it may be associated with adverse clinical and laboratory parameters but its effect on overall outcome remains unclear [12,19,20]. Deletion of *TP53* occurs in a minority of patients but appears to define patients with a poor outcome [20].

IGH sequence analysis has been performed by a number of investigators and this typically shows evidence of somatic hypermutation without intraclonal diversity consistent with an origin in a post-germinal centre B cell. These studies have also demonstrated preferential use of *VH3* segments and the *VH3–23* in particular [21–23].

IgM MGUS. It is important that IgG and IgA MGUS is distinguished from IgM MGUS as the former is a precursor of myeloma and the latter a precursor of WM or other B cell lymphoproliferative disorders. IgM MGUS is defined by the presence of IgM monoclonal gammopathy without morphological evidence of marrow infiltration or other features of an underlying lymphoma such as lymphadenopathy [1]. It is, however, recognized that clonal B cells are demonstrable in a significant proportion of patients without morphological evidence of marrow disease [24]. It is unclear whether the rate of progression to symptomatic disease is greater in such patients. The role of marrow assessment in asymptomatic individuals is not established but an arbitrary cut-off of 10 g/l has been proposed in some guidelines [25]. Bone marrow examination should, however, be considered at lower IgM concentrations particularly if the patient is suspected of having an IgM related syndrome such as peripheral neuropathy or cold agglutinin disease or AL amyloidosis.

If marrow examination is performed it is important that a trephine biopsy be obtained as well as a marrow aspirate. Flow cytometry may identify small clonal B cell populations but plasma cell phenotyping is rarely if ever informative.

There is very limited cytogenetic data in IgM MGUS but recent studies have failed to demonstrate 6q deletions suggesting that this abnormality is a secondary abnormality rather than an initiating event in IgM MGUS/WM [26,27].

Assessment of bone marrow response. The assessment of therapeutic response in WM relies heavily upon changes in the serum concentration of the IgM paraprotein. It has, however, become clear that there may be discrepancies between serum IgM and bone marrow responses. IgM responses are typically slow with purine analog and monoclonal antibody-based therapy as it appears these agents selectively deplete the CD20+ B cell component with sparing of the CD138+ plasma cell component of the disease [10,28]. In this context it is possible to demonstrate significant B cell depletion in the marrow but suboptimal IgM responses. Satisfactory IgM responses are subsequently documented in the majority of patients with maximum responses documented at a median of six months following the completion of therapy in fludarabine treated patients for instance [28]. Conversely bortezomib-containing regimens and other novel agents such as the mTOR inhibitor everolimus (RAD001) may demonstrate excellent IgM responses but suboptimal bone marrow responses [29].

Repeat marrow assessments can therefore provide significant value in the routine management of individual patients. In order to make a detailed assessment of residual infiltrates, it is recognized that both bone marrow aspirate and trephine biopsies should be obtained and that these should be routinely supplemented by flow cytometric and immunohistochemistry studies. Attempts should be made to characterize residual infiltrates with respect to their B cell and plasma cell content and immunohistochemical assessment of trephine biopsy sections provides the optimal method. CD138 and/or MUM1/IRF4 may be used to demonstrate residual plasma cells while CD20 may be used to define residual B cell infiltration, although additional markers such as PAX5 may be necessary in rituximab treated patients owing to the loss of antigen expression which is sometimes seen in post-treatment specimens.

There are very limited data on minimal residual disease (MRD) assessment in WM but these are likely to become more relevant as therapeutic strategies improve and the incidence of complete responses increases.

Histological transformation. Histological transformation, primarily to diffuse large B cell lymphona (DLBCL) is a well recognized phenomenon in indolent lymphoproliferative disorders. It has been reported to occur in 5%–10% of patients with WM which is very similar to the incidence reported in chronic lymphocytic leukemia (CLL). The pathobiologic events underlying histological transformation events are poorly characterized but recent studies have highlighted a potential role for the nucleoside analogs [30]. Histological transformation events have been thought traditionally to occur within the original B cell clone as a consequence of the acquisition of additional genetic events. Recent data, however, have demonstrated the potentially diverse nature of transformation events and in particular the role of Epstein–Barr virus (EBV). These latter events include EBV-positive but clonally unrelated diffuse large B cell lymphoma and spontaneously resolving EBV-positive mucocutaneous ulcer [31,32].

References

1. Owen, R. G., Treon, S. P., Al-Katib, A. *et al.* Clinicopathological definition of Waldenstrom's macroglobulinemia: consensus panel recommendations from the Second International Workshop on Waldenstrom's Macroglobulinemia. *Semin. Oncol.* 2003;**30**: 110–15.

2. Kyle, R. A., Garton, J. P. The spectrum of IgM monoclonal gammopathy in 430 cases. *Mayo. Clin. Proc.* 1987;**62**:719–31.

3. Owen, R. G., Parapia, L. A., Higginson, J. *et al.* Clinicopathological correlates of IgM paraproteinemias. *Clin. Lymphoma* 2000;**1**: 39–43.

4. Lin, P., Hao, S., Handy B. C. *et al.* Lymphoid neoplasms associated with IgM paraprotein: a study of 382 patients. *Am. J. Clin. Pathol.* 2005;**123**:200–5.

5. Owen, R. G., Barrans, S. L., Richards, S. J. *et al.* Waldenstrom macroglobulinemia. Development of diagnostic criteria and identification of prognostic factors. *Am. J. Clin. Pathol.* 2001;**116**:420–8.

6. Pasricha, S. R., Junega, S. K., Westerman, D. A. *et al.*

Chapter

3

Imaging of myeloma

Nicola Mulholland and Ming Young Simon Wan

Introduction

Multiple myeloma and its related entities (Table 3.1) are a spectrum of disorders characterized by monoclonal proliferation of plasma cells, usually with associated excessive production and secretion of monoclonal proteins detectable in serum or urine. While their management relies much on clinical and laboratory derived parameters, imaging also plays an important role. The suspicion of myeloma may be raised when an incidental lytic bone lesion is identified on a radiological examination performed for other purposes. Skeletal survey with plain radiographs is one of the initial screening tests performed when there is a suspicion of myeloma. Imaging is essential in accurately characterizing the disease entity within the spectrum. In some circumstances, such as in solitary plasmacytoma, diagnosis may be confidently achieved only with bone or soft tissue biopsy under image guidance. In addition, imaging may provide important staging and prognostic information and allow evaluation of response to treatment.

The use of X-rays in the evaluation of myeloma has been documented as early as 1900. To this date, the skeletal survey has remained the first line imaging investigation of choice. The introduction of CT and body MRI systems in the 1970s and hybrid PET/CT imaging systems in the 1990s have expanded the armament of the radiologist. Paralleling these developments

Table 3.1 Multiple myeloma and related disorders

Monoclonal gammopathy of uncertain significance (MGUS).
Smoldering/asymptomatic multiple myeloma.
Solitary plasmacytoma.
Extramedullary plasmacytoma.
Multiple solitary plasmacytomas.

is our improving understanding of the pathophysiology of myeloma and the on-going development and refinement of therapeutic strategies. These advances have necessitated continual evolution and standardization of diagnostic, staging and response evaluation criteria. This chapter reviews the imaging techniques currently available in routine clinical practice.

Plain radiography

Conventional radiography has been the workhorse for imaging myeloma for many years. Bone lesions identified on conventional radiographs is one of the defining characteristics of (symptomatic) myeloma, distinguishing this from smoldering myeloma and MGUS. The landmark study by Durie and Salmon in 1975 demonstrated an association between the extent of bone lesions identified on radiographs and tumor burden. This led to the incorporation of plain film findings into the original Durie/Salmon staging system, which has subsequently been widely adopted. Skeletal survey remains currently the first line imaging investigation of choice for the screening, diagnosis and staging of myeloma in various contemporary national and international guidelines, such as by the International Myeloma Working Group and the British Committee for Standards in Haematology.

A complete skeletal survey should include a postero-anterior (PA) view of the chest, anteroposterior (AP) and lateral views of the cervical spine, thoracic spine, lumbar spine, humeri and femora, AP and lateral views of the skull and AP view of the pelvis to provide adequate coverage of the skeleton; other symptomatic areas should be specifically visualized with appropriate views.

It is recognized that up to 80% of newly diagnosed patients with multiple myeloma will have radiological

Myeloma, ed. Stephen A. Schey, Kwee L. Yong, Robert Marcus and Kenneth C. Anderson. Published by Cambridge University Press. © Cambridge University Press 2014.

(a)

(b)

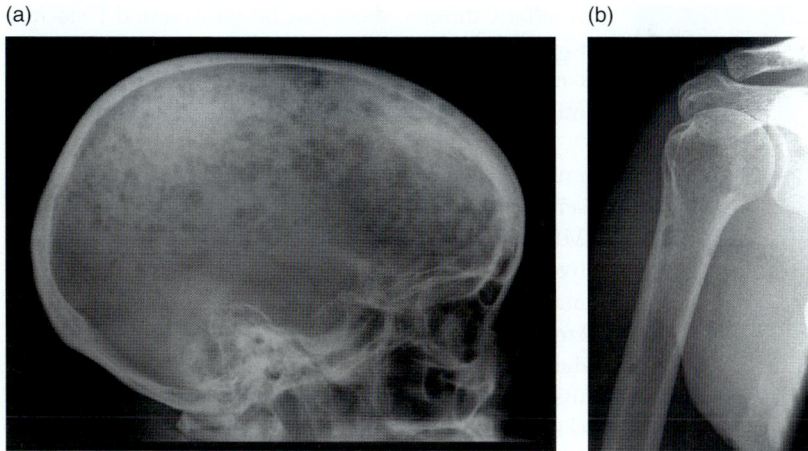

Figure 3.1 Multiple well-defined radiolucent lesions in the skull (a) and in the humerus (b). The appearances are classically described as "punched out."

evidence of skeletal involvement in skeletal surveys (the rest have their diagnoses established on the basis of raised M-protein in the serum +/− urine, bone marrow biopsy, and other related organ or tissue impairment such as hypercalcemia, renal insufficiency, anemia and amyloidosis). The radiographic findings may be focal or diffuse, with generalized osteopenia being the only findings in up to 15% of patients. Complicating pathological fractures are not uncommon. Focal lesions can be of varying sizes and are typically well-defined lucent areas with no sclerotic rim, classically described as "punched out lesions" (Figure 3.1a,b). The lytic lesions are often central in distribution, involving the vertebrae in 65% of patients, ribs in 45%, skull in 40%, shoulders in 40%, pelvis in 30% and proximal long bones in 25%. Lesions distal to the elbows and knees are uncommon. Bone destruction by myeloma may also present as having a permeated/moth-eaten pattern on radiographs. Osteosclerotic myelomatous lesions are rare and may be seen as isolated lesions in patients with POEMS syndrome (polyneuropathy, organomegaly, endocrinopathy, monoclonal gammopathy and skin changes). Myeloma with diffuse osteosclerosis has been reported but it has been argued by some that this represents a separate entity from POEMS syndrome.

The main differential diagnosis of myeloma on plain radiography would be metastatic bone disease, in cases of (multi-)focal lytic lesions, and osteoporosis, in cases where radiographs show diffuse osteopenia. Distinction between these may not be possible on skeletal survey but serum/urine protein measurements and identification of any separate primary malignancy would clarify.

Skeletal survey is widely available with relatively low cost and radiation burden. However, there are several disadvantages. The sensitivity and specificity are less, compared with other imaging techniques. It is recognized that conventional radiography is insensitive to bone marrow/early bone disease, requiring at least 30% of cancellous bone loss before a lytic lesion is perceptible. Overlapping structures and composite shadowing often obscure smaller lytic lesions. Distinguishing myeloma deposits from other metastatic bone deposits, vertebral fractures secondary to myelomatous infiltration from non-myelomatous causes are often not possible on plain radiography. In addition, bone lesions seldom show evidence of healing. Therefore evaluation of treatment response and disease restaging is not possible. On the other hand, new vertebral fractures in patients known to have myeloma cannot be relied upon to define disease progression, as this may be due to reduction of tumor mass to support the bone cortex. The reproducibility of skeletal survey findings has also been shown to be low between centers.

Computed tomography

Computed tomography (CT) is an X-ray based technique, where specialized X-ray tubes and detectors housed opposite to each other in the scanner gantry (ring) revolves around the patient. The innumerable projections acquired are reconstructed by computers into axial (or transverse) "slices," showing the cross-sectional anatomy of the patient. Recent development of multidetector row CT (MDCT) allows for faster image acquisition and with higher resolution. The

29

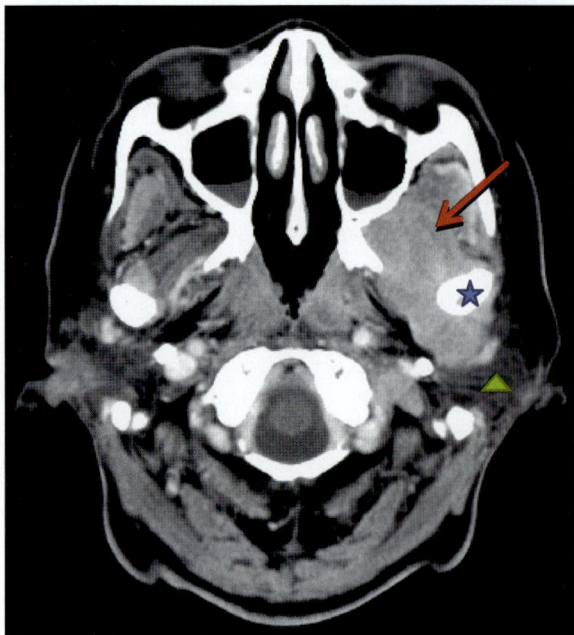

Figure 3.2 Contrast enhanced CT image (axial) at the level of the mandibular condyle (*). This known myeloma patient presented with left-sided facial nerve palsy. CT demonstrates a soft tissue mass (arrow) infiltrating the masticator space and involving the deep lobe of left parotid gland (triangle), causing the facial nerve palsy.

resultant thinner slices can be reformatted ("stacked together") and displayed in other planes, such as the coronal and sagittal images often seen presented at multidisciplinary meetings.

The strength of CT rests on its excellent ability to image bones with exquisite details. It has a high sensitivity in demonstrating early small lytic lesions. MDCT in particular has been shown to be very sensitive for detecting lytic lesions <5 mm, compared to magnetic resonance imaging (MRI) and positron emission tomography (PET). CT is much better at demonstrating extra-osseous lesions and defining soft tissue extension of disease than plain radiography (Figures 3.2 and 3.3). For these reasons, it has been recommended that CT is used to complement skeletal survey to assess sites not accurately assessed by plain radiography (e.g. ribs, sternum and scapula), and where the plain film finding is ambiguous. It may also be used to clarify situations where patients remain troubled by local symptoms despite negative results from other imaging modalities (e.g. pain despite unremarkable MRI of the spine).

CT is quick to perform, with a complete whole body diagnostic acquisition in seconds. The examination can be performed in a third of the time required

(a)

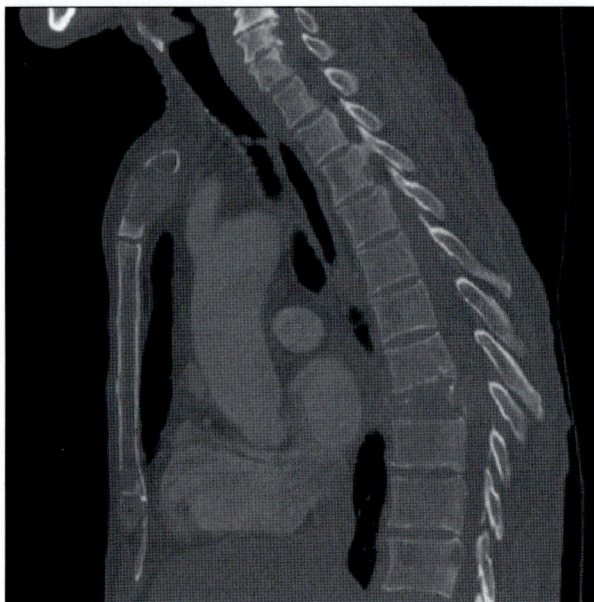

(b)

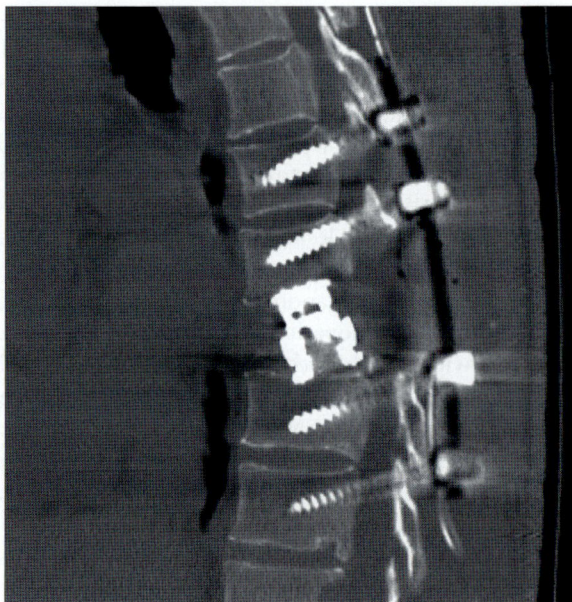

Figure 3.3 This patient without a previous diagnosis of myeloma presented with acute cord compression. CT demonstrated a destroyed T8 vertebral body, which was subsequently fixated by surgery. Further smaller lytic lesions can be seen in some of the other vertebral bodies on the pre-operative CT. Histology confirmed a plasma cell tumor.

for a complete skeletal survey and without having to reposition the patient multiple times. This can be an important consideration when patients with myeloma can sometimes be suffering from severe pain. Acquisition times for MRI and PET/CT are also much longer, with the examination time usually in the order of around half an hour, which may not be tolerated by some patients. In addition, CT is widely available, even outside of normal working hours and would give useful information at times when MRI is not readily available, for example, in urgent cases of suspected acute spinal fracture.

Beyond diagnostic studies, CT is an essential tool for directing percutaneous needle biopsy of soft tissue or bone lesions for histological diagnosis. CT is currently the basis of radiotherapy planning. CT's ability to image bone details makes it the choice for planning orthopedic fixation of established or impending pathological fractures (Figure 3.3).

Despite these advantages, radiation dose is a drawback, limiting its wider use and in screening for bone lesions in suspected myeloma cases. A typical dose for an adult body CT from thorax to pelvis would be in the order of 20–30 mSv (for comparison, the annual background radiation from natural sources is around 2 mSv; that of a chest radiograph is 0.02 mSv). With myeloma patients potentially requiring multiple examinations during the course of their disease, the accumulative dose would be considerable. Intravenous iodinated contrast media is required to optimally visualize soft tissue extent of disease. However, the use of these agents is associated with contrast induced nephropathy. This is of particular relevance as many myeloma patients may also have a degree of renal impairment. Like skeletal survey, CT is of little use for response evaluation as lytic lesions often remain radiolucent despite a biological response.

Magnetic resonance imaging

For magnetic resonance imaging (MRI), the patient is placed inside a strong magnetic field (usually generated by a superconductor magnet). Radiofrequency pulses are "fired" at the patient in a controlled fashion, which perturbs the proton spins in the tissues. Protons in different tissues become excited and relax at different rates – these differences are detected, localized and used to construct the images. T1 and T2 are fundamental properties of tissues corresponding to their response to the pulse sequences and these

are used to reconstruct the basic T1 and T2 "weighted" images. As a general rule, water is bright on T2 and dark on T1 weighted images, whereas fat is bright on both T1 and T2 weighted images. Further tissue characteristics can be probed by different and more sophisticated pulse sequence design. For instance, images can be generated that are "fat suppressed," "edema sensitive" (e.g. STIR), or to reflect diffusivity of water within tissues (diffusion weighted imaging, DWI). Like CT, contrast agents can be used to demonstrate enhancement but these are generally gadolinium based. Their use should also be cautious in patients with renal impairment due to its link with "nephrogenic systemic fibrosis."

Compared to other modalities (plain film/ CT / PET), MRI does not involve radiation and has true multiplanar imaging capability. It offers excellent delineation of soft tissue structures and pathologies, giving complementary information to CT. It is the imaging technique of choice in cases of suspected cord compression, giving information regarding the level of cord and nerve roots involvement and the extent of tumor extension into the epidural space.

With MRI, we are able to image marrow infiltration directly, before plain film or CT changes occur. Marrow signal depends on the fat, water and cellular contents and these changes with age. Normal adult patients have marrow signal that is high (bright) on T1 and T2 weighted images, reflecting the replacement of hematopoetic red marrow with predominant fat content. On the other hand, myelomatous deposits typically appear as areas which are darker on T1 weighted images due to cellular infiltration of the normally fatty marrow and they may show variable enhancement post contrast depending on vascularity. With this premise, different patterns of marrow infiltration in untreated disease have been described on MRI : (1) normal, (2) focal, (3) homogeneously and diffusely abnormal, (4) both focal and diffuse involvement and (5) "salt and pepper" pattern with heterogenous patchy appearance, corresponding to bone marrow with circumscribed fat islands beside normal bone marrow and minor infiltration of plasma cells. Several studies have suggested that the MRI pattern reflects the extent of tumor burden. Normal marrow pattern is present in 50%–75% of Salmon–Durie stage I disease at diagnosis whereas it is only present in 20% of stage III disease. The "salt and pepper" pattern tends to show signs of lower tumor burden compared to focal or diffuse patterns of infiltration.

(a)   (b)

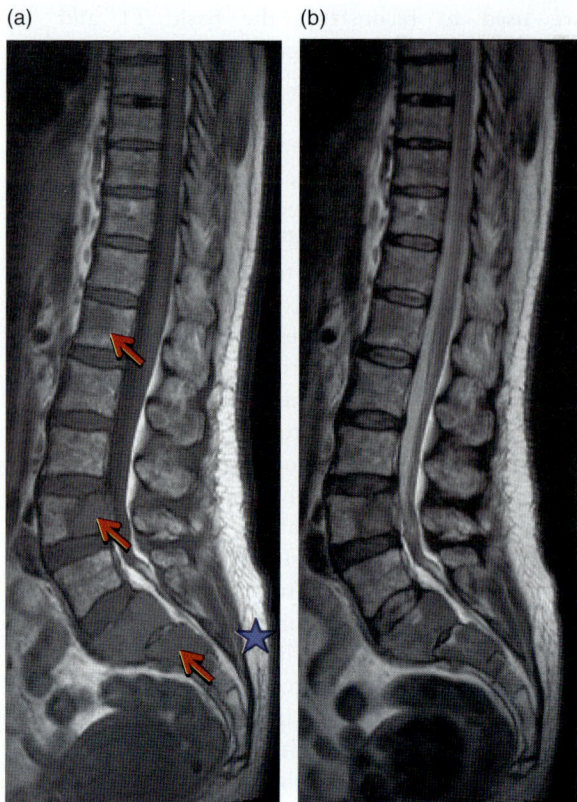

Figure 3.4 Focal and diffuse pattern. T1 weighted sagittal image of this patient's lumbar spine demonstrates numerous small foci of low T1 signal throughout the lumbar spine, with more discrete focal low T1 signal lesions in L1, L4 vertebral bodies and in the sacrum (arrows). Normal fat signal on T1 weighted images can be appreciated in the subcutaneous tissue (*). Contemporaneous bone marrow trephine demonstrates numerous plasma cells constituting >10% of total nucleated cells. The corresponding T2 weighted image is also shown.

On the other hand, the focal and diffuse pattern has been shown to correlate with low serum hemoglobin and high percentage of marrow plasmacytosis, supporting that this pattern correlates with a high tumor burden (Figure 3.4). A homogeneously diffuse abnormal marrow pattern also indicates high tumor load and is associated with poor prognosis (Figure 3.5). Caution should be exercised in the interpretation as these MRI findings are not completely specific, with some of these changes reflective of other pathological or physiological processes such as with iron overload, amyloid infiltration or reactive bone marrow hyperplasia.

MRI has been demonstrated to show more lesions than that apparent on skeletal surveys. In addition, MRI findings have also been shown to be of prognostic values. Patients with an apparent single lytic lesion on plain film but further lesions found on MRI have a shorter time to disease progression and need for therapy compared to those with normal MRI pattern. Patients with normal MRI findings are associated with a better response to conventional chemotherapy compared to those with focal or diffuse infiltration. In the context of tandem autologous transplantation based protocol, focal lesions defined on MRI, but not conventional radiography, have been shown to independently affect survival. The number of MRI lesions demonstrated in advanced stage myeloma has also been shown to predict fracture risk, with a six–ten fold increased risk if more than ten lesions are present.

MRI is a useful problem solving tool. In attempts to distinguish vertebral fractures secondary to osteoporosis from those due to malignant aetiology such as myeloma, demonstration on MRI of a convex border towards the spinal canal, an epidural mass and enhancement or abnormal signal characteristics, compatible with infiltration of the vertebral body would be suggestive of a malignant cause (Figure 3.6).

Distinction between MGUS and early myeloma can be difficult. Demonstration of normal marrow signal would be a useful piece of information to support a diagnosis of MGUS. On the other hand, one study has shown that in a small proportion of patients believed to have MGUS or monogammaglobulinemia of borderline significance, MRI abnormalities may be present. It has also shown that these patients had a shorter time to progression to multiple myeloma. In the context of suspected solitary plasmacytoma, detection of further bone lesions would prompt a significant change in diagnosis and management. Exclusion of further bone lesions to a high degree of certainty would be prudent before consideration of local therapy. To this end, MRI has been proposed to become part of routine staging in patients suspected of having solitary plasmacytoma.

Response assessment is limited on CT and plain film, but emerging evidence has shown that this may be possible with MRI. Responding lesions may reduce in size, T2 signal (i.e. becomes less bright on T2 weighted images) and enhancement. Some responding lesions may remain unchanged, however. Response assessment can be confounded by treatment induced inflammation or necrosis. Diffusion weighted imaging (DWI) is a well-established technique in neuroimaging and it is being increasingly

(a)   (b)

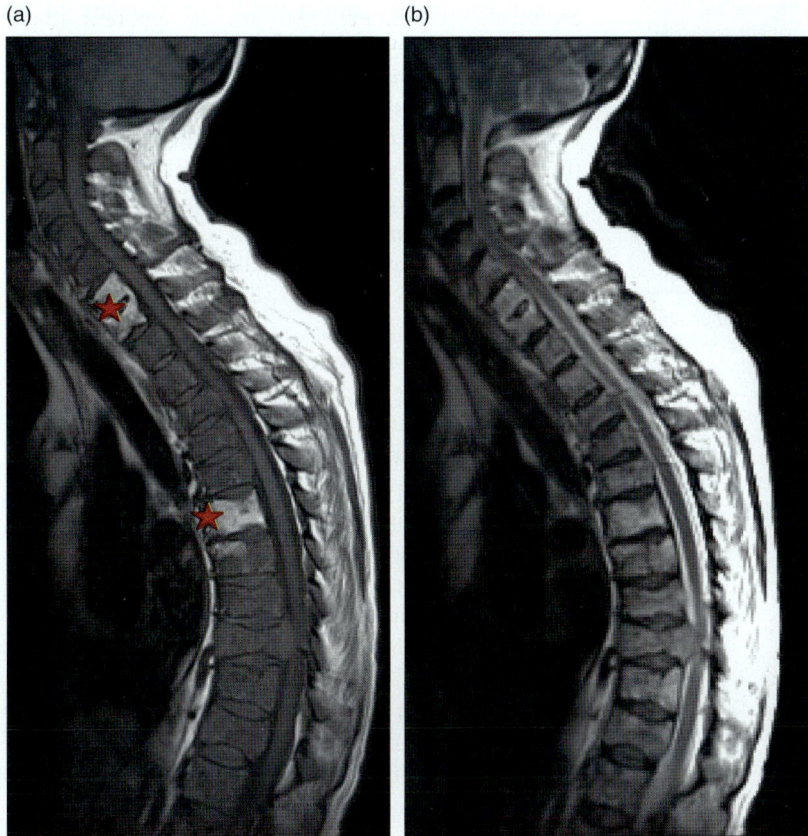

Figure 3.5 Diffusely abnormal marrow signal. T1 weighted sagittal image of the cervicothoracic spine of this patient shows a diffusely low T1 signal. Relatively normal marrow is present in only a handful of vertebral bodies (*). Contemporaneous bone marrow trephine demonstrates numerous plasma cells constituting 12%–36% of total nucleated cells. The corresponding T2 weighted image is also shown.

used in the oncological setting. In solid tumors, diffusivity of water within tissues is thought to be a surrogate marker of cellularity – water diffusion is "restricted" in a highly cellular environment due to cellular boundaries and the region would show high signal on the DWI images (Figure 3.7) and low signal on the apparent diffusion coefficient (ADC) map. However, in bone marrow, the relationship between diffusivity, marrow fat and changes in marrow cellularity is not straight forward, making the interpretation of DWI for response assessment complex. Nevertheless, studies are emerging to suggest that it could be useful for response assessment.

On the down side, MRI can be a lengthy procedure, lasting at least around 15–20 min but can be up to 1 h depending on coverage required, the complexity and number of sequences used. The central bore of the scanner is narrower and much noisier than that of CT. It is not infrequent that patients cannot tolerate an MRI examination due to claustrophobia. Metallic implants (pacemaker, older-generation aneurysm clips are common examples) and foreign body (for example in the eyes) are contraindications of MRI examinations. MRI is also relatively costly and not as widely available as plain radiography and CT.

Radionuclide imaging and hybrid imaging

Radionuclide imaging involves administration of a tiny amount of radiolabeled "tracer" into the patient. The tracer contains a radioactive isotope bound to a functional moiety, which determines its behavior in the body. The most commonly used isotopes are technetium-99m (Tc-99m) for conventional γ-emitting radionuclide studies and fluorine-18 (F-18) for positron emission tomography (PET). Physiological processes can be imaged by detecting, localizing and analyzing the radiation emitted from the patient inside dedicated scanners. More recently, technological advances have allowed the construction of hybrid scanners, enabling synergistic acquisition of functional data by nuclear medicine techniques and anatomical information by structural imaging, which

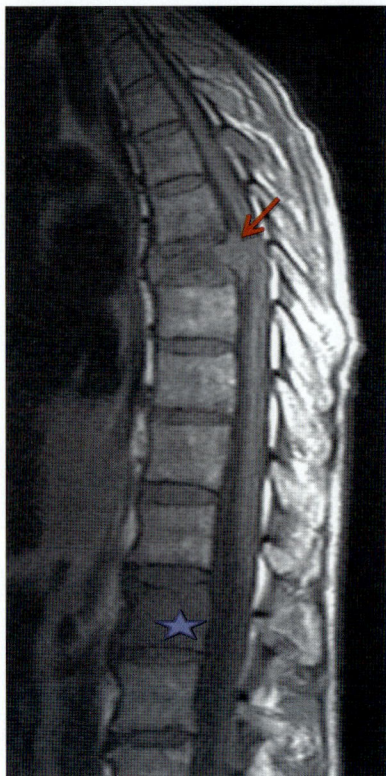

Figure 3.6 This patient presented with thoracic cord compression. Sagittal T1 weight image shows a fracture of an upper thoracic vertebral body which has been replaced by soft tissue mass. The epidural component of this mass demonstrates a convex border posteriorly (arrow), typical of malignant infiltration. Further abnormal marrow signal is observed in other vertebral bodies (*).

complement each other. PET/CT for PET tracers and SPECT/CT for γ-emitting tracers have become more widely available over the last decade, with whole-body PET/MRI systems emerging in the market in the last couple of years.

A number of radiotracers have been used in imaging myeloma over the years. Bone-seeking agents such as strontium-85, strontium-87m, non-specific tumor seeking agents such as Tc-99m V-DMSA, thallium-201 and gallium-67 citrate have been tried. These have not left long-lasting clinical impact. The currently commonly performed bone scans using technetium-99m diphosphonates compounds have been disappointing in the detection of myeloma lesions. These accumulate at sites of osteoblastic activity, which is lacking in myeloma, resulting in a normal bone scan or subtle focal areas of low uptake (photopenia). It has been shown that bone scans detect less lesions than skeletal survey (apart from at specific sites where lesions are difficult to appreciate on plain film, such as the sternum) and the sensitivity is in the range of 40%–60%.

Technetium-99m labeled sestamibi (MIBI) is a γ-emitting tracer for which the mechanism of action is not completely understood but thought to be related to mitochondrial activity. It is used extensively in myocardial perfusion imaging but it is also recognized to have tumor seeking properties. It had been used in the context of sarcoma, breast, brain, lung and thyroid cancers, with a body of literature supporting its use in plasma cell tumors. Studies have shown that it has a superior sensitivity in detecting myeloma lesions than conventional radiography but inferior to that of FDG PET/CT (F-18 flurodeoxyglucose PET/CT).

F-18 FDG is a commonly used PET tracer. It is a positron emitting, radiolabeled glucose analog which enters cells through active transporters and remains trapped in cells without undergoing further metabolism after initial phosphorylation. It is variably taken up by different tissues reflecting their glucose metabolism, demonstrating high uptake in organs like brain and in pathological tissues with high metabolic activity (e.g. inflammatory tissues and some tumors). Unlike MRI, which is still largely a regional imaging technique, PET/CT examinations provide whole body coverage (Figure 3.8). Studies have confirmed that FDG PET/CT is more sensitive in detecting myeloma deposits in the context of primary staging and disease relapse, compared to plain radiography and MRI. This is thought especially due to its wider coverage, "upstaging" what would otherwise be thought of as limited disease or solitary plasmacytoma. On the contrary, some studies have concluded that MRI performs better in detecting small lesions and in diffuse marrow infiltration. There is some evidence to suggest that FDG PET/CT can be useful in the distinction of MGUS from myeloma. In addition, studies have suggested a role of FDG PET/CT in evaluation of treatment response, demonstrating that active myeloma lesions show positive FDG uptake, which decreases with effective therapy, and that persistent FDG positivity correlates with likely earlier relapses.

Several non-FDG PET tracers have been studied in humans, including F-18 sodium fluoride (a bone-seeking agent), 3′-[18F]fluoro-3′-deoxythymidine (F-18 FLT, an analog of a DNA nucleoside hypothesized to be a "proliferation" marker) and carbon-11 methionine (an amino-acid analog). These tracers are not widely available and data regarding their use in myeloma are limited. It remains to be seen whether they will be translated into routine clinical use.

PET/MRI is a recent introduction, combining the exquisite sensitivity of functional and molecular

(a)

(b)

(c)

(d)

(e)

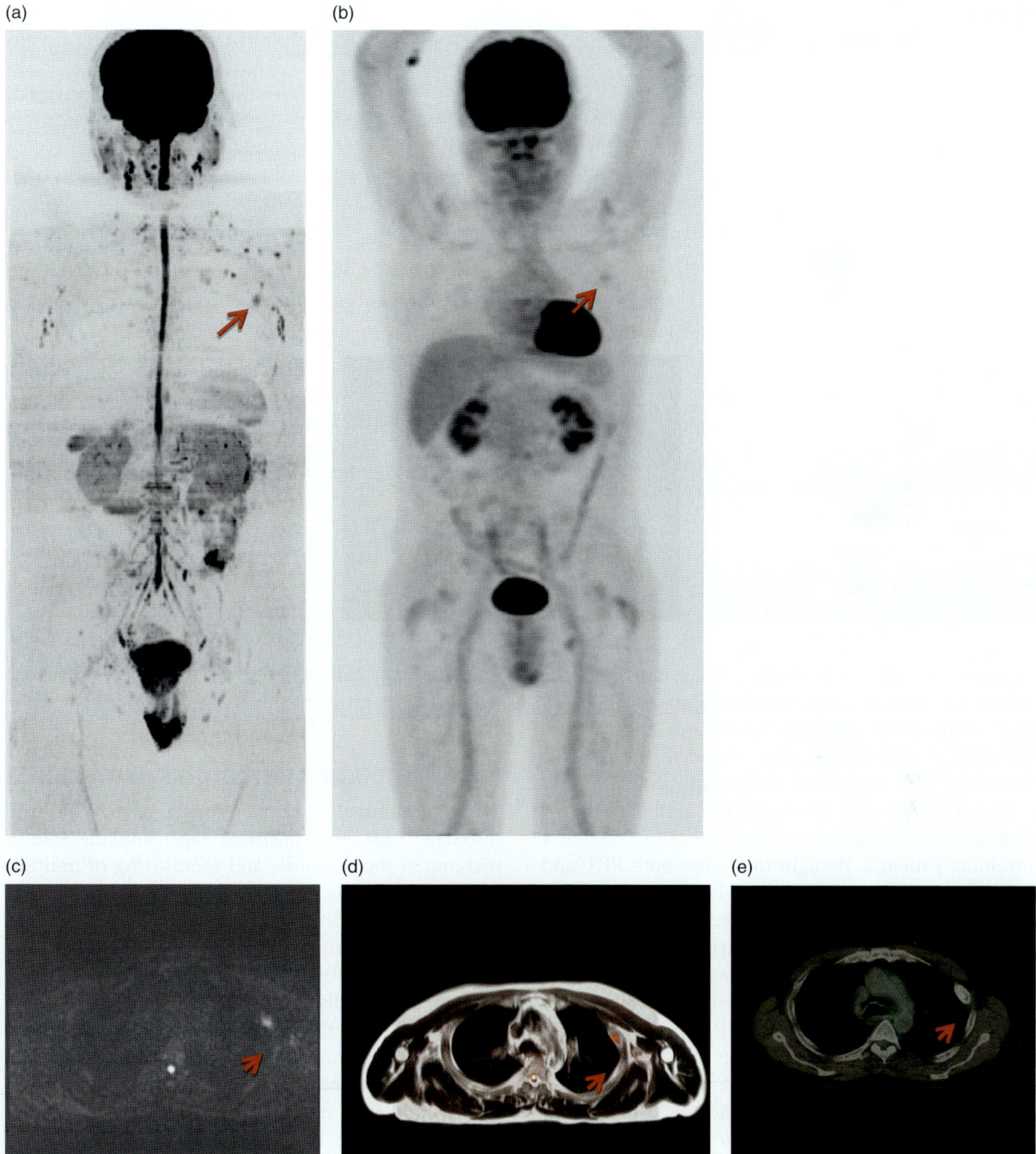

Figure 3.7 A patient with a slight rise in serum light chains and percentage of bone marrow plasma cells several years following autologous stem cell transplant for non-secretory myeloma. Whole-body DWI images (top left) displayed as maximum intensity projection (MIP), show a focus of altered diffusion in a left sided rib (arrow). This is confirmed on the axial MRI images (DWI image, bottom right; the same DWI image is colour coded and co-registered to a T2 weighted image in the middle, for better anatomical localization). The lesion correlates to a mildly FDG avid focus in a contemporaneous FDG PET/CT (top and bottom right), which on CT demonstrates an expanded appearance with some sclerosis. This is interpreted as representing residual active disease.

(a)

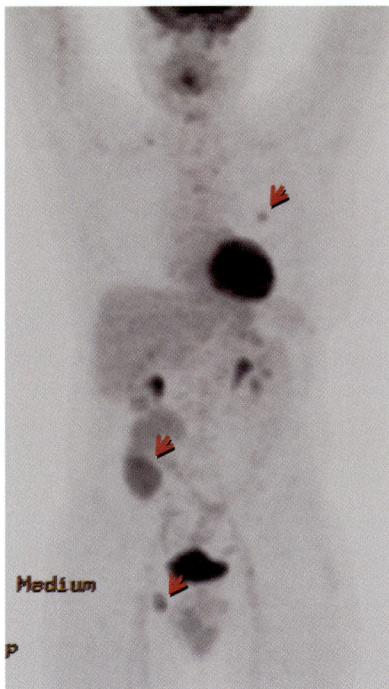

(b)

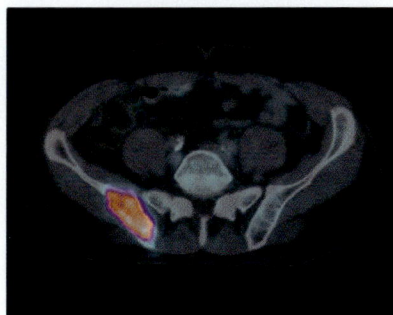

Figure 3.8 Whole-body MIP image of the FDG PET component of the PET/CT study showing multiple FDG avid lesions in a left-sided rib, right ilium and ischium (arrows), with corresponding axial fused PET/CT demonstrating the localization of the PET signal to a lytic lesion in the right ilium on CT.

imaging with PET and the excellent soft tissue resolution and emerging functional imaging capability of MRI (Figures 3.8 and 3.9). An obvious advantage is the comfort and convenience offered to the patients requiring PET and MRI, who can undergo both during a single visit. Currently the vast majority of clinical PET systems are in the form of PET/CT. If a myeloma patient is thought to require both PET and MRI, a CT study would inevitably be acquired as a "by-product" from PET/CT. Nevertheless, this would still give valuable complementary information (as described in the CT section above), even when the CT may not be of prime interest in the particular circumstance. Combined PET/MRI now allows PET and MRI examinations without the CT, offering potentially superior temporal and spatial registration of the PET and MRI datasets and a reduction of radiation burden. Advocates for PET/MRI would need to identify the cohort of patients and exact indications for which these advantages would outweigh the extra information gained from the CT generated by existing workflow. Radiotherapy planning for solitary plasmacytoma may be one such indication where the excellent spatial and temporal

image registration offered by the PET/MRI scan would be superior but this remains to be proven.

Current imaging paradigms in myeloma

The International Myeloma Working Group has produced a consensus statement regarding the role of imaging in the diagnosis and monitoring of multiple myeloma and this can be considered as the current standard of practice. It is recommended that skeletal survey be mandatory at the time of new diagnosis of myeloma as the first line staging modality. If only a solitary site of disease is identified irrespective of location, making the diagnosis of solitary plasmacytoma a possibility, an MRI of at least the whole spine should be performed. If the skeletal survey is normal, whole-body MRI may give complementary information. MRI is the method of choice if spinal cord compression is suspected. CT has complementary roles to MRI and may help clarify the presence or absence of bone destruction and the extent of any soft tissue disease if there is clinical concern and to guide biopsy. As described in earlier sections, response evaluation in bone lesions is difficult on imaging,

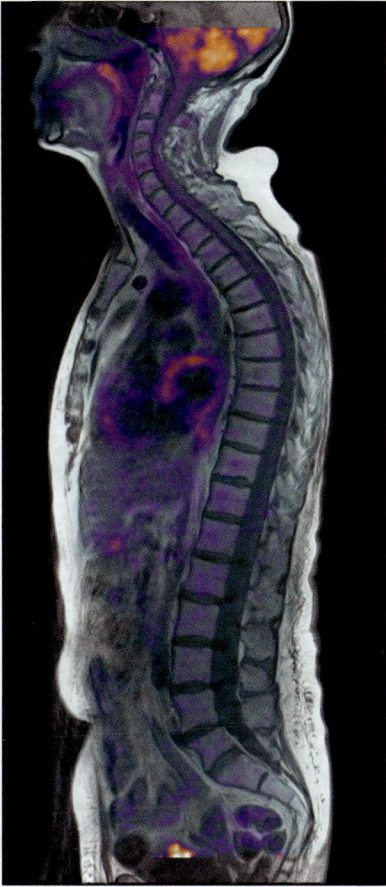

Figure 3.9 Sagittal fused FDG PET and T1 weighted MRI images of the whole body from a simultaneous acquisition, demonstrating no tracer avid disease in this patient suspected of having POEMS, with sclerotic lesions in the bones (not shown).

but CT and MRI can be used to monitor the response of soft tissue masses to therapy. Repeat skeletal survey should be used as the tool for restaging. Despite the emerging evidence for the use of FDG PET/CT and some authors proposing its usefulness (e.g. in Durie's Plus staging system), it is concluded that there is currently insufficient evidence to support its routine use. However, it is recognized that it may serve as a useful problem solving tool to clarify other imaging findings.

Conclusion

Imaging plays an important and supplementary role to other laboratory tests in the management of myeloma and its related disorders. Multiple imaging modalities are currently available for clinical use. Plain film and skeletal survey remains a time tested mainstay, with other modalities playing complementary roles in specific circumstances. Optimal choice of imaging test may also be influenced by local expertise and availability. Emerging techniques, such as advanced MRI techniques, FDG PET/CT, PET/MRI are exciting developments but their precise roles in imaging pathways are still to unravel.

Acknowledgement

The authors acknowledge Dr. Jamshed Bomanji (Consultant Nuclear Medicine Physician and Head of Department, Institute of Nuclear Medicine, University College Hospital, London) for providing the PET/MRI images and some of the MRI images.

Bibliography

1. The International Myeloma Working Group. Criteria for the classification of monoclonal gammopathies, multiple myeloma and related disorders: a report of the International Myeloma Working Group. *Br. J. Haematol.* 2003;**131**:749–57.

2. Weber, F. P., Hutchison, R., Macleod, J. J. R. Multiple myeloma (Myelomatosis) with Bence–Jones proteid in the urine. *Am. J. Med. Sci.* 1903;**126**(4):644–65.

3. Durie, B. G., Salmon, S. E. A clinical staging system for multiple myeloma. correlation of measured myeloma cell mass wth presenting clinical features, response to treatment and survival. *Cancer* 1975;**36**:842–54.

4. Kyle, R. A., Rajkumar, S. V. Criteria for diagnosis, staging, risk stratification and response assessment of multiple myeloma. *Leukemia* 2009;**23**(1):3–9.

5. D'Sa, S., Abildgaard, N., Tighe, J., Shaw, P., Hall-Craggs, M. Guidelines for the use of imaging in the management of myeloma. *Br. J. Haematol.* 2007;**137**(1): 49–63.

6. Bird, J. M., Owen, R. G., D'Sa, S. *et al.* Guidelines for the diagnosis and management of multiple myeloma 2011. *Br. J. Haematol.* 2011;**154**(1):32–75.

7. Dimopoulos, M., Terpos, E., Comenzo, R. L. *et al.* International myeloma working group consensus statement and guidelines regarding the current role of imaging techniques in the diagnosis and monitoring of multiple myeloma. *Leukemia* 2009;**23**(9):1545–56.

8. Collins, C. D. Multiple myeloma. *Cancer Imaging.* 2004;**4** Spec. No. A:S47–53.

9. Lacy, M. Q., Gertz, M. A., Hanson, C. A., Inwards, D., Kyle, R. Multiple myeloma associated with diffuse osteosclerotic bone lesions:

a clinical entity distinct from osteosclerotic myeloma (POEMS syndrome). *Am. J. Haematol.* 1997;**56**:288–93.

10. Fujii, K., Aoyama, T., Yamauchi-Kawaura, C., *et al.* Radiation dose evaluation in 64-slice CT examinations with adult and paediatric anthropomorphic phantoms. *Br. J. Radiol.* 2009;**82**(984): 1010–18.

11. Padhani, A. R., Gogbashian, A. Bony metastases: assessing response to therapy with whole-body diffusion MRI. *Cancer*

Imaging 2011;**11** Spec. No. A: S129–45.

12. Durie, B. G. The role of anatomic and functional staging in myeloma: description of Durie/Salmon plus staging system. *Eur. J. Cancer* 2006;**42** (11):1539–43.

13. Even-Sapir, E., Mishani, E., Flusser, G., Metser, U. 18F-Fluoride positron emission tomography and positron emission tomography/computed tomography. *Seminars Nuclear Med.* 2007;**37** (6):462–9.

14. Agool, A., Schot, B. W., Jager, P. L., Vellenga, E. 18-F-FLT PET in hematologic disorders: a novel technique to analyze the bone marrow compartment. *J. Nuclear Med.* 2006;**2006**(47):1592–8.

15. Dankerl, A., Liebisch, P., Glatting, G., *et al.* Multiple myeloma: molecular imaging with 11C-methionine PET/CT–initial experience. *Radiology* 2007;**242**(2):498–508.

16. Tan, E., Weiss, B. M., Mena, E., *et al.* Current and future imaging modalities for multiple myeloma and its precursor states. *Leukemia Lymphoma* 2011;**52**(9):1630–40.

4

Cell cycle regulation and myeloma precursor cells

John Quinn and Kwee L. Yong

Introduction

Unlike normal terminally differentiated plasma cells, MM cells are capable of self-renewal and proliferation. The direct impact of MM genetics on the expression and function of cell cycle proteins has provided the starting point for recent studies investigating the manner in which neoplastic plasma cells are able to bypass the cell cycle exit that is a prerequisite for terminal plasma cell differentiation. The search for tumor-initiating "stem" or "progenitor" cells is a current area of intense activity, and multiple myeloma, with its pre-malignant phase (MGUS), its derivation from an memory B cell compartment, and the (sometimes long) periods of disease quiescence termed the "plateau phase" offers unique opportunities to test certain hypotheses regarding these elusive cells. This chapter summarizes the current state of knowledge regarding cell cycle dysregulation in MM, and the existence and properties of myeloma precursor cells.

Cell cycle control

The mammalian cell cycle is tightly regulated through "checkpoints" to ensure that the cell enters S-phase undamaged. The transition between G1 and S-phase is regulated by the interaction between the major G1 cyclins – the D-type cyclins and the cyclin-dependent kinases (CDKs). The three D-type cyclins (D1, D2 and D3) control entry to the cell cycle and are usually induced in response to mitogens i.e. micro-environmental cytokines. D-type cyclins then bind to and activate CDK4 and -6 and these complexes phosphorylate retinoblastoma protein (phospho-pRb), thus allowing S-phase entry by releasing the E2F transcription factors which regulate genes controlling DNA synthesis [1] (Figure 4.1). The interaction between CDK2 and cyclin E also contributes to G1–S progression by phosphorylating pRb and the cyclin E/CDK2 complex is activated once the cyclin D-CDK4/6 complexes bind p21^{Cip1} and p27^{Kip1} [2]. G1–S progression is subject to further regulation by the cyclin-kinase inhibitor proteins (CKIs),

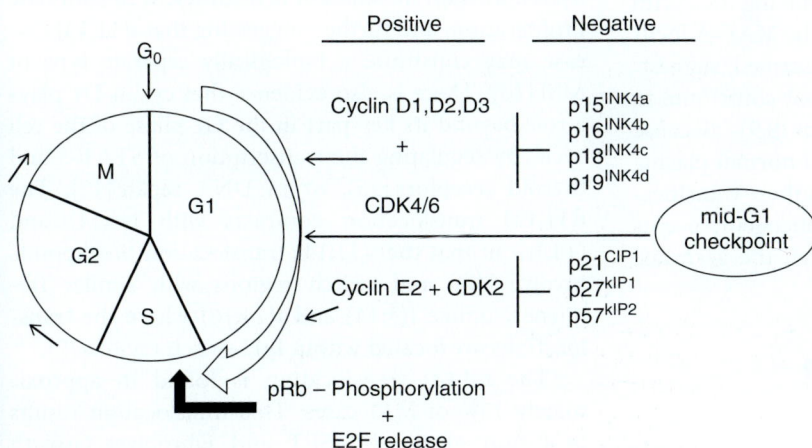

Figure 4.1 Control of G1-to-S phase cell cycle progression. In early G1, D-type cyclins are induced in response to mitogens to bind to and activate CDKs 4/6. These complexes then phosphorylate pRb allowing S-phase entry through release of E2F transcription factors. The INK4 and WAF/CIP families of CKIs inhibit the action of the CDKs as shown (adapted from Chan, Kiang S. Biology of plasma cells. *Best Pract. Res. Clin. Haematol.* 2005;**18**(4):493–507).

Myeloma, ed. Stephen A. Schey, Kwee L. Yong, Robert Marcus and Kenneth C. Anderson. Published by Cambridge University Press. © Cambridge University Press 2014.

which inhibit the actions of the CDKs. The INK4 family of proteins (p15 [INK4a], p16 [INK4b], p18 [INK4c], p19 [INK4d]) negatively regulates the effects of the cyclin-D/CDK complexes, whilst the WAF/CIP family of CKIs (p21 [Cip1], p27 [Kip1] and p57 [Kip2]) regulates the late G1 phase actions of cyclin-E and CDK2 [1]. In contrast, CKIs may also act as positive cell cycle regulators by stabilizing the cyclin-CDK complexes [3].

Cell cycle dysregulation in multiple myeloma

MM is a tumor with a low proliferative rate, thus it was surprising when gene-expression profiling experiments involving two large groups of MM patients showed that D-type cyclin expression was aberrantly increased in nearly all cases of MM [4,5]. These findings are partly explained by the fact that one of five recurrent translocations involving the IgH locus on 14q32 (IgH/TCs) is found in 40%–50% of MM cases [6]. It is thought that these errors occur during IgH switch recombination during B-cell maturation in germinal centers [7]. These IgH/TCs result in the dysregulation or increased expression of a D-type cyclin gene. The partner genes in these translocations include the cyclin D1 or D3 genes (11q13 or 6p21 respectively) that are positioned near the strong immunoglobin gene enhancers, those encoding the c-maf (16q23) and B-maf (20q11) transcription factors that target the cyclin D2 gene, or FGFR3/MMSET (4p16), also targeting the cyclin D2 gene via an unknown mechanism. More recently, translocations involving the cyclin D2 gene on chromosome 12p13 and the MAF-A locus on chromosome 8q24.3 have been described, suggesting further mechanisms may exist that contribute to the overexpression of D-type cyclins [8,9]. Because these mechanisms are not a feature of normal plasma cell biology, it has been suggested that these translocations represent tumor-initiating or oncogenic events in normal B cells as they pass through the germinal centers of lymph node tissue [6].

Impact of genetic lesions on cell cycle proteins

IgH translocations

The demonstration of near universal D-type cyclin mRNA overexpression in MM was emphasized by several subsequent studies confirming expression of cyclin D1, D2 and D3 proteins in addition to CDK 4/6 and phospho-pRb confirming cell cycle progression in primary MM cells [10,11,12]. However, whether IgH/TCs are necessary for progression of MM has not been fully resolved, although there is now increasing in vitro evidence that this may be the case. For example, when KMS12BM MM cells were transfected to overexpress cMAF, this lead to increased expression of the cyclin D2 and B7-integrin genes suggesting a mechanism whereby overexpression of cMAF leads to increased MM cell proliferation and also alters integrin-mediated interactions between MM cells and microenvironmental factors [13]. These findings were recently confirmed in a transgenic murine model of MM with t(14;16), where increased expression of the cyclin D2 and Integrin-B-7 genes was observed [14].

The role of cyclin D1 overexpression in the context of t(11;14) is less clear. SiRNA-mediated knockdown of the cyclin D1 gene lead to cell cycle arrest in KMS12BM cells which carry a t(11;14) translocation, providing evidence that the cyclin D1 protein plays an important functional role in MM cells with this translocation [11]. On the other hand, cyclin D1 overexpression in transgenic mice does not lead to the development of lymphoid tumors suggesting that cooperation between cyclin D1 and other factors such as Myc or Ras may be necessary to drive oncogenesis [15]. In fact, the percentage of S-phase tumor cells in MM cases expressing t(11;14) was lower than that in other subtypes of MM, again indicating that cyclin D1 overexpression in isolation is insufficient to stimulate proliferation, and further suggesting that t(11;14) disease may constitute a biologically separate type of MM [16]. There is also evidence that cyclin D1 plays a role beyond its key part in the G1 phase of the cell cycle, by regulating the transcription of STAT-3 and thyroid receptors [15], or in DNA repair [17]. The t(11;14) translocation contrasts with t(4;14) and (14;16) in that the t(11;14) translocation breakpoints involve VDJ and switch regions with similar frequency, unlike t(4;14) and t(14;16) where the translocations are located within IgH switch regions [7].

The t(4;14) translocation is found in approximately 15% of MM cases. This translocation results in fusion of the MMSET and Fibroblast Growth Factor Receptor-3 (FGFR3) genes resulting in their overexpression. However, in 30% of cases with t(4;14) MMSET overexpression is found without increased expression of FGFR3, suggesting a pivotal role for the

MMSET gene in MM pathogenesis. The possible epigenetic role for MMSET [18] is discussed in Chapter 5. A possible role in DNA damage response is also suggested by the observation that MMSET accumulates at the site of DNA damage and that knockdown of MMSET resulted in enhanced sensitivity to radiation. This may explain to some degree why MM patients with t(4;14) are less responsive to alkylator therapy [19]. On the other hand, the importance of FGFR3 in MM tumor initiation is emphasized by a study which showed that FFGFR3 cooperated with MYC to promote B cell tumor development in mice overexpressing both FGFR3 and MYC [20].

Dysregulation of CKIs

Although much of the focus has been on the increased expression of the "positive" regulators of the cell cycle in MM, several studies have highlighted dysregulation in the genes encoding the CKIs. A recent study, using single nucleotide polymorphism (SNP) analysis, found that the CDKN2C gene (encoding p18) was deleted in 4.5% MGUS cases and 15% of MM cases. Furthermore, deletion of CDKN2C was associated with an adverse outcome, suggesting that absence of p18 is an important factor in cell cycle progression in MM cells [21]. In addition, biallelic deletion of p18 is found in approximately 40% of HMCLs suggesting that this finding is associated with disease progression and increasing proliferative potential [22]. However, a separate study found a paradoxical increase in p18 expression in 60% of MM cases with a high proliferation index, perhaps suggesting that some MM cases may become less responsive to the anti-proliferative effects of p18 [23]. Both p27 and p21 (p27 ^{Kip1}, p21 $^{Waf/Cip1}$) interact with complexes containing cyclins D, E and A and regulate CDK activity during G1–S phase transition. The role of p27 may depend on the cellular context of individual MM cells within the BM microenvironment. For example, the induction of drug resistance following adhesion to extracellular matrix proteins such as fibronectin is accompanied by increased p27 expression, as discussed in Chapter 6. The poor overall survival of MM patients with 17pdel or p53 mutations suggests an important role for p21 in MM cells, as the expression of this protein is regulated by p53 expression. A recent study suggested a functional role for p21 in inhibiting G1–S progression in the setting of a novel anti-MM agent, whereas p27 expression was unaltered.

Induction of p21 expression has also been observed in the setting of treating MM cells with histone-deacetylase inhibitors [24,25].

1q gain and CKS1B overexpression

More recently, it has been proposed that amplification of the chromosomal region 1q21 (1q21 gain), which is found in approximately 30% of newly diagnosed MM cases, may contribute to cell cycle progression in MM. Importantly, 1q21 gain is not seen in MGUS, but is present in a proportion of smoldering MM cases where it is a risk factor for early disease progression and in MM and has been shown to be a poor prognostic factor [26,27]. CKS1B is member of the Cks/Suc1 family of proteins that bind to the catalytic subunit of CDKs and regulates their function whilst also playing a role in protein catabolism as an accessory protein for the Skp-Cul-F-box protein-SKP2 (SCF^{Skp2}) ubiquitin ligase. It has been suggested that increased expression of CKS1B may accelerate the degradation of p27, thus promoting cell cycle progression. Consistent with this hypothesis, it has recently been shown that knockdown of CKS1B in 3 different HMCLs led to stabilization of the p27 protein, cell cycle arrest and apoptosis [26].

Cell cycle progression in MM

The difficulty of maintaining primary MM cells in culture has made cell cycle experiments involving primary MM cells very challenging; thus, only a small number of studies have sought to examine the functional aspects of D-type cyclins and related cell cycle regulatory proteins in primary MM cells. Ludwig et al. reported that interferon stimulation of primary MM cells in vitro led to a significant increase in the incorporation of thymidine in a minority of samples, indicating that it was possible to increase the percentage of primary MM cells in S-phase following cytokine stimulation in vitro [28]. In further studies, MM cell lines were found to exhibit differential responsiveness to interferon-alpha and interleukin-6 (IL-6) whilst in a further study with MM cell lines, interferon stimulation led to increased expression of cyclin D2 and CDK2 and -4 proteins [29,30]. In more recent work from our laboratory, Glassford et al. showed that IGF-I stimulation of primary MM cells led to cell cycle progression, evidenced by increased thymidine incorporation and upregulation of cyclin D2, CDK4, CDK6 and phospho-pRb proteins [11]. Recently, we

41

reported that APRIL stimulation of primary MM cells increased the proportion of cells in S/G2/M phase, together with induction of cyclin D2, CDK4 and -6 and phospho-pRb expression in primary MM cells. These cell cycle responses were seen only in MM cells expressing cyclin D2, via t(14;16) or t(4;14), while MM cells expressing cyclin D1 with t(11;14) were unresponsive to growth factor stimulation [11,12,31]. These findings suggest that perhaps MM cells with t(11;14) may be less reliant upon mitogenic stimulation by growth factors such as IGF-I for cell cycle progression. The reasons for this are unclear; however, it is worth noting that cyclin D2 is up-regulated in normal B-lineage cells in response to mitogens and mediates cell cycle entry; hence it is not surprising that primary MM cells expressing cyclin D2, via t(4;14) or t(14;16), are growth factor responsive as the cyclin D2 gene in these cells is under the control of its natural promoter.

Targeting cell cycle regulatory proteins in multiple myeloma

Not surprisingly, D-type cyclins, and other cell cycle regulatory proteins, have now emerged as potential therapeutic targets in MM. In contrast to normal tissue where all three D-type cyclins are co-expressed and can function interchangeably [32], primary MM tumors demonstrate dysregulation of one single D-type cyclin. This characteristic of MM cells may render them susceptible to the targeting of one particular overexpressed D-type cyclin. Tiedemann and colleagues investigated the susceptibility of MM cells to individual D-type cyclin knockdown, via shRNA-mediated silencing cyclin D1 and D2 expression, and found that knockdown of each of these two cyclins in turn led to cell cycle arrest and cytotoxicity after prolonged in vitro culture [33]. By screening a chemical library for agents that could inhibit transactivation of the cyclin D2 gene, they identified kinetin riboside (a synthetic cytokinin) as an agent that suppressed cyclin D1 and D2 expression and led to early G1 - phase arrest in MM cell lines as well as inducing MM apoptosis in primary M cells and inhibiting tumor growth in MM xenograft models. However, a recent study emphasizes the complexity of targeting individual D-type cyclin proteins, even in the case of mantle cell lymphoma (MCL), which is characterized by a t(11;14) translocation and overexpression of cyclin D1. Klier and colleagues performed shRNA-mediated knockdown of cyclin D1 in MCL lines and observed a reduction in the percentage of cells in S-phase and increased expression of p27(Kip1). However, they also observed a consistent compensatory upregulation of cyclin D2 protein and disappointingly combined inhibition of both cyclins D1 and D2 did not further enhance the modest effects seen with cyclin D1 knockdown alone [34]. In addition, similar knockdown experiments in the U266 MM cell line led to a decrease in S-phase percentage cells but had no effect on cell survival, an effect that was posssibly explained by a compensatory increase in cyclin D2 protein [35]. Together, these results suggest that targeting cyclin D1 in isolation in MM (and MCL) may not result in a meaningful clinical result.

This has prompted other groups to focus on the CDK4 and -6 proteins as they form complexes with all three of the D-type cyclins. In vitro treatment of primary MM cells with PD0332991, a highly selective, orally active inhibitor of CDK4 and -6, led to early G1 arrest and also inhibited tumor growth in a MM xenograft model [36]. In a follow-up study, this agent was investigated as a combination treatment with bortezomib, with the combined treatment showing enhanced activity over single-agent treatment [37]. The sensitization to bortezomib-induced tumor cell killing was associated with induction of the pro-apoptotic protein, Bim, and with loss of insulin-response factor-4 (IRF4) [38]. More recently, another CDK-inhibitor (P276–00) that targets CDK9 and CDK1 in addition to CDK4 was shown to induce cell cycle arrest and cytotoxicity in MM cell lines and an RPMI8226 xenograft model [39]. Overall, the specific targeting of both CDKs and D-type cyclins in MM is at an early stage of development, and the results of early phase clinical studies of CDK4/6-inhibitors are awaited.

Myeloma precursor cells

The mechanisms that trigger relapse from plateau phase remain poorly understood, thus the cancer stem cell (CSC) hypothesis, which suggests that minor subpopulations of tumor cells possessing the stem cell properties of self-renewal and differentiation along with drug resistance are ultimately responsible for disease relapse is an understandably appealing one. Such cells have been identified in acute myeloid leukemia (AML), breast cancer, prostate cancer and melanoma and in recent years much effort has focused on the identification and characterization of

MM stem cells (MMSCs) [40,41]. Several independent groups have now identified MM cells with some or all of these features of CSCs; however, the exact phenotype and the frequency of such cells in MM remains controversial and is the subject of ongoing debate [42].

A role for clonotypic B cells

The possibility that a distinct subpopulation of cells, other than terminally differentiated plasma cells, might be part of the "MM clone" was suggested by the demonstration, by polymerase chain reaction (PCR), that MM cells possess immunoglobulin heavy chain genes that are somatically hypermutated and remain constant throughout the disease course, in keeping with the disease having arisen from a post-germinal center B cell [43]. Using PCR-based assays, several groups showed that a small population of B-lymphocytes from MM patients were clonally related to the main tumor bulk, i.e. contained identical immunoglobulin gene rearrangements to the malignant plasma cells comprising the main tumor bulk (i.e. clonotypic) [44,45,46]. This was followed by the demonstration that clonotypic B cells were capable of myelomagenesis upon transplantation into non-obese, diabetic, severe combined immunodeficient (NOD/SCID) mice [47,48,49]. These studies mainly used blood samples from MM patients, and more recent studies employing bone marrow material have not confirmed that B-lymphocytes are capable of initiating disease in immunodeficient animal models [50].

Cell surface marker expression

These reports lent weight to the notion that MM precursor cells belong to a pre-plasma cell compartment expressing B cell antigens including CD20, CD19 and CD27, but lacking CD138. (Figure 4.2). Work from the Matsui group [49] has provided most of the data on CD138− MM cells. This group initially reported that clonogenic MM cells lacked expression of CD138, and that small populations (2%–5%) of CD138− cells in the H929 and RPMI8226 MM cell lines had greater clonal expansion during serial re-plating experiments, and expressed CD19, CD20 and Ki67, in contrast to the CD138+ fraction. Bone marrow samples depleted of CD138 and CD34-expressing cells generated colonies containing mature plasma cells, whilst CD138+ cells did not. Importantly, depletion of cells expressing CD45, CD22 and CD19 reduced the growth of MM colonies, as did pre-treatment of MM BM, suggesting that MM progenitors have a B-cell phenotype [49]. The same group later reported on the stem cell features of CD138− cells from the RPMI8226 and H929 cell lines, including efflux of the DNA-binding dye Hoechst 33342, drug resistance, high expression of aldehyde dehydrogenase (ALDH) and tumorigenicity [51]. Finally, clonally related CD19+CD27+ cells isolated from the peripheral blood of MM patients were found to be myelomagenic as they led to a MM phenotype when injected into NOD/SCID mice, unlike CD138+ cells which did not engraft. A novel three-dimensional culture system provided some functional evidence to support the hypothesis that clonotypic B cells are MM

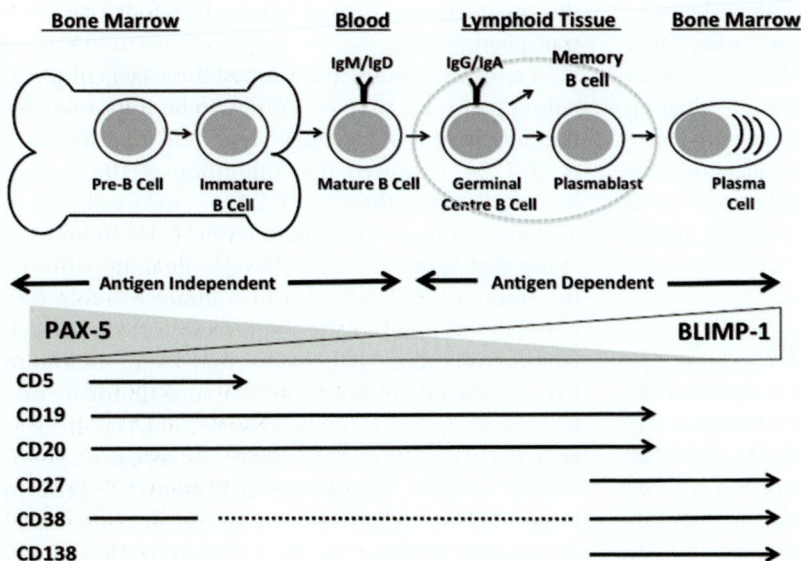

Figure 4.2 B cell development and plasma cell differentiation. Mature B cells leaving the bone marrow express the B-cell antigens CD19 and CD20, and bear surface IgM and IgD. Activated B cells in germinal centers upregulate CD38 and CD27, while CD138 is upregulated in the terminal stages of B cell differentiation into plasma cells. These surface phenotype changes are orchestrated by reciprocal down-regulation of the B cell transcription factor, Pax-5, and up-regulation of Blimp-1, and occur coordinately with the increase in immunoglobulin secretion capacity and exit from the cell cycle.

43

progenitors [52]. This system allowed the identification of a population of cells that retained CFSE, and therefore were quiescent, in keeping with a stem-cell phenotype. These cells were further shown to have a B cell phenotype whilst bearing identical immunoglobulin heavy chain gene sequences to the main plasma cell tumor, as well as displaying drug resistance and an ability to generate CD138+ cells during serial replating experiments.

More recently, however, evidence has accumulated to suggest CD138+ MM cells *are* capable of colony formation and display CSC characteristics. Injection of CD138-selected cells from MM patients directly in to rabbit bones implanted in SCID mice (SCID-rab model) led to successful engraftment in 81% of cases along with MM disease characteristics such as paraproteinemia and lytic bone disease [53]. The "side population" (SP) cells in both MM cell lines and primary MM cells that possessed "stem cell properties" were reported to express CD138 [54]. Purified CD138+ cells from patients with plasma cell leukemia (PCL) were found to be capable of colony formation, in contrast to the CD138− fraction, which were not [55]. Both CD138+ and CD138− cells from the murine 5T33MM model were found to be tumorigenic in c57BIKaLwRij mice; whilst CD138− cells showed slower engraftment, they were also found to be more resistant to bortezomib treatment. In another recent study, Hosen and colleagues used a cell fractionation method to demonstrate that clonogenic MM cells from the bone marrow are not CD19+, and moreover, that while both CD138+ and CD138− cells engrafted in the SCID-Rab model, CD19 + cells failed to do so. This report was followed closely by a report from the Weisman laboratory, who, using the same *in vivo* model of human bone grafts in immune-deficient animals, found that tumor-initiating cells from the bone marrow of MM patients were CD138+, but CD19− [56]. A possible explanation for such discrepant results is that clonotypic tumor cells bearing B cell antigens, but not CD138, circulate mainly in the peripheral blood.

Targeting MM progenitor cells

Following on from the studies that have explored the functional aspects of putative MM SCs have been several efforts to selectively target these cells. As a number of studies have identified CD20-expression on the surface of MM cells with stem-cell characteristics, this became an obvious target for immunotherapy and one

study showed that *in vitro* rituximab treatment of MM BM that had been depleted of CD34+ and CD138+ cells led to a reduction in clonogenic growth, which was further reduced by the addition of complement [49]. However, it is uncertain if rituximab has a role in this setting as the clinical experience with rituximab in MM is limited to studies and reports of small numbers of patients at varying disease stages. Overall, these studies would suggest a limited role for rituximab, as objective responses have been seen in just a handful of patients, an effect that may be partially explained by the low frequency of CD20-expression seen in MM [57]. Furthermore, another study that analyzed 2 MM patients for the presence of clonotypic B cells before, during, and after rituximab treatment found that these cells persisted despite rituximab treatment [58].

Other studies have focused on a possible interaction between MM progenitors and the BM microenvironment. Co-culturing primary MM cells with dendritic cells was found to enhance the clonogenic growth of the MM cells, whilst the inhibition of APRIL (A Proliferation-inducing Ligand), BAFF (B cell activating factor) and RANK (Receptor activator of NFκB) interactions led to reduced clonogenic growth [53]. More recently, it has been reported that the interaction between MM SP cells and BM stromal cells led to increased proliferation and viability of MM SP cells [54]. Importantly, lenalidomide was found to reduce the clonogenic ability of MM SP cells suggesting a role for lenalidomide in targeting MM progenitors, and also highlighting the recently published studies documenting the effect of lenalidomide in the maintenance setting post-autologous stem-cell transplant [59,60].

Yet other studies have focused on targeting signaling pathways that are known to be important for the regulation of normal stem fate and Peacock *et al.* (2007) showed that inhibition of the Hedgehog signaling pathway in CD138− MM cells led to a reduction in clonogenic potential [61]. In another study that focused on the Notch signaling pathway, the ability of HMCLs to form colonies was found to correlate strongly with expression of the Notch ligand JAG2 and furthermore that JAG2 inhibition led to reduced colony formation and tumor formation *in vivo*, suggesting a crucial for JAG2 in MM growth [62]. Other emerging therapeutic possibilities include employing autologous T cells to target MM progenitors, or using immune-based approaches to target the SOX-2 transcription factor, that was shown to be more highly expressed in the CD138− fraction in MGUS patients [63,64].

Conclusions regarding MM precursor cells

Evidence from several groups supports the notion that small populations of MM cells possess some CSC characteristics but the phenotype and the functional relevance of these cells remains to be fully defined. Divergent results have emerged from different studies; however, this is likely to be because of differences in culture methods, assay systems and animal models used, none of which faithfully recapitulates the human MM bone marrow environment, on which these tumor cells are so dependent. Disease heterogeneity, well recognized to be based on underlying molecular lesions, almost certainly contributes to these differences. The source of cells used for *in vivo* assay may also be important, as most of the data on the myelomagenic properties of clonotypic CD19+ B lymphocytes are derived from studies using peripheral blood, while the data on tumorigenic CD138+ cells have employed bone marrow. It is conceivable that MM precursor clonotypic B lymphocytes circulate in the blood to disseminate disease but, once in the bone marrow, these cells differentiate into more mature tumor cells. Perhaps future attempts to further characterize these cells should not be based on cell surface immunophenotype alone, if they are to be effectively targeted. In fact, there is now intriguing evidence of "plasticity" amongst CSCs that might also give some insight into why divergent results have been achieved by different groups [63,65]. In conclusion, the study of putative MMSCs continues to provoke debate and controversy, and the results of further studies in the area will be awaited with much interest.

References

1. Sherr, C. J. D-type cyclins. *Trends Biochem. Sci.* 1995;**20**:187–90.

2. Cheng, M., Olivier, P., Diehl, J. A. *et al.* The p21Cip1 and p27Kip1 CDK 'inhibitors' are essential activators of cyclin D-dependent kinases in murine fibroblasts. *EMBO J.* 1999;**18**:1571–83.

3. Sherr, C. J., Roberts, J. M. CDK inhibitors: positive and negative regulators of G1-phase progression. *Genes Development* 1999;**13**:1501–12.

4. Bergsagel, P. L., Kuehl, W. M., Zhan, F. *et al.* Cyclin D dysregulation: an early and unifying pathogenic event in multiple myeloma. *Blood* 2005;**106**:296–303.

5. Zhan, F., Huang, Y., Colla, S. *et al.* The molecular classification of multiple myeloma. *Blood* 2006;**108**:2020–8.

6. Kuehl, W. M., Bergsagel, P. L. Early genetic events provide the basis for a clinical classification of multiple myeloma. *ASH Education Program Book* 2005(1):346–52.

7. Bergsagel, P. L., Kuehl, W. M. Critical roles for immunoglobulin translocations and cyclin D dysregulation in multiple myeloma. *Immunological Reviews*, 2003;**194**:96–104.

8. Bergsagel, P. L., Kuehl, W. M. Chromosome translocations in multiple myeloma. *Oncogene*, 2001;**20**:5611–22.

9. Chng, W. J., Glebov, O., Bergsagel, P. L., Kuehl, W. M. Genetic events in the pathogenesis of multiple myeloma. *Best Practice Res. Clin. Haematol.* 2007;**20**:571–96.

10. Ely, S., Di Liberto, M., Niesvizky, R. *et al.* Mutually exclusive cyclin-dependent kinase 4/cyclin D1 and cyclin-dependent kinase 6/cyclin D2 pairing inactivates retinoblastoma protein and promotes cell cycle dysregulation in multiple myeloma. *Cancer Research* 2005;**65**:11;345–53.

11. Glassford, J., Rabin, N., Lam, E. W. F., Yong, K. L. Functional regulation of D-type cyclins by insulin-like growth factor-I and serum in multiple myeloma cells. *Br. J. Haematol.* 2007;**139**:243–54.

12. Quinn, J., Glassford, J., Percy, L. *et al.* APRIL promotes cell-cycle progression in primary multiple myeloma cells: influence of D-type cyclin group and translocation status. *Blood* 2011;**117**:890–901.

13. Hurt, E. M., Wiestner, A., Rosenwald, A. *et al.* Overexpression of c-maf is a frequent oncogenic event in multiple myeloma that promotes proliferation and pathological interactions with bone marrow stroma. *Cancer Cell* 2004;**5**:191–9.

14. Morito, N., Yoh, K., Maeda, A. *et al.* A novel transgenic mouse model of the human multiple myeloma chromosomal translocation t(14;16)(q32;q23). *Cancer Research* 2011;**71**(2):339–48.

15. Lesage, D., Troussard, X., Sola, B. The enigmatic role of cyclin D1 in multiple myeloma. *Int. J. Cancer* 2005;**115**(2):171–6.

16. Fonseca, R., Blood, E. A., Oken, M. M. *et al.* Myeloma and the t(11;14)(q13;q32); evidence for a biologically defined unique subset of patients. *Blood* 2002;**99** (10):3735–41.

17. Jirawatnotai, S., Hu, Y., Michowski, W. *et al.* A function for cyclin D1 in DNA repair uncovered by protein interactome

analyses in human cancers. *Nature* 2011;**474**(7350):230–4.

18. Martinez-Garcia, E., Popovic, R., Min, D. J. *et al*. The MMSET histone methyl transferase switches global histone methylation and alters gene expression in t(4;14) multiple myeloma cells. *Blood* 2011;**117**(1):211–20.

19. Pei, H., Zhang, L., Luo, K. *et al*. MMSET regulates histone H4K20 methylation and 53BP1 accumulation at DNA damage sites. *Nature* 2011;**470** (7332):124–8.

20. Zingone, A., Cultraro, C. M., Shin, D. M. *et al*. Ectopic expression of wild-type FGFR3 cooperates with MYC to accelerate development of B-cell lineage neoplasms. *Leukemia* 2010;**24**(6):1171–8.

21. Leone, P. E., Walker, B. A., Jenner, M. W. *et al*. Deletions of CDKN2C in multiple myeloma: biological and clinical implications. *Clinical Cancer Research* 2008;**14**(19):6033–41.

22. Kulkarni, M. S., Daggett, J. L., Bender, T. P. *et al*. Frequent inactivation of the cyclin-dependent kinase inhibitor p18 by homozygous deletion in multiple myeloma cell lines: ectopic p18 expression inhibits growth and induces apoptosis. *Leukemia* 2002;**16**(1):127–34.

23. Dib, A., Peterson, T. R., Raducha-Grace, L. *et al*. Paradoxical expression of INK4c in proliferative multiple myeloma tumors: bi-allelic deletion vs increased expression. *Cell Div.* 2006;**1**:23.

24. Streetly, M. J., Maharaj, L., Joel, S. *et al*. GCS-100, a novel galectin-3 antagonist, modulates MCL-1, NOXA, and cell cycle to induce myeloma cell death. *Blood*, 2010;**115**:3939–48.

25. Mandl-Weber, S., Meinel, F. G., Jankowsky, R. *et al*. The novel inhibitor of histone deacetylase resminostat (RAS2410) inhibits proliferation and induces apoptosis in multiple myeloma

(MM) cells. *Br. J. Haematol.* 2010;**149**:518–28.

26. Hanamura, I., Stewart, J. P., Huang, Y. *et al*. Frequent gain of chromosome band 1q21 in plasma-cell dyscrasias detected by fluorescence in situ hybridization: incidence increases from MGUS to relapsed myeloma and is related to prognosis and disease progression following tandem stem-cell transplantation. *Blood* 2006;**108**(5):1724–32.

27. Zhan, F., Colla, S., Wu, X. *et al*. CKS1B, overexpressed in aggressive disease, regulates multiple myeloma growth and survival through SKP2- and p27Kip1-dependent and -independent mechanisms. *Blood* 2007;**109**(11):4995–5001.

28. Ludwig, C. U., Durie, B. G. M., Salmon, S. E., Moon, T. E. Tumor growth stimulation in vitro by interferons. *Eur. J. Cancer Clinical Oncol.* 1983;**19**:1625–32.

29. Jelinek, D. F., Aagaard-Tillery, K. M., Arendt, B. K. *et al*. Differential human multiple myeloma cell line responsiveness to interferon-alpha. Analysis of transcription factor activation and interleukin 6 receptor expression. *J. Clin. Invest.* 1997;**99**:447–56.

30. Arora, T., Jelinek, D. F. Differential myeloma cell responsiveness to interferon-alpha correlates with differential induction of p19INK4d and cyclin D2 expression. *J. Biol. Chem.* 1998;**273**:11 799–805.

31. Glassford, J., Kassen, D., Quinn, J. *et al*. Inhibition of cell cycle progression by dual phosphatidylinositol-3-kinase and mTOR blockade in cyclin D2 positive multiple myeloma bearing IgH translocations. *Blood Cancer Journal*, 2012;**2**:e50

32. Lahti, J. M., Li, H., Kidd, V. J. Elimination of cyclin D1 in vertebrate cells leads to an altered cell cycle phenotype, which is rescued by overexpression of

murine cyclins D1, D2, or D3 but not by a mutant cyclin D1. *J. Biol. Chem.* 1997;**272**:10,859–69.

33. Tiedemann, R. E., Mao, X., Shi, C. X. *et al*. Identification of kinetin riboside as a repressor of CCND1 and CCND2 with preclinical antimyeloma activity. *J. Clin. Invest.* 2008;**118**:1750–64.

34. Klier, M., Anastasov, N., Hermann, A. *et al*. Specific lentiviral shRNA-mediated knockdown of cyclin D1 in mantle cell lymphoma has minimal effects on cell survival and reveals a regulatory circuit with cyclin D2. *Leukemia* 2008;**22**:2097–105.

35. Tchakarska, G., Le Lan-Leguen, A., Roth, L., Sola, B. The targeting of the sole cyclin D1 is not adequate for mantle cell lymphoma and myeloma therapies. *Haematologica* 2009;**94**:1781–2.

36. Baughn, L., Di Liberto, M., Wu, K. *et al*. A novel orally active small molecule potently induces G1 arrest in primary myeloma cells and prevents tumor growth by specific inhibition of cyclin-dependent kinase 4/6. *Cancer Research* 2006;**66**:7661–7.

37. Menu, E., Garcia, J., Huang, X. *et al*. A novel therapeutic combination using PD 0332991 and bortezomib: study in the 5T33MM myeloma model. *Cancer Research* 2008;**68**:5519–23.

38. Huang, X., Di Liberto, M., Jayabalan, D. *et al*. Prolonged early G1 arrest by selective CDK4/CDK6 inhibition sensitizes myeloma cells to cytotoxic killing through cell cycle-coupled loss of IRF4. *Blood* 2012;**120**(5):1095–106.

39. Manohar, S. M., Rathos, M. J., Sonawane, V., Rao, S. V., Joshi, K. S. Cyclin-dependent kinase inhibitor, P276–00 induces apoptosis in multiple myeloma cells by inhibition of Cdk9-T1 and RNA polymerase II-dependent transcription. *Leuk. Res.* 2011;**35** (6):821–30.

40. Rosen, J. M., Jordan, C. T. The increasing complexity of the cancer stem cell paradigm. *Science* 2009;**324**:1670–3.

41. Dean, M., Fojo, T., Bates, S. Tumour stem cells and drug resistance. *Nat. Rev. Cancer* 2005;**5**:275–84.

42. Brennan, S., Matsui, W. Cancer stem cells: controversies in multiple myeloma. *J. Molec. Med.* 2009;**87**:1079–85.

43. Bakkus, M. H., Heirman, C., Van Riet, I., Van Camp, B., Thielemans, K. Evidence that multiple myeloma Ig heavy chain VDJ genes contain somatic mutations but show no intraclonal variation. *Blood* 1992;**80**:2326–35.

44. Billadeau, D., Ahmann, G., Greipp, P., Van Ness, B. The bone marrow of multiple myeloma patients contains B cell populations at different stages of differentiation that are clonally related to the malignant plasma cell. *J Experimental Med.* 1993;**178**:1023–31.

45. Bergsagel, P. L., Smith, A. M., Szczepek, A. *et al.* In multiple myeloma, clonotypic B lymphocytes are detectable among CD19+ peripheral blood cells expressing CD38, CD56, and monotypic Ig light chain [published erratum appears in *Blood* 1995;**85**(11):436–47].

46. Rasmussen, T., Jensen, L., Johnsen, H. E. Levels of circulating CD19+ cells in patients with multiple myeloma. *Blood* 2000;**95**:4020.

47. Pilarski, L. M., Hipperson, G., Seeberger, K. *et al.* Myeloma progenitors in the blood of patients with aggressive or minimal disease: engraftment and self-renewal of primary human myeloma in the bone marrow of NOD SCID mice. *Blood* 2000;**95**:1056–65.

48. Pilarski, L. M., Belch, A. R. Clonotypic myeloma cells able to xenograft myeloma to nonobese diabetic severe combined immunodeficient mice copurify with CD34+ hematopoietic progenitors. *Clinical Cancer Research* 2002;**8**:3198–204.

49. Matsui, W., Huff, C. A., Wang, Q. *et al.* Characterization of clonogenic multiple myeloma cells. *Blood* 2004;**103**:2332–6.

50. Hosen, N., Matsuoka, Y., Kishida, S. *et al.* CD138-negative clonogenic cells are plasma cells but not B cells in some multiple myeloma patients. *Leukemia* 2012; e-pub ahead of print 20 April; doi:10.1038/leu.2012.80

51. Matsui, W., Wang, Q., Barber, J. P. *et al.* Clonogenic multiple myeloma progenitors, stem cell properties, and drug resistance. *Cancer Research* 2008;**68**(1):190–7.

52. Kirshner, J., Thulien, K. J., Martin, L. D. *et al.* A unique three-dimensional model for evaluating the impact of therapy on multiple myeloma. *Blood* 2008;**112**:2935–45.

53. Yata, K., Yaccoby, S. The SCID-rat model: a novel in vivo system for primary human myeloma demonstrating growth of CD138-expressing malignant cells. *Leukemia* 2004;**18**(11):1891–7.

54. Jakubikova, J., Adamia, S., Kost-Alimova, M. *et al.* Lenalidomide targets clonogenic side population in multiple myeloma: pathophysiologic and clinical implications. *Blood* 2011;**117**:4409–19.

55. Chiron, D., Surget, S., Maga, S. *et al.* The peripheral CD138+ population but not the CD138− population contains myeloma clonogenic cells in plasma cell leukaemia patients. *Br. J. Haematol.* 2012;**156**:679–83.

56. Kim, D., Park, C. Y., Medeiros, B. C., Weissman, I. L. CD19-CD45low/-CD38high/CD138+ plasma cells enrich for human tumorigenic myeloma cells. *Leukemia* 2012; e-pub head of print May 30, 2012.

57. Kapoor, P., Greipp, P. T., Morice, W. G. *et al.* Anti-CD20 monoclonal antibody therapy in multiple myeloma. *Br. J. Haematol.* 2008;**141**:135–48.

58. Pilarski, L. M., Baigorri, E., Mant, M. J. *et al.* Multiple myeloma includes phenotypically defined subsets of clonotypic CD20+ B cells that persist during treatment with rituximab. *Clinical Medicine Oncology* 2008;**2**: 275–87.

59. McCarthy, P. L., Owzar, K., Hofmeister, C. C. *et al.* Lenalidomide after stem-cell transplantation for multiple myeloma. *New Engl. J. Med.* 2012;**366**(19):1770–81.

60. Attal, M., Lauwers-Cances, V., Marit, G. *et al.* Lenalidomide maintenance after stem-cell transplantation for multiple myeloma. *New Engl. J. Med.* 2012;**366**(19):1782–91.

61. Peacock, C. D., Wang, Q., Gesell, G. S. *et al.* Hedgehog signaling maintains a tumor stem cell compartment in multiple myeloma. *Proc. Natl. Acad. Sci.* 2007;**104**:4048–53.

62. Chiron, D., Maga, S., Descamps, G. *et al.* Critical role of the NOTCH ligand JAG2 in self-renewal of myeloma cells. *Blood Cells Molecules Dis.* 2012;**48**:247–53.

63. Matsui, W., Borrello, I., Mitsiades, C. Autologous stem cell transplantation and multiple myeloma cancer stem cells. *Biol. Blood Marrow Transplant* 2012;**18**:S27–S32.

64. Spisek, R., Kukreja, A., Chen, L. C. *et al.* Frequent and specific immunity to the embryonal stem cell-associated antigen SOX2 in patients with monoclonal gammopathy. *J. Exp. Med.* 2007;**204**:831–40.

65. He, K., Xu, T., Goldkorn, A. Cancer cells cyclically lose and regain drug-resistant highly tumorigenic features characteristic of a cancer stem-like phenotype. *Molecular Cancer Therapeut.* 2011;**10**(6):938–48.

47

Chapter

5

The genetic and epigenetic mechanisms underlying the behavior of myeloma

Martin F. Kaiser, Kevin D. Boyd and Gareth J. Morgan

Background

Multiple myeloma is characterized by a clonal expansion of terminally differentiated plasma cells that reside at multiple sites in the bone marrow where they interact with different cell types of the bone marrow micro-environment. The clinical picture is heterogeneous and many of the past and present research efforts have aimed at identifying the underlying factors for this diversity. Furthermore, clinical outcome differs dramatically with a median overall survival (OS) of less than two years for a group of ultra-high risk patients in contrast to patients that achieve durable remissions for many years. Novel treatment approaches have significantly improved survival and intensively treated patients now have an overall median survival between five and nine years [1]. However, myeloma still remains an incurable disease with frequent relapses and development of drug resistance occurring in virtually every patient.

Despite the heterogeneity in disease biology, treatment decisions today are made on the basis of age and performance status rather than individual features of the disease. Understanding the genetics and epigenetics of myeloma should enable us to develop specific therapeutic strategies for individual patients but to achieve this will require the development of robust prognostic and therapeutic biomarkers to identify patient subgroups for study in well-designed clinical trials.

In this chapter, we present a model of myeloma pathogenesis, give a summary of our current understanding of the genetic alterations in myeloma and highlight links to tumor biology or patient prognosis. In addition, we will present an overview of the

epigenetic modifications in myeloma and their possible implications for biology and therapy.

The model of myeloma pathogenesis

Multiple myeloma evolves in a multi-step process during which the cumulative acquisition of genetic and epigenetic hits leads to the transformation of a benign plasma cell to a myeloma cell. Relevant genetic hits equip the cell with features that provide a selection benefit either immediately or in combination with a subsequent hit. Monoclonal gammopathy of undetermined significance (MGUS) is the earliest recognizable phenotype in the stepwise pathogenesis of myeloma that has gained features of malignant behavior without causing clinical symptoms. MGUS has a high prevalence of ~2% in individuals over the age of 50 and progresses to symptomatic myeloma at a rate of 1% per year [2]. Asymptomatic myeloma differs from MGUS by an increased bone marrow plasma cell burden (>10%) and a higher rate of progression to symptomatic myeloma. At the active, symptomatic stage the malignant plasma cell clone further expands in the bone marrow and causes irreversible end organ damage. The last phenotype of the disease is plasma cell leukemia (PCL), in which the myeloma clone has acquired genetic changes that permit proliferation outside of the bone marrow niche. Studying DNA mutations and epigenetic modifications present at different stages of this multi-step process allows an archeological reconstruction of their role in disease development (Figure 5.1). This has led to the definition of primary and secondary genetic events in myeloma that are described below. Ideally, identification of essential events in disease

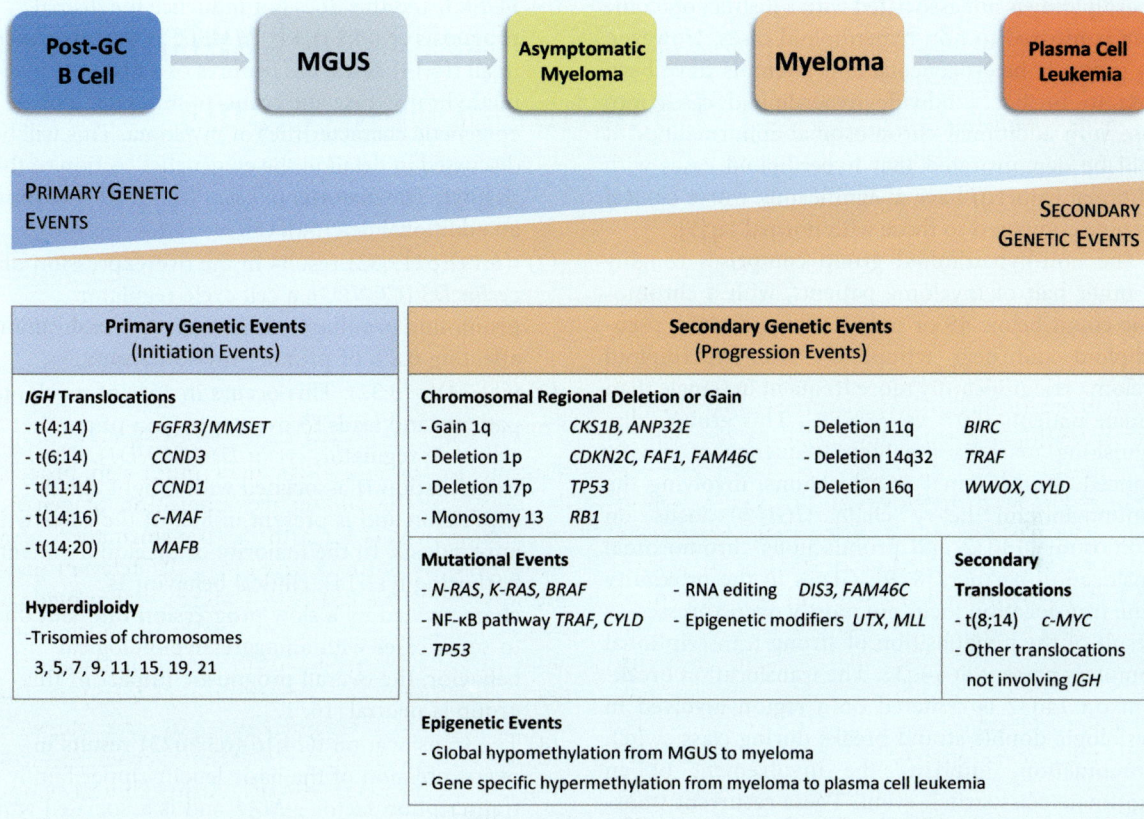

| Post-GC B Cell | → | MGUS | → | Asymptomatic Myeloma | → | Myeloma | → | Plasma Cell Leukemia |

PRIMARY GENETIC EVENTS

SECONDARY GENETIC EVENTS

Primary Genetic Events (Initiation Events)		Secondary Genetic Events (Progression Events)			
IGH Translocations		**Chromosomal Regional Deletion or Gain**			
- t(4;14)	FGFR3/MMSET	- Gain 1q	CKS1B, ANP32E	- Deletion 11q	BIRC
- t(6;14)	CCND3	- Deletion 1p	CDKN2C, FAF1, FAM46C	- Deletion 14q32	TRAF
- t(11;14)	CCND1	- Deletion 17p	TP53	- Deletion 16q	WWOX, CYLD
- t(14;16)	c-MAF	- Monosomy 13	RB1		
- t(14;20)	MAFB				

Mutational Events		**Secondary Translocations**
- N-RAS, K-RAS, BRAF	- RNA editing DIS3, FAM46C	- t(8;14) c-MYC
- NF-κB pathway TRAF, CYLD	- Epigenetic modifiers UTX, MLL	- Other translocations not involving IGH
- TP53		

Hyperdiploidy
-Trisomies of chromosomes
  3, 5, 7, 9, 11, 15, 19, 21

Epigenetic Events
- Global hypomethylation from MGUS to myeloma
- Gene specific hypermethylation from myeloma to plasma cell leukemia

Figure 5.1 The multi-step model of myeloma pathogenesis. The upper part of the diagram depicts the distinguishable entities of the step-wise transformation process in multiple myeloma. A post-germinal-center B cell is assumed to clonally evolve and result in MGUS following a first genetic hit. Accumulation of subsequent genetic and epigenetic aberrations results in the expansion of the plasma cell clone, leading from asymptomatic to symptomatic myeloma and to an aggressive type of disease that becomes independent of the bone marrow micro-environment (PCL). An individual patient can be diagnosed at any stage of this process. Accordingly, the genetic lesions detectable in an individual's myeloma cell clone at the time of diagnosis can predominantly consist of primary or secondary genetic events, as shown in the middle part of the diagram. Primary and secondary genetic events are summarized in the lower part of the diagram.

progression would make the development of specific therapies targeting these aberrations possible.

Primary genetic events in multiple myeloma

The genetic lesions identified in multiple myeloma are complex and comprise patterns of chromosomal gains and losses, non-random reciprocal chromosomal translocations, sub-chromosomal amplifications, deletions and point mutations. Although some of these lesions are present at high frequencies, our knowledge about how these lesions occur and the mechanisms by which they contribute to myeloma pathogenesis remains limited. Nevertheless, a molecular classification based on the association of certain

mutations with biological or prognostic features of myeloma has been proposed [3]. At the topmost level of this classification, myeloma can be divided in two overlapping genetic subgroups: Hyperdiploid and non-hyperdiploid.

Hyperdiploid myeloma is characterized by gain of the odd numbered chromosomes (3, 5, 7, 9, 11, 15, 19 and X in female patients) in the plasma cell clone, resulting in a chromosome count of 48–72 [4]. Hyperdiploidy is found in about 55% of all myeloma cases; it is more frequent in the male population (68% of cases) and there is an increasing proportion of hyperdiploidy with advanced age at the time of diagnosis [5, 6]. The primary pathogenetic event leading to an illegitimate non-random accrual of multiple entire chromosomes is unknown. Clinically,

49

hyperdiploidy is not associated with a distinct outcome when compared to non-hyperdiploid cases. However, this group is heterogeneous and attempts have been made to further subdivide hyperdiploid cases into those with additional chromosomal abnormalities. It could be demonstrated that hyperdiploid cases with additional gain(1q) have a significantly worse clinical outcome compared to those with normal 1q [7].

The non-hyperdiploid group comprises roughly the other half of myeloma patients, with a chromosome count below 48 or over 72 (hypodiploid, pseudodiploid and near tetraploid). Non-hyperdiploid myeloma is significantly more frequent in female than in male patients (50% vs. 38%)[6]. This group's distinguishing mark is the high frequency of mostly balanced chromosomal translocations, involving the immunoglobulin heavy chain (*IGH@*) locus on chromosome 14q32 and promiscuous chromosomal translocation partners [8, 9]. Genes in the proximity of the translocation locus are mostly overexpressed as a result of the juxtaposition of strong transcriptional promoters present at 14q32. The translocation breakpoint on 14q32 is centered on a region involved in physiologic double strand breaks during class switch recombination, implying the involvement of an illegitimate class switch event. These recurrent translocations occur in the physiologically inactivated *IGH@* allele, and an entire, class switched antibody is normally transcribed and translated from the other, non-translocated allele [10].

Five recurrent translocations can be detected at relatively high frequencies (Table 5.1).

(1) t(4;14)(p16;q32). This translocation is present in about 10% of myeloma patients. It is positively associated with IgA myeloma and an independent predictor of poor outcome. t(4;14) results in increased expression of two genes: *fibroblast growth factor receptor 3* (*FGFR3*), a tyrosine kinase on der (14), and *MMSET* (also termed *WHSC1*) on der(4) [11]. The *FGFR3* gene can carry activating mutations in a small set of patients but is otherwise not expressed in myeloma without t(4;14)[12]. Overexpression of *FGFR3* has been shown to increase myeloma cell proliferation in experimental models and *FGFR3* can be therapeutically targeted [13]. However, the impact of the other overexpressed gene, *MMSET*, on disease biology might be dominating in t(4;14) since about 25% of t(4;14) cases show a loss of der(14), containing *FGFR3*, and this does not influence the dismal prognosis of t(4;14)[14]. *MMSET* is overexpressed in all t(4;14) cases, has features of a histone methyltransferase and seems to influence global epigenetic characteristics of myeloma. This will be discussed in detail in the epigenetics section of this chapter. The majority of cases with t(4;14) harbor an additional del(13q)[15].

(2) t(6;14)(p21;q32) results in the overexpression of *cyclin D3* (*CCND3*), a cell cycle regulator promoting proliferation. It is a rare translocation, affecting 0.8% of primary myeloma samples.

(3) t(11;14)(q13;32). This occurs in 15% of myeloma patients and leads to overexpression of another cell cycle regulator, *cyclin D1* (*CCND1*). The translocation is associated with λ light chain expression and is present in half of the cases with amyloidosis. In the majority of myeloma patients harboring t(11;14), clinical behavior is characterized by a slow progression rate, but due to some cases with an aggressive biological behavior, the overall prognostic impact of this group is neutral [16, 17].

(4) The translocation t(14;16)(q32;q23) results in overexpression of the basic leucin-zipper family transcription factor *c-MAF* and is associated with poor prognosis [18, 19]. Gene expression array analysis has identified upregulation of *cyclin D2* (*CCND2*) as a downstream effect of this translocation.

(5) t(14;20)(q32;q21) results in the overexpression of *MAFB*, a transcription factor that has similar downstream targets to *c-MAF* including upregulation of *CCND2*. This translocation group is associated with poor prognosis. [20, 21].

Hyperdiploidy and recurrent translocations are thought to be primary events in the multi-step transformation process of myeloma since virtually all cases can be assigned to at least one of the two groups. In addition, hyperdiploidy and *IGH@* translocations can be detected in a substantial proportion of MGUS plasma cells, in contrast to other secondary genetic events that are predominantly present in advanced cases of myeloma or in PCL. It is assumed that myeloma cells retain these basic genetic features throughout the course of the disease. Hyperdiploidy and recurrent translocations generally occur in a mutually exclusive manner, but it is important to bear

Table 5.1 Recurrent genetic events in myeloma and their impact on biology.

Molecular Hallmarks of myeloma	Genes	Chromo some	IGH@ TL	CNA	SNV
Immortalization	CCND1	11q13	X (14%)		X (3%)
	CCND3	6p21	X (<1%)		
	RB1	13q14		X (45%)	X (3%)
	CDKN2C	1p32		X (30%)	X
G1/S abnormality proliferation	NRAS	1p13			X (21%)
	KRAS	12p12			X (28%)
	BRAF	7q34			X (5%)
	c-MYC	8q24	X†	X	X (1%)
Interaction with the microenvironment	MAF	16q22	X (3%)		
	MAFB	20q11	X (1%)		
NF-κB pathway	TRAF3	14q32		X (38%)	X (3%)
	CYLD	16q12		X (35%)	X (3%)
Abnormal DNA repair	TP53	17p13			X (6%)
RNA editing	DIS3	13q22		X (45%)	X (13%)
	FAM46C	1p12		X (17%)	X (10%)
Epigenetic abnormalities	KDM6A (UTX)	Xp11			X (10%)
	MLL	11q23			X (1%)
	MMSET	4p16	X (11%)		X (8%)

† Translocations of c-MYC are considered late genetic events and rarely involve the IGH@ locus.

in mind that cases demonstrating both genetic aberrations do exist.

Secondary genetic events

Secondary genetic events are mutations that occur during the progression of myeloma. They are middle or late stage events in the multi-step evolution of the malignant plasma cell clone. The exact occurrence and the biological implications of secondary genetic events are often not well defined.

MYC translocations

Examples of secondary genetic events are translocations that involve the c-MYC gene. These activating c-MYC translocations are typically complex mutations, involving for example three chromosomes, duplications, amplifications or inversions [22]. They often do not target the breakpoint at the switch region at 14q32, typical for primary translocations, but various other non-recurrent chromosomal loci. Translocations of c-MYC are rare or absent in MGUS, but occur at a rate of 15% in presentation myeloma [23]. Their incidence increases to 44% in advanced disease and to nearly 90% in myeloma cell lines.

Some secondary genetic events may contribute to the critical malignant transformation from MGUS to myeloma whereas others might reduce the bone marrow niche dependency of the tumor clone, inducing the progression to PCL. One way to identify genes or genetic regions of interest is the analysis of copy number alterations (CNA) using high resolution single nucleotide polymorphism (SNP) arrays. With these arrays, genomic deletions or amplifications, as well as regions with uniparental disomy (UPD; that is, loss of one allele with subsequent duplication of the corresponding allele, resulting in copy number neutral loss of genetic information) can be detected at high resolution.

Copy number alterations in myeloma

Our group, among others, recently performed high resolution SNP arrays on presentation myeloma samples [7]. This work combined the information on genetic gains or losses with mRNA gene expression array datasets in order to identify genes of interest within deleted or amplified genetic areas. We will specifically highlight CNAs that correlate with a favorable or dismal prognosis in myeloma patients.

CNA with prognostic impact

Genetic regions that have been demonstrated to have an impact on prognosis are del(1p), gain(1q), del (17p), gain(5q) and del(12p).

Deletion 1p

Hemizygous deletion of 1p is a common event in myeloma, affecting 30% of patients in our dataset with the majority of cases harboring interstitial deletions, some in the form of UPD, and some cases with loss of the whole chromosomal arm. There are four minimally deleted regions (MDR), of which deletion of 1p32.3 confers an adverse prognosis with an OS of 34.5 months in patients with the deletion versus more than 70 months OS in those without. A study by the Mayo Clinic using array comparative genomic hybridization (aCGH) also identified frequently deleted regions located at 1p32.2–p32.1 and 1p31.1 to be of negative prognostic significance [24]. Two genes with potential tumor suppressor function are located in this region and are downregulated by deletion of 1p32.2: CDKN2C and FAF1. The cell cycle regulator CDKN2C (also known as p18 or INK4c) controls G1/S cell cycle transition and inactivation of CDKN2C is associated with increased cell proliferation [22]. FAF1 inhibits the function of protein chaperones HSC70 and HSP70 and interacts with the ubiquitin–proteasome pathway [25]. Depletion of FAF1 activates NF-κB signalling via increased IκB kinase complex activity [26].

Another frequently deleted region is 1p12, which is hemizygously deleted in 17% of cases in our dataset. Homozygous deletions have been mapped to the FAM46C gene located at 1p12. Having deletion of this locus showed a tendency towards an adverse outcome (P = 0.06), and with accrual of more cases FAM46C deletions may acquire prognostic significance. Interestingly, FAM46C mutations have been identified in 13% of myeloma patients in a recent genome-wide sequencing analysis (see section "Mutational events in myeloma"), further highlighting the potential importance of this gene.

Gain of 1q

Gain of 1q is frequent in primary myeloma with about 39% of presentation samples harboring this aberration. In specific translocation groups such as t(4;14) and t(14;16), up to 70% of patients present with an additional gain(1q), which may be important for disease progression in these primary translocation groups. Increased expression of genes mapping to 1q has for the first time been associated with a patient group with unfavorable prognosis in a gene expression array unsupervised clustering analysis of the University of Arkansas Medical School (UAMS) group [27]. Patients with amplification of 1q21 detected by FISH had an inferior OS in our cohort (52 vs. 70 months for patients without gain(1q21)). A minimally amplified region mapping to 1q21.1-q23.3 contains the potential candidate gene ANP32E, and we have found that upregulation of ANP32E is associated with an inferior OS. Another gene at this locus is CKS1B, and overexpression of this gene has been linked to cell cycle progression and aggressive behavior in several tumors. The strong association of gain(1q21) with an unfavorable prognosis means that it is central to a risk-adapted therapeutic approach.

Amplification of 5q and deletion of 12p

Gain(5q31.3) and del(12p13.31) were recently reported to have an impact on patient prognosis. In this analysis, frequent genetic lesions were identified by using high resolution SNP arrays in a cohort of 192 newly diagnosed patients treated in the French IFM99 trial and tested against defined prognostic factors in a multivariate analysis [28]. Gain(5q31.3) was nearly exclusively present in hyperdiploid samples and patients carrying this mutation had an improved OS in comparison to patients lacking it. However, no minimally amplified region for 5q31.3 was defined.

Presence of del(12p13.31) was correlated with a dismal prognosis in the same initial analysis. Gene expression analysis showed that the gene CD27, encoding a tumor necrosis factor receptor superfamily member, was downregulated in the del(12p13.31) group in comparison to samples not carrying this mutation. However, in a different patient cohort (MRC Myeloma IX trial) that was treated differently, presence of del(12p) detected by FISH was not associated with an unfavorable prognosis [29].

Deletion of 17p

In about 10% of myeloma cases deletion of 17p is present and in most of these cases the whole short arm of chromosome 17 is deleted. The adverse prognostic effect of this lesion has been described by several groups [30]. TP53 is a potent tumor suppressor gene on 17p. In our FISH analysis of 1080 cases using a TP53 probe, loss of 17p was associated with an adverse OS (median OS 27 vs. 49 months). Samples with LOH at the *TP53* locus showed a high mutation rate of about 25% of the remaining *TP53* allele, compared to a background rate of <1% in cases without del(17p), underlining that *TP53* is the crucial gene in this region [31].

Other frequent CNA

Deletion of 6q

Thirty-three percent of our cases had deletion of 6q, the majority being interstitial deletions with the most commonly deleted region centred on 6q25.3, containing 32 genes and the fragile site FRA6E. The three genes with the greatest reduction of expression in cases with a deletion were *IGF2R*, *TFB1M* and *WTAP*.

Gains of chromosomal regions occurred in 23% of our samples and were predominantly located on the short arm of chromosome 6. Minimally amplified regions consisted of a 3.1 Mb are at 6p22.3 and a neighboring, larger region spanning from 6p22.3–p21.31. When a gain was present, 34 genes in the latter region were differentially expressed.

Deletion of chromosome 13

Chromosome 13 deletions are the commonest genetic alteration in myeloma cells and are present in about 50% of cases. Monosomy of chromosome 13 is the most frequent event with interstitial deletions occurring to a much lesser extent. Chromosome 13 abnormalities are closely associated with unfavorable translocation groups, deletions or gains like t(4;14), t(14;16), t(14;20), del(17p) or gain(1q) and when those cases are excluded from the analysis, the effect of del(13q14) on clinical outcome becomes neutral. Still, the association of del(13) with high risk cytogenetic groups implicates a role in disease biology. In our dataset, an MDR at 13q14.11–q14.3 encompassing 68 genes could be detected and of these, *RB1* was the most downregulated gene in deleted vs. non-deleted samples. *RB1* is a well-characterized tumor suppressor gene and plays an essential role in DNA-damage induced cell cycle arrest via inhibition of E2F family transcription factors.

Deletion of 16q

Deletions of the entire long arm of chromosome 16 as well as interstitial deletions are frequent, affecting an estimated 43% of patients with additional cases harboring UPD [32]. The tumor suppressor gene *WWOX*, located at the common fragile site (FRA16D)

at 16q23 is downregulated in del(16q) samples [33]. In addition, *WWOX* becomes frequently disrupted by t(14;16) since the translocation breakpoint on 16q is located in the region of FRA16D. Three other genes on 16q, namely *CHD9*, *MAF* and *CDH1*, were also underexpressed in patients with del16q.

An MDR at 16q12.1 contains the gene *CYLD*, which was also downregulated upon deletion of the locus. *CYLD* is a negative regulator of NF-κB and a tumor suppressor in neoplasias that are dependent on active NF-κB signaling [34]. Inactivating mutations of *CYLD* have been detected in myeloma samples with UPD of 16q [32], which confirms the important role of *CYLD* as a myeloma tumor suppressor gene.

Mutational events in myeloma

Knowledge about mutation status was, until very recently, limited to single candidate genes in myeloma due to technical limitations. Recent next-generation sequencing analyses of myeloma patient samples using either whole-genome or whole-exome sequencing demonstrated that each sample carried an average of 35 point mutations that changed the amino acid sequence of the encoded protein [35, 36]. As expected, genes that had been previously reported to be frequently mutated in myeloma, like *K-RAS*, *N-RAS* and *TP53*, were detected by these analyses. Mutations previously undetected in myeloma are affecting, for example, the genes *BRAF*, *FAM46C*, *DIS3* and histone modifying enzymes. Numerous mutations in non-coding sequences that are likely to influence gene expression as well as a high number of previously unknown translocations were shown to be present in the analyzed myeloma samples.

The high number of mutations identified per sample in the first whole-genome sequencing approaches makes the challenge of identifying the essential "driver" mutations against the background noise of thousands of non-essential mutations obvious. Identification of therapeutically targetable mutations in a tumor will, in addition, require an understanding of the interactions between mutations to be able to target the vulnerable factors in a mutational interaction network [37].

We will highlight some mutations that may have implications for tumor biology or treatment approaches. Mutations affecting histone modifying enzymes will be discussed in the "Myeloma epigenetics" section.

Activating RAS and BRAF mutations

Activating *KRAS* and *NRAS* mutations are virtually absent in MGUS but can be found in 30%–50% of newly diagnosed myeloma and it has been hypothesized that *RAS* may play a role in the process of malignant transformation of the plasma cell clone. The prevalence of *RAS* mutations is relatively high in t(11;14) myeloma and particularly low in cases carrying t(4;14) or del(17p). Patients with *RAS* mutations have an inferior clinical outcome than those without [38]. *RAS* encodes for a small GTPase family member protein that can activate the RAS/RAF/MEK/ERK pathway. The biological consequences of *RAS* mutations for disease development are poorly understood, mostly because of a lack of specific inhibitors for *RAS*.

Mutations of *BRAF* in myeloma were first identified by whole-genome sequencing and are present in 5% of patient samples [35,36]. The majority of the mutations were V600E, the most common *BRAF* mutation in melanoma, with the remainder leading to K601N or G469A substitutions. This finding could be of immediate clinical importance since specific BRAF inhibitors are currently in clinical development and have been shown to improve the survival of melanoma patients carrying the V600E *BRAF* mutation [39]. In addition, inhibitors acting downstream of BRAF (e.g. MEK) may show activity in this group of myeloma patients.

TP53 mutations

Deletion of 17p, where the *TP53* gene is located, is associated with an unfavorable prognosis in myeloma. In samples with a hemizygous del(17p), the remaining *TP53* allele has been shown to be frequently mutated (about 20%–40%), leading to a complete functional abrogation of TP53 function as a DNA damage response protein and cell cycle regulator [31, 40, 41]. *TP53* mutations in the absence of del(17p) are very rare events (<1%). It is suggestive that especially bi-allelic functional loss of *TP53* may contribute to the aggressive phenotype associated with del(17p) myeloma, but the impact of mutations of *TP53* on myeloma tumor biology remains to be elucidated.

Mutations of genes involved in RNA processing

Recent next-generation sequencing approaches revealed frequent mutations in two genes that are involved in RNA processing: *DIS3* and *FAM46C*, a gene on 1p initially identified to be deleted in myeloma by ourselves [35,36]. In 13% of patients, the *DIS3* gene harbored assumed loss-of-function mutations in an important catalytic domain of the gene. Mutations were frequently accompanied by hemizygous deletion of the remaining *DIS3* allele and by deletion of the *RB1* region (13q14), suggesting that these may be collaborating events. The *DIS3* gene encodes a highly conserved RNA exonuclease that serves as a key component in the exosome complex. This complex regulates processing and abundance of the RNA pool and, consequently, plays an important role for translation. Mutations of *FAM46C* were present in 10% of patients and although the precise function of the encoded protein is unknown, it is assumed that it is involved in modulating mRNA stability and translation. The identification of these mutations suggests that alterations in RNA processing and translation may play a role in myeloma pathogenesis and that the proteins involved could be potential therapeutic targets.

Mutations in NF-κB related genes

The NF-κB (nuclear factor kappa-light-chain-enhancer of activated B cells) pathway is involved in normal plasma cell development. Activation of this pathway via extrinsic ligands, secreted by bone marrow stromal cells, like BAFF and APRIL finally results in dimerization and nuclear translocation of transcription factors of the Rel/NF-κB family. It has been shown by gene expression profiling that myeloma cells express an NF-κB target gene signature indicative of constitutive activation of NF-κB signaling in myeloma. Recent in-depth analyses demonstrated that several components of the NF-κB pathway are mutated in various myeloma cell lines and in about 15% of presentation myeloma patient samples [42,43]. Frequent mutations comprise inactivating mutations in NF-κB suppressors like *TRAF3* or *CYLD*, a gene located on 16q and picked up by our CNA screen, and activating mutations of NF-κB activators, i.e. *NIK*. These mutations have been shown to activate canonical as well as non-canonical NF-κB signaling in cell lines, contributing to improved cell survival. Several inhibitors targeting NF-κB are under development and a recent report demonstrated that tumor cells arising from the background of germline *CYLD* deletions could be effectively inhibited by the multikinase inhibitor lestaurtinib [44].

Gene expression and micro RNA profiling

Some of the genetic lesions described above have been linked to specific gene expression patterns by microarray gene expression profiling (GEP). The recurrent translocations lead to overexpression of genes that are directly affected by the translocations, like *CCND1*, *CCND3*, *FGFR3*, *MMSET*, *MAF* and *MAFB*. In addition, there are genes that are overexpressed as a downstream effect of a translocation, like *ITGB7* or *CX3CR1* in t(14;16) and *DSG2* in t(4;14) myeloma [45, 46]. These effector genes are known to functionally contribute to the specific biology of the translocation groups. The Translocation and Cyclin D (TC) classification was the first to classify patient samples based on GEP data regarding overexpression of translocation genes. It also identified overexpression of cyclin D genes as a unifying molecular event in myeloma [45]. Based on the TC classification, targeted expression qPCR assays can be used to predict the presence of translocations [47]. Genomic gains or losses can also result in specific gene expression patterns and accordingly be predicted by GEP, with the exception of the prognostically important del(17p) [48].

In addition, specific gene expression profiles have been defined that are linked to short patient survival. The first prognostic signature in myeloma was a 70 gene signature defined by the UAMS which was later refined to a 17 gene signature with equal performance [27]. It was followed by a 15 gene signature by the IFM trial group, a 6 gene signature based on the MRC Myeloma IX trial data and a 92-gene high-risk signature by the HOVON65/GMMG-HD4 group [49–51]. Interestingly, there is little overlap of the genes comprising the different signatures, which can be explained by differences in patient selection, treatment modalities or methods. However, unless common genes with a well-defined function in myeloma biology are identified, GEP risk profiling is likely to remain limited to individual specialized treatment centers.

MicroRNAs (miRs) are small RNAs (17–25 base pairs) that do not encode for proteins themselves, but regulate other protein coding RNAs (mRNA) by inducing their degradation or inhibiting their translation. MiRs are potent regulators of gene expression networks because of their ability specifically to bind and inhibit several mRNA targets per individual miR.

Several miRs have been associated with disease pathogenesis, with genetic lesions or with patient prognosis in myeloma. For example, miR-32 and the miR-17–92 cluster were shown to be overexpressed in symptomatic myeloma compared to MGUS. The miR-17–92 cluster has been associated with *MYC* dysregulation, suggestive of a functional involvement of miRs in the malignant transformation of plasma cells [52, 53]. Specific miRs have been associated with chromosomal translocations, e.g. overexpression of miR-1 and miR-133a in t(14;16) or silencing of miR-24, miR-152 and miR-425 in cases with hyperdiploidy [54, 55]. Also, miRs were shown to modulate the biologically important MDM2/p53 axis, as well as STAT3 signaling [52, 56]. A global increase in miR expression has been linked with shorter survival in myeloma and amplification of genes encoding for the master miR regulator complex EIF2C2/AGO2 [57]. Defining the impact of miRs on the biology of myeloma will require further investigation. However, the complex role of miRs in combination with the recently discovered mutations in the RNA editing genes *DIS3* and *FAM46C* suggest an important role for post-transcriptional RNA editing in myeloma.

Myeloma epigenetics

Epigenetic modifications are dynamic covalent changes to chromatin or DNA that do not alter the primary DNA sequence. These changes are largely maintained throughout cell division and cell lineage specific epigenetic patterns can be observed. Two classes of epigenetic marks have been shown to be perturbed in cancer: histone modifications and DNA methylation. Both these epigenetic marks change globally during tissue specific cell differentiation and are involved in the control of transcriptional activity. Histone modifying proteins (e.g. histone methyltransferases) physically interact with DNA methyltransferases (DNMTs) in multi-protein complexes, implicating that histone modifications can induce DNA methylation changes and vice versa. The combined effects of both mechanisms are assumed to result in the fine-tuning of mRNA transcription (Figure 5.2) [58].

Histone proteins are the main protein components of the chromatin structure and can be dynamically modified by acetylation, methylation, phosphorylation, ubiquitination and SUMOylation of specific lysine or arginine residues located on

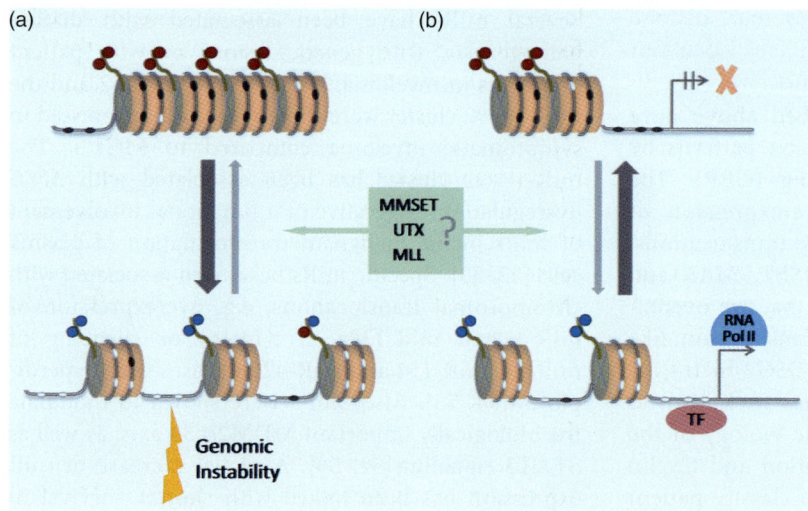

Figure 5.2 Epigenetic modifications in myeloma. (a) DNA methylation globally decreases during the transition from MGUS to myeloma. Loss of methylation predominantly occurs outside of CpG islands and in non-coding areas. DNA demethylation in cancer has been related to genomic instability, in part due to a higher exposure of uncondensed chromatin to DNA damaging mechanisms. (b) Several genes become hypermethylated with the progression from myeloma to plasma cell leukemia, leading to a more condensed chromatin conformation. Chromatin condensation decreases the accessibility of the DNA for transcription factors (TF) and RNA polymerase II (RNA Pol II). The combination of DNA methylation and histone modifications can ultimately result in transcriptional silencing of genes. *MMSET*, *UTX* and *MLL* are genes that are putatively involved in the epigenetic modifications in myeloma, but the exact mechanisms are unknown. White and black ovals = unmethylated and methylated CpG cytosine residues, respectively; red and blue circles = repressive and activating histone modifications, respectively.

histone tails. The two histone modifications that have been most widely studied in the context of neoplasia are acetylation and methylation.

Histone acetylation

Histone acetylation most often occurs at lysine residues of histone tails and is believed to decrease the affinity of the specific histone complex to its attached supercoiled DNA molecule. The DNA thus becomes more accessible to transcription factors and polymerases, resulting in increased transcriptional activity. Histone acetylation is modulated by two sets of proteins, histone acetyltransferases (HATs) and histone deacetylases (HDACs), and an imbalance of these antagonistic enzymes has been associated with cancer. To date, 18 HDACs belonging to four subclasses have been identified, and although the different HDAC members may share common features, each HDAC seems to have specific substrates and thus functional implications, as has been shown in more detail for HDAC6 [59, 60].

Overexpression of different classes of HDACs has been linked to the transcriptional silencing of tumor suppressor genes in several disease entities like breast, colorectal or esophageal cancer. In addition, translocation fusion proteins in hematological malignancies like PML-RARA and AML1-ETO in acute myeloid leukemia have been shown to recruit HDACs to specific tumor suppressor target genes.

Thus far, genome-wide histone acetylation patterns have not been studied in myeloma because of technical limitations. Most of our knowledge about the role of this type of epigenetic modification results from pharmacologic inhibition of HDAC functions. Several highly potent HDAC inhibitors like vorinostat or panobinostat have been developed. Many of these inhibitors have a broad spectrum and inhibit HDACs belonging to different classes. In myeloma, HDAC inhibitors have been shown to lead to hyperacetylation of histones and up-regulation of the cell cycle regulator protein p21, among other factors, with subsequent induction of cell cycle arrest and apoptosis. HDAC inhibitors have successfully been tested in numerous early phase clinical studies in myeloma [61] and several phase III studies are currently underway. However, the impact of HDAC inhibition on tumor biology goes beyond the simple concept of hyperacetylation of histones and subsequent de-silencing of tumor suppressor genes. There are far more targets for HATs and HDACs than histone molecules, and recent studies have identified about 3600 acetylation sites in various functional protein classes like transcription factors (e.g. MYC), cell cycle regulators (e.g. p53) and heat shock proteins (e.g. HSP90)[62]. In addition, it has been shown that HDAC inhibition potently interferes with DNA replication, leading to increased double strand breaks and the mechanism for this is not completely understood [63]. Further insights into epigenetic acetylation patterns and their functional effects in myeloma are necessary, ever more since HDAC inhibitors are probably to enter daily clinical practice soon.

Histone methylation

Aberrant histone methylation is regarded as an important pathophysiologic mechanism in myeloma and has possible therapeutic implications. Methyl groups are transferred by histone methyltransferases to specific lysine residues on histone tails and different patterns of histone methylation are associated with transcriptional activity. In this context, trimethylation of histone 3 lysine 4 residues (H3K4me3) and H3K36me3 are commonly associated with actively transcribed genes, whereas H3K27me3 and H3K9me3 are more frequently associated with transcriptionally repressed genes.

Several lines of evidence support a role for aberrant histone methylation in myeloma biology. The translocation t(4;14) leads to overexpression of MMSET, which has histone methyltransferase activity, and implicates a potential tumor initiating role for aberrant epigenetic modifications in myeloma. In addition, aberrant overexpression of the polycomb group gene EZH2 in myeloma cell lines has been associated with aberrant H3K27me3 patterns, increased proliferation and independence from external growth factors [64, 65]. Very recently, mutations in several histone methyltransferases have been identified in a whole-genome sequencing approach, and MMSET, MLL, MLL2, MLL3 and UTX were shown to be mutated in myeloma, although at low frequencies [35]. The MLL gene encodes a DNA-binding protein that methylates histone H3 lysine 4 (H3K4), generally promoting gene transcription. MLL fusion proteins that lead to loss of the histone methyltransferase capability play a role in acute leukemia pathogenesis. The significance of MLL mutations for myeloma biology is not clear. UTX is a large gene located on Xp11.2 consisting of 29 exons. It encodes for JmjC and tricopeptide protein domains that are implicated in histone demethylation and polycomb protein interactions. Experimental knockdown of UTX was shown to promote cell proliferation, and re-expression of UTX in mutated samples reduced cell growth. Interestingly, genome-wide chromatin immunoprecipitation studies have shown that UTX specifically accumulates at genes belonging to the RB cell cycle control network [66]. In a Drosophila study, UTX suppressed the development of Notch- and Rb-dependent tumors [67]. However, the functional role of UTX needs to be further defined in patients with myeloma.

MMSET has been studied in more detail in the context of myeloma. The full-length MMSET II isoform contains domains that suggest a role in DNA binding and chromatin modification like PWWP domains; moreover it includes a HMG domain, PHD zinc fingers, and a C-terminal SET domain characteristic of histone methyltransferases. There are two shorter isoforms: MMSET I, which shares the N-terminal sequence with MMSET II but lacks the SET-domain, and REII-BP, which contains only the C-terminal domains of the full-length isoform. Depending on their location, translocation breakpoints in t(4;14) can either produce unaltered MMSET isoforms or cause truncations at the N-terminus of MMSET I and MMSET II. Truncation of MMSET may lead to an altered sub-cellular localization of the translated protein, but the functional role of these truncated proteins is yet unknown [68]. A recent publication highlighted a role for MMSET in DNA repair by inducing 53BP1 foci formation at double strand break sites, suggesting that overexpression of MMSET might contribute to rapid disease progression due to altered DNA repair in response to conventional chemotherapy in the t(4;14) subgroup [69]. This hypothesis has not been confirmed by experimental data so far.

MMSET knockdown in t(4;14) myeloma cell lines leads to reduced proliferation, cell cycle arrest and apoptosis, implicating a major pathogenic role for this protein [70]. The current assumption is that MMSET overexpression results in an increased H3K36 tri-methylation and a decrease in H3K27 methylation marks, thereby acting as a transcriptional activator [71]. There have been other reports that associated the isoforms MMSET I or REII-BP with an increase in H3K27 tri-methylation and transcriptional silencing [72, 73]. Further genome-wide studies of chromatin modifications comparing different *MMSET* isoform effects will probably further elucidate the impact of these proteins on histone modifications. In addition to its histone methyltransferase activity, *MMSET* has been shown to interact with HDAC1, HDAC2 and mSin3a, implicating a cross-talk of different layers of epigenetic modifications in t(4;14) myeloma. We have found evidence that *MMSET* influences the global DNA methylation status in myeloma, as samples with t(4;14) had a distinct methylation pattern that was different from cases without this translocation [74]. It is unclear by which mechanism *MMSET* modifies DNA methylation, but it is known that repressive histone methylation marks are associated with DNA methyltransferases (DNMTs). We and others speculate that the *SET* domain with its methyltransferase property is responsible for the changes in chromatin architecture and for aggressive disease features in the t(4;14) myeloma subgroup. This makes the *SET* domain of *MMSET* an interesting target for the development of specific inhibitors.

DNA methylation

DNA methylation changes in cancer generally occur at CpG dinucleotides and are mediated by DNMTs. Three DNMTs have been characterized in humans: DNMT1, which maintains DNA methylation in the context of replication; and DNMT3A and B, which are both involved in *de novo* methylation. In normal cells, about 70% of all CpGs in the genome are methylated and these CpGs are mostly located in intergenic, repetitive non-coding or intronic sequences. Methylation of these non-coding regions is associated with condensation of DNA to a heterochromatic state, which is assumed to maintain genomic stability by decreased exposition to mutational processes (e.g. by reactive oxygen species) and an inactivation of endogenous transposable elements. CpG islands (CGI) are short regions of DNA that have a high content of CpG dinucleotides and are mostly localized in gene promoters or at transcription start sites. A relatively small fraction of CGI CpGs is methylated and dynamic changes in this methylation, together with histone modifications, are involved in transcriptional regulation of genes. DNA methylation changes in cancer are characterized by a demethylation of non-coding regions, which has been correlated with

an increased genomic instability. Subsequently, selective gene promoter regions become hypermethylated and this has often been associated with transcriptional silencing of tumor suppressor genes (reviewed in [75]).

With the exception of two recent studies, DNA methylation changes in myeloma have mostly been studied on a gene-by-gene basis. Hypermethylation in myeloma samples has been reported for *VHL, XAF1, IRF8, TP53, DAPK, CDH1, PTGS2, DCC, CCND2, TGFBR2, CDKN2A* and *CDKN2B* (reviewed in [76]). Of these, promoter hypermethylation of *CDKN2A* and *TGFBR2* have been shown to correlate with poor prognosis in myeloma patients. In a recent study, methylation levels in repetitive elements in myeloma samples were investigated by using the sensitive method of bisulfite pyrosequencing and decreased methylation levels of *Alu, LINE-1* and *SAT-α* were detected in myeloma samples in comparison to healthy controls [77].

Robust techniques for the study of entire methylomes have become commercially available in the past few years and we have used a bead-based methylation array that interrogates ~27 000 CpGs to identify global methylation patterns in multiple myeloma. We first focused on methylation changes associated with disease progression and analyzed B cells, normal plasma cells, MGUS, myeloma and PCL samples. We observed a global decrease in methylation in the malignant phenotypes (myeloma and PCL) compared to non-malignant or pre-malignant samples (normal plasma cells and MGUS). These differences imply that the transition from MGUS to myeloma is accompanied by a massive loss of methylation. The methylation changes mainly affected CpG dinucleotides outside of CpG islands and gene promoter regions. This finding resembles the global hypomethylation patterns of non-coding regions observed in other malignancies. Simultaneously, we identified focal hypermethylation of 77 genes in the transition from MGUS to myeloma. Pathway analysis of the hypermethylated genes demonstrated involvement of developmental, cell cycle and transcriptional regulation processes. The transition from myeloma to PCL involves further focal, gene-specific hypermethylation, but no further demethylation, as might have been expected. We found 1803 genes to be hypermethylated in PCL in comparison to myeloma and these were enriched for cell signaling and cell adhesion processes. This finding is consistent with the

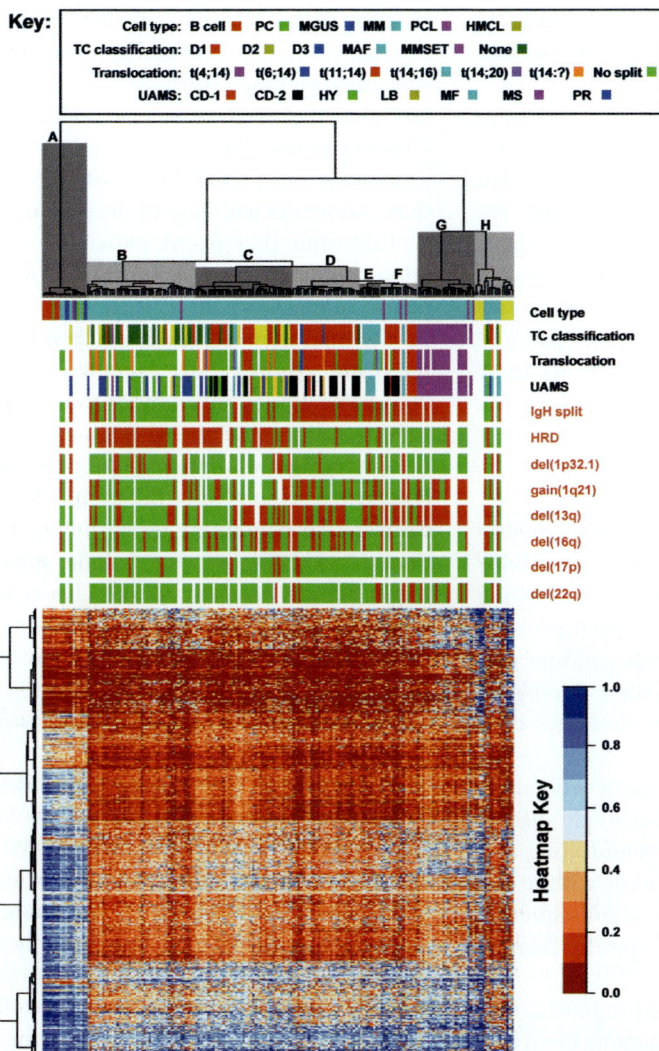

Figure 5.3 Discrete methylation patterns of non-malignant B cells, MGUS, myeloma subgroups and human myeloma cell lines. Unsupervised hierarchical clustering of genome-wide methylation data per sample was performed for a group consisting of normal B cells, normal plasma cells (PCs), MGUS, presentation myeloma, PCL, and human myeloma cell lines (HMCLs). A "non-malignant" clade encompassing B cells, normal PCs and most MGUS samples was clearly separated from the group of presentation myeloma samples and from a third clade containing HMCL samples. The presentation myeloma samples segregated into five clades that correlated with the presence of the following cytogenetic aberrations: t(4;14), t(11;14), t(14;16) and hyperdiploidy (split in two separate clades). Cytogenetic data are coded as red for present, green for absent, and white for no data available. Heatmap key indicates methylation level (deep red = 0%, deep blue = 100% methylated). UAMS subgroups: CD-1/CD-2, cyclin D1 subgroups; HY, hyperdiploid; LB, low bone disease; MF, MAF; MS, MMSET/FGFR3; PR, proliferation. TC subgroups: D1, cyclin D1; D2, cyclin D2; D3, cyclin D3; MAF, MAF/MAFB; MMSET, MMSET/FGFR3.

biological features of the PCL cell, characterized by a decreased homing to the bone marrow niche and the ability to proliferate in peripheral blood.

A second analysis identified specific methylation patterns within the myeloma patient samples. Methylation pattern subgroups identified by unsupervized clustering overlapped with genetic subgroups defined by primary genetic events. Samples clustered in a t(4;14) group, two separate t(11;14) groups, and two separate hyperdiploid groups, as shown in Figure 5.3. Other chromosomal abnormalities, such as del(1p32.1), gain 1q, del(13q), del(16q), del(17p), or del(22) did not affect clustering of the samples. The most distinct methylation profile belonged to samples in the t(4;14) groups, showing an increased

methylation in comparison to other cytogenetic groups. This is probably due to overexpression of *MMSET*, which has histone methyltransferase properties and induces chromatin changes that may subsequently lead to accrual and activation of DNMTs. However, no conclusive functional experiment has verified this hypothesis yet. We identified genes that were hypermethylated only in the t(4;14) subgroup, and these included *PAX1*, *CDKN2A*, *APC* and *SOCS2*. Gene expression changed only in a subset of the genes hypermethylated in t(4;14), suggesting that expression of the majority of genes might be regulated by other epigenetic modifications like histone methylation or acetylation. The fact that subgroups that are associated with a dismal prognosis can be characterized by specific methylation patterns could make methylation analysis a useful tool for diagnostic purposes.

Interestingly, hyperdiploid patient samples were clustered in two groups with differential methylation patterns and one of these groups was associated with a significantly worse OS. Hyperdiploid patients are known to be clinically heterogeneous; attempts have been made to sub-classify this group using genetic abnormalities, i.e. gain(1q), or gene expression patterns. Determination of DNA methylation patterns might be useful as a prognostic biomarker in the large group of hyperdiploid patients.

Conclusions

It is important to understand the genetic and epigenetic abnormalities associated with malignant behavior in myeloma cells as they ultimately define the individual's course of disease. We have given an overview of the anatomy of the myeloma genome and epigenome and demonstrated that these biological features can serve as disease classifiers that have clinical significance.

The diversity of the genetic and epigenetic alterations suggests that myeloma is not a single disease but rather a series of related entities manifesting as a clonal proliferation of plasma cells, each with a distinct biologic and clinical course. As a consequence, each entity should be treated with a specific therapy tailored to its molecular properties.

This highlights the importance of prognostic biomarkers and the importance of implementing them into clinical trials of risk-adapted treatment strategies. The simultaneous occurrence of more than one genetic lesion associated with an unfavorable prognosis, namely t(4;14), t(14;16), t(14;20), gain(1q) and del(17p), defines an ultra-high risk group that should be considered for alternative innovative treatment approaches [78].

A plethora of different formerly unknown mutations in myeloma has been found by an initial whole-genome sequencing approach and will very probably be further expanded by whole-genome sequencing

study analyses of larger patient populations. This high number of new candidate genes will require genetic screening methods, such as RNA interference, to differentiate between passenger and driver mutations. Understanding the interactions of different driver mutations and identification of vulnerable targets in these networks will help to develop novel therapies.

Tailoring therapy to individual molecular alterations requires the establishment of specific therapeutic biomarkers. It is likely that the pathobiology in the majority of myeloma patients is complex, requiring combination therapies, targeting several vulnerable nodes in mutational networks as well as tumor–stroma interactions simultaneously.

Emerging data demonstrate that intra-clonal heterogeneity results in different, related myeloma clones, each containing a unique repertoire of mutations, co-existing in one tumor. Specific therapies might select for resistant sub-clones that were pre-existing but represented only a minor fraction of the original tumor that may initiate disease relapse and may be more difficult to target during the course of the disease due to additionally acquired genetic aberrations.

Mutations in key targetable oncogenes like *BRAF* have recently been identified in myeloma patients. The therapeutic use of specific *BRAF* inhibitors in this subgroup will have to be investigated and may open novel, individualized treatment options. In patients with t(4;14), the subsequently overexpressed epigenetic modifier *MMSET* has evolved as a potential therapeutic target, and specific inhibitors of *MMSET* are under development. The t(4;14) subgroup is defined by specific DNA methylation patterns, which could potentially be used as therapeutic biomarkers for *MMSET*-targeted therapies.

Genotyping of individual tumor genomes might become part of the routine diagnostic workup in the future and will allow for the identification of deregulated oncogenic networks of an individual tumor. Thus, understanding the biologic principals of disease is likely to be utilized in order to target the biologic basis of an individual tumor.

References

1.   Barlogie, B., Attal, M., Crowley, J. *et al.* Long-term follow-up of autotransplantation trials for multiple myeloma: update of protocols conducted by the intergroupe francophone du myelome, southwest oncology group, and university of arkansas for medical sciences. *J. Clin. Oncol.* 2010;**28**:1209–14.

2.   Kyle, R. A., Rajkumar, S. V., Larson, D. R. *et al.* Prevalence of monocloncal gammopathy of

undetermined significance. *New Engl. J. Med.* 2006;**354**:1362–9.

3. Fonseca, R., Bergsagel, P. L., Drach, J. *et al.* International Myeloma Working Group molecular classification of multiple myeloma: spotlight review. *Leukemia* 2009;**23**: 2210–21.

4. Debes-Marun, C. S., Dewald, G. W., Bryant, S. *et al.* Chromosome abnormalities clustering and its implications for pathogenesis and prognosis in myeloma. *Leukemia* 2003;**17**:427–36.

5. Ross, F. M., Ibrahim, A. H., Vilain-Holmes, A. *et al.* Age has a profound effect on the incidence and significance of chromosome abnormalities in myeloma. *Leukemia* 2005;**19**:1634–42.

6. Boyd, K. D., Ross, F. M., Chiecchio, L. *et al.* Gender disparities in the tumor genetics and clinical outcome of multiple myeloma. *Cancer Epidemiol Biomarkers Prev.* 2011;**20**: 1703–7.

7. Walker, B. A., Leone, P. E., Chiecchio, L. *et al.* A compendium of myeloma-associated chromosomal copy number abnormalities and their prognostic value. *Blood* 2010;**116**: e56–65.

8. Fonseca, R., Debes-Marun, C. S., Picken, E. B. *et al.* The recurrent IgH translocations are highly associated with nonhyperdiploid variant multiple myeloma. *Blood* 2003;**102**:2562–7.

9. Avet-Loiseau, H., Li, J. Y., Facon, T. *et al.* High incidence of translocations t(11;14)(q13;q32) and t(4;14)(p16;q32) in patients with plasma cell malignancies. *Cancer Res.* 1998;**58**:5640–5.

10. Gonzalez, D., van der Burg, M., Garcia-Sanz, R. *et al.* Immunoglobulin gene rearrangements and the pathogenesis of multiple myeloma. *Blood* 2007;**110**: 3112–21.

11. Chesi, M., Nardini, E., Lim, R. S. *et al.* The t(4;14) translocation in myeloma dysregulates both FGFR3 and a novel gene, MMSET, resulting in IgH/ MMSET hybrid transcripts. *Blood* 1998;**92**:3025–34.

12. Onwuazor, O. N., Wen, X. Y., Wang, D. Y. *et al.* Mutation, SNP, and isoform analysis of fibroblast growth factor receptor 3 (FGFR3) in 150 newly diagnosed multiple myeloma patients. *Blood* 2003;**102**:772–3.

13. Chen, J., Lee, B. H., Williams, I. R. *et al.* FGFR3 as a therapeutic target of the small molecule inhibitor PKC412 in hematopoietic malignancies. *Oncogene* 2005;**24**:8259–67.

14. Keats, J. J., Reiman, T., Maxwell, C. A. *et al.* In multiple myeloma, t(4;14)(p16;q32) is an adverse prognostic factor irrespective of FGFR3 expression. *Blood* 2003;**101**:1520–9.

15. Fonseca, R., Griepp, P. R. The t(4;14)(p16.3;q32) is strongly associated with chromosome 13 abnormalities in both multiple myeloma and monoclonal gammopathy of undetermined significance. *Blood.* 2001;**98**: 1271–2.

16. Fonseca, R., Blood, E. A., Oken, M. M. *et al.* Myeloma and the t(11;14)(q13;q32); evidence for a biologically defined unique subset of patients. *Blood* 2002;**99**: 3735–41.

17. Garand, R., Avet-Loiseau, H., Accard, F. *et al.* t(11;14) and t(4;14) translocations correlated with mature lymphoplasmacytoid and immature morphology, respectively, in multiple myeloma. *Leukemia* 2003;**17**:2032–5.

18. Chesi, M., Bergsagel, P. L., Shonukan, O. O. *et al.* Frequent dysregulation of the c-maf proto-oncogene at 16q23 by translocation to an Ig locus in multiple myeloma. *Blood* 1998;**91**:4457–63.

19. Hurt, E. M., Wiestner, A., Rosenwald, A. *et al.* Overexpression of c-maf is a frequent oncogenic event in multiple myeloma that promotes proliferation and pathological interactions with bone marrow stroma. *Cancer Cell* 2004;**5**:191–9.

20. Boersma-Vreugdenhil, G. R., Kuipers, J., Van Straler, E. *et al.* The recurrent translocation t(14;20)9q32;q12) in multiple myeloma results in aberrant expression of MAFB: a molecular and genetic analysis of the chromosomal breakpoint. *Br. J. Haematol.* 2004;**126**:355–63.

21. van Stralen, E., van de Wetering, M., Agnelli, L. *et al.* Identification of primary MAFB target genes in multiple myeloma. *Exp. Hematol.* 2009;**37**:78–86.

22. Dib, A., Gabrea, A., Glebov, O. K., Bergsagel, P. L., Kuehl, W. M. Characterization of MYC translocations in multiple myeloma cell lines. *J. Natl Cancer Inst. Monogr.* 2008:25–31.

23. Avet-Loiseau, H., Gerson, F., Magrangeas, F. *et al.* Rearrangements of the c-myc oncogene are present in 15% of primary human multiple myeloma tumors. *Blood* 2001;**98**:3082–6.

24. Chng, W. J., Gertz, M. A., Chung, T. H. *et al.* Correlation between array-comparative genomic hybridization-defined genomic gains and losses and survival: identification of 1p31–32 deletion as a prognostic factor in myeloma. *Leukemia* 2010;**24**:833–42.

25. Kim, H. J., Song, E. J., Lee, Y. S., Kim, E., Lee, K. J. Human Fas-associated factor 1 interacts with heat shock protein 70 and negatively regulates chaperone activity. *J. Biol. Chem.* 2005;**280**:8125–33.

26. Park, M. Y., Moon, J. H., Lee, K. S. *et al.* FAF1 suppresses IkappaB kinase (IKK) activation by disrupting the IKK complex

assembly. *J. Biol. Chem.*
2007;**282**:27 572–7.

27. Shaughnessy, J. D., Jr., Zhan, F.,
Burington, B. E. *et al.* A validated
gene expression model of high-
risk multiple myeloma is defined
by deregulated expression of genes
mapping to chromosome 1. *Blood*
2007;**109**:2276–84.

28. Avet-Loiseau, H., Li, C.,
Magrangeas, F. *et al.* Prognostic
significance of copy-number
alterations in multiple myeloma.
J. Clin. Oncol. 2009; **27**:4585.

29. Tapper, W., Chiecchio, L.,
Dagrada, G. P. *et al.* Heterogeneity
in the prognostic significance of
12p deletion and chromosome 5
amplification in multiple
myeloma. *J. Clin. Oncol.* 2011;**29**:
e37–9; author reply e40–1.

30. Avet-Loiseau, H., Leleu, X.,
Roussel, M. *et al.* Bortezomib plus
dexamethasone induction
improves outcome of patients
with t(4;14) myeloma but not
outcome of patients with del(17p).
J. Clin. Oncol. 2010;**28**:4630–4.

31. Boyd, K. D., Ross, F. M., Tapper,
W. J. *et al.* The clinical impact and
molecular biology of del(17p) in
multiple myeloma treated with
conventional or Thalidomide-
based therapy. *Genes
Chromosomes Cancer*
2011;**50**:765–74.

32. Jenner, M. W., Leone, P. E.,
Walker, B. A. *et al.* Gene mapping
and expression analysis of 16q loss
of heterozygosity identifies
WWOX and CYLD as being
important in determining clinical
outcome in multiple myeloma.
Blood 2007;**110**:3291–300.

33. Qin, H. R., Iliopoulos, D.,
Semba, S. *et al.* A role for the
WWOX gene in prostate cancer.
Cancer Res. 2006;**66**:6477–81.

34. Kovalenko, A., Chable-Bessia, C.,
Cantarella, G. *et al.* The tumour
suppressor CYLD negatively
regulates NF-kappaB signalling by
deubiquitination. *Nature*
2003;**424**:801–5.

35. Chapman, M. A., Lawrence, M. S.,
Keats, J. J. *et al.* Initial genome
sequencing and analysis of
multiple myeloma. *Nature*
2011;**471**:467–72.

36. Walker, B. A., Wardell, C. P.,
Melchor, L. *et al.* Intraclonal
heterogeneity and distinct
molecular mechanisms
characterize the development of
t(4;14) and t(11;14) myeloma.
Blood 2012;**120**:1077–86.

37. Ashworth, A., Lord, C. J., Reis-
Filho, J. S. Genetic interactions in
cancer progression and treatment.
Cell 2011;**145**:30–8.

38. Chng, W. J., Gonzalez-Paz, N.,
Price-Troska, T. *et al.* Clinical and
biological significance of RAS
mutations in multiple myeloma.
Leukemia 2008;**22**:2280–4.

39. Chapman, P. B., Hauschild, A.,
Robert, C. *et al.* Improved survival
with vemurafenib in melanoma
with BRAF V600E mutation.
N. Engl. J. Med. 2011;**364**:
2507–16.

40. Chng, W. J., Price-Troska, T.,
Gonzalez-Paz, N. *et al.* Clinical
significance of TP53 mutation
in myeloma. *Leukemia*
2007;**21**:582–4.

41. Lode, L., Eveillard, M., Trichet, V.
et al. Mutations in TP53 are
exclusively associated with del
(17p) in multiple myeloma.
Haematologica 2010;**95**:1973–6.

42. Annunziata, C. M., Davis, R. E.,
Demchenko, Y. *et al.* Frequent
engagement of the classical and
alternative NF-kappaB pathways
by diverse genetic abnormalities
in multiple myeloma. *Cancer Cell*
2007;**12**:115–30.

43. Keats, J. J., Fonseca, R., Chesi, M.
et al. Promiscuous mutations
activate the noncanonical NF-
kappaB pathway in multiple
myeloma. *Cancer Cell*
2007;**12**:131–44.

44. Rajan, N., Elliott, R., Clewes, O.
et al. Dysregulated TRK signalling
is a therapeutic target in CYLD

defective tumours. *Oncogene*
2011;**30**:4243–60.

45. Bergsagel, P. L., Kuehl, W. M.,
Zhan, F. *et al.* Cyclin
D dysregulation: an early and
unifying pathogenic event in
multiple myeloma. *Blood*
2005;**106**:296–303.

46. Brito, J. L., Walker, B., Jenner, M.
et al. MMSET deregulation affects
cell cycle progression and
adhesion regulons in t(4;14)
myeloma plasma cells.
Haematologica 2009;**94**:78–86.

47. Kaiser, M. F., Walker, B. A.,
Hockley, S. L. *et al.* A TC
classification based predictor for
multiple myeloma using
multiplexed real-time quantitative
PCR. *Leukemia* 2013. (In the
press.)

48. Zhou, Y., Zhang, Q., Stephens, O.
et al. Prediction of cytogenetic
abnormalities with gene
expression profiles. *Blood*
2012;**119**:e148–50.

49. Decaux, O., Lode, L., Magrangeas,
F. *et al.* Prediction of survival in
multiple myeloma based on gene
expression profiles reveals cell
cycle and chromosomal instability
signatures in high-risk patients
and hyperdiploid signatures in
low-risk patients: a study of the
Intergroupe Francophone du
Myeloma. *J. Clin. Oncol.*
2008;**26**:4798–805.

50. Dickens, N. J., Walker, B. A.,
Leone, P. E. *et al.* Homozygous
deletion mapping in myeloma
samples identifies genes and an
expression signature relevant to
pathogenesis and outcome. *Clin.
Cancer Res.* 2010;**16**:1856–64.

51. Kuiper, R., Broyl, A., de Knegt, Y.
et al. A gene expression signature
for high-risk multiple myeloma.
Leukemia 2012;**26**:2406–13.

52. Pichiorri, F., Suh, S. S., Ladetto,
M. *et al.* MicroRNAs regulate
critical genes associated with
multiple myeloma pathogenesis.
Proc. Natl Acad. Sci. USA
2008;**105**:12,885–90.

53. Chesi, M., Robbiani, D. F., Sebag, M. *et al.* AID-dependent activation of a MYC transgene induces multiple myeloma in a conditional mouse model of post-germinal center malignancies. *Cancer Cell* 2008;**13**:167–80.

54. Rio-Machin, A., Ferreira, B. I., Henry, T. *et al.* Downregulation of specific miRNAs in hyperdiploid multiple myeloma mimics the oncogenic effect of IgH translocations occurring in the non-hyperdiploid subtype. *Leukemia* 2012; **27**(4):925–31.

55. Gutierrez, N. C., Sarasquete, M. E., Misiewicz-Krzeminska, I. *et al.* Deregulation of microRNA expression in the different genetic subtypes of multiple myeloma and correlation with gene expression profiling. *Leukemia* 2010;**24**: 629–37.

56. Pichiorri, F., Suh, S. S., Rocci, A. *et al.* Downregulation of p53-inducible microRNAs 192, 194, and 215 impairs the p53/MDM2 autoregulatory loop in multiple myeloma development. *Cancer Cell* 2010;**18**:367–81.

57. Zhou, Y., Chen, L., Barlogie, B. *et al.* High-risk myeloma is associated with global elevation of miRNAs and overexpression of EIF2C2/AGO2. *Proc. Natl Acad. Sci. USA* 2010;**107**:7904–9.

58. Kalari, S., Pfeifer, G. P. Identification of driver and passenger DNA methylation in cancer by epigenomic analysis. *Adv. Genet.* 2010;**70**:277–308.

59. Kovacs, J. J., Murphy, P. J., Gaillard, S. *et al.* HDAC6 regulates Hsp90 acetylation and chaperone-dependent activation of glucocorticoid receptor. *Mol. Cell* 2005;**18**:601–7.

60. Marks, P., Rifkind, R. A., Richon, V. M. *et al.* Histone deacetylases and cancer: causes and therapies. *Nat. Rev. Cancer* 2001;**1**: 194–202.

61. Smith, E. M., Boyd, K., Davies, F. E. The potential role of epigenetic therapy in multiple myeloma. *Br J Haematol.* 2010;**148**:702–13.

62. Choudhary, C., Kumar, C., Gnad, F. *et al.* Lysine acetylation targets protein complexes and co-regulates major cellular functions. *Science* (New York, NY) 2009;**325**:834–40.

63. Namdar, M., Perez, G., Ngo, L., Marks, P. A. Selective inhibition of histone deacetylase 6 (HDAC6) induces DNA damage and sensitizes transformed cells to anticancer agents. *Proc. Natl Acad. Sci. USA* 2010;**107**:20 003–8.

64. Croonquist, P. A., Van Ness, B. The polycomb group protein enhancer of zeste homolog 2 (EZH 2) is an oncogene that influences myeloma cell growth and the mutant ras phenotype. *Oncogene* 2005;**24**:6269–80.

65. Kalushkova, A., Fryknas, M., Lemaire, M. *et al.* Polycomb target genes are silenced in multiple myeloma. *PLoS One* 2010;**5**:e11 483.

66. Wang, J. K., Tsai, M. C., Poulin, G. *et al.* The histone demethylase UTX enables RB-dependent cell fate control. *Genes Dev.* 2010;**24**:327–32.

67. Herz, H. M., Madden, L. D., Chen, Z. *et al.* The H3K27me3 demethylase dUTX is a suppressor of Notch- and Rb-dependent tumors in Drosophila. *Mol. Cell Biol.* 2010;**30**:2485–97.

68. Keats, J. J., Maxwell, C. A., Taylor, B. J. *et al.* Overexpression of transcripts originating from the MMSET locus characterizes all t(4;14)(p16;q32)-positive multiple myeloma patients. *Blood* 2005;**105**:4060–9.

69. Pei, H., Zhang, L., Luo, K. *et al.* MMSET regulates histone H4K20 methylation and 53BP1 accumulation at DNA damage sites. *Nature* 2011;**470**:124–8.

70. Lauring, J., Abukhdeir, A. M., Konishi, H. *et al.* The multiple myeloma associated MMSET gene contributes to cellular adhesion, clonogenic growth, and tumorigenicity. *Blood* 2008;**111**:856–64.

71. Martinez-Garcia, E., Popovic, R., Min, D. J. *et al.* The MMSET histone methyl transferase switches global histone methylation and alters gene expression in t(4;14) multiple myeloma cells. *Blood* 2011;**117**:211–20.

72. Kim, J. Y., Kee, H. J., Choe, N. W. *et al.* Multiple-myeloma-related WHSC1/MMSET isoform RE-IIBP is a histone methyltransferase with transcriptional repression activity. *Mol. Cell Biol.* 2008;**28**:2023–34.

73. Todoerti, K., Ronchetti, D., Agnelli, L. *et al.* Transcription repression activity is associated with the type I isoform of the MMSET gene involved in t(4;14) in multiple myeloma. *Br. J. Haematol.* 2005;**131**:214–18.

74. Walker, B. A., Wardell, C. P., Chiecchio, L. *et al.* Aberrant global methylation patterns affect the molecular pathogenesis and prognosis of multiple myeloma. *Blood* 2011;**117**:553–62.

75. Ehrlich, M. DNA methylation in cancer: too much, but also too little. *Oncogene* 2002;**21**:5400–13.

76. Sharma, A., Heuck, C. J., Fazzari, M. J. *et al.* DNA methylation alterations in multiple myeloma as a model for epigenetic changes in cancer. *Wiley Interdiscip. Rev. Syst. Biol. Med.* 2010;**2**:654–69.

77. Bollati, V., Fabris, S., Pegoraro, V. *et al.* Differential repetitive DNA methylation in multiple myeloma molecular subgroups. *Carcinogenesis* 2009;**30**:1330–5.

78. Boyd, K. D., Ross, F. M., Chiecchio, L. *et al.* A novel prognostic model in myeloma based on co-segregating adverse FISH lesions and the ISS: analysis of patients treated in the MRC Myeloma IX trial. *Leukemia* 2012;**26**:349–55.

Chapter

6

The myeloma bone marrow environment and survival signaling

Asim Khwaja, John Quinn and Kwee L. Yong

Introduction

The interactions of clonal cells with the bone marrow begin with the initial establishment of transformed precursor MM cells in specialized niches, and their survival and persistence in such niches during the disease stage termed MGUS. During this stage, which can last for years, the bone marrow is gradually "re-modeled" to provide a permissive environment for the self-renewal of these (pre)malignant PC, with acquisition of (further) genetic lesions that trigger progression from MGUS to MM, accompanied by clonal expansion. Release of clonal cells into the circulation, and their homing to and establishment in other sites of hemopoietic bone marrow, with disruption of the bone homeostasis and angiogenesis, characterize the mature malignancy we call multiple myeloma (MM).

A multitude of players feature in these interactions (Table 6.1). Soluble factors direct migration and homing into bone marrow, upregulate anti-apoptotic pathways for drug resistance, modulate immune responses, act as mitogens to induce self-renewal and clonal expansion and function in many autocrine and paracrine loops to maintain survival, angiogenesis and bone destruction. Reciprocal interactions between MM cells and other cell types in the BM such as osteoblasts, osteoclasts, stromal cells and endothelial cells are mediated by some of these soluble factors, as well as by cell–cell contact dependent mechanisms such as adhesion molecules. Cell contact is also important for interactions with extracellular matrix proteins resulting in anti-apoptotic signaling and consequent drug resistance. This chapter will discuss these players in the context of each stage or component of disease pathogenesis, highlighting

key players, and will consider in more detail the biochemical pathways that orchestrate survival and drug resistance of MM cells.

Homing and migration: role of MMPs and chemokines

The selective localization of MM cells in the bone marrow is orchestrated by the actions of matrix metalloproteinases (MMPs), that are secreted in latent form, that is cleaved to active form, or expressed as integral membrane proteins (membrane-type MMPs, MT-MMPs), chemokines and their cognate receptors, and adhesion molecules. Although roles have been suggested for several MMPs, there is most evidence for MMP9 [1]. MMP9 is secreted by MM cells in response to SDF-1 or to contact with BM endothelium, and functions in promoting transendothelial migration and, by inference, the extravasation of circulating MM cells into the BM [2,3]. MMPs are also important in the invasion into ECM proteins such as collagen, encountered in the sub-endothelial space. Much of the *in vivo* evidence for the role of MMPs derives from work in the murine 5T2MM model. Here, systemically infused murine MM cells that have localized to the BM are found to have upregulated MMP9. Considering their prominent role in the extravasation of other hemopoietic cells, chemokines are also likely to direct the migration of MM cells into and within the BM. MCP-1 is secreted by BM endothelium, and is a chemo-attractant for MM cells [4]. SDF-1 (CXCL12) is present at high concentrations in the BM, where it is produced by stromal cells and has a physiological role in the establishment of

Myeloma, ed. Stephen A. Schey, Kwee L. Yong, Robert Marcus and Kenneth C. Anderson. Published by Cambridge University Press. © Cambridge University Press 2014.

Table 6.1 Players involved in homing, migration and adhesive interactions of MM cells in the bone marrow environment

Soluble factors	Cell types	Cell surface receptors
IL-6	Osteoblasts	Integrins
IGF-1	Osteoclasts	• LFA-1
VEGF	Endothelial cells	• VLA-4
HGF	Mesenchymal	• Integrin β7
MIP-1α	stromal cells	CD44
TNFα	(MSC)	CXCR4
SDF-1	T cells	CCR2, 7
APRIL	Dendritic cells	N- and E-Cadherin
BAFF	Monocytes/	
MMP2, 7, 9	macrophages	**Extracellular matrix**
		Collagen
		Laminin
		Fibronectin

IGF-I = Insulin-like growth factor-I, VEGF = vascular endothelial growth factor, HGF = hepatocyte growth factor, MIP-1α = macrophage inflammatory protein-1 alpha, SDF-1 = stromal derived growth factor-1, LFA-1 = lymphocyte function-associated antigen-1, VLA-4 = very late antigen-4

hemopoiesis. SDF-1 is chemo-attractant for MM cells and mediates *in vivo* homing to the BM [5], as well as tumor growth and stromal cell-mediated drug protection, perhaps by modulating integrin-mediated adhesion [6]. MM cell derived SDF-1 may also contribute to bone disease by attracting osteoclast precursors to MM cell foci [7]. As well as mediating homing and migration of MM cells, SDF-1 may also have a role in drug resistance, as revealed by the ability of the CXCR4 antagonist, AMD100 to sensitize MM cells in vitro to bortezomib [8]. The central role of the SDF-1/CXCR4 axis in MM and other hematological malignancies has led to strategies aimed at disrupting this axis [9]. Another key cytokine in myelomagenesis is IGF-1, which has a major role in promoting survival of MM cells (see below), but also induces migration of tumor cells [10,11] a function of especial importance because it is sequestered in bone, from whence it is released by osteoclastic activity.

Finally, adhesion receptors also provide anchorage for migrating MM cells, and certain isoforms of CD44 have been described to play a role in marrow homing and the tumor load [12]. In the murine 5T33MM model, for example, CD44v6 becomes upregulated after contact with the marrow endothelium [13], and mediates the binding of tumor cells to marrow stromal cells [14]. CD44 binds to several ligands in the bone marrow, the most important of which are hyaluronic acid, a glycosaminoglycan that is present as an extracellular matrix component, and osteopontin, also known

as bone sialoprotein protein-1 that is produced by osteoblasts and is hence found close to the endosteal surface. The VLA-4/VCAM adhesion receptor/ligand pair mediates adhesion of myeloma cells to stromal cells (see below), while the fibronectin-binding integrin, β7, is expressed on MM cells, mediates binding to fibronectin and may have a role in the homing and recirculation of tumor cells *in vivo* [15]. A role has also been described for N-cadherin in the homing of systemically injected MM cells into immunodeficient hosts [16]. These authors also showed that primary MM cells express N-cadherin. Recently, the selectin ligand, PSGL-1, expressed on MM cells, was observed to mediate binding to endothelial and stromal cells, transendothelial migration and homing *in vivo* [17].

Survival and drug resistance: soluble factors and adhesion molecules

The propensity of MM tumor cells to die rapidly when removed from the bone marrow, the extreme difficulty associated with culturing these cells *in vitro* for any length of time [18], and the predominantly intramedullary location of this tumor lend support to the prevailing view that these tumor cells are critically dependent on the bone marrow environment for survival, drug resistance and expansion. Cytokines that act to promote MM cell survival include interleukin-6 (IL-6), Insulin-like growth factor-I (IGF-I), Vascular endothelial growth factor (VEGF), B - cell activating factor (BAFF), A Proliferation-Inducing Ligand (APRIL), hepatocyte growth factor (HGF) and, as indicated above, Stromal-derived factor-I (SDF-1). Soluble factors mediate the protective effect of stromal and other cells, via autocrine and paracrine loops that lead not only to the growth and survival of MM cells but also to the development of both cytokine-mediated drug resistance (CM-DR) and cell-adhesion mediated drug resistance (CAM-DR). Surface adhesion molecules on MM cells mediate not only extravasation and homing, but also cellular adhesion molecule (CAM)-mediated drug resistance (DR) [19]. The multiple interactions within the MM micro-envionment are also believed to be important in the pathogenesis of myeloma bone disease, stimulating osteoclastic activity and inhibiting osteoblast activity, and this is dealt with in more detail in Chapter 8. The key BM microenvironment components and their interactions are depicted in Figure 6.1.

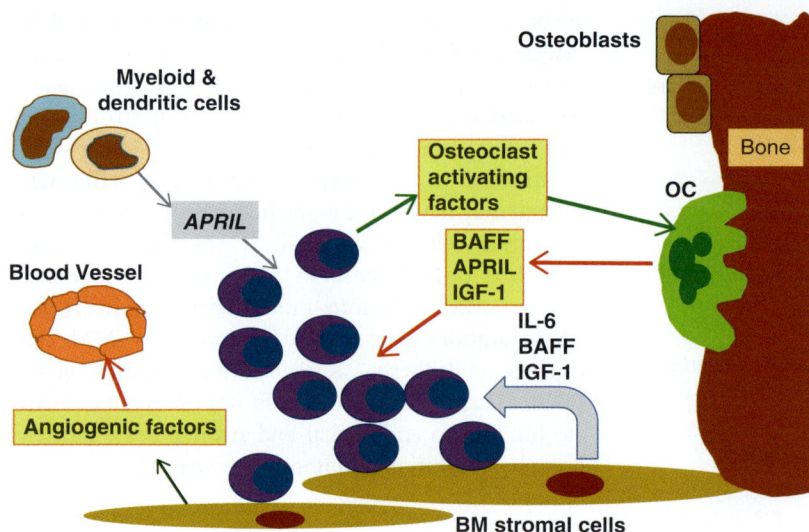

Figure 6.1 Schematic representation of major cellular interactions within the myeloma bone marrow. Myeloma plasma cells reside in close proximity to other cells of hemopoietic lineages, as well as osteoblasts, osteoclasts, stromal cells and endothelial cells. Production of growth factors, angiogenic factors and bone cytokines occurs in a paracrine as well as autocrine fashion to maintain and expand the malignant plasma cell clone, as well as disrupting bone physiology. Abbreviations: BAFF = B - cell activating factor; APRIL = A proliferation-inducing ligand; IL-6 = interleukin 6; IGF-I = Insulin-like growth factor-I; OC = osteoclast.

Cytokines in the myeloma bone marrow microenvironment

The following soluble factors have been shown to be important in disease pathogenesis on the basis of (a) *in vitro* studies demonstrating their ability to promote MM cell survival, (b) studies reporting increased circulating levels in MM patients' sera, along with expression of cytokine receptors by MM cells, and (c) effect of blockade *in vitro* and, in some cases, *in vivo*.

IL-6

Often regarded as the most important MM growth factor, IL-6 was one of the first myeloma growth factors described and since then many studies have confirmed a key role for IL-6 in MM pathogenesis [20]. The role of IL-6 as an MM growth factor is highlighted by the development of many HMCLs that are IL-6 dependent (e.g. XG named HMCLs), and IL-6 deficient mice do not develop MM [21,22]. Although originally thought to be produced mainly in an autocrine fashion it has more recently been shown that IL-6 is also produced in a paracrine fashion by monocytes and bone marrow stromal cells [23]. IL-6 also inhibits dexamethasone-induced apoptosis in MM cells in a dose dependent-fashion and interacts with fibronectin in the BM micro-environment to promote drug-resistance [24,25]. These actions of IL-6 are mediated by the Janus Kinase and signal transducers and activation of transcription 3 (JAK/STAT3), extracellular signal-related kinase 1/2 (ERK 1/2) and phosphatidyl-inositol-3-kinase/AKT (PI3K/AKT) signaling pathways (see also Chapter 7).

From a clinical perspective, MM patients have elevated serum levels of IL-6 and IL-6R, which are features associated with a poor prognosis [26]. Given its prominent role in MM pathogenesis, much effort has been directed at targeting IL-6 as an anti-MM strategy. Although anti-IL-6 antibodies have been shown to inhibit myeloma cell proliferation *in-vitro*, and also in a MM patient with end-stage disease, a significant anti-MM effect was not seen in early phase clinical trials in MM patients [27,28]. Nevertheless this cytokine remains an attractive target, and a recent study has suggested that the anti-IL-6R monoclonal antibody, siltuximab, may enhance melphalan-induced cytotoxicity in MM cells [29]. Intriguingly, it has also been shown that myeloid engraftment following high-dose melphalan and autologous stem cell transplantation results in the increased concentrations of IL-6 in the MM bone marrow micro-environment, which may promote the survival of drug resistant MM cells, thus presenting a possible therapeutic window. Accordingly, treating patients with IL-6 blocking agents is currently being investigated in this setting [30].

IGF-I

Along with IL-6, IGF-I is regarded as one of the two most critical MM growth factors. IGF-I stimulation of HMCLs led to a growth effect in all HMCLs treated, in contrast to cytokines such as APRIL and HGF which induced a growth response in less than one third of cell lines treated [31]. Furthermore, recent work from our laboratory has shown that IGF-I promotes cell cycle progression in HMCLs and MM cells bearing t(4;14) and t(4;16) with increased expression of cyclin D2 protein [32]. IGF-I predominantly activates both the PI3K/AKT and MAPK signaling pathways but, unlike IL-6, does not appear to activate the JAK/STAT pathway [31]. IGF-I attenuates dexamethasone induced apoptosis in HCMLs and cooperates with IL-6 to enhance the growth and survival of MM cells [33,34].

In MM patients, expression of the IGF-I receptor (IGF-IR) is found in 30%–50% of cases and is associated with a poor prognosis, particularly when found to co-exist with the t(4;14) translocation in MM patients [32]. Furthermore, although plasma levels of IGF-I were not found to be elevated in the sera of MM patients when compared with controls, elevated individual IGF-I serum levels in MM patients were found to be predictive of poor outcome [35]. The abundant in - vitro evidence demonstrating a key role for IGF-I in promoting MM cell growth and survival has prompted investigators to attempt to block its actions in vivo. To date, a small molecule IGF-IR tyrosine kinase inhibitor (NVP-ADW742) has shown promising pre-clinical activity and the results of clinical studies are awaited [36].

APRIL and BAFF

APRIL and the closely related B-cell activating factor (BAFF) are members of the tumor necrosis factor (TNF) superfamily of cytokines, and play key roles in normal B-cell and plasma cell development as well as in an increasing number of autoimmune disorders and malignant diseases [37,38]. The importance of APRIL in the development of normal immune function is underscored by the demonstration that APRIL-deficient (−/−) mice have significantly reduced IgA levels despite having normal B and T-lymphocyte development [39]. In contrast, transgenic mice overexpressing APRIL developed lymph node hyperplasia and lymphoid infiltration of kidneys and liver [40]. Several lines of evidence have confirmed that APRIL is an important survival factor for BM plasmablasts, as well as tissue-resident plasma cells [41]. APRIL is a type II membrane protein that is released by proteolytic cleavage in the Golgi apparatus to form active soluble homotrimers; this prevents its expression on the cell surface. APRIL and BAFF share two common receptors: B-cell maturation antigen (BCMA) and transmembrane activator, calcium modulator, and cyclophilin ligand interactor (TACI). In addition APRIL also binds to heparin sulfate proteoglycans (HSPGs), whilst BAFF (but not APRIL) binds to BAFF-receptor (BAFF-R) [42] (Figure 6.2). Increasing evidence points to a role for APRIL in MM pathogenesis. Both BCMA and TACI are expressed

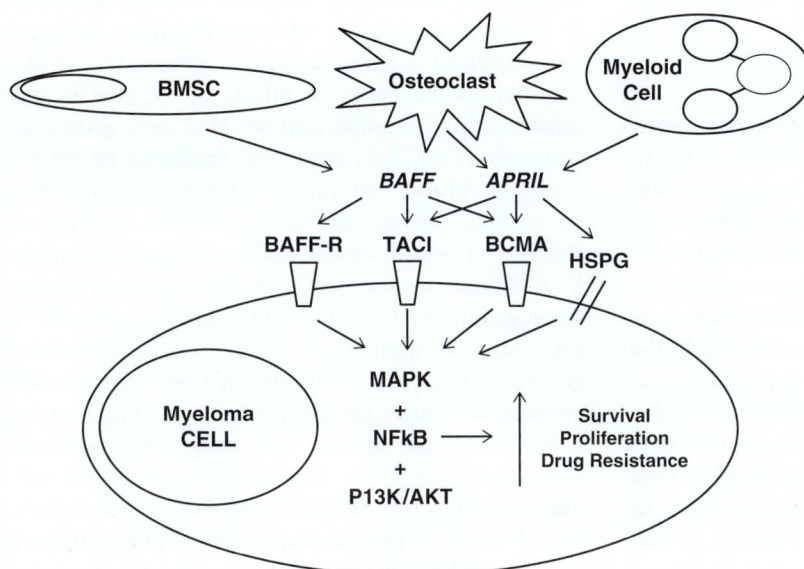

Figure 6.2 The BAFF and APRIL receptor–ligand complex. These ligands share three receptors, BAFF-R, TACI and BCMA. BAFF is produced mainly by bone marrow stromal cells and binds all three receptors, whilst APRIL is produced mainly by osteoclasts and myeloid cells in the bone marrow, and binds to BCMA and TACI, and is also able to interact with cell-surface HSPGs. Receptor–ligand binding activates MAPK, NFκB and PI3K/AKT signaling pathways leading to the upregulation of genes controlling MM cell survival and drug resistance. Abbreviations: BAFF-R = B - cell activating factor receptor; TACI = transmembrane activator, calcium modulator, and cyclophilin ligand interactor; HSPG = heparin sulfate proteoglycans; BMSC = bone marrow stromal cells; MAPK = mitogen-activated protein kinase; NFkB = nuclear factor kappa-light-chain-enhancer of activated B cells; PI3K/Akt = phosphoinositide-3-kinase/Akt.

67

on HMCL and primary MM cells [43,44] and APRIL also binds proteoglycans [45]. APRIL is produced mainly by myeloid-lineage cells in the bone marrow [46], and is present in abundance in MM bone marrow [47]. MM patients have higher circulating serum levels of APRIL in comparison to normal controls. APRIL protects IL-6 dependent HMCL from dexamethasone-induced apoptosis, and rescued IL-dependent MM cell lines from IL-6 withdrawal. In MM cells, APRIL has been shown to activate the MAPK, PI3K/AKT and NFκB signaling pathways and to upregulate the expression of the anti-apoptotic protein PIM-2, particularly in cooperation with IL-6 [43,48].

The therapeutic potential of APRIL blockade has been explored by employing TACI-Fc, a fusion protein consisting of the extracellular domain of TACI fused with human IgG1. TACI-Fc overcomes the anti-apoptotic effect of APRIL in the presence of dexamethasone and inhibits the growth of TACI^{high} MM cells in a murine model [49]. Furthermore, TACI-Fc was shown to inhibit the dendritic cell-mediated clonogenic growth of HMCLs [50]. Recently, Atacicept was used to treat patients with MM and Waldenstrom's Macroglobulinemia in a Phase I clinical trial. In this study Atacicept treatment was well tolerated and led to disease stabilization in five out of 25 patients treated [51]. Alternative approaches utilizing specific anti-APRIL monoclonal antibodies has the theoretical advantage of inhibiting APRIL but not BAFF, which plays a critical role in normal B cell development [52].

VEGF

There is evidence that angiogenesis plays an important role in the growth and survival of MM cells [53]. In fact, angiogenesis appears to be associated with disease activity as one study showed that BM angiogenesis was correlated with plasma cell labeling index (PCLI), whilst another showed that increased serum levels of VEGF portended poor prognosis when combined with HGF levels in MM patients [54,55]. In the MM BM micro-environment, VEGF is produced not only by bone marrow stromal cell (BMSCs) but also by MM cells. VEGF has been shown to interact with several other BM factors such as IGF-I, IL-6, stromal derived factor-1 (SDF-1) and fibronectin (FN) in paracrine loops to promote MM cell survival, as well as attenuating MM cell apoptosis through increased expression of Mcl-1 in MM cells [56,57,58].

Hepatocyte Growth Factor (HGF)

Like VEGF, HGF is secreted in the MM BM micro-environment by BM stromal cells and also by MM cells, and is found at increased concentrations in the sera of MM patients, higher levels being associated with a poor prognosis [59] [60]. HGF binds to its receptor c-Met and cooperates with IL-6 to promote MM cell growth [61]. Importantly, HGF activity also appears to rely to some degree on syndecan-1 (CD138) to signal through c-Met and it is possible that this interaction may be inhibited by heparatinase which promotes syndecan-1 shedding thus offering a potential therapeutic target [62].

In addition to those discussed above, several other cytokines have been shown to be present at increased concentrations in the MM bone marrow micro-environment and to promote the survival of MM cells. These include TNFα, IL-4, IL-10, Transforming Growth Factor-β (TGF-β) and Fibroblast Growth Factor (FGF). Establishing a hierarchy of MM cytokines is difficult but overall, IGF-I and IL-6 are still considered to be among the major MM growth factors [63].

Adhesion to extracellular matrix proteins

MM cells express a range of adhesion receptors including CD29, CD44, CD49d (VLA-4), CD54, CD138 and CD184, with variable expression of CD49e (VLA-5), CD11a and CD18 [64,65]. The engagement of integrin receptors confers resistance to MM cells exposed to cytotoxic therapies. MM cell lines adhering to fibronectin were observed to be less sensitive to the cytotoxic effects of melphalan and doxorubicin in comparison to MM cells grown in suspension [66]. This effect was mediated by the β1 integrins, VLA-4 and VLA-5. VLA-4 binds to fibronectin and to vascular cell adhesion molecule-1 (VCAM-1), which is expressed on stromal cells, while VLA-5 binds to fibronectin. A later report from the same group implicated the upregulation of p27^{kip1} expression to induce cell cycle arrest and chemoresistance [67]. The addition of IL-6 to MM cell cultures overcame the cell cycle arrest imposed by adhesion to fibronectin, but drug resistance was maintained, suggesting that dual stimulation by soluble growth factors and anchorage to integrin ligands would serve to protect tumor cells from cytotoxic therapies whilst maintaining clonal expansion [68]. Another adhesion pathway that has been implicated in drug resistance mechanism for MM cells is CD44, a receptor already mentioned earlier in the context of migration and homing.

Cellular interactions

Bone marrow stromal cells

Multiple studies indicate that co-culture of MM cells with bone marrow stromal cells (BMSCs) promotes survival and, in particular, drug resistance in MM cells [69]. At least part of this effect is related to the engagement of integrin receptors, in particular, VLA-4 on MM cells. Exposure to bortezomib downregulates VLA-4 expression on MM cells and reverses the drug resistance conferred by stromal cells to dexamethasone. Adhesion to stromal cells also stimulates autocrine and paracrine secretion of growth factors that play an important role in mediating protection from drug-induced apoptosis. Thus, adhesion of MM cells to bone marrow stromal cells stimulates the production of IL-6 [70,71]. Alternatively, direct contact between MM cells and BMSCs via VLA-4 or VLA-5 may induce MM cell "quiescence" thus rendering MM cells less chemosensitive [72]. Interrupting the BMSC-MM cell interaction is an attractive therapeutic target, and a recent study suggests that blocking the interaction between the chemokine, stromal derived factor-1 (SDF-1) and its receptor CXCR4 with AMD3100 (Plerixafor) increases the sensitivity of MM cells to anti-MM agents *in vitro* [8].

Whilst many of the earlier studies on stromal cell mediated drug resistance in MM have employed immortalized (MM) cell lines, these reports have been confirmed in a few studies on primary MM cells isolated from patient bone marrow samples [73].

Osteoblasts and mesenchymal stem cells

The early stages of MM are characterized by osteoblast expansion, keeping pace with osteoclast activity [74]. These observations, and the localization of MM cells near the endosteal surface, suggest that osteoblasts, or their precursors, may play a role in maintenance of the malignant plasma cell clone. Osteoblasts are derived by differentiation from multi-potential progenitor cells, termed mesenchymal stromal cells (MSC) resident in the bone marrow [75]. These cells are described in more detail in Chapter 8. Because MSC are a minority population, *ex-vivo* culture and expansion are required, yielding a mixed population with varying cellular functions. This

makes it difficult to interpret reports on the abnormalities of MSC derived from patients with MM [76,77]. A recent study that utilized minimal cell expansion to obtain MSC and osteoblasts from patient and normal bone biopsies reported that the gene expression profile of MSC, but not osteoblasts, differed between patients and controls [78]. Likewise, there are conflicting reports with regard to the suppressive or promoting effects of MSC on MM growth *in vitro*, or *in vivo* [79,80,81]. Taken as a whole, current evidence supports the notion that MSC and osteoblast progenitors undergo functional changes as a result of the presence of MM cells; however, the exact nature of these changes and the impact on MM disease course remain to be clarified.

Osteoclasts

Osteoclasts are derived from CD14+ monocyte/macrophages under the influence of M-CSF and RANK-ligand. The data on osteoclast effects on MM cell growth seem clearer and more consistent. For example, co-culturing primary MM cells with osteoclast precursors has been shown on one hand to promote osteoclast differentiation to multinucleated cells, whilst in turn the direct contact between MM cells and osteoclasts significantly improved the viability of MM cells in comparison with control samples as well as promoting cell cycle progression as shown by increased uptake of bromodeoxyuridine (BrdU) in the MM cells. [82] A more recent study focusing on the expression of growth factors by osteoclasts from MM patients has shown that these osteoclasts express APRIL, IGF-I and IL-10 in large amounts but show lesser expression of BAFF and IL-6 [83]. This study also demonstrated a role for the chemo-attractant receptor chemokine C-C motif receptor 2 (CCR2) as an anti-CCR2 monoclonal antibody blocked osteoclast chemo-attractant activity for MM cells.

Plasmacytoid dendritic cells and macrophages

The number of cellular components within the BM micro-environment shown to be important in promoting MM cell survival has expanded to include accessory cells such as macrophages and plasmacytoid dendritic cells (pDCs). One recent study showed that the immune function of pDCs was defective in MM and that interaction between MM cells and pDCs stimulated MM cell growth and drug resistance [84]. Furthermore, this study showed that although pDCs were relatively resistant to novel anti-myeloma agents, targeting toll-like receptors abrogated the growth effect of pDCs on MM cells and also restored the immune function of pDCs. In another recent study, macrophages were shown to be more plentiful in the MM BM micro-environment in comparison with the BM from healthy controls. In addition, the interaction between MM cells and macrophages stimulated increased secretion of IL-6 and also attenuated drug-induced apoptosis of MM cells [85].

Hypoxia in the MM bone marrow

The contribution of hypoxia to tumor growth and dissemination has long been recognized, but only recently have researchers focused on the hypoxic bone marrow environment in MM. Hypoxia leads to the stabilization of the hypoxia-inducible transcription factors, HIF-1 and HIF-2, which then orchestrate a transcriptional cellular adaptive program that, for tumor cells, includes genes for survival, migration and decreased adhesion, and in general correlating with a poorer outcome. MM in bone marrow biopsies have been demonstrated to express both HIF-1 and HIF-2 [86,87]. Exposure of MM cells to hypoxia increased expression of CXCR4, reduced expression of E-cadherin, reduced adhesion to stromal cells and increased migration towards SDF-1, functional changes suggestive of a more invasive phenotype. The impact of altered adhesive behavior on tumor pathogenesis is complex, however, and whilst reduced adhesion may promote invasion and metastatic behavior, particular adhesive interactions may promote drug resistance. Thus, a recent study in which NOD/SCID/gammaC^{null}(NOG) animals engrafted with the MM cell line, U266, were treated with bendamustine, reported that drug resistance was associated with expression of VE-cadherin and HIF-2 [88].

Biochemical pathways that mediate survival and drug resistance

Thus a complex array of cellular and non-cellular interactions are implicated in promoting myeloma cell survival and resistance to chemotherapy [89]. In addition to the soluble factors and adhesive pathways mentioned above, ligands normally involved in developmental pathways (Wnt, Jagged/Notch) may also be important [90]. Cell intrinsic features of myeloma, for example chromosomal translocations and oncogenic mutations, may also influence the response of the tumor cell to the micro-environment. For example,

c-Maf overexpressing tumors show elevated levels of integrin beta 7 and enhanced stromal interaction that can promote chemoresistance [91], and MM responses to IGF-1 and APRIL are determined by D-type cyclin grouping and IgH translocation status [31,48]. Identification of biomarkers that could enrich for patients likely to respond to a given therapy is a major goal of current research efforts.

This section will describe in more detail what is known about the biochemical pathways that mediate tumor survival, drug resistance and growth. Although the potential combinations of external factors regulating myeloma cell growth and survival are bewildering in their complexity, a number of core signaling pathways are employed repeatedly by different stimuli. These include the NF-kB, PI3K, RAS and STAT modules. Several of these pathways are also repeatedly targeted by genetic aberrations (eg RAS and NF-kB pathway component mutations), and they may be associated with advanced stages of the disease when there is less dependence on the BM micro-environment. This gives rise to the possibility that targeting such core molecules may be able to enhance current therapies in both early and late phases of disease.

One of the difficulties in evaluating the potential for targeting micro-environmental signaling pathways in myeloma is developing appropriate model systems. Much pre-clinical work relies on myeloma cell lines that have acquired a mutational load that allows them to thrive in the absence of a micro-environment. It should be preferable to study primary tumor cells but these are difficult to maintain *ex - vivo* and it is not a trivial undertaking to devise a model system that is truly representative of the BM milieu in the patient. *In vivo* xenograft model systems can suffer from the lack of activity of murine micro-environmental factors on human cells, although attempts to overcome this by engrafting human bone in mice have been made. In the following section, the major biochemical pathways activated by factors present in the bone marrow milieu will be discussed, with particular emphasis on targeting them for therapy.

NF-kB

NF-kB signaling results in the transcription of a number of genes whose products are predominantly involved in immunity and the inflammatory response [92]. In cancer, NF-kB has been shown to regulate cell proliferation, survival, metastasis and

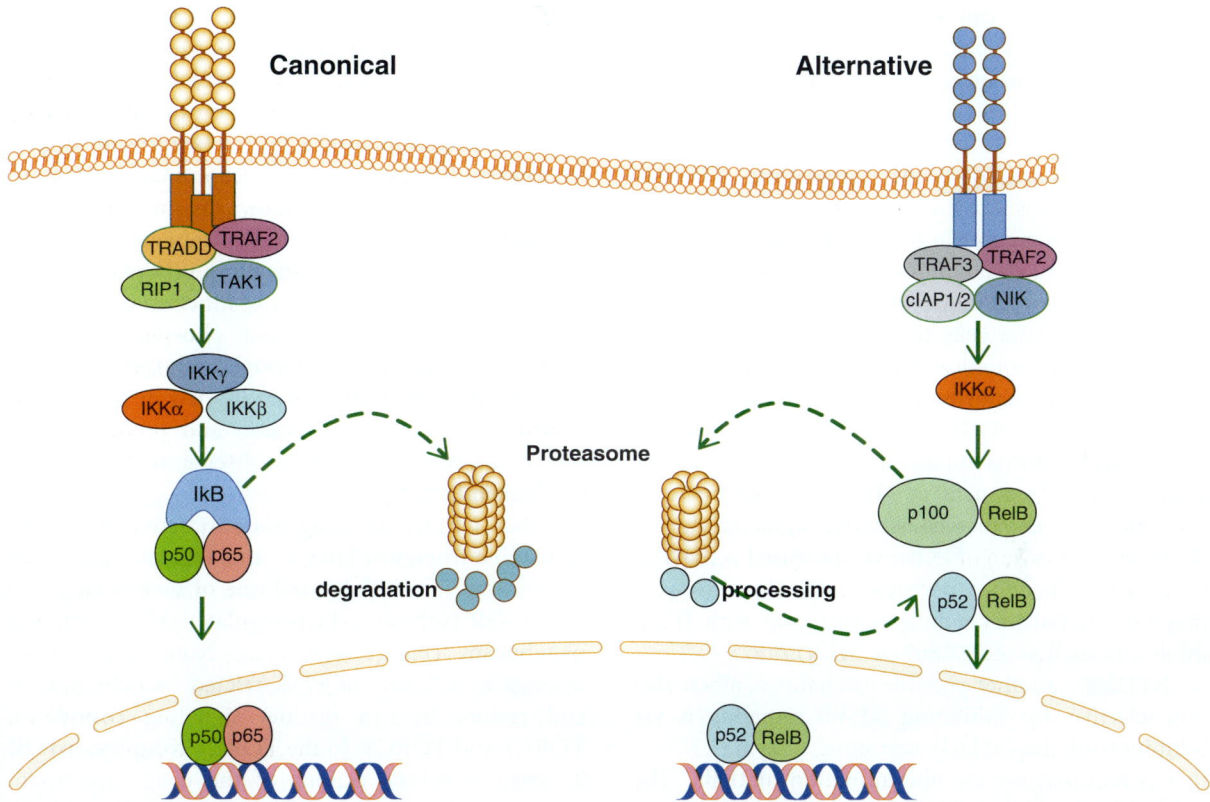

Figure 6.3 NF-kB signaling. The canonical pathway, activated by ligands such as TNF, results in the phosphorylation of IkB proteins by IKKβ leading to their ubiquitination and degradation via the proteasome. This releases p50/p65 complexes to translocate to the nucleus where they regulate gene transcription. The alternative pathway, engaged by ligands such as BAFF, results in the activation of IKKα via the NIK kinase leading to phosphorylation of p100, which undergoes proteolytic processing to generate p52. This translocates to the nucleus in a complex with RelB to activate gene transcription. Abbreviations: TRADD = tumor necrosis factor receptor associated DEATH domain protein; TRAF2 and 3 = TNF receptor-associated factor 2 and 3; TAK1 = TGF-beta activated kinase 1; RIP1 = receptor-interacting protein 1; cIAP1 and 2 = cellular inhibitor of apoptosis 1 and 2.

angiogenesis. NF-kB activation can occur via two routes, the classical (canonical) and alternative (non-canonical) pathways. – In the classical pathway, IkB kinase beta (IKKβ or IKK2), which is present in a complex that includes IKKα and IKKγ, phosphorylates inhibitory IkB proteins leading to their ubiquitination and degradation via the proteasome [93] (Figure 6.3). This releases IkB-associated p50/p65 and p50/c-Rel dimers to translocate to the nucleus and regulate transcription. In the alternative pathway, phosphorylation of p100 by IKKα results in its proteolytic processing and the generation of p52/relB dimers. The NIK kinase predominantly acts in the alternative or non-canonical pathway but can also act as an upstream positive regulator of classical NF-kB signaling. The importance of the NF-kB pathway to myeloma pathophysiology is illustrated by the presence of a variety of genetic abnormalities in

NF-kB pathway components – these include NIK amplification, TRAF3 deletion and inactivation of the negative regulator CYLD [94,95,96].

In addition to myeloma cell-intrinsic abnormalities in NF-kB, a number of components of the BM micro-environment are known to activate NF-kB signaling. Both BAFF and APRIL are potent activators of the non-canonical pathway via activation of NIK and may also activate canonical signaling [97]. Adhesion to fibronectin has been shown to activate NF-kB dependent gene transcription [72]. In addition to effects within the tumor cells, MM cell adhesion to BMSC results in NF-kB activation within the stromal cells, leading to increased transcription and subsequent secretion of cytokines, including IL-6 and BAFF – these feed back to promote myeloma cell growth and survival. NF-kB can upregulate a variety of anti-apoptotic targets including BCL2, BCL-XL and BCL2A1 and can repress pro-apoptotic genes such as BIM. Upregulation of cyclin D1, CDK2 and MYC contribute to increased proliferation [98].

Targeting NF-kB

Proteasomal inhibition – the degradation of inhibitory IkB proteins via the proteasome and resulting NF-kB activation contributed to the rationale of utilizing proteasomal inhibitors to block this pathway. Indeed, proteasomal inhibitors can reduce NF-kB signaling in myeloma cells that is induced via ligands that activate the canonical pathway, such as TNF [99]. However, in the majority of primary samples, constitutive NF-kB activity is resistant to bortezomib and culture with stroma further enhances this resistant activity [100]. Treatment of MM cells with bortezomib may even enhance constitutive signaling due to decreased expression of IKBa, via increased activity of IKKb [101]. Therefore, perhaps counter-intuitively, it may be rational to combine bortezomib with IKKβ inhibitors such as AS602808 or MLN120B.

NEDD8 – another possible mechanism, albeit also non-selective, for inhibiting NF-kB signaling is via inhibition of the NEDD8-activating enzyme (NAE), that is required for the ubiquitination of IKBa. The NAE inhibitor MLN4924 has activity against MM cells in stromal contact [102].

Inhibition of IKKβ – this has the potential to inhibit signaling via the classical pathway and a number of compounds have been developed, including AS602808 and MLN120B. Such compounds can directly inhibit growth and diminish the survival of MM cells and also inhibit canonical signaling in stromal cells, for example decreasing their secretion of the paracrine growth factor IL-6 [103,104]. In MM cells that express high levels of the IGF1 receptor, the combination of IKKb inhibition and an IGF1R monoclonal antibody shows enhanced activity [105]. No selective IKKα inhibitors are reported but combined inhibition of both IKKs via a combination of RNAi and small molecule inhibition, or by the use of dual inhibitors, can overcome the myeloma-protective effect of stroma and enhance the effect of bortezomib [106,107].

PI3K and mTOR

PI3Ks catalyze the phosphorylation of phosphoinositide lipids at the $3'$ position of the inositol ring and contribute to the regulation of various cell functions including proliferation and survival [108,109]. Mammals have eight distinct catalytic isoforms of PI3K, divided into three classes, of which the class I catalytic subunits (p110α, p110β, p110γ and p110δ) produce PIP$_3$, are acutely activated by extracellular stimuli and also signal downstream of Ras; p110a, b and d are predominantly activated by tyrosine kinases whereas p110γ and p110β (predominantly in non-hematopoietic cells), signal downstream of G-protein coupled receptors [111]. PI3K signaling can be enhanced by mutational activation, reported only for p110α (PIK3CA), and by loss of function of the negative regulator PTEN, a lipid phosphatase which dephosphorylates PIP$_3$. Although both these mechanisms for PI3K activation are reported in plasma cell disorders, they are uncommon and predominantly seen in advanced stages of the disease, such as plasma cell leukemia [110].

Class I PI3K signaling leads to activation of the Akt serine/threonine kinase – this regulates a number of downstream modules and one of its key targets is the mTOR pathway, which regulates cell growth and metabolism (Figure 6.4) [111]. Note that mTOR belongs to a family of PI3K-related Ser/Thr kinases and resides in two distinct signaling complexes, TORC1 and TORC2. In the TORC1 complex, mTOR is sensitive to the actions of the drug rapamycin; mTOR is also regulated by other signaling inputs including Ras/MAPK signaling, nutrient and energy levels. Akt also regulates a number of targets known to be important for cell proliferation and survival including GSK3, BAD and the Forkhead family of transcription factors [112].

PI3K is activated by the majority, if not all, of the key BM micro-environmental factors relevant to MM pathophysiology including IGF-1, IL-6, BAFF, APRIL and chemokines [113,114,115,116,117]. PI3K signaling is also activated by integrin binding to a variety of ligands including fibronectin and collagen [118]. In the past few years, a large number of novel therapeutics that target PI3K, Akt and mTOR signaling have been developed, in addition to more established compounds such as Rapamycin and its analogs. These new agents include inhibitors of individual (p110α, p110β or p110δ) or all class 1 PI3K isoforms, steric or ATP-competitive Akt inhibitors and ATP-competitive inhibitors of mTORC1 and TORC2 signaling. In addition, pan-class 1 PI3K inhibitors with dual mTOR kinase inhibitory activity are available [119,120].

Several investigators have shown that targeting PI3K or Akt can induce responses in MM even in the presence of stromal factors. The dual PI3K and

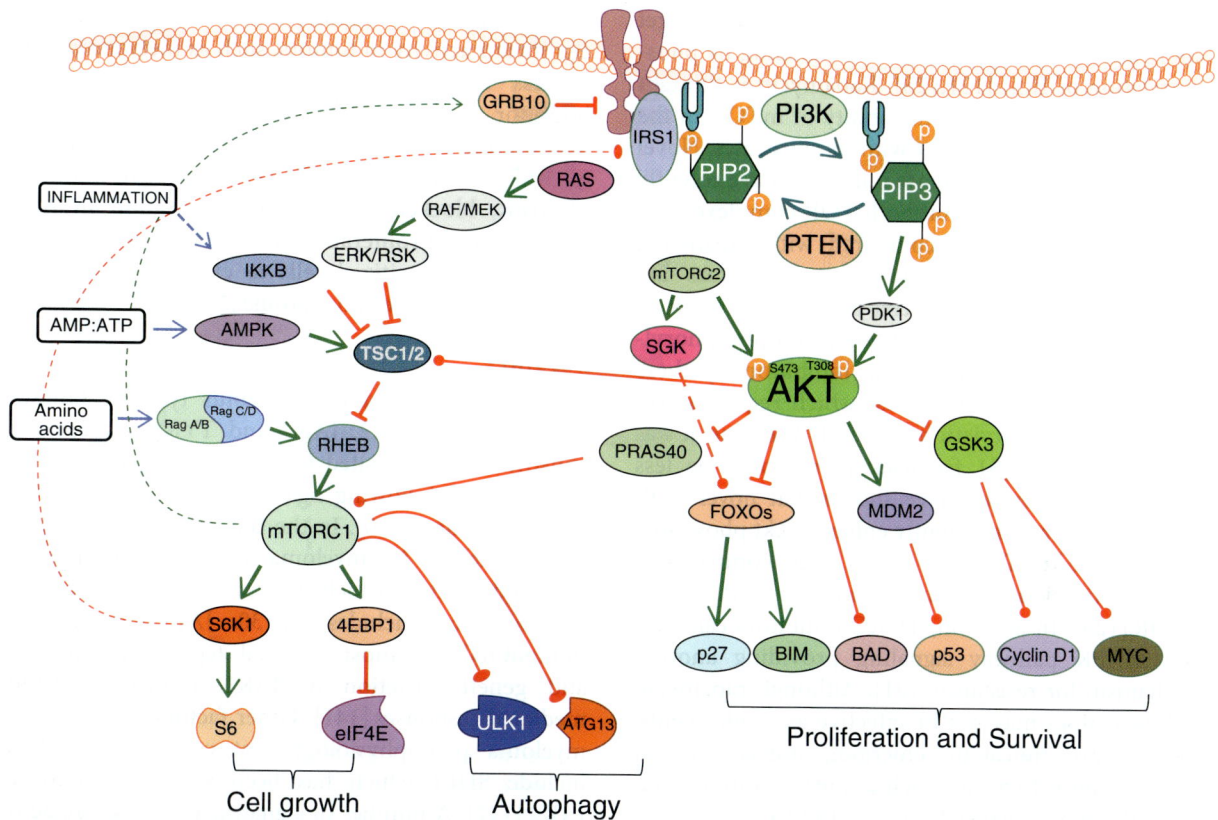

Figure 6.4 PI3-kinase and mTOR signaling. Activation of growth factor receptors by ligand leads to PI3K recruitment and phosphorylation of phosphatidylinositol-4,5-bisphosphate (PIP2) to PIP3, a process that is reversed by PTEN. Subsequent phosphorylation of Akt leads to the regulation of a number of downstream effectors which control cell growth, proliferation and survival. Akt regulates mTOR complex 1 (mTORC1) activation via inhibitory phosphorylation of negative regulators such as TSC2 and PRAS40. However, mTORC1 can also be regulated via input from a number of pathways including those that sense nutrient and energy levels. Note that mTORC1 can negatively regulate PI3K signaling through phosphorylation of IRS1 and GRB10. Abbreviations: GSK3 = glycogen synthase kinase 3; MDM2 = murine double minute 2; FOXO = forkhead box O; PRAS40 = proline-rich Akt substrate, 40 kDa; SGK = serum/glucocorticoid regulated kinase; ERK = extracellular signal-regulated kinase; RSK = ribosomal S6 kinase; TSC1/2 = tuberous sclerosis 1/2; Rheb = Ras homolog enriched in brain; AMPK = 5'-AMP-activated protein kinase; S6K1 = p70 ribosomal S6 kinase; 4EBP1 = eukaryotic translation initiation factor 4E binding protein 1; eIF4E = eukaryotic translation initiation factor 4E; ULK1 = unc-51-like kinase-1; ATG13 = autophagy-related protein 13.

mTOR inhibitor BEZ235 can induce an anti-proliferative response in the majority of myeloma cells. Much work has been carried out using the alklyl-phospholipid perifosine and related compounds [121]. Perifosine can inhibit the phosphorylation and activation of Akt by poorly understood mechanisms. Although its effects are usually attributed to its anti-Akt activity, it is likely that other pathways are also affected. Perifosine induces cytotoxicity in cells adherent to BM stroma and cooperates with MEK inhibitors and more standard anti-myeloma therapies [122]. Several early phase studies with perifosine have been carried out and have shown that the drug is well tolerated and can be combined with lenalidomide and bortezomib based regimens [123,124]. Myeloma

cells showing increased Akt activity are more likely to respond to pathway blockade. We have recently shown that cells from patients with t(4;14) or t(14;16) are more likely to respond to PI3K pathway inhibitors than those with t(11;14) [125]. Strong co-operativity is seen with other anti-myeloma agents, in particular with glucocorticoids.

Although pre-clinical studies have shown that rapamycin can inhibit constitutive or growth factor induced MM cell proliferation [126], this has largely not been borne out in single agent studies of rapamycin analogs such as temsirolimus in relapsed disease [127]. Although rapamycin inhibits mTOR, it has been shown to increase PI3K/Akt signaling in myeloma – this is likely due to the repression of a

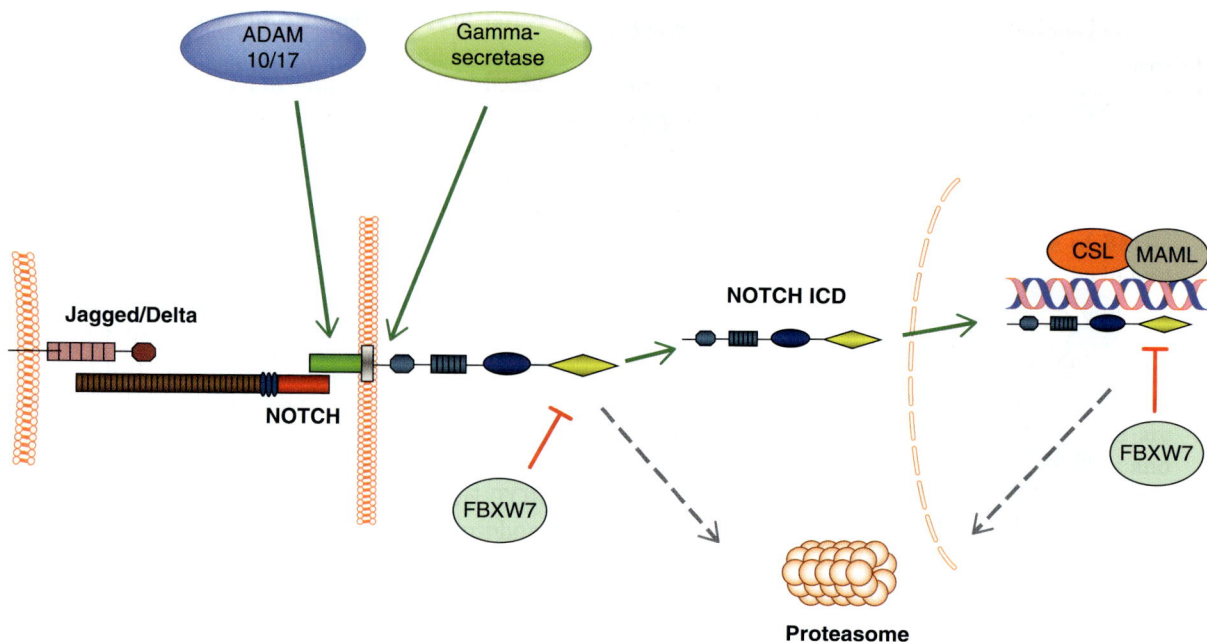

Figure 6.6 Notch signaling. Ligands of the Jagged and Delta families, present as transmembrane proteins on "sending" cells, engage heterodimeric NOTCH receptors on "receiving" cells. NOTCH intracellular domain (ICD) is released by sequential cleavage involving ADAM proteases and gamma-secretase. NOTCH ICD translocates to the nucleus where it interacts with the CSL (CBF-1/RBP-jκ, Su(H), Lag-1) transcription factor in a complex with Mastermind-like proteins (MAML). NOTCH is negatively regulated by proteasomal degradation mediated via F-box and WD repeat domain containing 7 (FBXW7), an E3 ubiquitin protein ligase.

including Jagged and Delta, bind to the Notch extracellular domain – this interaction leads to two successive cleavage events of Notch. Firstly, ligand binding results in a conformational change that exposes a cleavage site for proteases of the ADAM metalloprotease family in the extracellular negative regulatory region of Notch (Figure 6.6). This leads to cleavage and release of the Notch intracellular domain (ICD) by the gamma-secretase complex. The free Notch ICD translocates to the nucleus, associates with the CSL transcription factor, displaces co-repressors and recruits co-activators that include the Mastermind-like protein (MAML). This results in the activation of transcription of target genes.

Myeloma cells express NOTCH receptors which can respond to ligands expressed on stromal and myeloma cells themselves, which frequently express Jagged 2 [158,159]. Interaction of MM cells with BM stroma can lead to activation of Notch signaling [160] – this resulted in growth inhibition (via p21 induction) and protection from the cytotoxic effects of melphalan and mitoxantrone. In contrast, Jagged ligand mediated NOTCH activation has been shown to increase MM cell proliferation and Dll1 mediated

Notch activation results in enhanced proliferation and clonogenic growth. At present, it is not completely clear how much of a role NOTCH signaling from the BM micro-environment plays in MM.

NOTCH signaling can be inhibited by blocking the activity of the gamma-secretase complex. This prevents cleavage and processing of NOTCH to its active form [161]. Several studies have investigated the effects of GSIs in myeloma and have shown activity [162], albeit at high concentrations that may be difficult to sustain *in vivo*, as previous clinical trials have shown marked GI toxicity due to inhibition of NOTCH signaling in intestinal stem and progenitor cells. Other means of targeting NOTCH signaling such as antibodies to NOTCH1 and DLL and peptide inhibitors of transcriptional mediators are also in development.

Targeting multiple signaling pathways

Myeloma cells in the BM micro-environment may have cell-intrinsic activation of cell signaling pathways and be simultaneously influenced by a large variety of extracellular stimuli that activate multiple pathways (e.g. IL6-STAT3, IGF1-PI3K, BAFF-NF-kB, integrin-MAPK). It is probable that inhibition of single pathways would be insufficient to overcome the protective effects of the micro-environment. One possible approach, that has already shown some success, is to target chaperone proteins that regulate multiple clients. Heat shock protein 90 (Hsp90) is known to be involved in protein folding, assembly and maintenance of conformational stability for a number of client molecules including Akt and RAF [163]. Geldanamycin and its analog 17-AAG have been shown to be effective in pre-clinical studies and in early trials and a number of novel Hsp90

inhibitors with better pharmacological profiles are in development.

A number of studies across tumor types have shown that dual inhibition of the MEK/ERK MAPK module and of the PI3K/Akt/mTOR pathway results in synergistic responses [164]. Both pathways converge on regulation of a number of proteins including the pro-apoptotic BIM, which is regulated transcriptionally by a PI3K/Akt/FOXO pathway and post-translationally by MAPK-controled proteasomal degradation. [165] A number of clinical trials are underway in solid tumors using this combination and full results for tolerability are awaited.

References

1. Barillé, S., Akhoundi, C., Collette, M. et al. Metalloproteinases in multiple myeloma: production of matrix metalloproteinase-9 (MMP-9), activation of proMMP-2, and induction of MMP-1 by myeloma cells. *Blood* 1997;**90**(4):1649–55.

2. Vande Broek, I., Asosingh, K., Allegaert, V. et al. Bone marrow endothelial cells increase the invasiveness of human multiple myeloma cells through upregulation of MMP-9: evidence for a role of hepatocyte growth factor. *Leukemia* 2004; **18**(5):976–82.

3. Menu, E., Asosingh, K., Indraccolo, S. et al. The involvement of stromal derived Factor 1alpha in homing and progression of multiple myeloma in the STMM model. *Haematologica* 2006;**91**:605–12.

4. Vanderkerken, K. et al. Monocyte chemoattractant protein-1 (MCP-1), secreted by bone marrow endothelial cells, induces chemoattraction of 5TMM cells. *Clin. Exp. Metastasis* 2002; **19**:87–90.

5. Alsayed, Y., Ngo, H., Runnels, J. et al. Mechanisms of regulation of CXCR4/SDF-1 (CXCL12)-dependent migration and homing in multiple myeloma. *Blood* 2007;**109**(7):2708–17.

6. Sanz-Rodriguez, F., Hidalgo, A., Teixido, J. Chemokine stromal cell-derived factor-1α modulates VLA-4 integrin-mediated multiple myeloma cell adhesion to CS-1/fibronectin and VCAM-1. *Blood* 2001;**97**:346–51.

7. Diamond, P., Labrinidis, A., Martin, S. K. et al. Targeted disruption of the CXCL12/CXCR4 axis inhibits osteolysis in a murine model of myeloma-associated bone loss. *J. Bone Miner. Res.* 2009;**24**:1150–61.

8. Azab, A. K., Runnels, J. M., Pitsillides, C. et al. CXCR4 inhibitor AMD3100 disrupts the interaction of multiple myeloma cells with the bone marrow microenvironment and enhances their sensitivity to therapy. *Blood* 2009;**113**(18):4341–5.

9. O'Callaghan, K., Lee, L., Nguyer, N. et al. Targeting CXCR4 with cell-penetrating pepducins in lymphoma and lymphocytic leukemia *Blood* 2012; **119**:1717–25.

10. Asosingh, K. et al. In vivo induction of insulin-like growth factor-I receptor and CD44v6 confers homing and adhesion to murine multiple myeloma cells. *Cancer Res.* 2000;**60**:3096–104.

11. Tai, Y. T. et al, Insulin-like growth factor-1 induces adhesion and migration in human multiple myeloma cells via activation of

beta1-integrin and phosphatidylinositol 3′-kinase/AKT signaling. *Cancer Res.* 2003;**63**:5850–8 (Erratum: *Cancer Res.* 2003;63:7543).

12. Asosingh, K., Günthert, U., De Raeve, H. et al. A unique pathway in the homing of murine multiple myeloma cells: CD44v10 mediates binding to bone marrow endothelium. *Cancer Res.* 2001;**61**(7):2862–5.

13. Van Valckenborgh, E., Matsui, W., Agarwal, P. et al. Tumor-initiating capacity of CD138- and CD138+ tumor cells in the 5T33 multiple myeloma model. *Leukemia* 2012;**26**:1436–9.

14. Van Driel, M. et al. CD44 variant isoforms are involved in plasma cell adhesion to bone marrow stromal cells. *Leukemia* 2002;**16**:135–43.

15. Neri, P., Ren, L., Azab, A. K. et al. Integrin-β7 mediated regulation of multiple myeloma cell adhesion, migration, and invasion. *Blood* 2011;**117**(23):6202–13.

16. Groen, R. W. J., de Rooij, M. F. M., Kocemba, K. A. et al. N-cadherin-mediated interaction with multiple myeloma cells inhibits osteoblast differentiation. *Haematologica* 2011; **96**(11):1653–61.

17. Azab, A. K., Quang, P., Azab, F. et al. P-selectin glycoprotein ligand regulates the interaction of

multiple myeloma cells with the bone marrow microenvironment. *Blood* 2012;**119**(6):1468–78.

18. Zlei, M., Egert, S., Wider, D. *et al.* Characterization of in vitro growth of multiple myeloma cells. *Experimental Hematol.* 2007;**35**[10]:1550–61. (Abstract.)

19. Katz, B. Z. Adhesion molecules. The lifelines of multiple myeloma cells. *Seminars in Cancer Biology* 2010;**20**(3):186–95.

20. Klein, B., Zhang, X. G., Lu, Z. Y., Bataille, R. Interleukin-6 in human multiple myeloma. *Blood* 1995 Feb 15;**85**(4):863–72.

21. Zhang, X. G., Gaillard, J. P., Robillard, N. *et al.* Reproducible obtaining of human myeloma cell lines as a model for tumor stem cell study in human multiple myeloma. *Blood* 1994; **83**(12):3654–6.

22. Hilbert, D. M., Kopf, M., Mock, B. A., Kuhler, G., Rudikoff, S. Interleukin 6 is essential for in vivo development of B lineage neoplasms. *J. Experimental Med.* 1995;**182**(1):243–8.

23. Mahtouk, K., Moreaux, J., Hose, D. *et al.* Growth factors in multiple myeloma: a comprehensive analysis of their expression in tumor cells and bone marrow environment using Affymetrix microarrays. *BMC Cancer* 2010;**10**:198.

24. Hardin, J., MacLeod, S., Grigorieva, I. *et al.* Interleukin-6 prevents dexamethasone-induced myeloma cell death. *Blood* 1994; **84**(9):3063–7.

25. Shain, K. H., Yarde, D. N., Meads, M. B. *et al.* Integrin adhesion enhances IL-6 mediated STAT3 signaling in myeloma cells: implications for microenvironment influence on tumor survival and proliferation. *Cancer Research* 2009; **69**(3):1009–15.

26. Bataille, R., Jourdan, M., Zhang, X. G., Klein, B. Serum levels of

interleukin-6, a potent myeloma cell growth factor, as a reflect of disease severity in plasma cell dyscrasias. *J. Clin. Invest.* 1989;**84**:2008–11.

27. Klein, B., Wijdenes, J., Zhang, X. G. *et al.* Murine anti-interleukin-6 monoclonal antibody therapy for a patient with plasma cell leukemia. *Blood* 1991;**78**:1198–204.

28. Trikha, M., Corringham, R., Klein, B., Rossi, J. F. Targeted anti-interleukin-6 monoclonal antibody therapy for cancer. *Clinical Cancer Research* 2003; **9**(13):4653–65.

29. Hunsucker, S. A., Magarotto, V., Kuhn, D. J. *et al.* Blockade of interleukin-6 signalling with siltuximab enhances melphalan cytotoxicity in preclinical models of multiple myeloma. *Br. J. Haematol.* 2011;**152**(5):579–92.

30. Condomines, M., Veyrune, J. L., Larroque, M. *et al.* Increased plasma-immune cytokines throughout the high-dose melphalan-induced lymphodepletion in patients with multiple myeloma: a window for adoptive immunotherapy. *J. Immunol.* 2010;**184**(2):1079–84.

31. Sprynski, A. C., Hose, D., Caillot, L. *et al.* The role of IGF-1 as a major growth factor for myeloma cell lines and the prognostic relevance of the expression of its receptor. *Blood* 2009;**113**(19):4614–26.

32. Glassford, J., Rabin, N., Lam, E. W., Yong, K. L. Functional regulation of D-type cyclins by insulin-like growth factor-I and serum in multiple myeloma cells. *Br. J. Haematol.* 2007; **139**(2):243–54.

33. Xu, F., Gardner, A., Tu, Y. *et al.* Multiple myeloma cells are protected against dexamethasone-induced apoptosis by insulin-like growth factors. *Br. J. Haematol.* 1997;**97**(2):429–40.

34. Abroun, S., Ishikawa, H., Tsuyama, N. *et al.* Receptor

synergy of interleukin-6 (IL-6) and insulin-like growth factor-I in myeloma cells that highly express IL-6 receptor. *Blood* 2004; **103**(6):2291–8.

35. Standal, T., Borset, M., Lenhoff, S. *et al.* Serum insulin-like growth factor is not elevated in patients with multiple myeloma but is still a prognostic factor. *Blood* 2002;**100**(12): 3925–9.

36. Mitsiades, C. S., Mitsiades, N. S., McMullan, C. J. *et al.* Inhibition of the insulin-like growth factor receptor-1 tyrosine kinase activity as a therapeutic strategy for multiple myeloma, other hematologic malignancies, and solid tumors. *Cancer Cell* 2004; **5**(3):221–30.

37. Roosnek, E., Burjanadze, M., Dietrich, P. Y. *et al.* Tumors that look for their springtime in APRIL. *Crit. Rev. Oncol./Hematol.* 2009;**72**(2):91–7.

38. Rickert, R. C., Jellusova, J., Miletic, A. V. Signaling by the tumor necrosis factor receptor superfamily in B-cell biology and disease. *Immunol. Rev.* 2011; **244**(1):115–33.

39. Castigli, E., Scott, S., Dedeoglu, F. *et al.* Impaired IgA class switching in APRIL-deficient mice. *Proc. Natl. Acad. Sci. USA* 2004; **101**(11):3903–8.

40. Planelles, L., Carvalho-Pinto, C. E., Hardenberg, G. *et al.* APRIL promotes B-1 cell-associated neoplasm. *Cancer Cell* 2004; **6**[4]:399–408.

41. Belnoue, E., Pihlgren, M., McGaha, T. L. *et al.* APRIL is critical for plasmablast survival in the bone marrow and is poorly expressed by early life bone marrow stromal cells. *Blood* 2008;**111**(5):2755–64.

42. Bossen, C., Schneider, P. BAFF, APRIL and their receptors: structure, function and signaling. *Semin. Immunol.* 2006; **18**(5):263–75.

43. Moreaux, J., Legouffe, E., Jourdan, E. *et al*. BAFF and APRIL protect myeloma cells from apoptosis induced by interleukin 6 deprivation and dexamethasone. *Blood* 2004;**103**(8):3148–57.

44. Novak, A. J., Darce, J. R., Arendt, B. K. *et al*. Expression of BCMA, TACI, and BAFF-R in multiple myeloma: a mechanism for growth and survival. *Blood* 2004;**103**(2):689–94.

45. Moreaux, J., Sprynski, A. C., Dillon, S. R. *et al*. APRIL and TACI interact with syndecan-1 on the surface of multiple myeloma cells to form an essential survival loop. *Eur. J. Haematol.* 2009; **83**(2):119–29.

46. Matthes, T., Dunand-Sauthier, I., Santiago-Raber, M. L. *et al*. Production of the plasma-cell survival factor a proliferation-inducing ligand (APRIL) peaks in myeloid precursor cells from human bone marrow. *Blood* 2011;**118**(7):1838–44.

47. Quinn, J., Glassford, J., Percy, L. *et al*. APRIL promotes cell-cycle progression in primary multiple myeloma cells: influence of D-type cyclin group and translocation status. *Blood* 2011;**117**:890–901.

48. Moreaux, J., Cremer, F. W., Reme, T. *et al*. The level of TACI gene expression in myeloma cells is associated with a signature of microenvironment dependence versus a plasmablastic signature. *Blood* 2005;**106**(3):1021–30.

49. Yaccoby, S., Pennisi, A., Li, X. *et al*. Atacicept (TACI-Ig) inhibits growth of TACI high primary myeloma cells in SCID-hu mice and in coculture with osteoclasts. *Leukemia* 2007;**22**(2):406–13.

50. Kukreja, A., Hutchinson, A., Dhodapkar, K. *et al*. Enhancement of clonogenicity of human multiple myeloma by dendritic cells. *J. Exp. Med.* 2006; **203**(8):1859–65.

51. Rossi, J. F., Moreaux, J., Hose, D. *et al*. Atacicept in relapsed/ refractory multiple myeloma or active Waldenström's macroglobulinemia: a phase I study. *Br. J. Cancer* 2009; **101**(7):1051–8.

52. Guadagnoli, M., Kimberley, F. C., Phan, U. *et al*. Development and characterization of APRIL antagonistic monoclonal antibodies for treatment of B-cell lymphomas. *Blood* 2011; **117**(25):6856–65.

53. Hose, D., Moreaux, J., Meissner, T. *et al*. Induction of angiogenesis by normal and malignant plasma cells. *Blood* 2009;**114**(1):128–43.

54. Iwasaki, T., Sano, H. Predicting treatment responses and disease progression in myeloma using serum vascular endothelial growth factor and hepatocyte growth factor levels. *Leuk. Lymphoma* 2003;**44**(8):1275–9.

55. Vacca, A., Ribatti, D., Roncali, L. *et al*. Bone marrow angiogenesis and progression in multiple myeloma. *Br. J. Haematol.* 1994;**87**(3):503–8.

56. Gupta, D., Treon, S. P., Shima, Y. *et al*. Adherence of multiple myeloma cells to bone marrow stromal cells upregulates vascular endothelial growth factor secretion: therapeutic applications. *Leukemia* 2001; **15**(12):1950–6.

57. Dankbar, B., Padró, T., Leo, R. *et al*. Vascular endothelial growth factor and interleukin-6 in paracrine tumor–stromal cell interactions in multiple myeloma. *Blood* 2000;**95**(8):2630–6.

58. Le Gouill, S., Podar, K., Amiot, M. *et al*. VEGF induces Mcl-1 up-regulation and protects multiple myeloma cells against apoptosis. *Blood* 2004;**104**(9):2886–92.

59. Borset, M., Hjorth-Hansen, H., Seidel, C., Sundan, A., Waage, A. Hepatocyte growth factor and its receptor c-met in multiple myeloma. *Blood* 1996; **88**(10):3998–4004.

60. The Nordic Myeloma Study Group. Seidel, C., Børset, M., Turesson, I. *et al*. Elevated serum concentrations of hepatocyte growth factor in patients with multiple myeloma. *Blood* 1998; **91**(3):806–12.

61. Hov, H., Tian, E., Holien, T. *et al*. c-Met signaling promotes IL-6-induced myeloma cell proliferation. *Eur. J. Haematol.* 2009;**82**(4):277–87.

62. Seidel, C., Børset, M., Hjertner, O. *et al*. High levels of soluble syndecan-1 in myeloma-derived bone marrow: modulation of hepatocyte growth factor activity. *Blood* 2000;**96**(9):3139–46.

63. Klein, B., Seckinger, A., Moehler, T., Hose, D. Molecular pathogenesis of multiple myeloma: chromosomal aberrations, changes in gene expression, cytokine networks, and the bone marrow microenvironment. *Recent Results Cancer Res.* 2011;**183**:39–86.

64. Pellat-Deceunynck, C., Barille, S., Puthier, D. *et al*. Adhesion molecules on human myeloma cells: significant changes in expression related to malignancy, tumor spreading, and immortalization. *Cancer Res.* 1995;**55**(16):3647–53.

65. Noborio-Hatano, K., Kikuchi, J., Takatoku, M. *et al*. Bortezomib overcomes cell-adhesion-mediated drug resistance through downregulation of VLA-4 expression in multiple myeloma. *Oncogene* 2009;**28**(2):231–42.

66. Damiano, J. S., Cress, A. E., Hazlehurst, L. A., Shtil, A. A., Dalton, W. S. Cell adhesion mediated drug resistance (CAM-DR): role of integrins and resistance to apoptosis in human myeloma cell lines. *Blood* 1999; **93**(5):1658–67.

67. Hazlehurst, L. A., Damiano, J. S., Buyuksal, I., Pledger, W. J., Dalton, W. S. Adhesion to fibronectin via beta1 integrins

regulates p27kip1 levels and contributes to cell adhesion mediated drug resistance (CAM-DR). *Oncogene* 2000;**19** (38):4319–27.

68. Shain, K. H., Yarde, D. N., Meads, M. B. *et al.* Integrin adhesion enhances IL-6 mediated STAT3 signaling in myeloma cells: implications for microenvironment influence on tumor survival and proliferation. *Cancer Research* 2009;**69**(3):1009–15.

69. Abe, M. Targeting the interplay between myeloma cells and the bone marrow microenvironment in myeloma. *Int. J. Hematol.* 2011;**94**(4):334–43.

70. Perez, L. E., Parquet, N., Meads, M., Anasetti, C., Dalton, W. Bortezomib restores stroma-mediated APO2L/TRAIL apoptosis resistance in multiple myeloma. *Eur. J. Haematol.* 2010;**84**(3):212–22.

71. Landowski, T. H., Olashaw, N. E., Agrawal, D., Dalton, W. S. Cell adhesion-mediated drug resistance (CAM-DR) is associated with activation of NF-kappaB (RelB/p50) in myeloma cells. *Oncogene* 2003; **22**(16):2417–21.

72. Dalton, W. S. The tumor microenvironment: focus on myeloma. *Cancer Treatment Rev.* 2003;**29**(Suppl. 1):11–19.

73. Zlei, M., Egert, S., Wider, D. *et al.* Characterization of in vitro growth of multiple myeloma cells. *Exp. Hematol.* 2007;**35**[10]: 1550–61.

74. Bataille, R., Chappard, D., Marcelli, C. *et al.* Recruitment of new osteoblasts and osteoclasts is the earliest critical event in the pathogenesis of human multiple myeloma. *J. Clin. Invest.* 1991; **88**(1):62–6.

75. Aubin, J. E. Regulation of osteoblast formation and function. *Rev. Endocr. Metab. Disord.* 2001;**2**:81094.

76. Corre, J., Mahtouk, K., Attal, M. *et al.* Bone marrow mesenchymal stem cells are abnormal in multiple myeloma. *Leukemia* 2007;**21**:1079–88.

77. Garderet, L., Mazurier, C., Chapel, A. *et al.* Mesenchymal stem cell abnormalities in patients with multiple myeloma. *Leuk. Lymphoma* 2007;**48**:2032–41.

78. Todoerti, K., Lisignoli, G., Storti, P. *et al.* Distinct transcriptional profiles characterize bone microenvironment mesenchymal cells rather than osteoblasts in relationship with multiple myeloma bone disease. *Exp. Hematol.* 2010;**38**(2): 141–53.

79. Yaccoby, S., Wezeman, M. J., Zangari, M. *et al.* Inhibitory effects of osteoblasts and increased bone formation on myeloma in novel culture systems and a myelomatous mouse model. *Haematologica* 2006;**91**(2):192–9.

80. Reagan, M. R., Ghobrial, I. M. Multiple myeloma mesenchymal stem cells: characterization, origin, and tumor-promoting effects. *Clinical Cancer Research* 2012;**18**(2):342–9.

81. Li, X., Ling, W., Khan, S., Yaccoby, S. Therapeutic effects of intrabone and systemic mesenchymal stem cell cytotherapy on myeloma bone disease and tumour growth. *J. Bone Mineral. Res.* 2012;**27**:1635.

82. Yaccoby, S., Wezeman, M. J., Henderson, A. *et al.* Cancer and the microenvironment: myeloma-osteoclast interactions as a model. *Cancer Res.* 2004;**64**(6):2016–20.

83. Moreaux, J., Hose, D., Kassambara, A. *et al.* Osteoclast-gene expression profiling reveals osteoclast-derived CCR2 chemokines promoting myeloma cell migration. *Blood* 2011; **117**(4):1280–90.

84. Chauhan, D., Singh, A. V., Brahmandam, M. *et al.* Functional interaction of plasmacytoid dendritic cells with multiple myeloma cells: a therapeutic target. *Cancer Cell* 2009; **16**(4):309–23.

85. Zheng, Y., Cai, Z., Wang, S. *et al.* Macrophages are an abundant component of myeloma microenvironment and protect myeloma cells from chemotherapy drug-induced apoptosis. *Blood* 2009; **114**(17):3625–8.

86. Martin, S. K., Diamond, P., Williams, S. A. *et al.* Hypoxia-inducible factor-2 is a novel regulator of aberrant CXCL12 expression in multiple myeloma plasma cells. *Haematologica* 2010;**95**:776–84.

87. Giatromanolaki, A., Bai, M., Margaritis, D. *et al.* Hypoxia and activated VEGF/ receptor pathway in multiple myeloma. *Anticancer Res.* 2010;**30**:2831–6.

88. Iriuchishima, H., Takubo, K., Miyakawa, Y. *et al.* Neovascular niche for human myeloma cells in immunodeficient mouse bone. *PloS One* 2012;**7**(2):e30557.

89. Shain, K. H., Dalton, W. S. Environmental-mediated drug resistance: a target for multiple myeloma therapy. *Expert. Rev. Hematol.* 2009;**2**(6):649–62.

90. Grivennikov, S. I., Greten, F. R., Karin, M. Immunity, inflammation, and cancer. *Cell* 2010;**140**(6):883–99.

91. Hurt, E. M., Wiestner, A., Rosenwald, A. *et al.* Overexpression of c-maf is a frequent oncogenic event in multiple myeloma that promotes proliferation and pathological interactions with bone marrow stroma. *Cancer Cell* 2004; **5**(2):191–9.

92. DiDonato, J. A., Mercurio, F., Karin, M. NF-kappaB and the link between inflammation and cancer. *Immunol. Rev.* 2012; **246**(1):379–400.

93. Rickert, R. C., Jellusova, J., Miletic, A. V. Signaling by the tumor necrosis factor receptor superfamily in B-cell biology and disease. *Immunol. Rev.* 2011; **244**(1):115–33.

94. Keats, J. J., Fonseca, R., Chesi, M. *et al.* Promiscuous mutations activate the noncanonical NF-kappaB pathway in multiple myeloma. *Cancer Cell* 2007; **12**(2):131–44.

95. Annunziata, C. M., Davis, R. E., Demchenko, Y. *et al.* Frequent engagement of the classical and alternative NF-kappaB pathways by diverse genetic abnormalities in multiple myeloma. *Cancer Cell* 2007;**12**(2):115–30.

96. Chapman, M. A., Lawrence, M. S., Keats, J. J. *et al.* Initial genome sequencing and analysis of multiple myeloma. *Nature* 2011;**471**(7339):467–72.

97. Endo, T., Nishio, M., Enzler, T. *et al.* BAFF and APRIL support chronic lymphocytic leukemia B-cell survival through activation of the canonical NF-kappaB pathway. *Blood* 2007;**109**(2):703–10.

98. Baud, V., Karin, M. Is NF-kappaB a good target for cancer therapy? Hopes and pitfalls. *Nat. Rev. Drug Discov.* 2009;**8**(1):33–40.

99. Hideshima, T., Chauhan, D., Schlossman, R., Richardson, P., Anderson, K. C. The role of tumor necrosis factor alpha in the pathophysiology of human multiple myeloma: therapeutic applications. *Oncogene* 2001; **20**(33):4519–27.

100. Markovina, S., Callander, N. S., O'Connor, S. L. *et al.* Bortezomib-resistant nuclear factor-kappaB activity in multiple myeloma cells. *Mol. Cancer Res.* 2008;**6**(8): 1356–64.

101. Hideshima, T., Ikeda, H., Chauhan, D. *et al.* Bortezomib induces canonical nuclear factor-kappaB activation in multiple myeloma cells. *Blood* 2009;**114** (5):1046–52.

102. McMillin, D. W., Jacobs, H. M., Delmore, J. E. *et al.* Molecular and cellular effects of NEDD8-activating enzyme inhibition in myeloma. *Mol. Cancer Ther.* 2012;**11**(4):942–51.

103. Romagnoli, M., Desplanques, G., Maiga, S. *et al.* Canonical nuclear factor kappaB pathway inhibition blocks myeloma cell growth and induces apoptosis in strong synergy with TRAIL. *Clin. Cancer Res.* 2007;**13**(20): 6010–18.

104. Hideshima, T., Neri, P., Tassone, P. *et al.* MLN120B, a novel IkappaB kinase beta inhibitor, blocks multiple myeloma cell growth in vitro and in vivo. *Clin. Cancer Res.* 2006;**12**(19):5887–94.

105. Tagoug, I., Sauty De Chalon, A., Dumontet, C. Inhibition of IGF-1 signalling enhances the apoptotic effect of AS602868, an IKK2 inhibitor, in multiple myeloma cell lines. *PLoS One* 2011;**6**(7): e22641.

106. Fabre, C., Mimura, N., Bobb, K. *et al.* Dual inhibition of canonical and non-canonical NF-kappaB pathways demonstrates significant anti-tumor activities in multiple myeloma. *Clin. Cancer Res.* 2012; **18**(17): 4669–81.

107. Hideshima, T., Chauhan, D., Kiziltepe, T. *et al.* Biologic sequelae of I{kappa}B kinase (IKK) inhibition in multiple myeloma: therapeutic implications. *Blood* 2009; **113**(21):5228–36.

108. Khwaja, A. PI3K as a target for therapy in haematological malignancies. *Curr. Top. Microbiol. Immunol.* 2010;**347**:169–88.

109. Vanhaesebroeck, B., Stephens, L., Hawkins, P. PI3K signalling: the path to discovery and understanding. *Nat. Rev. Mol. Cell Biol.* 2012;**13**(3):195–203.

110. Tiedemann, R. E., Gonzalez-Paz, N., Kyle, R. A. *et al.* Genetic aberrations and survival in plasma cell leukemia. *Leukemia* 2008; **22**(5):1044–52.

111. Laplante, M., Sabatini, D. M. mTOR signaling in growth control and disease. *Cell* 2012; **149**(2):274–93.

112. Manning, B. D., Cantley, L. C. AKT/PKB signaling: navigating downstream. *Cell* 2007; **129**(7):1261–74.

113. Tai, Y. T., Podar, K., Mitsiades, N. *et al.* CD40 induces human multiple myeloma cell migration via phosphatidylinositol 3-kinase/AKT/NF-kappa B signaling. *Blood* 2003;**101**(7):2762–9.

114. Mitsiades, C. S., Mitsiades, N., Poulaki, V. *et al.* Activation of NF-kappaB and upregulation of intracellular anti-apoptotic proteins via the IGF-1/Akt signaling in human multiple myeloma cells: therapeutic implications. *Oncogene* 2002; **21**(37):5673–83.

115. Hideshima, T., Nakamura, N., Chauhan, D., Anderson, K. C. Biologic sequelae of interleukin-6 induced PI3-K/Akt signaling in multiple myeloma. *Oncogene* 2001;**20**(42):5991–6000.

116. Moreaux, J., Legouffe, E., Jourdan, E. *et al.* BAFF and APRIL protect myeloma cells from apoptosis induced by interleukin 6 deprivation and dexamethasone. *Blood* 2004;**103**(8):3148–57.

117. Ge, N. L., Rudikoff, S. Insulin-like growth factor I is a dual effector of multiple myeloma cell growth. *Blood* 2000;**96**(8):2856–61.

118. Khwaja, A., Rodriguez-Viciana, P., Wennstrom, S., Warne, P. H., Downward, J. Matrix adhesion and Ras transformation both activate a phosphoinositide 3-OH kinase and protein kinase B/Akt cellular survival pathway. *EMBO J.* 1997;**16**(10):2783–93.

119. McNamara, C. R., Degterev, A. Small-molecule inhibitors of the PI3K signaling network. *Future Med. Chem.* 2011;**3**(5):549–65.

81

120. Willems, L., Tamburini, J., Chapuis, N. *et al.* PI3K and mTOR signaling pathways in cancer: new data on targeted therapies. *Curr. Oncol. Rep.* 2012;**14**(2):129–38.

121. Richardson, P. G., Eng, C., Kolesar, J., Hideshima, T., Anderson, K. C. Perifosine, an oral, anti-cancer agent and inhibitor of the Akt pathway: mechanistic actions, pharmacodynamics, pharmacokinetics, and clinical activity. *Expert Opin. Drug Metab. Toxicol.* 2012;**8**(5):623–33.

122. Hideshima, T., Catley, L., Yasui, H. *et al.* Perifosine, an oral bioactive novel alkylphospholipid, inhibits Akt and induces in vitro and in vivo cytotoxicity in human multiple myeloma cells. *Blood* 2006;**107**(10):4053–62.

123. Jakubowiak, A. J., Richardson, P. G., Zimmerman, T. *et al.* Perifosine plus lenalidomide and dexamethasone in relapsed and relapsed/refractory multiple myeloma: a Phase I Multiple Myeloma Research Consortium study. *Br. J. Haematol.* 2012; **158**(4):472–80.

124. Richardson, P. G., Wolf, J., Jakubowiak, A. *et al.* Perifosine plus bortezomib and dexamethasone in patients with relapsed/refractory multiple myeloma previously treated with bortezomib: results of a multicenter phase I/II trial. *J. Clin. Oncol.* 2011;**29**(32):4243–9.

125. Stengel, C., Cheung, C. W., Quinn, J., Yong, K., Khwaja, A. Optimal induction of myeloma cell death requires dual blockade of phosphoinositide 3-kinase and mTOR signalling and is determined by translocation subtype. *Leukemia* 2012 (epub Mar 14).

126. Frost, P., Moatamed, F., Hoang, B. *et al.* In vivo antitumor effects of the mTOR inhibitor CCI-779 against human multiple myeloma cells in a xenograft model. *Blood* 2004;**104**(13):4181–7.

127. Farag, S. S., Zhang, S., Jansak, B. S. *et al.* Phase II trial of temsirolimus in patients with relapsed or refractory multiple myeloma. *Leuk. Res.* 2009;**33**(11):1475–80.

128. Shi, Y., Yan, H., Frost, P., Gera, J., Lichtenstein, A. Mammalian target of rapamycin inhibitors activate the AKT kinase in multiple myeloma cells by up-regulating the insulin-like growth factor receptor/insulin receptor substrate-1/phosphatidylinositol 3-kinase cascade. *Mol. Cancer Ther.* 2005;**4**(10):1533–40.

129. Hoang, B., Frost, P., Shi, Y. *et al.* Targeting TORC2 in multiple myeloma with a new mTOR kinase inhibitor. *Blood* 2010; **116**(22):4560–8.

130. Maiso, P., Liu, Y., Morgan, B. *et al.* Defining the role of TORC1/2 in multiple myeloma. *Blood* 2011;**118**(26):6860–70.

131. Hoang, B., Benavides, A., Shi, Y. *et al.* The PP242 mammalian target of rapamycin (mTOR) inhibitor activates extracellular signal-regulated kinase (ERK) in multiple myeloma cells via a target of rapamycin complex 1 (TORC1)/ eukaryotic translation initiation factor 4E (eIF-4E)/RAF pathway and activation is a mechanism of resistance. *J. Biol. Chem.* 2012;**287**(26):21 796–805.

132. Ghobrial, I. M., Weller, E., Vij, R. *et al.* Weekly bortezomib in combination with temsirolimus in relapsed or relapsed and refractory multiple myeloma: a multicentre, phase 1/2, open-label, dose-escalation study. *Lancet Oncol.* 2011;**12**(3):263–72.

133. Hofmeister, C. C., Yang, X., Pichiorri, F. *et al.* Phase I trial of lenalidomide and CCI-779 in patients with relapsed multiple myeloma: evidence for lenalidomide-CCI-779 interaction via P-glycoprotein. *J. Clin. Oncol.* 2011;**29**(25):3427–34.

134. Steinbrunn, T., Stuhmer, T., Gattenlohner, S. *et al.* Mutated RAS and constitutively activated Akt delineate distinct oncogenic pathways, which independently contribute to multiple myeloma cell survival. *Blood* 2011; **117**(6):1998–2004.

135. Lentzsch, S., Chatterjee, M., Gries, M. *et al.* PI3-K/AKT/FKHR and MAPK signaling cascades are redundantly stimulated by a variety of cytokines and contribute independently to proliferation and survival of multiple myeloma cells. *Leukemia* 2004;**18**(11):1883–90.

136. Sousa, S. F., Fernandes, P. A., Ramos, M. J. Farnesyltransferase inhibitors: a detailed chemical view on an elusive biological problem. *Curr. Med. Chem.* 2008;**15**(15):1478–92.

137. Yauch, R. L., Settleman, J. Recent advances in pathway-targeted cancer drug therapies emerging from cancer genome analysis. *Curr. Opin. Genet. Dev.* 2012; **22**(1):45–9.

138. Ramakrishnan, V., Timm, M., Haug, J. L. *et al.* Sorafenib, a dual Raf kinase/vascular endothelial growth factor receptor inhibitor has significant anti-myeloma activity and synergizes with common anti-myeloma drugs. *Oncogene* 2010;**29**(8):1190–202.

139. Tai, Y. T., Fulciniti, M., Hideshima, T. *et al.* Targeting MEK induces myeloma-cell cytotoxicity and inhibits osteoclastogenesis. *Blood* 2007;**110**(5):1656–63.

140. Kontzias, A., Kotlyar, A., Laurence, A., Changelian, P., O'shea, J. J. Jakinibs: a new class of kinase inhibitors in cancer and autoimmune disease. *Curr. Opin. Pharmacol.* 2012(Jul 19).

141. Khwaja, A. The role of Janus kinases in haemopoiesis and haematological malignancy. *Br. J. Haematol.* 2006;**134**(4): 366–84.

142. Vila-Coro, A. J., Rodriguez-Frade, J. M., Martin De Ana, A. *et al.* The chemokine SDF-1alpha triggers CXCR4 receptor dimerization and activates the JAK/STAT pathway. *FASEB J.* 1999;**13**(13):1699–710.

143. Frank, D. A. STAT3 as a central mediator of neoplastic cellular transformation. *Cancer Lett.* 2007;**251**(2):199–210.

144. Chen, E., Staudt, L. M., Green, A. R. Janus kinase deregulation in leukemia and lymphoma. *Immunity* 2012;**36**(4):529–41.

145. Galm, O., Yoshikawa, H., Esteller, M., Osieka, R., Herman, J. G. SOCS-1, a negative regulator of cytokine signaling, is frequently silenced by methylation in multiple myeloma. *Blood* 2003;**101**(7):2784–8.

146. Pedranzini, L., Dechow, T., Berishaj, M. *et al.* Pyridone 6, a pan-Janus-activated kinase inhibitor, induces growth inhibition of multiple myeloma cells. *Cancer Res.* 2006;**66**(19):9714–21.

147. Kockeritz, L., Doble, B., Patel, S., Woodgett, J. R. Glycogen synthase kinase-3 – an overview of an over-achieving protein kinase. *Curr. Drug Targets* 2006;**7**(11):1377–88.

148. Hoeflich, K. P., Luo, J., Rubie, E. A. *et al.* Requirement for glycogen synthase kinase-3beta in cell survival and NF-kappaB activation. *Nature* 2000;**406**(6791):86–90.

149. Zhou, Y., Uddin, S., Zimmerman, T. *et al.* Growth control of multiple myeloma cells through inhibition of glycogen synthase kinase-3. *Leuk. Lymphoma* 2008;**49**(10):1945–53.

150. Gunn, W. G., Krause, U., Lee, N., Gregory, C. A. Pharmaceutical inhibition of glycogen synthetase kinase-3beta reduces multiple myeloma-induced bone disease in a novel murine plasmacytoma xenograft model. *Blood* 2011;**117**(5):1641–51.

151. Busino, L., Millman, S. E., Scotto, L. *et al.* Fbxw7alpha- and GSK3-mediated degradation of p100 is a pro-survival mechanism in multiple myeloma. *Nat. Cell Biol.* 2012;**14**(4):375–85.

152. Herr, P., Hausmann, G., Basler, K. WNT secretion and signalling in human disease. *Trends Mol. Med.* 2012(Jul 13).

153. Derksen, P. W., Tjin, E., Meijer, H. P. *et al.* Illegitimate WNT signaling promotes proliferation of multiple myeloma cells. *Proc. Natl. Acad. Sci. USA* 2004;**101**(16):6122–7.

154. Qiang, Y. W., Shaughnessy, J. D., Jr., Yaccoby, S. Wnt3a signaling within bone inhibits multiple myeloma bone disease and tumor growth. *Blood* 2008;**112**(2):374–82.

155. Edwards, C. M., Edwards, J. R., Lwin, S. T. *et al.* Increasing Wnt signaling in the bone marrow microenvironment inhibits the development of myeloma bone disease and reduces tumor burden in bone in vivo. *Blood* 2008;**111**(5):2833–42.

156. Pinzone, J. J., Hall, B. M., Thudi, N. K. *et al.* The role of Dickkopf-1 in bone development, homeostasis, and disease. *Blood* 2009;**113**(3):517–25.

157. Ferrando, A. A. The role of NOTCH1 signaling in T-ALL. *Hematology Am. Soc. Hematol. Educ. Program* 2009:353–61.

158. Houde, C., Li, Y., Song, L. *et al.* Overexpression of the NOTCH ligand JAG2 in malignant plasma cells from multiple myeloma patients and cell lines. *Blood* 2004;**104**(12):3697–704.

159. Chiron, D., Maiga, S., Descamps, G. *et al.* Critical role of the NOTCH ligand JAG2 in self-renewal of myeloma cells. *Blood Cells Mol. Dis.* 2012;**48**(4):247–53.

160. Nefedova, Y., Cheng, P., Alsina, M., Dalton, W. S., Gabrilovich, D. I. Involvement of Notch-1 signaling in bone marrow stroma-mediated de novo drug resistance of myeloma and other malignant lymphoid cell lines. *Blood* 2004;**103**(9):3503–10.

161. Groth, C., Fortini, M. E. Therapeutic approaches to modulating Notch signaling: Current challenges and future prospects. *Semin. Cell Dev. Biol.* 2012;**23**(4):465–72.

162. Nefedova, Y., Sullivan, D. M., Bolick, S. C., Dalton, W. S., Gabrilovich, D. I. Inhibition of Notch signaling induces apoptosis of myeloma cells and enhances sensitivity to chemotherapy. *Blood* 2008;**111**(4):2220–9.

163. Jhaveri, K., Taldone, T., Modi, S., Chiosis, G. Advances in the clinical development of heat shock protein 90 (Hsp90) inhibitors in cancers. *Biochim. Biophys. Acta* 2012;**1823**(3):742–55.

164. Castellano, E., Downward, J. RAS interaction with PI3K: more than just another effector pathway. *Genes Cancer* 2011;**2**(3):261–74.

165. Gillings, A. S., Balmanno, K., Wiggins, C. M., Johnson, M., Cook, S. J. Apoptosis and autophagy: BIM as a mediator of tumour cell death in response to oncogene-targeted therapeutics. *FEBS J.* 2009;**276**(21):6050–62.

Chapter

7

Immune dysfunction in multiple myeloma

Guy Pratt and Paul Moss

Introduction

Immune dysfunction is an important feature of multiple myeloma and infection remains a major cause of morbidity and mortality. Numerous defects of the immune system occur in multiple myeloma and can also be observed in monoclonal gammopathy of uncertain significance. Indeed, evidence suggests that immune deficiency and infection may serve to promote progression to MM.

There has also been considerable interest in the identification of an autologous response against myeloma. Although cellular and humoral responses directed against myeloma-associated antigens have been described, it remains somewhat uncertain if the immune system plays a significant role in preventing or controlling myeloma cell growth. Despite this, there is an increasing interest in the potential role of immunotherapeutic approaches to treatment paraproteinemia although the immunologically hostile environment associated with multiple myeloma remains a major challenge.

An improved understanding of the mechanisms that mediate immune surveillance and tumor immunity in myeloma are important as a basis for improving patient outcome and are the subject of this review (Table 7.1).

The burden of infectious disease in multiple myeloma

A variety of factors underlie the increased susceptibility of myeloma patients to infectious disease. These include hypogammaglobulinemia, impaired lymphocyte function, steroid-related immunosuppression, neutropenia and physical factors such as vascular catheters, impaired mucosal integrity and

respiratory compromise. The risk of infection is highest in patients with active disease and a characteristic feature is the relatively poor association with neutropenia. Grade 3 infections occur in around 5%–15% of patients treated with lenalidomide or thalidomide-based regimens in association with dexamethasone and present a novel challenge for immune function. A retrospective analysis of 3107 myeloma patients registered onto MRC trials showed that 10% of patients died within 60 days of trial entry and that 45% of these deaths were due to infection [1]. *Streptococcus pneumoniae*, *Haemophilus influenzae* and *Escherichia coli* are the most frequent causes of infection in myeloma patients [2]. The benefit of prophylactic antibiotics in patients with multiple myeloma is unclear. Modest benefit was observed for cotrimoxazole in a small randomized trial, although a recent study of 212 myeloma patients randomized equally between ciprofloxacin, cotrimoxazole or placebo revealed no apparent value [3,4]. Further studies are now under way. Bortezomib-based regimens appear to be associated with impairment in cellular immunity and associated with a significantly higher incidence of varicella zoster infections. As such, prophylactic acyclovir is generally recommended in this setting.

The role and cost effectiveness of both vaccination and prophylactic immunoglobulin are currently unclear [5] (unpublished data; placebo-controlled randomized MRC trial). Prophylactic immunoglobulin may possibly reduce the frequency of infections in patients with recurrent infections but there is a paucity of data and no evidence of a survival benefit.

There is increasing interest in the potential role of infections in stimulation of growth and survival

Table 7.1 Soluble molecules, receptors and immune cells relevant to the immune dysfunction in multiple myeloma

Soluble molecules and receptors	Abnormalities in myeloma	Function
TGF-β	Increased	Globally immunosuppressive cytokine inhibiting B and T cell function
IL-10	Increased	Inhibits dendritic cell function and skews CD4+ T cells to CD4+ Th2 cell differentiation
IL-6	Increased	Inhibits dendritic cell function and skews CD4+ T cells to Th2 cell differentiation
VEGF	Increased	Inhibits dendritic cell function, promotes production of IL-6
Muc-1	Increased surface expression and shedding	Inhibits dendritic cell maturation
β2-microglobulin	Increased	Possibly inhibits dendritic cell function
Cyclo-oxygenase-2	Increased	Skews CD4+ T cells to Th2 cell differentiation, inhibits macrophage and T cell killing
Chemokine CXCL12/stromal-derived factor-1α (SDF-1α)	Increased	Important in T cell migration and CD4+ T cell memory development
Chemokines CCL4 (MIP-1b), CCL5 (RANTES), CXCL9 (MIG), CXCL10 (IP10), CXCL8 (IL8)	Increased marrow/blood chemokine gradients	Altered T cell migration
IL-1β, IL-6, IL-23	Increased	IL-1β, IL-6, IL-23 and possibly TGF-β drive CD4+ Th 17 development
NKG2D2B4/CD244/CD16/ NCAM140 MHC class I chain-related protein A (MICA)	Down regulated on tumor cells; MICA actively shed with MGUS to MM progression	NK cell activatory receptors
HLA-DR, MHC class I, CD40, CD28 and CD80	Down regulated on tumor cells and antigen presenting cells	Antigen presenting and co-stimulatory molecules on myeloma plasma cells and antigen presenting cells
PD-1/PDL1 CTLA-4	PD-1 increased signaling implicated in NK cell defect in MM. CTLA-4 unclear. Both being targeted for inhibition in other malignancies	Important inhibitory pathways for cytotoxic immune cells
Fas/Fas ligand	Possibly defective, implicated in other malignancies	Important in tumor cell killing and apoptosis of T cells
Toll like receptors	Expressed on MM plasma cells	Stimulated by microbes. May promote tumor pathogenesis
Indoleamine 2, 3-dioxygenase	Unclear in MM, implicated in other malignancies	Immunosuppressive particularly for dendritic cells
April/Baff	Increased	Unclear but possibly immunomodulatory (important for normal B cell function)
Matrix-metalloproteinases (MMPs)	Increased	MM9 increases TGFβ. MMPs possibly immunomodulatory
Hepatocyte growth factor (HGF)	Increased	Immunosuppressive in mouse models

85

Table 7.1 *(cont.)*

Soluble molecules and receptors	Abnormalities in myeloma	Function
IMMUNE CELLS		
Dendritic cells	Inhibited function, poor maturation, reduced number, poorly co-stimulatory with reduced co-stimulatory molecule expression (HLA-DR, CD40, CD80)	Specialized antigen presenting cells
CD8 T cells	Numerical and functional defects, oligoclonal expansions. Loss of T cell immunity to tumor antigens such as SOX2 seen in MGUS to MM progression	Cytotoxic T cells
CD4 T reg	Conflicting data on changes in T reg numbers and function	Immunosuppressive regulatory T cells
CD4 helper cells	Possibly altered Th1/Th2 balance with increased Th2 cytokines and reduced Th1 cytokines	Altered Th1/T cell cytotoxic activity
CD4 Th17	Increased in the bone marrow	Inflammatory T cell subset with uncertain effects on myeloma biology. Possibly implicated in bone disease
γδ T cells	Inhibited function	Cytotoxic T cells
NK cells	Inhibited function	Cytotoxic NK immune cells
NK T cells	Increasingly inhibited in transition from MGUS to MM	Cytotoxic NK T immune cells
B cells	Inhibited function and reduced numbers resulting in immunoparesis	Antibody production

of myeloma cells possibly through the activity of pathogen associated molecular patterns (PAMP) on micro-organisms triggering Toll-like receptors (TLR) [6]. There is an increased history of pneumonia in the five years preceding the development of multiple myeloma and MGUS individuals have a reduced survival compared to the general population that includes, amongst other causes, an excess mortality due to bacterial infections [7,8]. These studies suggest that the increased susceptibility to infection occurs at the MGUS stage. Further evidence is required to support a role for infections in directly driving myeloma pathogenesis.

The immunologically hostile microenvironment

The relationship between myeloma plasma cells and the bone marrow microenvironment is critical for maintenance of disease. Tumor cells and stromal cells interact via adhesion molecules and cytokine networks to simultaneously promote such diverse effects as tumor cell survival, drug resistance, angiogenesis and disordered bone metabolism. A number of immunologically active compounds are increased including transforming growth factor-beta (TGF-β), interleukin-10 (IL-10), interleukin-6 (IL-6), vascular endothelial growth factor (VEGF), Fas ligand, Muc-1, cyclooxygenase-2 and related prostanoids, matrix metalloproteinases, APRIL and BAFF (Figure 7.1).

Transforming growth factor-β (TGF-β)

Myeloma cells produce excess TGF-β an immunosuppressive cytokine with global effects on immune cells, suppressing normal B cell and T cell responses and promoting T regulatory cell and possibly Th17 cell differentiation. Myeloma plasma cells appear resistant to the inhibitory effects of TGF-β.

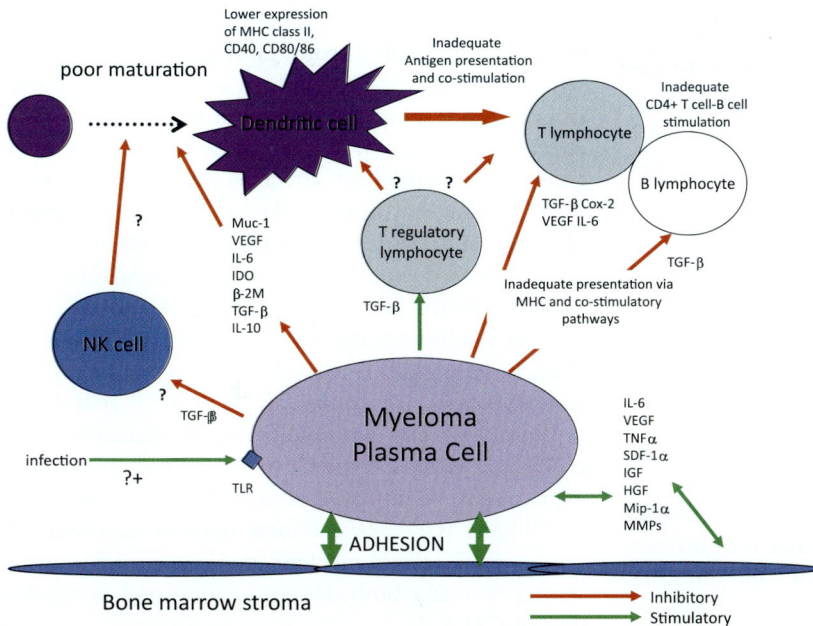

Figure 7.1 Interaction between tumor cells and the host immune system VEGF – vascular endothelial growth factor; IL6 – interleukin-6; IDO – indoleamine 2,3-dioxygenase; b2M – b-2 microglobulin; TGFb – transforming growth factor b; IL10 – interleukin-10; TNFa – tumor necrosis factor a; SDF-1a – stromal derived factor 1a; IGF – insulin growth factor; HGF- hepatocyte growth factor; MMPs- matrix metalloproteases; TLR- Toll-like receptors.

Interleukin-10 (IL-10)

Interleukin-10 (IL-10) is implicated in myeloma pathogenesis but its role in the immune dysfunction of multiple myeloma is unclear with possible suppressive effects on dendritic cells and Cox-2.

Muc-1

Muc-1 is a membrane bound mucin glycoprotein that is overexpressed by myeloma plasma cells acting as a potential tumor-associated antigen in immunotherapy studies. Muc-1 has suppressive effects on differentiation of dendritic cells (DCs) and possibly has a pro-apoptotic effect on T cells.

Vascular endothelial growth factor (VEGF)

VEGF is an important cytokine in the myeloma micro-environment where it can augment pro-inflammatory T cell differentiation, inhibit maturation of dendritic cells and promotes the production of IL-6.

Interleukin 6 (IL-6)

In the myeloma micro-environment IL-6 is produced in excess primarily by bone marrow stromal cells and mediates paracrine myeloma growth. IL-6 promotes CD4+ T cell Th2 differentiation at the expense of the

Th1 anti-tumor and inhibits dendritic cell maturation and function [9].

Fas/FasL

The Fas/FasL apoptotic pathway is important for T cell mediated lysis of virally infected or transformed cells, in the acquisition of self-tolerance and when expressed by tumor cells as a mechanism for killing tumor specific T cells. Myeloma cell lines do express FasL on their surface and can induce T cell apoptosis *in vitro* but the role of FasL expression by tumors remains unclear given that additional pathways exist that can lead to either tumor death or escape from immunosurveillance.

Cyclooxygenase-2 (Cox-2) and prostanoids

Overexpression of Cox-2 is a feature of many tumors including multiple myeloma leading to suppression of macrophage mediated or T cell mediated tumor killing and skewing T cells towards T_H 2 cell responses.

Matrix metalloproteinases

Martix metalloproteinases (MMPs) facilitate tumor invasion and have immunomodulatory properties through MMP9 mediated cleavage of CD25 and activation of TGFβ.

APRIL and BAFF

APRIL and BAFF are two related members of the TNF ligand superfamily with protumor effects including in multiple myeloma and also modulate T and B cell function although their role in the immune dysfunction in myeloma is unclear.

The cellular immune defects in multiple myeloma

A decrease in CD19+ B cells, CD4+ and CD8+ T cells in multiple myeloma has been shown to negatively correlate with survival [10] and in peripheral blood hematopoietic stem cell transplantation (PBSCT), both the dose of infused lymphocytes and early lymphocyte recovery correlate with positive clinical outcome indicating a potential positive relationship between the cellular components of the immune system and disease control.

Dendritic cell dysfunction in multiple myeloma

Dendritic cells (DCs) are highly specialized antigen presenting cells that play a critical role in the activation and potentiation of antigen specific responses. Defects in the DCs of patients with multiple myeloma include reduced overall number, defective maturation, lower expression of co-stimulatory molecules such as HLA-DR, CD40, and CD80, and impaired induction of allogeneic T cell proliferation [9]. A number of components within the myeloma microenvironment can inhibit dendritic cell function including transforming growth factor-beta (TGF-β), interleukin-10 (IL-10), interleukin-6 (IL-6), vascular endothelial growth factor (VEGF), Muc-1, PGE$_2$, Cox-2, β-2 microglobulin and indoleamine 2,3-dioxygenase (IDO). Increased numbers of plasmacytoid dendritic cells are found in the bone marrow in myeloma and, as well as promoting tumor growth and survival, have a reduced ability to induce T cell responses although this is potentially reversible using CpG-containing oligodeoxynucleotides to stimulate Toll-like receptors [11].

T cell dysfunction in multiple myeloma

Patients with multiple myeloma exhibit a variety of numerical and functional abnormalities of T cells. T cell subsets are frequently abnormal with inversion of the CD4:CD8 ratio, abnormal Th1/Th2 CD4+ ratios and a severe disruption of global T cell diversity. The exact extent to which alterations in T cell subsets result from direct generating or suppressing effects on T cells in the tumor micro-environment compared to migratory effects is unclear. Our recent studies show that at least part of the T cell changes observed in patients with myeloma and MGUS result from increased expression of chemokines within bone marrow leading to migration of CCR4 and CXCR3-bearing T cells from the blood into marrow (Goodyear et al., unpublished) (Figure 7.2). Abnormal functional responses are also commonly seen in T cells from myeloma patients, with alterations in signaling molecules and virus-specific CD8+ T cell responses often appearing to be impaired in myeloma. The expression of CTLA-4 (CD152), a critical negative regulator of T cells, on T cells in myeloma patients is unclear with studies showing both downregulation and upregulation of CTLA-4.

Oligoclonal expansions of CD4+ and CD8+ T cells that occur in healthy individuals with increasing age are much more marked and frequent in patients with a paraproteinemia [12]. These oligoclonal expansions display a cytotoxic T cell phenotype, have a higher frequency in bone marrow, correlate with prolonged survival but their target antigens remain unclear. Persistent herpes virus infections such as cytomegalovirus and Epstein Barr virus are likely to be important candidates.

γδ T cells in multiple myeloma

γδ T cells constitute 1%–5% of peripheral T cells and recognize families of unprocessed non-peptide compounds such as pyrophosphomonoesters and alkylamines. They have cytotoxic activity against myeloma cells, and bisphosphonates are known to be able to stimulate γδ T cell expansion [13,14] both by accumulation of upstream isoprenoid intermediates [13] and enhancement of signaling through the activating receptor NKG2D [14]. Administration of zoledronate activated Vγ9γδ T cells is safe and currently being investigated in immunotherapy strategies.

T regulatory cells in multiple myeloma

The role of T regulatory cells in multiple myeloma remains unclear but clearly may be of importance to the immune dysregulation found in this disorder. The data on regulatory T cells in multiple is

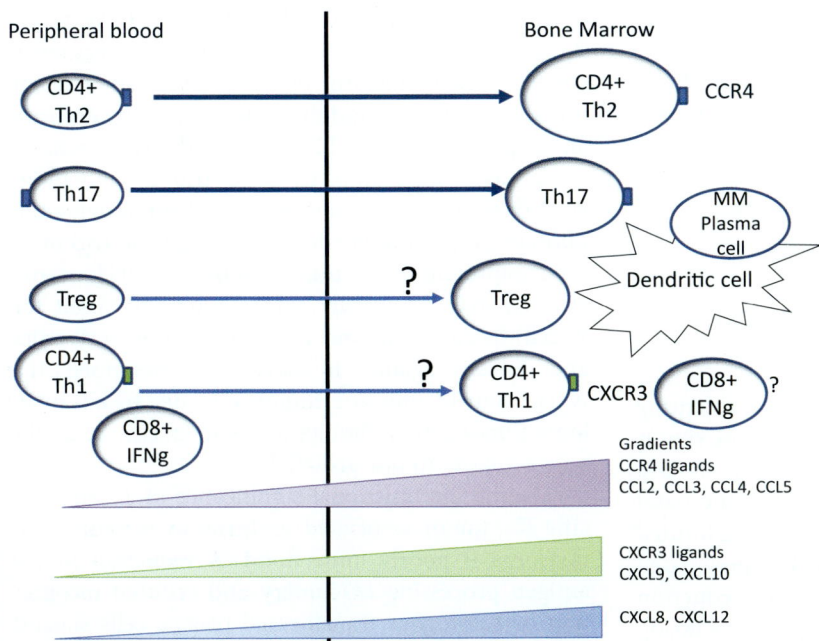

Figure 7.2 T cell dysfunction is due to chemokine gradients and direct effects of tumor micro-environment.

conflicting with reports of elevated levels of functional CD4(+)CD25(+)FoxP3(+) [15,16] and conversely reports of reduced numbers in the peripheral blood [17]. More recently Noonan *et al.* [18] showed that in bone marrow CD4+ CD25 + T cell lymphocytes in myeloma patients display an activated phenotype, lack suppressive function and a regulator T cell phenotype.

Th17 cells in multiple myeloma

The role of Th17 and IL-17 in tumor biology is complex with both antitumor and protumor effects reported and a range of solid tumors have an increased Th17 cell population in the tumor environment.

Cytokines thought to be important in Th17 differentiation and maintenance, namely IL-1β, IL-6, IL-23 and possibly TGF-β, are known to be increased in the bone marrow micro-environment in multiple myeloma. Th17 cells are increased in the peripheral blood and bone marrow in myeloma and increased Th17-related cytokines (IL-17, IL-21, IL-22 and IL-23) have been shown to promote myeloma cell growth and survival [18–20]. IL-17 is implicated in osteoclast maturation and elevated Th-17 cytokines correlate with the extent of lytic bone disease [18].

B cells in multiple myeloma

A reduced level of polyclonal immunoglobulin is a consistent feature of active multiple myeloma. This hypogammaglobulinemia reflects a suppression of CD19+ B lymphocytes that correlates inversely with disease stage and specifically affects the early and late stages of normal B cell differentiation. Possible contributory factors to B cell dysfunction in myeloma are the immunosuppressive B cell effects of TGF-β, lack of B cell accessory signals from helper T cells and altered transcription factors.

Natural killer cell function in multiple myeloma

Natural killer cells have an important role in the lysis of tumor cells or virally infected cells and are activated predominantly by recognition of downregulation of HLA class I expression. NK cells have anti-myeloma activity [21] and thalidomide and related immunomodulatory drugs can augment this effect [22]. However, escape mechanisms may exist in myeloma by downregulation of receptors such as 2B4/CD244 and CD16 and the NK receptor NCAM140. Changes in activatory and inhibitory NK receptors have been implicated in the transition form MGUS to myeloma [23]. In addition aberrant PD-1/PD-L1 signaling inhibits the NK-cell immune response against MM and inhibition of PD-1 may enhance the NK-cell versus myeloma effect [24].

Dhodapkar *et al.* [25] studied natural killer T (NKT) cells that recognize glycolipids presented by CD1d and showed an acquired functional defect that was potentially reversible in progressive multiple myeloma but not in MGUS or non-progressive myeloma.

Myeloma bone marrow plasma cells as antigen presenting cells

Myeloma plasma cells may act as antigen presenting cells *in vitro* [26] but their ability to do this in vivo is unclear. Myeloma plasma cells express HLA-DR, MHC class I, CD40, CD28 and CD80 but the basal expression of these molecules is often weak and limited to a part of the clone. Expression may be upregulated by cytokines such as IFN-γ and TNF-α [26]. Reduction in the components involved in antigen processing machinery is seen in multiple myeloma and reflects reduced recognition by CD8+ T cells [27]. Transduction of co-stimulatory molecules B7–1 and 4–1BB ligand into human myeloma cell lines transforms them into antigen presenting cells capable of expanding autologous tumor specific cytotoxic T cells *in vitro* [28].

Tumor-specific immune responses

The identification of T cell immunity against tumor-associated antigens is a major goal of cancer immunology and such responses have been reported in myeloma against cancer testis antigens [29,30], Muc-1 and idiotype protein [31]. Using a sensitive clonotypic assay, persistent tumor-reactive T cells can be found at low frequencies in the majority of myeloma patients, demonstrate cytotoxic activity and their presence reduces with disease progression [32].

Cancer testis antigens (CTAgs) are a family of proteins that are expressed in the testis, supposedly an immune privileged site, and are aberrantly expressed in many cancers including the majority of multiple myeloma tumors where they may provoke an immune response [33,34]. Van Rhee *et al.* [30] showed a correlation between expression of the cancer testis antigen, NY-ESO-1, and abnormal metaphase cytogenetic abnormalities, a poor prognostic marker. CD8+ T cells responses against the MAGE cancer testis antigens are frequently found in myeloma, at a frequency ranging from 0.0004% to 0.1% of the total CD8+ T cell pool, are persistent, correlate with disease burden, have an effector memory phenotype and their presence correlates with an improved survival [29]. Antibody responses to tumor associated antigens have also been demonstrated in myeloma and MGUS. Immunoglobulin idiotype (Id) is the portion of the variable region of the paraprotein that is unique to that B cell clone and as such may potentially act as a unique target for B cell specific immune responses. Both antibodies and T cells against Id have been described [31]. A Th1 anti-Id immune response is able to kill myeloma tumor cells, although idiotype specific Th2 cells may promote tumor growth [35].

Overall the functional significance of T cells specific for tumor-associated antigens in patients with myeloma is poorly understood. A reduction in the antigen processing machinery and reduced recognition of autologous transformed plasma cells suggest escape from immunosurveillance with progressive disease [27]. The clear presence of these T cell populations at least raises the possibility that they may be exploited in future immunotherapy strategies.

Immune factors regulating the transformation of MGUS to myeloma

The principles that regulate the transformation of MGUS to multiple myeloma are poorly understood and the genetic defects and gene expression profile found in multiple myeloma and MGUS are remarkably similar. If immunosurveillance does indeed have a role in limiting development of disease then it would be expected that patients with pre-malignant MGUS would mount vigorous immune responses. Dhodapkar *et al.* [36] showed that patients with MGUS mount a vigorous T cell response to autologous premalignant plasma cells, whereas this was not observed in patients with myeloma. Serological analysis of a recombinant cDNA expression library identified ten antigens with tumor specific antibody responses in MGUS patients [37]. A specific functional defect in natural killer T (NKT) cells has also been shown in patients progressing with myeloma [25]. The same group looked at antibody responses to a panel of tumor antigens in myeloma and showed T cell immunity against SOX2 an embryonic stem cell antigen specifically in MGUS patients [38]. Plasma cells from patients with MGUS have higher expression of co-stimulatory molecules [39] and anti-gen processing machinery [27] compared to myeloma plasma cells. Expression of MHC class I chain-related protein A (MICA), an NKG2D ligand, which is important in stimulating anti-myeloma γδ T cells by the NKG2D receptor, inversely correlates with disease stage [14]. A further study also showed increased MICA expression on plasma cells from MGUS patients compared with normal donors, whereas myeloma patients display intermediate MICA levels and a high expression of ERp5, a protein disulfide isomerase linked to MICA shedding (sMICA). Myeloma, but not MGUS, patients have circulating sMICA, which triggers the down-regulation of NKG2D and impaired lymphocyte cytotoxicity. In contrast, MGUS, but not myeloma patients generate high-titer anti-MICA anti-bodies that antagonize the suppressive effects of sMICA and stimulate dendritic cell cross-presentation of malignant plasma cells [40]. Potentially bortezomib could activate the DNA damage response to augment MICA expression in myeloma plasma cells. These studies provide indirect evidence that the host immune system may be important in preventing the progression from MGUS to multiple myeloma.

Immunomodulatory drugs in multiple myeloma

Thalidomide was the first immunomodulatory drug widely used in myeloma and has promiscuous modes of action with anti-angiogenic activity, direct anti-tumor effects, modulates the cytokine milieu within the bone marrow microenvironment (downregulation of chemokines such as TNFα, IL-12 and IL-15) and has immunomodulatory properties [22]. Thalidomide has potent co-stimulatory activity on primary T cells and NK cell activity in vitro, acts via the B7-CD28 pathway and leads to increased IL-2 and IFN-γ production and increases virus-specific CD8+ T cell cytokine production [22]. However, current knowledge of thalidomide activity comes from ex vivo research and there is limited insight into the principal mechanisms of action in vivo. The immunomodulatory derivatives of thalidomide (IMiDS), lenalidomide and pomalidomide are far more potent than thalidomide at co-stimulation of CD4+ T cells, CD8+ T cells and NK T cells. Their effects on the immune system are broad with reduction in interleukin-2, interferonγ and IL-6 regulator suppressor of cytokine signaling (SOCS)1 expression in T cells [41], enhanced

presentation of glycolipid by CD1d to NK T cells and also enhance the anti-myeloma activity of a humanized anti-CD40 monoclonal antibody by enhancing NK cell activity. Lenalidomide and pomalidomide reverse both decreased T cell and humoral activity, have beneficial effects in immunotherapy approaches in murine tumor models and beneficially enhance cytoskeletal formation of T cells and monocytes via modulation of Rho GTPases [42]. Similar effects are being seen in related diseases like chronic lymphocytic leukemia and suggest that immunomodulatory effects are major modes of action of these drugs raising the question of whether such agents are best given separately from immunosuppressive chemotherapy treatments and further explored in combination immunotherapy strategies. Indeed Hsu et al. [43] showed that the immunostimulatory effect of lenalidomide on NK cell function is profoundly suppressed by concurrent dexamethasone (Dex) therapy in multiple myeloma patients.

Bortezomib is also immunomodulatory with affects on the survival and function of lymphocytes and dendritic cells [44]. Proteasome inhibition alters the spectrum of antigenic peptides presented to T cells opening up the possibility of immunotherapy targeted against proteasome independent tumor specific CTL epitopes [45].

Bisphosphonates are used primarily for reducing skeletal complications but, as indicated above, also stimulate γδ T cells [13]. Bisphosphonates act indirectly by inhibiting the mevalonate pathway, specifically through inhibition of farnesyl diphosphate, leading to the accumulation of upstream isoprenoid intermediates that are recognized by and stimulate γδ T cells [13]. Bisphosphonates also enhance signaling through the activating receptor NKG2D on γδ T cells following engagement with MICA, an MHC Class I homolog, which is induced at the cell surface during periods of cell stress.

The potential for immunotherapy in multiple myeloma

In a minority of patients with multiple myeloma, long-term disease-free survival has been achieved by the graft-versus-myeloma (GVM) effect induced through allogeneic hemopoietic stem cell transplantation or donor lymphocyte infusions following allogeneic transplants [46]. However, this approach has been challenging because of high levels of treatment-related morbidity/mortality and reduced intensity non-myeloablative conditioning regimens have yet to show an overall major clinical benefit. It is uncertain whether any GVM effect can be dissociated from graft versus host disease (GVHD) [46]. Interestingly syngeneic transplantation in multiple myeloma appears to have a better outcome and, although unproven, there may be a graft-versus-myeloma effect against myeloma associated antigens in this setting [47]. These observations have prompted research into mechanisms to enhance the autologous immune response to myeloma. The majority of vaccination studies in patients have targeted tumor derived idiotype (Id) protein delivered using DNA vaccines, purified Id protein or Id-derived regions linked to adjuvant molecules. Although Id-specific immune responses have been shown, the clinical results have been largely disappointing and have not replicated the promising results obtained in murine models. Cancer testis antigens (CTAGs) are a potential target for immunotherapy in myeloma and have been a target for immunotherapy protocols in melanoma for many years. Epigenetic manipulation with the hypomethylating agent 5-azacitidine (5AC) and the histone deacetylase inhibitors can enhance the expression of CTAGs, raising the possibility of combining these agents in CTAG based immunotherapy. A number of other tumor specific targets are currently being explored that include WT1, Muc-1, hTERT, RHAMM-R3, DKK1, Survivin, PAK2, CDKN1A, Hsp 70, PRD1-BF1 and XBP-1 and these are being investigated together with efforts to improve vaccine technology. Dendritic cell vaccination has exploited DCs that have been pulsed with tumor derived peptides, such as Id, or have generated dendritic cell–tumor cell fused cells [48]. All these approaches may generate immune responses but their clinical effectiveness remains unproven and induction of tumor specific cytotoxic T lymphocyte and humoral responses does not necessarily translate into clinical tumor efficacy.

Vaccination strategies after autologous PBSCT in myeloma suggests that a combination approach using infusion of *in vivo* vaccine-primed and *ex vivo* co-stimulated T cells followed by post-transplant immunizations are most likely to induce clinically relevant immunity [49,50]. The timing of immunotherapy is important and it is generally believed that immunization strategies will be most effective in the setting of minimal residual disease. The period following autologous transplantation may offer the optimal timing in myeloma given the low tumor burden and more favorable immunological environment.

The development of anti-myeloma monoclonal antibody therapy, such as anti-CD138, anti-CD38 and anti-HM1.24 monoclonal antibodies, has been so far largely disappointing. However, this approach continues to gain interest in light of its proven value in other malignancies and a number of early phase trials are currently ongoing with several antibodies including the following: anti-CS1 monoclonal antibody elotuzumab (HuLuc63), anti-IL 6 antibody (siltuximab), anti-insulin-like growth factor 1 receptor antibody (AVE 1642), humanized anti-CD40 monoclonal antibody (SGN-40), anti-KIR antibodies (IPH 2101) and anti-CD74 antibody (milatuzumab). Other immunotherapeutic approaches that are currently being explored are T cell receptor therapies, either using TCR transduced T cells or TCR conjugates, and oncolytic measles virus therapy.

Discussion

Despite increasing information in this field some fundamental questions remain unanswered. A number of areas require particular focus if we are able to take advantage of current opportunities.

(a) The role of infections in promoting myeloma pathogenesis. Large epidemiological studies of infection rates in MGUS and myeloma patients, particularly in progressing MGUS patients, will improve our understanding in this area. Laboratory work which addresses the role of Toll-like receptors in promoting plasma cell survival may offer novel therapeutic targets.

(b) The role of prophylactic antibiotics and immunoglobulin replacement in multiple myeloma. This can only be addressed by large prospective randomized trials which must address the optimal timing, duration and nature of prophylaxis.

(c) The potential role of natural immune surveillance in controlling disease progression. Although humoral and T cell responses have been identified, it is unclear which responses, if any, have a role in immunosurveillance. Theoretically responses in early stage disease may be particularly important. Further immunotherapy strategies to optimize these responses *in vivo* will help in addressing this issue.

(d) Optimization of immunotherapy strategies. Improving strategies to enhance tumor specific immune responses requires a better understanding of many aspects of fundamental immunology including T cell tolerance, vaccine development, dendritic cell function and manipulation of the cytokine microenvironment to promote anti-tumor activity. Immunotherapy strategies in human cancer patients using single strategies have shown little clinical efficacy and

there is a belief that a combination approach is required as recently demonstrated in melanoma. This may be improved by the addition of immunomodulatory agents such as thalidomide, lenalidomide and possibly bortezomib.

Trying to dissect out the most important pathways in the immune dysfunction in myeloma is difficult but clearly of huge relevance given the increasing interest in the role of immunotherapy, immunomodulatory drugs and in enhancing the graft versus myeloma effect in some patients post-allogeneic transplantation.

References

1. Augustson, B. M., Begum, G., Dunn, J. A., *et al*. Early mortality after diagnosis of multiple myeloma: analysis of patients entered onto the United Kingdom Medical Research Council trials between 1980 and 2002–Medical Research Council Adult Leukaemia Working Party. *J. Clin. Oncol.* 2005;**23**:9219–26.

2. Rayner, H. C., Haynes, A. P., Thompson, J. R., Russell, N., Fletcher, J. Perspectives in multiple myeloma: survival, prognostic factors and disease complications in a single centre between 1975 and 1988. *Quarterly J. Med.* 1991;**79**:517–25.

3. Oken, M., Pomeroy, C., Weisdorf, D., Bennett, J. Prophylactic antibiotics for the prevention of early infection in multiple myeloma. *Am. J. Med.* 1996;**100**:624–8.

4. Vesole, D. H., Oken, M. M., Heckler, C. *et al*. Oral antibiotic prophylaxis of early infection in multiple myeloma: a URCC/ECOG Phase III study. *Blood* 2010;**116** (abstract 3017).

5. Raanani, P., Gafter-Gvili, A., Paul, M. *et al*. Immunoglobulin prophylaxis in chronic lymphocytic leukemia and multiple myeloma: systematic review and meta-analysis. *Leuk. Lymphoma* 2009;**50**:764–72.

6. Chiron, D., Jego, G., Pallat-Deuceunynck, C. Toll-like receptors: expression and involvement in multiple myeloma. *Leuk. Res.* 2010;**34**:1545–50.

7. Landgren, O., Rapkin, J. S., Mellemkjaer, L. *et al*. Respiratory tract infections in the pathway to multiple myeloma: a population-based study in Scandinavia. *Haematologica* 2006;**91**:1697–700.

8. Kristinsson, S. Y., Bjorkholm, M., Andersson, T. M. *et al*. Patterns of survival and causes of death following a diagnosis of monoclonal gammopathy of undetermined significance: a population based study. *Haematologica* 2009;**94**:1641–4.

9. Ratta, M., Fagnoni, F., Curti, A. *et al*. Dendritic cells are functionally defective in multiple myeloma: the role of interleukin-6. *Blood* 2002;**100**:230–7.

10. Kay, N. E., Leong, T. L., Bone, N. *et al*. Blood levels of immune cells predict survival in myeloma patients: results of an Eastern Cooperative Oncology Group phase 3 trial for newly diagnosed multiple myeloma patients. *Blood* 2001;**98**:23–8.

11. Chauhan, D., Singh, A. V., Brahmandam, M. *et al*. Functional interaction of plasmacytoid dendritic cells with multiple myeloma cells: a therapeutic target. *Cancer Cell* 2009;**16**:309–23.

12. Moss, P., Gillespie, G., Frodsham, P., Bell, J., Reyburn, H. Clonal populations of CD4+ and CD8+ T cells in patients with multiple myeloma and paraproteinemia. *Blood* 1996;**87**:3297–306.

13. Thompson, K., Rojas-Navea, J., Rogers, M. J. Alkylamines cause Vgamma9Vdelta2 T-cell activation and proliferation by inhibiting the mevalonate pathway. *Blood* 2006;**107**:651–4.

14. Girlanda, S., Fortis, C., Belloni, D. *et al*. MICA expressed by multiple myeloma and monoclonal gammopathy of undetermined significance plasma cells costimulates pamidronate-activated gammadelta lymphocytes. *Cancer Res.* 2005;**65**:7502–8.

15. Beyer, M., Kochanek, M., Giese, T., *et al*. In vivo peripheral expansion of naive CD4+CD25high FoxP3+ regulatory T cells in patients with multiple myeloma. *Blood* 2006;**107**:3940–9.

16. Feyler, S., von Lilienfeld-Toal, M., Jarmin, S., *et al*. CD4(+)CD25(+)FoxP3(+) regulatory T cells are increased whilst CD3(+)CD4(-)CD8(-)alphabetaTCR(+) Double Negative T cells are decreased in the peripheral blood of patients with multiple myeloma which correlates with disease burden. *Br. J. Haematol.* 2009;**144**;686–95.

17. Prabhala, R. H., Neri, P., Bae, J. E. *et al.* Dysfunctional T regulatory cells in multiple myeloma. *Blood* 2006;**107**:301–4.

18. Noonan, K., Marchionni, L., Anderson, J. *et al.* A novel role of IL-17 producing lymphocytes in mediating lytic bone disease in multiple myeloma. *Blood* 2010;**116**:3554–63.

19. Dhodapkar, K. M., Barbuto, S., Matthews, P. *et al.* Dendritic cells mediate the induction of polyfunctional human IL17-producing cells (Th17–1 cells) enriched in the bone marrow of patients with myeloma. *Blood* 2008;**112**:2878–85.

20. Prabhala, R. H., Pelluru, D., Fulciniti, M. *et al.* Elevated IL-17 produced by TH17 cells promotes myeloma cell growth and inhibits immune function in multiple myeloma. *Blood* 2010;**115**:5385–92.

21. Carbone, E., Neri, P., Mesuraca, M. *et al.* HLA class I, NKG2D, and natural cytotoxicity receptors regulate multiple myeloma cell recognition by natural killer cells. *Blood* 2005;**105**:251–8.

22. Davies, F. E., Raje, N., Hideshima, T. *et al.* Thalidomide and immunomodulatory derivatives augment natural killer cell cytotoxicity in multiple myeloma. *Blood* 2001;**98**:210–16.

23. Bernal, M., Garrido, P., Jiménez, P. *et al.* Changes in activatory and inhibitory natural killer (NK) receptors may induce progression to multiple myeloma: implications for tumor evasion of T and NK cells. *Hum. Immunol.* 2009;**70**;854–7.

24. Benson, D. M., Jr, Bakan, C. E., Mishra, A. *et al.* The PD-1/PD-L1 axis modulates the natural killer cell versus multiple myeloma effect: a therapeutic target for CT-011, a novel monoclonal anti-PD-1 antibody. *Blood* 2010;**11**:2286–94.

25. Dhodapkar, M. V., Geller, M. D., Chang, D. H. *et al.* A reversible defect in natural killer T cell function characterizes the progression of premalignant to malignant multiple myeloma. *J. Exp. Med.* 2003;**198**:1667–76.

26. Yi, Q., Dabadghao, S., Osterborg, A., Bergenbrant, S., Holm, G. Myeloma bone marrow plasma cells: evidence for their capacity as antigen-presenting cells. *Blood* 1997;**90**:1960–7.

27. Racanelli, V., Leone, P., Frassanito, M. A. *et al.* Alterations in the antigen processing-presenting machinery of transformed plasma cells are associated with reduced recognition by CD8+ T cells and characterize the progression of MGUS to multiple myeloma. *Blood* 2010;**115**:1185–93.

28. Lu, Z. Y., Condomines, M., Tarte, K. *et al.* B7-1 and 4–1BB ligand expression on a myeloma cell line makes it possible to expand autologous tumor-specific cytotoxic T cells in vitro. *Exp. Hematol.* 2007;**35**:443–53.

29. Goodyear, O., Pratt, G., McLarnon, A. *et al.* Differential pattern of CD4+ and CD8+ T cell immunity to MAGE-A1/A2/A3 in patients with monoclonal gammopathy of undetermined significance (MGUS) and multiple myeloma. *Blood* 2008;**112**:3362–72.

30. van Rhee, F., Szmania, S. M., Zhan, F. *et al.* NY-ESO-1 is highly expressed in poor-prognosis multiple myeloma and induces spontaneous humoral and cellular immune responses. *Blood* 2005;**105**:3939–44.

31. Yi, Q., Osterborg, A., Bergenbrant, S. *et al.* Idiotype-reactive T-cell subsets and tumor load in monoclonal gammopathies. *Blood* 1995;**86**:3043–9.

32. Michalek, J., Ocadlikova, D., Matejkova, E. *et al.* Individual myeloma-specific T-cell clones eliminate tumour cells and correlate with clinical outcomes in patients with multiple myeloma. *Br. J. Haematol.* 2010;**148**:859–67.

33. Jungbluth, A. A., Ely, S., DiLiberto, M. *et al.* The cancer-testis antigens CT7 (MAGE-C1) and MAGE-A3/6 are commonly expressed in multiple myeloma and correlate with plasma-cell proliferation. *Blood* 2005;**106**:167–74.

34. Atanackovic, D., Arfsten, J., Cao, Y. *et al.* Cancer-testis antigens are commonly expressed in multiple myeloma and induce systemic immunity following allogeneic stem cell transplantation. *Blood* 2007;**109**:1103–12.

35. Hong, S., Qian, J., Yang, J. *et al.* Roles of idiotype-specific t cells in myeloma cell growth and survival: Th1 and CTL cells are tumoricidal while Th2 cells promote tumor growth. *Cancer Res.* 2008;**68**:8456–64.

36. Dhodapkar, M. V., Krasovsky, J., Osman, K., Geller, M. D. Vigorous premalignancy-specific effector T cell response in the bone marrow of patients with monoclonal gammopathy. *J. Exp. Med.* 2003;**198**:1753–7.

37. Blotta, S., Tassone, P., Prabhala, R. H. *et al.* Identification of novel antigens with induced immune response in monoclonal gammopathy of undetermined significance. *Blood* 2009;**114**:3276–384.

38. Spisek, R., Kukreja, A., Chen, L. C. *et al.* Frequent and specific immunity to the embryonal stem cell-associated antigen SOX2 in patients with monoclonal gammopathy. *J. Exp. Med.* 2007;**204**:831–40.

39. Pérez-Andrés, M., Almeida, J., Martín-Ayuso, M. *et al.* Clonal plasma cells from monoclonal gammopathy of undetermined significance, multiple myeloma and plasma cell leukemia show different expression profiles of molecules involved in the

interaction with the immunological bone marrow microenvironment. *Leukemia* 2005;**19**:449–55.

40. Jinushi, M., Vanneman, M., Munshi, N. C. *et al.* MHC class I chain-related protein A antibodies and shedding are associated with the progression of multiple myeloma. *Proc. Natl Acad. Sci. USA* 2008;**105**:1285–90.

41. Gorgun, G., Calabrese, E., Soydan, E. *et al.* Immunomodulatory effects of lenalidomide and pomalidomide on interaction of tumor and bone marrow accessory cells in multiple myeloma. *Blood* 2010;**116**:3227–37.

42. Xu, Y., Li, J., Ferguson, G. D. *et al.* Immunomodulatory drugs reorganize cytoskeleton by modulating Rho GTPases. *Blood* 2009;**114**:338–45.

43. Hsu, A. K., Quach, H., Tai, T. *et al.* The immunostimulatory effect of lenalidomide on NK-cell function is profoundly inhibited by concurrent dexamethasone therapy. *Blood* 2011;**117**:1605–13.

44. Nencioni, A., Grunebach, F., Patrone, F., Ballestro, A., Brossart, P. Proteasome inhibitors: antitumor effects and beyond. *Leukemia* 2007;**21**:30–6.

45. Luckey, C. J., Marto, J. A., Partridge, M. *et al.* Differences in the expression of human class I MHC alleles and their associated peptides in the presence of proteasome inhibitors. *J. Immunol.* 2001;**167**:1212–21.

46. Crawley, C., Iacobelli, S., Bjorkstrand, B. *et al.* Reduced-intensity conditioning for myeloma: lower nonrelapse mortality but higher relapse rates compared with myeloablative conditioning. *Blood* 2007;**109**:3588–94.

47. Gahrton, G., Svensson, H., Bjorkstand, B. *et al.* Syngeneic transplantation in multiple myeloma – a case-matched comparison with autologous and allogeneic transplantation. European Group for Blood and Marrow Transplantation. *Bone Marrow Transplant* 1999;**24**:741–5.

48. Rosenblatt, J., Vasir, B., Uhl, L. *et al.* Vaccination with dendritic cell/tumor fusion cells results in cellular and humoral antitumor immune responses in patients with multiple myeloma. *Blood* 2011;**117**:393–402.

49. Rapoport, A. P., Aqui, N. A., Stadtmauer, E. A. *et al.* Combination immunotherapy using adoptive T-cell transfer and tumor antigen vaccination on the basis of hTERT and survivin after ASCT for myeloma. *Blood* 2011;**117**:788–97.

50. Rapoport, A. P., Stadtmauer, E. A., Aqui, N. *et al.* Restoration of immunity in lymphopenic individuals with cancer by vaccination and adoptive T-cell transfer. *Nature Med.* 2005;**11**:1230–7.

Chapter

8

Myeloma bone disease – pathogenesis of bone destruction and therapeutic strategies

Andrew Chantry and Neil Rabin

Introduction

Myeloma bone disease is a major cause of morbidity in patients, the clinical manifestations of which include pain, cord compression, loss of mobility and deformity. The clinical features of myeloma bone disease are due to osteoporosis, or focal lytic lesions leading to pathological fractures, vertebral collapse and hypercalcemia (Figure 8.1). Neurological sequelae secondary to bone disease are commonly caused by compression of nerves by damaged and displaced bone and most dramatically include spinal cord compression, which often presents as a neurosurgical emergency occurring in up to 5% of patients with myeloma (Figure 8.2) [1]. Indeed, consequences of osteolytic bone disease are often the presenting features of myeloma. Approximately 67% of patients with myeloma present with bone pain and up to 90% of patients with myeloma exhibit features of myeloma bone disease at some stage of the disease course [2,3].

The bone marrow micro-environment has long been recognized as a hospitable locale for the growth and rapid expansion of myeloma and other hematological malignancies as well as the metastatic spread of solid tumors including breast and prostate cancers. However, myeloma is uniquely associated with an aggressive and destructive osteolytic bone disease, which not only causes substantial morbidity as a direct result of bone destruction but, owing to the destruction of boney barriers, enables rapid tumor expansion and spread to extra-medullary sites. Once myeloma has escaped from the bone marrow micro-environment, disease enters a leukemic phase and is rapidly fatal.

Pathophysiology of myeloma bone disease

Myeloma bone disease is driven by an increase in osteoclasts and bone resorption *and* a decrease in osteoblasts and bone formation. This is mediated by various secreted factors which stimulate osteoclastogenesis and inhibit osteoblastogenesis, as well as by cell:cell contact-activated pathways (Figure 8.3). Hence, myeloma bone disease is caused by disruption of physiological bone remodeling, specifically the uncoupling of the normal balance between bone resorption mediated by osteoclasts and bone formation mediated by osteoblasts resulting in net osteolysis [4–9].

Osteoclast activating factors

Over 30 years ago, in studies of myeloma, Mundy and co-workers (1974) suggested that increased osteoclastogenesis was mediated by secreted osteoclast activating factors (OAFs). Histological and biochemical analysis has confirmed increased bone resorption associated with tumor infiltration [10]. Initially, the identity of the OAFs was uncertain. Since then many factors have been confirmed to have osteoclastogenic effects including interleukin 1β (IL-1β) [11–13], interleukin-6 (IL-6) [14,15], interleukin-11 (IL-11) [16], tumor necrosis factor-α (TNF-α) [17], tumor necrosis factor-β (TNF-β) [18,19], macrophage inflammatory protein 1α (MIP 1-α) [20], and hepatocyte growth factor (HGF) [21]. It has been proposed that many of these osteoclast activating factors mediate their effects via the receptor activator of nuclear factor kappa B ligand/osteoprotegerin (RANKL/OPG) system, which acts as a final common pathway [22–25].

Myeloma, ed. Stephen A. Schey, Kwee L. Yong, Robert Marcus and Kenneth C. Anderson. Published by Cambridge University Press. © Cambridge University Press 2014.

(a)

(b)

(c)

(d)

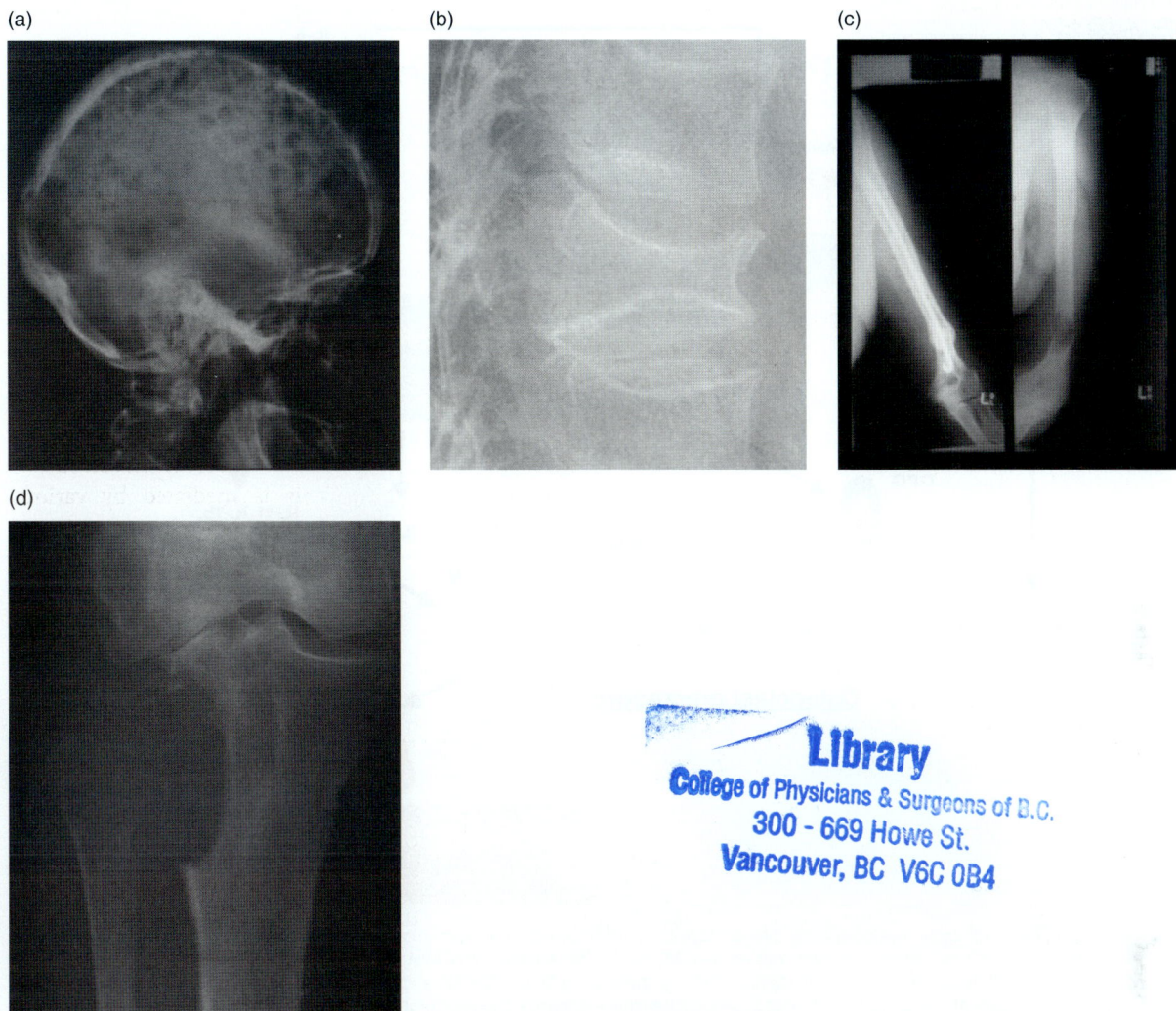

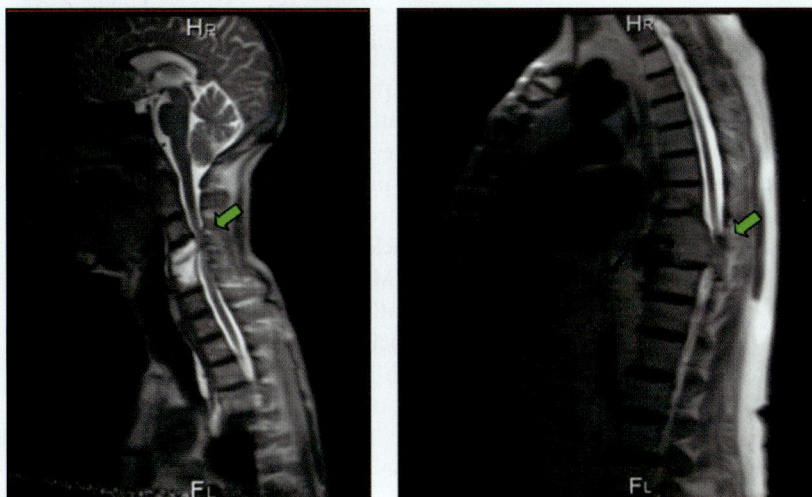

Figure 8.1 Radiological features of myeloma bone disease. Typical features of myeloma bone disease (a) "pepper pot" skull, (b) vertebral wedge fracture, (c) pathological fracture arising from a lytic lesion of the humerus, (d) large lytic lesion of the proximal tibia.

Figure 8.2 Spinal disease causing cord compression (arrowed) of the cervical spine (left) and the thoracic spine (right).

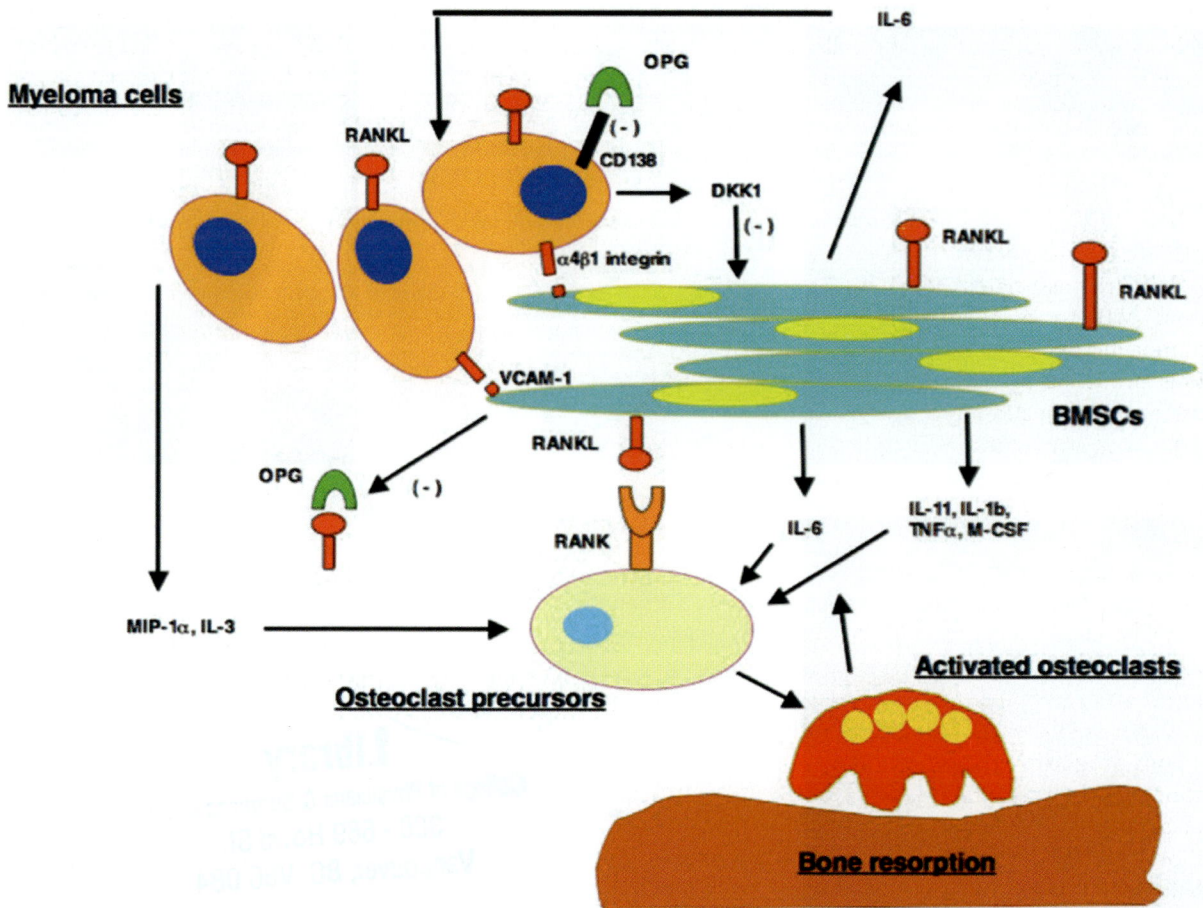

Figure 8.3 Pathophysiology of myeloma bone disease. Myeloma (MM) cells bind bone marrow stromal cells (BMSCs), through the interaction of the integrin α4β1 and vascular cell adhesion molecule-1 (VCAM-1). This adherence of MM cells to BMSCs enhances the production of receptor activator of NF$_k$B ligand (RANKL), macrophage colony stimulating factor (M-CSF) and other osteoclast activating factors (OAFs, see text for details). MM cells also express MIP-1α and IL-3. Together these enhance the proliferation and differentiation of osteoclast precursors leading to bone resorption. MM cells also express RANKL. Osteoprotegerin (OPG) binds RANKL inhibiting osteoclast development and bone resorption. OPG also binds syndecan 1 (CD138). Dickkop-1 (DKK1), expressed by MM cells, inhibits Wnt signaling, reducing osteoblast development. See text for other inhibitors of osteoblast development. Adapted from Terpos *et al.*, *Annals of Oncology* **16**:1223–31 (2005).

RANKL/RANK signaling pathway

The RANKL/RANK signaling pathway is the primary mediator of osteoclast induced bone resorption and is a critical determinant of bone remodeling. RANKL is a transmembrane protein, which is a member of the TNF superfamily and also exists in a soluble form. It binds RANK, activates TRAF1–6, and through downstream signaling activates osteoclasts. OPG is the natural decoy receptor for RANKL and prevents it binding to RANK.

Evidence to date indicates that a major cause of osteolytic bone disease in patients with MM is an imbalance in the ratio of RANKL to OPG. RANKL expression is increased in the bone marrow stroma of patients with MM [26]. Furthermore OPG is reduced in the bone marrow [26] and serum [27] of patients with MM. Circulating levels of soluble RANKL/OPG correlated with severity of bone disease, as well as conferring a poor prognosis [28]. RANKL is produced by bone marrow stroma as a result of interactions with MM cells. It is unclear whether MM cells also express RANKL. While MM cells have been reported to express RANKL [29,30], other groups have failed to corroborate these results, including one study employing microarray analysis in primary MM cells [31]. Other potential sources of RANKL in MM bone marrow are T cells [32]. The reduction in OPG observed in patients may be due to several factors. Binding of

OPG to CD138, syndecan-1, with internalization and subsequent degradation by MM cells [27] would serve to lower circulating levels. In addition, MM cells may also reduce OPG expression by bone marrow stromal cells [26].

MIP-1α

MIP-1α is a member of the CC chemokine family and is primarily associated with cell adhesion and migration. MIP-1α is chemotactic for monocytes and monocytic like cells, including osteoclast precursors. It is produced by MM cells and directly stimulates osteoclast formation and differentiation in a dose dependent way, through receptors CCR1 and CCR5, which are expressed on osteoclasts. Addition of a neutralizing antibody against MIP-1α to human marrow cultures treated with freshly isolated marrow from patients with MM blocked MIP-1α induced osteoclast formation [33]. MIP-1α mRNA has been detected in MM cells, and MIP-1α protein levels are elevated in bone marrow plasma of MM patients [34]. Furthermore MIP-1α serum levels correlate with severe bone disease, as well as being associated with a poor prognosis [35]. MIP-1α has also been found to stimulate the proliferation, migration and survival of plasma cells, both *in vitro* and *in vivo* [33]. In addition, MIP-1α enhanced adhesive interactions between MM cells and marrow stromal cells increasing expression of IL-6 and RANKL, which further increased bone destruction and tumor burden [36].

Other osteoclast activating factors

IL-6 is a potent inducer of human osteoclast formation [37]. Serum levels of IL-6 and its receptor (IL-6R) are increased in MM and correlate with MM stage, disease activity and disease free survival [38]. IL-6 can increase the effects of MIP-1α, IL-3 and RANKL on osteoclast formation in murine models, and can induce RANKL expression by murine stromal cells [39]. However, the precise role that IL-6 plays in osteoclast formation in MM remains to be defined. IL-3 is an inducer of human osteoclast formation, and both mRNA and protein levels are reported to be elevated in bone marrow from MM patients [40]. Furthermore, addition of IL-3 in combination with MIP-1α or RANKL significantly enhanced human osteoclast formation and bone resorption compared with MIP-1α or RANKL alone [39]. In addition IL-3 enhanced the growth of MM cells (independent of IL-6). This

suggests that IL-3 may increase both bone destruction and tumor growth. IL-1β has potent OAF activity, enhancing the expression of adhesion molecules and inducing paracrine IL-6 production, resulting in osteolytic disease. Increased levels of IL-1β were detected in the supernatant of cultures of freshly isolated MM cells, as well as the plasma of patients with MM [41]. TNF-α is found at high levels in the supernatant of plasma cell cultures from MM patients. The actions of TNF-α are mediated by stimulation of the proteolytic breakdown of I-kappa B (the inhibitor of nuclear factor-kappa B (NfkB), leading to NfkB activation and enhancement of gene transcription of IL-6, which promotes bone resorption [42].

Osteoblast inhibitory factors

In addition to increased recruitment and activity of osteoclasts, it has become apparent that osteoblast activity is also inhibited. Histomorphometric evidence suggests that early in the disease process there is an *increase* in the recruitment of both osteoclasts and osteoblasts. There are also well documented reports of MM bone disease with an osteosclerotic phenotype [43–45]. In 1991, Bataille and co-workers proposed that the early increased recruitment of osteoblast precursors is a critical step in the pathogenesis of MM mediated by the secretion of large amounts of IL-6 from these cells. Not only has IL-6 been identified as an important osteoclast activating factor, it is also recognized as a potent myeloma cell survival factor [46–48]. Other investigators have proposed that recruitment of osteoblast precursors may be mediated by soluble interleukin-6 receptor (IL-6R) shed from myeloma cells [49]. The authors suggest that sIL-6 receptor shed from the surface of myeloma cells binds to IL-6 released from mesenchymal stem cells/osteoblast precursors; this complex then binds gp130 on osteoblast precursors to activate the IL6 pathway, leading to osteoblast recruitment and differentiation.

Thus, an increase in early osteoblast recruitment may promote myeloma cell survival via the secretion of IL-6. However, typically as disease progresses osteoblast numbers decrease, and osteoclast activity is stimulated resulting in net osteolysis [6]. The molecular mechanism/s responsible for the inhibition of osteoblast number and function remain to be fully elucidated. Following biochemical analysis of markers of bone metabolism, Abildgaard and co-workers suggested that an unknown factor in myeloma was responsible for inhibition of later stage osteoblast differentiation and function leading to the uncoupling of osteoblast and osteoclast activity and net bone lysis [50].

The role of dickkopf-1 (Dkk-1)

Evidence is now accumulating to suggest that the Wnt/β-catenin signaling pathway inhibitor, *dickkopf* (Dkk-1) inhibits osteoblast differentiation and may be important in driving osteolytic bone disease. This was initially suggested following a study of genes upregulated in myeloma [51]. In this study, the authors screened patients with multiple myeloma who had radiological evidence of lytic lesions and compared them with those without lytic lesions, as well as patients with Waldenström macroglobulinemia, and monoclonal gammopathy of undetermined significance (MGUS). They identified overexpression of four genes associated with myeloma osteolytic bone disease, one of which encodes Dkk-1. These gene expression results correlated with the level of Dkk-1 protein in bone marrow plasma of patients from these different groups. Addition of recombinant Dkk-1 inhibited osteoblast differentiation of murine osteoblastic precursor cells, an effect that was reversed by an anti-Dkk-1 antibody. The correlation between serum Dkk-1 levels and osteolytic bone disease has been subsequently confirmed by other groups [52]. Since then a number of *in vivo* studies have demonstrated that targeting Dkk-1 in murine models of myeloma protects against myeloma bone disease [53–55].

The role of other inhibitors of Wnt/β-catenin signaling

Recent reports suggest that other inhibitors of Wnt/β-catenin signaling, including soluble frizzled related proteins 2 and 3, wise and sclerostin, may also play a role in the reduction of osteoblast numbers and inhibition of osteoblast function in myeloma bone disease and as such constitute potential therapeutic targets. Sclerostin is expressed by osteocytes and in a similar fashion to Dkk-1, binds to Lrp5, sequestering it away from association with frizzled and subsequent downstream Wnt/β-catenin signaling [56]. Recently, plasma cells obtained from myeloma patient bone marrows have been shown to overexpress sclerostin [57]. Furthermore, elevated levels of sclerostin in

serum have demonstrated in patients with advanced myeloma [58]. Sclerostin may prove to be a useful potential target in patients with myeloma bone disease.

Other postulated osteoblast inhibitors in myeloma bone disease

Interleukin-7 (IL-7)

IL-7 has also been implicated in osteoblast suppression; this evidence derives from *in vitro* studies where culturing myeloma cell lines with osteoblast precursors reduced markers of osteoblast differentiation, e.g. module formation, and the colony forming assay (colony forming unit – osteoblast, CFU-OB). This effect was reversed by anti-IL-7 antibodies, and was also observed to be contact-dependent effect with a role for very late antigen 4 (VLA-4) adhesion molecule. In this system, suppression of osteoblast differentiation was mediated via reduced expression of the transcription factor Runx2/Cbfa1 [59]. IL-7 is secreted by T-cells and is known to stimulate osteoclast activation via up regulation of RANKL [60] these on osteoblasts were previously unknown. IL-7 may act independently of the Wnt pathway.

Hepatocyte growth factor

Hepatocyte growth factor (HGF) is produced by osteoclasts, and may act in autocrine fashion, as well as regulating osteoblasts in a paracrine manner [61]. HGF has also been reported to be expressed by myeloma cell lines, and primary myeloma cell expression has also been reported [62]. Standal and co-workers have recently demonstrated that HGF inhibits BMP induced expression of alkaline phosphatase in human mesenchymal stem cells and the murine osteoblast precursor cell line C2C12.

Interleukin-3 (IL-3)

Similarly, recent studies have suggested that IL-3 plays a dual role in the pathogenesis of myeloma bone disease [40], both increasing tumor growth and osteoclastogenesis. More recently, the same group confirmed that IL-3 was significantly increased in the bone marrow plasma of patients with myeloma compared to healthy controls and that IL-3 was also able to inhibit basal and bone morphogenic protein (BMP) induced osteoblast differentiation [63].

TGF-β signaling also regulates osteoblast differentiation

Given the importance of osteoblast inhibition in the pathogenesis of myeloma bone disease, attention has also focused on other pathways that may regulate osteoblastogenesis. Transforming growth factor beta (TGF-β) signaling is one such pathway [64]. The TGF-β superfamily of cytokines, comprising TGF-βs, the bone morphogenic proteins (BMPs) and the activin/inhibin system, is a highly conserved system performing a wide variety of biological functions ranging from regulation of embryogenesis to regulation of reproduction and widespread tissue homeostasis [65].

Within the context of myeloma, investigators have recently suggested that TGF-β released from bone mineral matrix as a result of increased, myeloma driven osteoclastic resorption, inhibits osteoblast differentiation [66]. Recent studies inhibiting the TGF-β type I receptor in mice has demonstrated anabolic and anti-catabolic effects on bone mediated by increased osteoblast differentiation and bone formation and reducing osteoclast differentiation and resorption [67].

Activin-A regulates bone phenotype

Furthermore, recent studies have identified activin-A as an important regulator of bone phenotype. Activins are members of the transforming growth factor beta (TGF-β) superfamily closely related to their natural antagonists, the inhibins. Inhibins are comprised of a common α subunit coupled to one of two β subunits leading to inhibin-A (αβA) or inhibin-B (αβB). Activins are homo- or heterodimers of the β subunits. The most commonly occurring β subunits are βA and βB leading to the homodimers activin-A (βAβA), activin-B (βBβB) and the heterodimer activin-AB (βAβB). Activins and inhibins were first identified as important regulators of pituitary follicle stimulating hormone release [68–71]. Subsequent studies have demonstrated that activins are expressed in diverse tissues and play important roles in embryology, wound healing and tissue homeostasis [72–76].

Recently, a number of investigators have identified the activin/inhibin system as an important regulator of bone formation [77]. Specifically, activin-A has been shown to be abundantly expressed in bone [78]. Conversely, neither activin-B nor activin-AB has been detected in bone. Conflicting evidence exists concerning the role of activin-A in bone. It has been reported to both inhibit and stimulate osteoblastogenesis *in vitro*, and to promote osteoclast formation *in vitro* [77,79–81]. *In vivo*, direct administration of activin-A increases bone mineral density [82], whereas over-expression of inhibin-A, which blocks activin-A and other TGF-β family members, increases bone mass [83,84]. Other investigators have recently demonstrated that activin-A signalling can be blocked *in vivo* with a soluble ActRIIA.muFc fusion protein leading to increased bone mass and strength [85]. ACE-011, a soluble form of the extra-cellular domain of the human activin type II receptor, fused to a human IgG-Fc fragment, has also been shown to increase bone formation and decrease bone resorption markers in healthy, post-menopausal women [86].

Therapeutic strategies targeting bone resorption

Bisphosphonates

The dramatic increase in osteoclast activity seen in myeloma provides a rationale for the clinical use of bisphosphonates, which are potent inhibitors of osteoclasts. The three most commonly used bisphosphonates in patients with myeloma are the oral, daily, bisphosphonate, sodium clodronate, and the third generation nitrogen containing bisphosphonates, pamidronate and zoledronic acid, administered monthly via intravenous infusion.

Clodronate, given to patients with symptomatic myeloma reduced the development of new osteolytic lesions, the number of vertebral and non-vertebral fractures, and reduced the degree of hypercalcemia and bone pain [87,88]. Pamidronate, given to patients with evidence of bone disease, reduced the number of skeletal related events (SRE), and time to the next SRE, as well as improving pain scores and quality of life. Although the standard dose of pamidronate is 90 mg monthly, a recently published study comparing 30 mg versus 90 mg monthly in newly diagnosed symptomatic patients showed no difference in median time to SRE and median SRE survival between the groups [89]. A large phase 3 study, designed to test non-inferiority zoledronic acid to pamidronate in patients with myeloma showed that both reduced SRE, bone pain and need for radiotherapy in an equivalent manner, although zoledronic acid demonstrated clear benefit in patients treated for metastatic breast cancer [90]. The recently published Myeloma IX trial reports a significantly reduced rate of SRE in patients receiving zoledronic acid compared with clodronate in newly diagnosed symptomatic myeloma ($n = 1960$ evaluable patients) [91]. After a median follow up of 3.7 years, 35% patients receiving clodronate experienced an SRE versus 27% of patients receiving zoledronic acid ($p = 0.0004$). The benefit of bisphosphonates in symptomatic MM is clearly demonstrated. Bisphosphonates are not recommended for the treatment of patients with monoclonal gammopathy or asymptomatic MM. Zoledronic acid reduced the number of SRE at progression in a large phase 3 study of patients with asymptomatic myeloma, but had no affect on other disease parameters or indeed in survival of patients [92]. Bisphosphonates are therefore not recommended for asymptomatic patients outside of a clinical trial.

Several issues remain with regard to bisphosphonate therapy in patients with symptomatic disease.

(1)   Is there an anti-myeloma effect?

Intriguing evidence dating back over the past 15 years from animal models and *in vitro* studies have suggested that bisphosphonates also exert an anti-tumor effect. The MRC Myeloma IX trial is the first major randomized controlled trial to show an apparent anti-tumor effect in human subjects with myeloma, and was irrespective of whether the treatment was consolidated with an autologous stem cell transplant, or if bone disease was present at diagnosis [91]. However, despite this striking evidence, the mechanism of the anti-tumor effect is not entirely clear.

Various mechanisms have been proposed to account for the anti-tumor effects of bisphosphonates ranging from relatively simple mechanisms to more complex interactions. Perhaps most simply, it has been proposed that because less bone is destroyed following bisphosphonate treatment, there is less volume available for tumor expansion. Furthermore, bony barriers to tumor expansion remain intact, i.e. the tumor is less likely to break out of its locale, expand and spread [93]. Similarly, the bone marrow microenvironment has often been perceived as a hospitable environment for tumor growth especially when enriched by growth factors such as TGF-β, ILGF liberated from the bone matrix during bone resorption – the so-called "seed and soil" concept. Because treatment with bisphosphonates inhibits bone resorption, this favorable environment would be rendered relatively more inert [94]. It has also been

suggested that bisphosphonate treatment can inhibit tumor cell adhesion to mineralized surfaces [95]. Also, similar to their effects on osteoclasts, bisphosphonates have now been shown to have pro-apoptotic and anti-proliferative effects on myeloma cells [96]. Anti-angiogenic effects have also been proposed [97]. More complex interactions have also been proposed including enhanced $\gamma\delta$ T-cell mediated immunosurveillance [98].

Intriguing data have also emerged suggesting synergy between bisphosphonates and various chemotherapeutic agents including doxorubicin, paclitaxel and cyclophosphamide [99–101]. Most recently, sequential administration of doxorubicin followed 24 h later by zoledronic acid has been shown to decrease tumor burden in a mouse model of breast cancer. The authors propose that this is mediated by a complex interaction of increased pro-apoptotic factors and decreased cell cycle proteins [102]. Further studies are required to confirm which of these mechanisms are most important.

Most studies have focused on the nitrogen containing bisphosphonates. Most commentators now conclude that the anti-tumor effect of bisphosphonates is probably attributable to the inhibition of the mavelonate pathway unique to the nitrogen containing bisphosphonates and, in particular, to the inhibition of the enzyme farsenyl pyrophosphate synthase (FFP synthase), which prevents the formation of isoprenoid lipids e.g. geranyl geranyl pyrophosphate (GGPP); these are required for the post-translational prenylation (i.e. transfer of long-chain isoprenoid lipids) of proteins especially Ras, Rho, Rab, Rac – common intracellular proteins required for many cellular functions; reduction in these almost certainly interferes with cellular function and increases apoptosis and may well decrease concentrations of functional cell cycle proteins inhibiting proliferation [93]. Thus these pro-apoptotic and anti proliferative properties, first proposed to act on osteoclasts may well also act on tumor cells.

Other indirect anti-tumor mechanisms may also come into play. For example, it is known that osteoclasts secrete a number of tumor growth factors including IL-6, osteopontin, BAFF and APRIL. Hence reduction of osteoclast numbers caused by bisphosphonate therapy is likely to reduce the production of these tumor survival factors.

(2)   Adverse effects of bisphosphonates

Potential adverse reactions from bisphosphonates include gastrointestinal reactions after oral administration, acute phase reactions after intravenous administration, and hypocalcemia. Osteonecrosis of the jaw (ONJ) and renal impairment are rare but potentially serious complications of bisphosphonates. ONJ is dependent on potency of the bisphosphonate, is time dependent, age dependent and related to dental extractions [103,104]. Supportive care remains the cornerstone of management, whereas surgical therapy helps only a subset of patients. The incidence of ONJ in the prospective Myeloma IX study is 3.8% in the transplant and 3.3% in the non-transplant arm (after a median follow up of 3.7 years) [91]. Preventative measures include a comprehensive dental examination at the start of treatment, excellent dental hygiene, and avoiding dental procedures during bisphosphonate treatment. Initial treatment of ONJ includes discontinuation of bisphosphonates until healing occurs, and the decision to restart should be individualized until prospective studies are available, although the potential benefit of these drugs should not be ignored. There was no difference in renal impairment between zoledronic acid and clodronate in the Myeloma IX trial [91], and monitoring serum creatinine rates can help diagnose renal impairment at an early stage.

(3)   What is the optimal duration and dose of bisphosphonate?

There are several guidelines currently available (NCCN, ESMO, ASCO, MAYO, IMWG reply to MAYO). The majority suggest 2 years of treatment and after this at the physician's discretion. However, in light of the Myeloma IX trial, this may change in future, because zoledronic acid was given until disease progression, prompting many clinicians to consider indefinite treatment, thus exploiting an ongoing anti-tumor effect. The survival advantage of zoledronic acid may lead to its wider use, and survival data from comparison studies are awaited. A recent review of the Myeloma IX trial advises caution in this respect [105]. Rajkumar observes that, in non-UK countries, the alternative bisphosphonate to zoledronic acid is pamidronate, which is less expensive by a factor of ten than zoledronic acid, has not been associated with a survival disadvantage and may also have a lower incidence of ONJ. Secondly, he points out that it remains unclear whether patients without bone disease at presentation do better or not. The possibility of an anti-tumor effect does, however, raise the intriguing question of whether treating patients with asymptomatic myeloma with bisphosphonates (using an attenuated, e.g. yearly, schedule) may slow tumor progression and the development of myeloma bone disease. Thirdly, although the observation that most survival benefit appears to be derived early, i.e. within the first four months of treatment, is clearly important, mortality at this juncture in Myeloma IX is quoted at 8%. This compares less favorably with mortality at this juncture in patients treated with lenalidomide or bortezomib which is quoted as 1% or less. Finally, he observes that the median duration of treatment with zoledronic acid is 12 months; given that most benefit appears to be gained early, he suggests that this should not be used to justify indefinite treatment with zoledronic acid.

Novel therapies inhibiting osteoclastogenesis

Denosumab is a fully human monoclonal antibody that binds to RANKL with high affinity and specificity, inhibiting osteoclastogenesis. Denosumab was non-inferior to zoledronic acid in delaying time to first SRE in patients with advanced solid tumors and myeloma [106]. Denosumab was inferior to zoledronic acid in overall survival, and thus a large phase 3 randomized study is currently ongoing, and the results are eagerly awaited. Therapies using recombinant OPG and OPG mimetics are in development [107–109].

Therapeutic strategies targeting bone formation

Targeting Dkk-1

Although bisphosphonates and other therapies have demonstrated some protection against myeloma bone disease and a reduction in the incidence of subsequent skeletal events, protection is not complete and existing bone lesions do not heal. Attention has therefore shifted to anabolic strategies aiming to increase bone formation thus enhancing protection against the development of new osteolytic lesions, retarding progression of existing lesions and ultimately to stimulate repair of lesions. As an anabolic target, Dkk-1 in particular looks promising. Following on from *in vivo* murine studies, a humanized version of an antiDkk-1 antibody is currently the subject of a large, multi-centered phase 2 trial in patients with myeloma intolerant of bisphosphonates.

Targeting Activin-A

Recently, two studies have targeted activin-A in murine models of myeloma demonstrating substantial protection against osteolytic disease [110,111]. Specifically, activin-A has been targeted using a soluble decoy receptor in the 5T2MM and 5T33MM murine models of myeloma demonstrating not only prevention of osteolytic bone disease but also a survival advantage [111]. Given these promising results, targeting activin-A signaling may well be beneficial in myeloma bone disease. Clinical studies are also in progress using ActRIIA. muFc in combination with conventional chemotherapy regimens in patients with myeloma. Given the substantial protective effect against osteolytic bone disease following treatment with ActRIIA. muFc, it is hoped that these studies will result in a clinically relevant and effective new treatment for patients with myeloma.

Bone anabolic approaches may also inhibit tumor growth

Recent evidence has also emerged to suggest that agents that target bone formation also exhibit anti-tumor effects [112]. It has been proposed that the anti-tumor effect of bone anabolic approaches may be mediated by the osteogenic matrix factor, decorin, highly secreted by osteoblasts during bone formation, and which has anti-angiogenic, anti-tumor and anti-osteoclastogenic effects [113]. Furthermore, two other bone anabolic approaches, parathyroid hormone and mesenchymal stem cell therapy, have been shown to be not only effective bone anabolic strategies but also associated with anti-tumor properties [114,115].

New anti-myeloma drugs may also have bone protective effects

Evidence is now also accumulating to suggest that the newer anti-myeloma drugs may also have direct bone protective effects, for example, proteasome inhibitors. The proteasome is responsible for the suppression of the Wnt signaling pathway, by targeting β-catenin. Thus proteasome inhibition increases the stability of β-catenin, allowing translocation to the nucleus and the subsequent transcription of osteoblastogenic genes. Proteasome inhibition strategies would therefore be expected to lead to activation of Wnt signaling, in a similar manner to various bone anabolic strategies which target Wnt signaling [53,54,116]. This is supported by the observation that patients treated with bortezomib have increased levels of total and bone specific alkaline phosphatase. Furthermore, investigators have shown upregulation of the key osteoblastogenic transcription factor Runx2 and the subsequent increase in bone formation markers in patients treated with bortezomib. *In vitro* studies using cell contact co-culture systems suggest that thalidomide and lenalidomide act to reduce the production of RANKL by human osteoprogenitor cells, thus reducing osteoclastogenesis. Furthermore, this may be mediated by downregulation of certain critical adhesion molecules by myeloma cells including ITGA4 (CD49d), ITGA8 and ICAM2 (CD102) [117].

Concluding remarks

As the overall prognosis for patients with myeloma improves, especially with the arrival of novel therapies, improved treatment of myeloma bone disease remains a clinical priority. Considering the pathophysiology of myeloma bone disease, there is a strong rationale for targeting both increased bone resorption and decreased bone formation. Anti-resorptive therapies are well established, but the successful deployment of bone anabolic agents will represent a vital step forward.

References

1. Kyle, R. A. *et al.* Review of 1027 patients with newly diagnosed multiple myeloma. *Mayo Clin. Proc.* 2003;**78**:21–33.

2. Kariyawasan, C. C., Hughes, D. A., Jayatillake, M. M., Mehta, A. B. Multiple myeloma: causes and consequences of delay in diagnosis. *Q. J. M.* 2007;**100**:635–40.

3. Coleman, R. E. Skeletal complications of malignancy. *Cancer* 1997;**80**:1588–94.

4. Mundy, G. R., Raisz, L. G., Cooper, R. A., Schecter, G. P., Salmon, S. E. Evidence for the secretion of an osteoclast stimulating factor in myeloma. *N. Eng. J. Med.* 1974;**291**:1041–6.

5. Roodman, G. D. Interleukin-6: an osteotropic factor? *J. Bone Miner. Res.* 1992;**7**:475–8.

6. Bataille, R. *et al.* Recruitment of new osteoblasts and osteoclasts is the earliest critical event in the pathogenesis of human multiple

myeloma. *J. Clin. Invest.* 1991;**88**:62–6.

7. Bataille, R., Chappard, D., Basle, M. Excessive bone resorption in human plasmacytomas: direct induction by tumour cells in vivo. *Br. J. Haematol.* 1995;**90**:721–4.

8. Bataille, R., Chappard, D., Basle, M. F. Quantifiable excess of bone resorption in monoclonal gammopathy is an early symptom of malignancy: a prospective study of 87 bone biopsies. *Blood* 1996;**87**:4762–9.

9. Croucher, P. I., Apperley, J. F. Bone disease in multiple myeloma. *Br. J. Haematol.* 1998;**103**:902–10.

10. Taube, T. *et al.* Abnormal bone remodelling in patients with myelomatosis and normal biochemical indices of bone resorption. *Eur. J. Haematol.* 1992;**49**:192–8.

11. Cozzolino, F. *et al.* Production of interleukin-1 by bone marrow myeloma cells. *Blood* 1989;**74**:380–7.

12. Kawano, M. *et al.* Interleukin-1 beta rather than lymphotoxin as the major bone resorbing activity in human multiple myeloma. *Blood* 1989;**73**:1646–9.

13. Yamamoto, I. *et al.* Production of interleukin 1 beta, a potent bone resorbing cytokine, by cultured human myeloma cells. *Cancer Res.* 1989;**49**:4242–6.

14. Lowik, C. W. *et al.* Parathyroid hormone (PTH) and PTH-like protein (PLP) stimulate interleukin-6 production by osteogenic cells: a possible role of interleukin-6 in osteoclastogenesis. *Biochem. Biophys. Res. Commun.* 1989;**162**:1546–52.

15. Ishimi, Y. *et al.* IL-6 is produced by osteoblasts and induces bone resorption. *J. Immunol.* 1990;**145**:3297–303.

16. Paul, S. R., Bennett, F., Calvetti, J. A., *et al.* Molecular cloning of a cDNA encoding interleukin 11, a stromal cell-derived lymphopoietic and haematopoietic cytokine. *Proc. Natl Acad. Sci. USA* 1990;**98**:581–6.

17. Lichtenstein, A., Berenson, J., Norman, D., Chang, M. P., Carlile, A. Production of cytokines by bone marrow cells obtained from patients with multiple myeloma. *Blood* 1989;**74**:1266–73.

18. Garrett, I. R. *et al.* Production of lymphotoxin, a bone-resorbing cytokine, by cultured human myeloma cells. *N. Engl. J. Med.* 1987;**317**:526–32.

19. Bataille, R., Klein, B., Jourdan, M., Rossi, J. F., Durie, B. G. Spontaneous secretion of tumor necrosis factor-beta by human myeloma cell lines. *Cancer* 1989;**63**:877–80.

20. Wolpe, S. D. *et al.* Macrophages secrete a novel heparin-binding protein with inflammatory and neutrophil chemokinetic properties. *J. Exp. Med.* 1988;**167**:570–81.

21. Kukita, T. *et al.* Macrophage inflammatory protein-1 alpha (LD78) expressed in human bone marrow: its role in regulation of hematopoiesis and osteoclast recruitment. *Lab. Invest.* 1997;**76**:399–406.

22. Lacey, D. L. *et al.* Osteoprotegerin ligand is a cytokine that regulates osteoclast differentiation and activation. *Cell* 1998; **93**:165.

23. Hsu, H. *et al.* Tumor necrosis factor receptor family member RANK mediates osteoclast differentiation and activation induced by osteoprotegerin ligand. *Proc. Natl Acad. Sci. USA* 1999;**96**:3540–5.

24. Simonet, W. S. *et al.* Osteoprotegerin: a novel secreted protein involved in the regulation of bone density. *Cell* 1997; **89**:309.

25. Choi, S. J. *et al.* Macrophage inflammatory protein 1-alpha is a potential osteoclast stimulatory factor in multiple myeloma. *Blood* 2000;**96**:671–5.

26. Giuliani, N., Bataille, R., Mancini, C., Lazzaretti, M., Barille, S. Myeloma cells induce imbalance in the osteoprotegerin/ osteoprotegerin ligand system in the human bone marrow environment. *Blood* 2001;**98**:3527–33.

27. Seidel, C. *et al.* Serum osteoprotegerin levels are reduced in patients with multiple myeloma with lytic bone disease. *Blood* 2001;**98**:2269–71.

28. Terpos, E. *et al.* Soluble receptor activator of nuclear factor kappaB ligand-osteoprotegerin ratio predicts survival in multiple myeloma: proposal for a novel prognostic index. *Blood* 2003;**102**:1064–9.

29. Heider, U. *et al.* Expression of receptor activator of nuclear factor kappaB ligand on bone marrow plasma cells correlates with osteolytic bone disease in patients with multiple myeloma. *Clin. Cancer Res.* 2003;**9**: 1436–40.

30. Sezer, O., Heider, U., Jakob, C., Eucker, J., Possinger, K. Human bone marrow myeloma cells express RANKL. *J. Clin. Oncol.* 2002;**20**:353–4.

31. Shaughnessy, J. D., Jr., Barlogie, B. Interpreting the molecular biology and clinical behavior of multiple myeloma in the context of global gene expression profiling. *Immunol. Rev.* 2003;**194**:140–63.

32. Giuliani, N. *et al.* Human myeloma cells stimulate the receptor activator of nuclear factor-kappa B ligand (RANKL) in T lymphocytes: a potential role in multiple myeloma bone disease. *Blood* 2002;**100**:4615–21.

33. Choi, S. J. *et al.* Antisense inhibition of macrophage inflammatory protein 1-alpha

88. McCloskey, E. V. *et al.* A randomized trial of the effect of clodronate on skeletal morbidity in multiple myeloma. MRC Working Party on Leukaemia in Adults. *Br. J. Haematol.* 1998;**100**:317–25.

89. Gimsing, P. *et al.* Effect of pamidronate 30 mg versus 90 mg on physical function in patients with newly diagnosed multiple myeloma (Nordic Myeloma Study Group): a double-blind, randomised controlled trial. *Lancet Oncol.* 2010;**11**: 973–82.

90. Rosen, L. S. *et al.* Long-term efficacy and safety of zoledronic acid compared with pamidronate disodium in the treatment of skeletal complications in patients with advanced multiple myeloma or breast carcinoma: a randomized, double-blind, multicenter, comparative trial. *Cancer* 2003;**98**:1735–44.

91. Morgan, G. J. *et al.* First-line treatment with zoledronic acid as compared with clodronic acid in multiple myeloma (MRC Myeloma IX): a randomised controlled trial. *Lancet* 2010;**376**:1989–99.

92. Musto, P. *et al.* A multicenter, randomized clinical trial comparing zoledronic acid versus observation in patients with asymptomatic myeloma. *Cancer* 2008;**113**:1588–95.

93. Fleisch, H. Development of Bisphosphonates. *Breast Cancer Res.* 2001;**4**(1).

94. Mundy, G. R., Yoneda, T. Facilitation and suppression of bone metastasis. *Clin. Orthop. Relat. Res.* 1995;34–44.

95. van der Pluijm, G. *et al.* Bisphosphonates inhibit the adhesion of breast cancer cells to bone matrices in vitro. *J. Clin. Invest.* 1996;**98**:698–705.

96. Shipman, C. M., Croucher, P. I., Russell, R. G., Helfrich, M. H., Rogers, M. J. The bisphosphonate incadronate (YM175) causes apoptosis of human myeloma cells in vitro by inhibiting the mevalonate pathway. *Cancer Res.* 1998;**58**:5294–7.

97. Croucher, P. I., DeHendrik, R., Parry, M. J., *et al.* Zoledronic acid treatment of 5T2MM-bearing mice inhibits the development of myeloma bone disease: evidence for decreased osteolysis, tumour burden and angiogenesis, and increased survival. *J. Bone Miner. Res.* 2003;**18**:482–92.

98. Kunzmann, V., Bauer, E., Feurle, J., Tony, F. W. H.-P., Wilhelm, M. Stimulation of gamma delta T cells by aminobisphosphonates and induction of antiplasma cell activity in multiple myeloma. *Blood* 2000;**96**:384–92.

99. Neville-Webbe, H. L., Rostami-Hodjegan, A., Evans, C. A., Coleman, R. E., Holen, I. Sequence- and schedule-dependent enhancement of zoledronic acid induced apoptosis by doxorubicin in breast and prostate cancer cells. *Int. J. Cancer* 2005;**113**:364–71.

100. Neville-Webbe, H. L., Evans, C. A., Coleman, R. E., Holen, I. Mechanisms of the synergistic interaction between the bisphosphonate zoledronic acid and the chemotherapy agent paclitaxel in breast cancer cells in vitro. *Tumour Biol.* 2006;**27**: 92–103.

101. Vogt, U., Bielawski, K. P., Bosse, U., Schlotter, C. M. Breast tumour growth inhibition in vitro through the combination of cyclophosphamide/methotrexate/5-fluorouracil, epirubicin/cyclophosphamide, epirubicin/paclitaxel, and epirubicin/docetaxel with the bisphosphonates ibandronate and zoledronic acid. *Oncol. Rep.* 2004;**12**:1109–14.

102. Ottewell, P. D. *et al.* Anticancer mechanisms of doxorubicin and zoledronic acid in breast cancer tumor growth in bone. *Mol. Cancer Ther.* 2009;**8**:2821–32.

103. Dimopoulos, M. A. *et al.* Osteonecrosis of the jaw in patients with multiple myeloma treated with bisphosphonates: evidence of increased risk after treatment with zoledronic acid. *Haematologica* 2006;**91**: 968–71.

104. Zervas, K. *et al.* Incidence, risk factors and management of osteonecrosis of the jaw in patients with multiple myeloma: a single-centre experience in 303 patients. *Br. J. Haematol.* 2006;**134**:620–3.

105. Rajkumar, S. V. Zoledronic acid in myeloma: MRC Myeloma IX. *Lancet* 2010;**376**:1965–6.

106. Henry, D. H. *et al.* Randomized, double-blind study of denosumab versus zoledronic acid in the treatment of bone metastases in patients with advanced cancer (excluding breast and prostate cancer) or multiple myeloma. *J. Clin. Oncol.* 2011;**29**: 1125–32.

107. Body, J. J. *et al.* A phase I study of AMGN-0007, a recombinant osteoprotegerin construct, in patients with multiple myeloma or breast carcinoma related bone metastases. *Cancer* 2003;**97**: 887–92.

108. Rabin, N. *et al.* A new xenograft model of myeloma bone disease demonstrating the efficacy of human mesenchymal stem cells expressing osteoprotegerin by lentiviral gene transfer. *Leukemia* 2007;**21**:2181–91.

109. Heath, D. J. *et al.* An osteoprotegerin-like peptidomimetic inhibits osteoclastic bone resorption and osteolytic bone disease in myeloma. *Cancer Res.* 2007;**67**:202–8.

110. Vallet, S. *et al.* Activin A promotes multiple myeloma-induced osteolysis and is a promising target for myeloma bone disease.

Proc. Natl Acad. Sci. USA 2010;**107**(11):5124–9.

111. Chantry, A. D. *et al.* Inhibiting activin-A signaling stimulates bone formation and prevents cancer-induced bone destruction in vivo. *J. Bone Miner. Res.* 2010;**25**:2357–70.

112. Yaccoby, S. Bone anabolism and tumour growth in myeloma. *Haematologica* 2011;**96**(s1).

113. Li, X., Pennisi, A., Yaccoby, S. Role of decorin in the antimyeloma

effects of osteoblasts. *Blood* 2008;**112**:159–68.

114. Pennisi, A. *et al.* Consequences of daily administered parathyroid hormone on myeloma growth, bone disease, and molecular profiling of whole myelomatous bone. *PLoS One* 2010;**5**:e15233.

115. Li, X. *et al.* Human placenta-derived adherent cells prevent bone loss, stimulate bone formation, and suppress growth of multiple myeloma in bone.

Stem Cells 2011;**29**: 263–73.

116. Edwards C. M., Esparza, J., Oyajobi, B. O. *et al.* Lithium inhibits the development of myeloma bone disease in vivo (abstract). *J. Bone Miner. Res.* 2006; Abstracts 21, Suppl. 1.

117. Guiliani, N. Effect of new anti-myeloma drugs on bone microenvironment. *Haematologica* 2011; **96**(s1).

Chapter

9

Principles of pathway directed therapy

Yu-Tzu Tai and Kenneth C. Anderson

Introduction

One of the hallmarks of the malignant phenotype is the ability of cells to grow in an autonomous manner with minimal cell death. This has been linked to diverse machinery of the proliferative and/or survival signaling pathways that become constitutively activated or deregulated in all human cancers. The proto-oncogenic driver mutations of Ras (H-, N-, K-ras, depending on tissue origin) or Raf gene are frequently tied to constitutive mitogen activated protein kinases (MAPK)/the extracellular signal regulated kinase (ERK1/2) signaling in a variety of tumors (Figure 9.1). Since the ERK signaling pathway is involved in both physiological and pathological cell proliferation, ERK1/2 inhibitors represent a desirable class of anti-neoplastic agents. Accumulating results have independently supported the promising anti-cancer effects of this class of inhibitor in numerous pre-clinical and clinical studies, i.e. CI-1040 [1], selumetinib (AZD6244) [2–4], AS703026[5] and GSK1120212 [6]. In fact, the MEK1/2 inhibitor CI-1040 (Pfizer) was the first signal transduction inhibitor tested in clinical trials in various advanced solid tumors [7]. Although no MEK1/2 inhibitors are approved for clinical use, kinase inhibitors that also inhibit Raf and VEGFR kinases (e.g. Sorafenib inhibiting

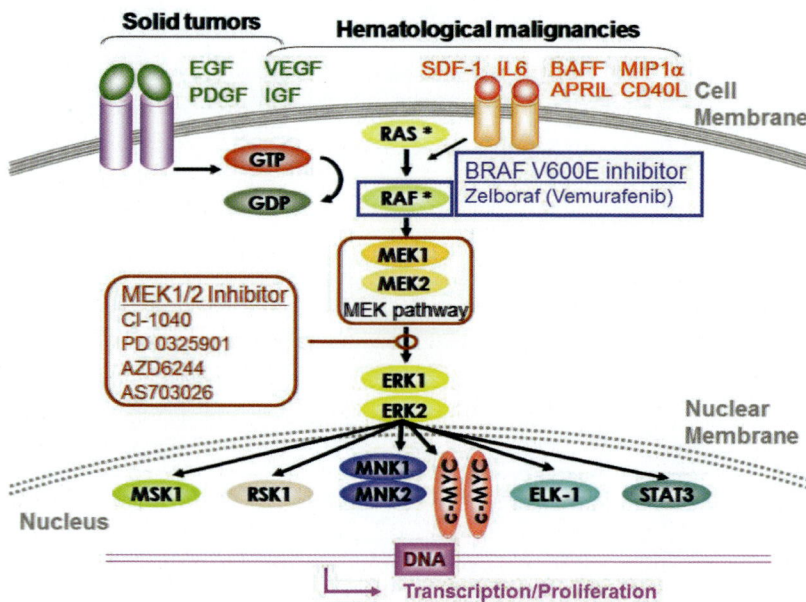

Figure 9.1 Therapeutic targeting mitogen activated protein kinase (MAPK) signaling cascades. Mitogens/growth/survival factors, upon binding to their cognate receptors frequently induce this signaling pathway in a variety of human cancers, supporting clinical development of specific inhibitors against individual components with identified genetic abnormalities. MEK1/2 inhibitors are under clinical evaluation, and specific BRAF V600E inhibition by Zelboraf/vemurafenib was the first FDA approved treatment for BRAF V600E mutation positive metastatic melanoma. Among further trials planned is the combination of vemurafenib with MEK1/2 inhibitor in this cancer.

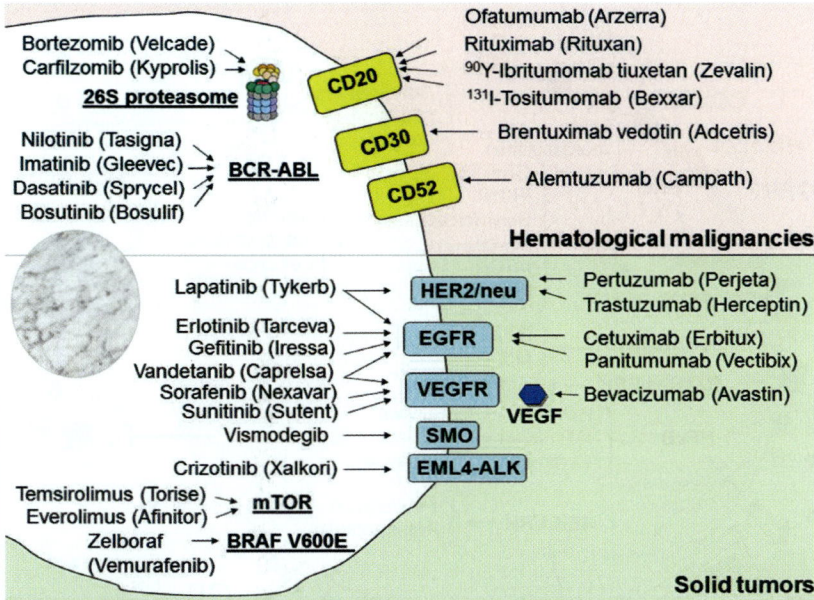

Figure 9.2 Current targeted cancer therapies approved by the FDA. Listed here are FDA-approved drugs, either small molecules (on the left) or monoclonal antibodies (on the right), which are targeted therapies to treat blood and solid cancers. They are based on the findings of commonly occurring oncogenic and abnormal surface receptors (shown in yellow and blue boxes) to constitutively augment signaling pathways predominantly regulated by tyrosine kinases. Targets in the cytoplasm are underlined, which include nonreceptor tyrosine kinases and 26S proteasomes. These targeted inhibitors block uncontrolled growth and survival of cancer cells via blockade of common downstream signaling cascades, i.e. MEK1/2, Akt, NFkB, and STAT3. They also directly induce cell death of tumors. For example, bortezomib and carfilzomib directly target 26 proteasomes and potently induce multiple myeloma cells to undergo apoptosis. Vismodegib is an inhibitor of Smoothened (SMO)-dependent Hedgehog signaling used in treating basal cell carcinoma [49].

multikinases) [8, 9] are successful anti-neoplastic agents against many types of cancer and FDA approved for the treatment of patients with unresectable hepatocellular carcinoma and advanced renal cell carcinoma [10, 11] (Figure 9.2). Such information support targeting this pathway, alone or in combination with other well-established growth and survival pathways, i.e. phosphoinositide 3-kinase (PI3K)/Akt/mTOR, STAT3, NFkB, heat shock proteins (Hsp90, Hsp70), histone deacetylases (HDAC), osteoblast (OB) as effective strategies across multiple cancers.

On the other hand, many studies have attempted to demonstrate that a given molecular mechanism is the key event involved in the pathogenesis of a specific cancer. Such information may not only provide a better understanding of cancer, but may also identify a novel target for therapeutic intervention. The best example is the mutation in B-Raf oncogene in >80% of melanoma, which has led to the development of the specific BRAF inhibitor zelboraf (vemurafenib) and successfully translated into the clinic. This inhibitor was approved for the treatment of metastatic melanoma harboring V600E mutation in 2011 [12] (Figure 9.2). Although also identified in human multiple myeloma (MM), only 7%–10% of MM patients have BRAF V600E mutation [13, 14] which might be targeted by this drug. Owing to the heterogeneity

of cancers, it is difficult to develop one such targeted therapy. This is especially true in MM, a malignancy of isotype-switched, bone marrow (BM)-localized plasma cells that frequently results in bone destruction, BM failure, and death. The molecular mechanisms underlying the development of this malignancy, which are complex and vary among individual tumors, include genetic and epigenetic alterations and resulting changes in the activity of signaling pathways. Specifically, BM stromal cells with defective OB differentiation are a major component of the MM niche, which produces various growth and anti-apoptotic factors for MM cells including IL-6, IGF-1, VEGF and SDF-1, while expressing the receptor activator of NFkB ligand (RANKL) to stimulate osteoclastogenesis (Figure 9.3). The BM microenvironment protects and supports MM cell proliferation, survival, and development of drug resistance [15]. In the era of targeted therapies, treatments combining a high specificity for neoplastic cells and the capability to interfere with environmental signals are most promising. Since there is no known genetic abnormality common to all patients with MM, it is crucial to understand how genetic heterogeneity in the BM milieu affects therapeutic responses, ultimately providing the framework for personalized medicine in MM.

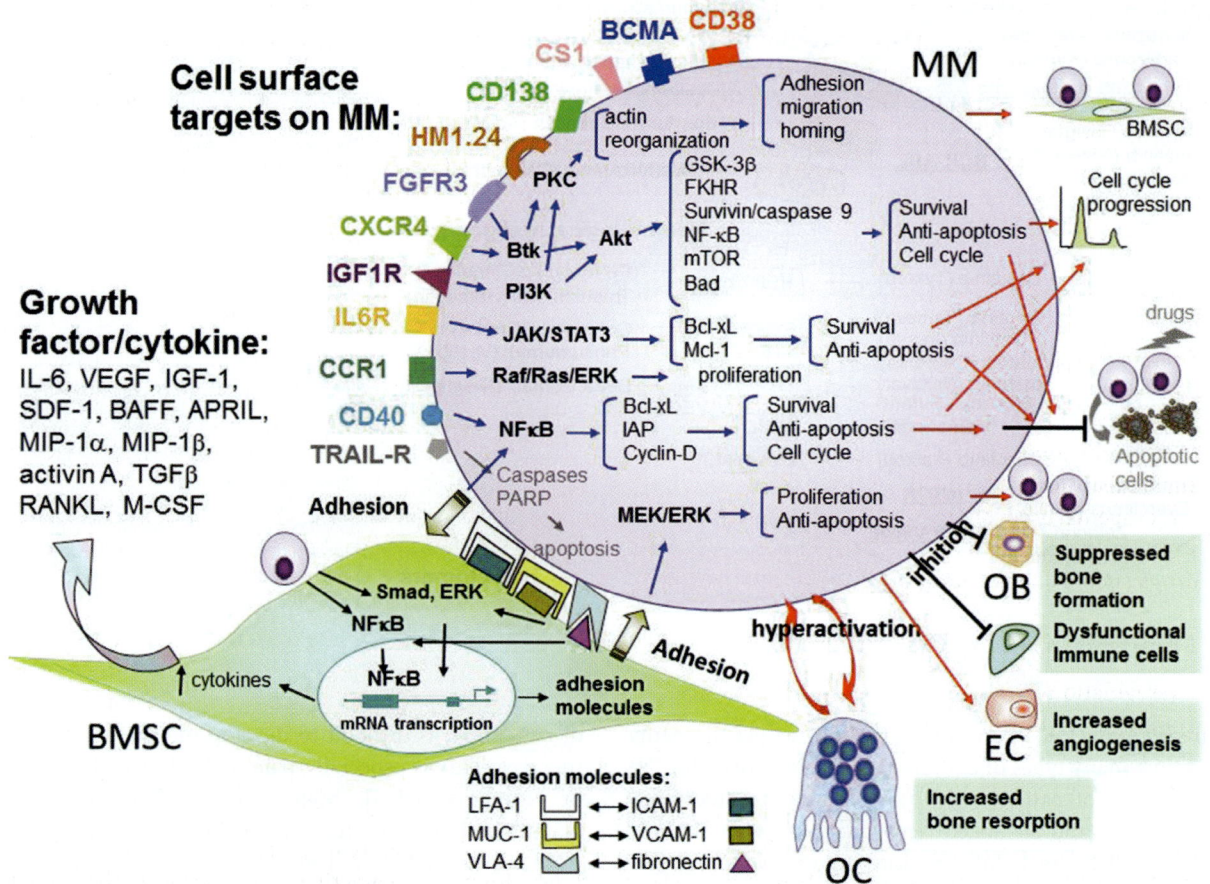

Figure 9.3 Complex interactions between tumor cell and its BM micro-environment in MM. Besides mutations in essential growth control genes within tumor cells, the BM micro-environment plays a pivotal role in tumor maintenance, progression and development of drug resistance. For example, growth and survival of human multiple myeloma (MM) cells in the bone marrow (BM) milieu are mediated via signaling cascades triggered by binding of receptors/antigens on MM cells and growth factors secreted by non-tumor cells, i.e. bone marrow stromal cells (BMSC), osteoclast (OC), osteoblast (OB), and endothelial cells (EC). BMSCs, inactive OB, over-reactive OC, increased angiogenesis induced by abnormal EC, and dysfunctional immune cells are major components of the MM niche. For example, BMSCs produce various growth and anti-apoptotic factors and cytokines for MM cells, i.e. IL-6, IGF-1, SDF1, BAFF, APRIL, as well as M-CSF, RANK ligand (RANKL), MIP-1α, TGFβ to stimulate OC differentiation leading to severe bone lysis. Elevated VEGF in MM enhances EC function and augments angiogenesis. Therapies which both directly target tumor cells and inhibit MM-promoting factors/cells in BM milieu are the most promising targets for future drug development, either as small molecules and/or monoclonal antibodies (mAb). Figure adapted [15].

Current key pathways for targeted therapeutics in cancers

MAPK and PI3K/Akt/mTOR signaling pathway

The MAPK/ERK1/2 pathway downstream of the IL-6 receptor family and other receptor tyrosine kinases (family of EGFR, VEGFR and IGFR) mediates cell proliferation, differentiation and survival (Figure 9.1). The PI3K/AKT/mammalian target of rapamycin (mTOR) pathway also plays a central role in cell proliferation, survival and motility, as well as angiogenesis and metabolism. This pathway often crosstalks with the MAPK/ERK1/2 pathway, which is stimulated by many MM growth and survival factors, i.e. IL-6, IGF-1, VEGF, APRIL, BAFF and SDF-1 (Figure 9.3). The PIK3CA gene encodes the PI3K catalytic subunit p110α, which is mutated in multiple cancers and results in constitutive activation of this pathway. Such mutations in breast cancer have been linked to resistance to therapy with anti-HER2 mAb trastuzumab [16]. On the other hand, when PTEN tumor suppressor gene is faulty or deficient, this pathway is activated in many cancer types. PI3K signaling also serves integral functions for non-cancerous cells in the tumor micro-environment. Consequently, therapeutics targeting the PI3K pathway are being developed at a rapid pace, and pre-clinical and early clinical studies are beginning to suggest specific strategies to use them effectively [17, 18]. However, the central role of PI3K signaling in a large array of diverse biologic processes also raises concerns about its use in therapeutics and increases the need to develop sophisticated strategies for its use. Some of these compounds target PI3K alone, while others target PI3K and mTOR [18, 19]. Promising results have been recently obtained with AKT inhibitors (perifosine) and mTOR inhibitors (everolimus and temsirolimus) in MM. However, the activity of these agents used alone is still limited, and can be strongly increased by their combination with other drugs such as bortezomib or dexamethasone [20].

Apoptosis signaling pathway

Dysregulation of apoptosis, the process of programmed cell death, plays a key role in tumorigenesis and resistance to anti-cancer treatments. This pathway is also governed by complex, gene-directed pathways. The rationale for targeting apoptosis in the treatment of cancers includes the overexpression of Bcl-2 protein family members like Bcl-2 and Mcl1 in many tumors, which confers resistance to chemotherapy. For example, there is a strong association of downregulation of Mcl1 with apoptosis induced by FDA approved and experimental drugs targeting multiple signaling pathways in MM. Loss of expression of the gene for the proapoptotic protein Bax and differential expression of tumor necrosis factor-related apoptosis-inducing ligand-receptor 2 have also been reported. In fact, the majority of drugs targeting pathways described in this chapter induce cancer cell death directly or indirectly via apoptosis.

Heat shock protein (Hsp) signaling pathway

Hsp90 is an ATP dependent molecular chaperone protein which integrates multiple oncogenic pathways. It acts as a regulator of many cancer-related receptors by functioning as a chaperone protein, binding to and maintaining client molecules in their active conformation. Hsp90 is overexpressed two- to tenfold in many human tumor cells and chaperones a number of cancer-related kinases, including HER2,

SRC, CRAF, CDK4 and WEE1. As such, Hsp90 inhibition is a promising anti-cancer strategy to target a diverse array of resistance mechanisms. For example, in resistance to BRAF inhibitors, it appears to be more effective at restoring BIM expression and down-regulating Mcl-1 expression than combined MEK/PI3K inhibitor therapy. There are many Hsp90 inhibitors currently under investigation [21]; to date, however, there is no FDA approved Hsp90 inhibitor nor standardized assay to ascertain Hsp90 inhibition [22]. Hsp90 inhibitor may be most active to treat cancers addicted to amplified, mutated or translocated driver oncogene products which are client proteins of Hsp90, including HER2, ALK, EGFR and BRAF. Additional cancers sensitive to Hsp90 inhibitors may include malignancies in which buffering of proteotoxic stress is essential for cancer cell survival, as exemplified by MM [23, 24]. Hsp90 is also a promising therapeutic target in JAK2-driven cancers, including those with genetic resistance to JAK enzymatic inhibitors [25].

Angiogenesis pathway

VEGF-A levels are increased in several hematologic malignancies in addition to many solid cancers [26]. Processes modulating VEGF secretion include: (A) secretion of IL-6, IGF-1, or VEGF by both BMSCs and tumor cells (paracrine/autocrine loop); (B) hypoxia and the presence of mutant oncogenes such as mutant Ras or BCR-Abl, up-regulating VEGF expression via HIF-1 protein); (C) c-maf–driven expression of tumor integrin; (D) tumor cell expression of ICAM1 and LFA1 modulating adhesion to ECM and BMSCs, thereby increasing VEGF production and secretion; and (E) CD40 activation, which induces p53-dependent VEGF secretion [27]. Furthermore, VEGFR-1 expression is regulated by IGF-1 via HIF-1. These data further support targeting angiogenesis via VEGF inhibition in cancers. Anti-VEGF antibody Bevacizumab (Avastin) was approved to treat multiple metastatic solid cancers in combination with chemotherapy (Figure 9.2).

The proteasome-ubiquitin pathway

Most intracellular proteins are degraded by the proteasome, a multicatalytic enzyme complex containing a 20S catalytic core and two 19S regulatory complexes. The ubiquitin-proteasome pathway plays a vital role in almost all cellular events, including cell cycle progression, transcription, DNA repair, signal transduction and immune response. Selective degradation of proteins by the ubiquitin-proteasome pathway is a critical determinant for maintaining cellular homeostasis. Thus, proteasome inhibition in cancer cells may lead to accumulation of pro-apoptotic target proteins followed by induction of cell death. In addition, ubiquitination (ligases) as well as deubiquitination (deubiquitylating enzymes, DUBs) offer numerous opportunities for therapeutic interventions for treating cancer, inflammation and metabolic diseases.

Drugs targeting the ubiquitin system are still relatively new. The first proteasome inhibitor approved by the FDA was velcade in MM in 2003 (Figure 9.2). Velcade is also the first successful targeted therapy against MM, which is now approved as frontline therapy as well as in relapsed refractory disease [28]. The clinical efficacy of velcade in MM and other hematologic malignancies (i.e. mantle cell lymphoma) provides the "proof of concept" that targeting the proteasome is a promising strategy for cancer treatment. Moreover, the approval of velcade for the treatment of MM has opened the way to the discovery of drugs targeting the proteasome and ubiquitinating and deubiquitinating enzymes, as well as the delivery system [29].

Multiple mechanisms mediate the anti-cancer activity induced by proteasome inhibition. Although velcade was quickly translated into clinical use to treat MM, its effect in solid tumors was less than encouraging. Additionally, dose-limiting toxicities, drug-resistance, and interference by some natural compounds hampered the extensive clinical use of velcade. These findings helped to guide physicians in refining the clinical use of velcade, and encouraged basic scientists to generate next-generation proteasome inhibitors that broaden the spectrum of efficacy and produce a more durable clinical response in cancer patients. Excitingly, second generation proteasome inhibitors carfilzomib (Kyprolis, Onyx) was approved by the FDA to treat velcade-resistant MM patients in July, 2012. Other members in the ubiquitin-proteasome pathway (i.e. E3 ligases, DUB USP7) have also emerged as novel therapeutic targets to directly induce MM cell death and overcome velcade resistance [29, 30]. Moreover, targeting cellular signaling pathways and targets such as the MAPK, PI3K/Akt, Hsp90/70 and HDAC pathways, in combination with proteasome inhibitors, predicted upon synergistic tumor cell cytotoxicity, holds great clinical promise.

Potential monocloncal antibody (mAb)-targeted therapies in MM

Although more than a dozen of monoclonal antibody (mAb)-targeted therapies have been approved for treating various solid and hematologic cancers (Figure 9.2), there is no mAb-based treatment modality approved for MM [31]. Nonetheless, many potential mAbs for MM are under intensive clinical development, either fully human mAbs or mAbs conjugated to chemoreagents (Figure 9.4). These mAb targets are either expressed on the surface of MM cells or ligands secreted in the BM microenvironment important for MM cell growth, survival and adhesion/migration (Figure 9.3). Drug-conjugated mAbs like huN901-DM1 (CD56), nBT062-maytansinoid (CD138), and Milatuzumab-DOX (CD74) directly induce specific killing against antigen-expressing target cells while sparing surrounding normal cells, as in the case of brentuximab (SGN-35, cAC10-vcMMAE DKK-1), the first antibody–drug conjugate approved to treat CD30-positive Hodgkin lymphoma (Figure 9.2).

Some potential mAb therapies block important signaling transduction in MM. For example, siltuximab (CNTO 328) and single-chain fragment NRI (a humanized anti-IL-6 receptor monoclonal antibody) inhibit IL-6-mediated phosphorylation of ERK1/2, STAT1, and STAT3 in myeloma cells. Lucatumumab (HCD122), an antagonistic anti-CD40 mAb, blocked CD40L-induced phosphorylation of AKT, IκBα, and ERK, thereby inhibiting CD40L-induced viability and growth in patient myeloma cells. Dalotuzumab acts by inhibiting IGF-1- and IGF-2-mediated tumor cell proliferation, IGFR1 autophosphorylation, and Akt phosphorylation. Anti-CD74 mAb milatuzumab (hLL-1), which lacks complement dependent cytotoxicity (CDC) or antibody-dependent cellular cytotoxicity (ADCC) activity, has been combined with a cross-linking antibody to induce direct cytotoxicity in vitro in chronic lymphocytic leukemia (CLL) and MM cells in vitro. In addition to inducing ADCC and CDC, daratumumab (CD38), when cross-linked in vitro, also triggers MM cell death via upregulating annexin V+ and annexin V+/PI+ MM cells and caspase 3/7 activation. Encouraging early responses with manageable toxicity has been reported in a recent phase I clinical trial of daratumumab, supporting further investigations in MM [23]. XmAb5592, a Fc-engineered HM1.24 human mAb, has enhanced binding to effector cells

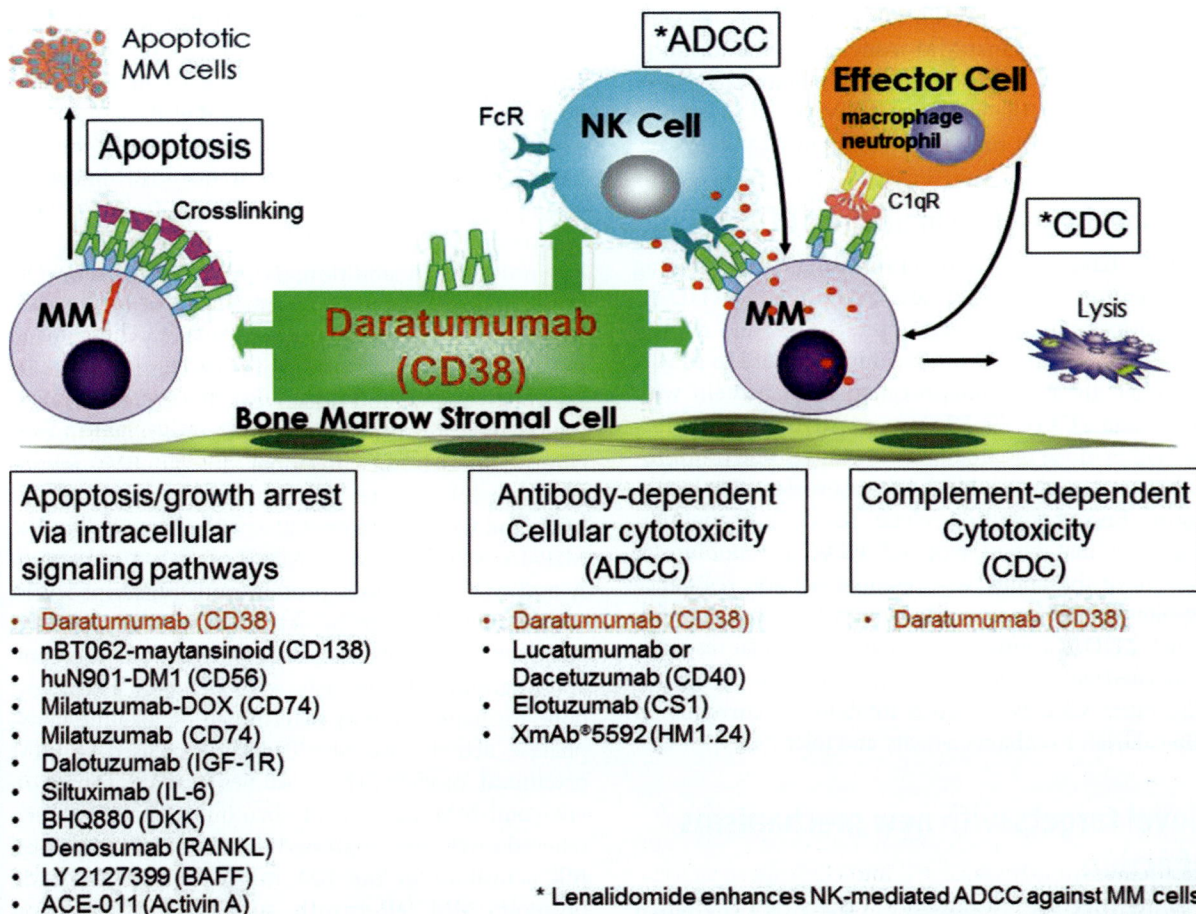

Figure 9.4 Potential monoclonal antibody (mAb)-based targeted therapies against MM. Therapeutic mAbs mediate antibody-dependent cellular cytotoxicity (ADCC) or complement-mediated cytotoxicity (CDC), and can also directly inhibit growth or trigger apoptotic signaling pathways [31]. They are designed to target receptors/cell surface proteins and extracellular factors in Figure 9.2. Although no mAb therapy for MM is approved by the FDA, many of mAbs have been evaluated in preclinical studies and clinical trials. For example, shown here are cellular mechanisms whereby anti-CD38 mAb Daratumumab kills MM cells, alone and in the contact with BMSCs. It has shown great promise with manageable toxicity in relapsed refractory MM [23]. Immunomodulatory reagents, i.e. lenalidomide, enhance natural killer/ NK-mediated ADCC and CDC to eliminate MM cells and the combination of elotuzumab, lenalidomide and low-dose dexamethasone has shown encouraging response rates in recent clinical trials [50].

(e.g. NK, macrophage) and demonstrated superior MM cell lysis than HM1.24 mAb with normal human Fc, both *in vivo* and *in vitro* [32]. Another Fc-engineered mAbs targeting B cell maturation antigen (BCMA), either as a naked Ab or drug conjugate, also hold great promise against all MM cells since this antigen is very highly and selectively expressed on patient MM cells (Tai *et al.*, unpublished data).

In addition, MM is commonly associated with bone destruction due to overactive osteoclasts (OC) and severely inhibited OB. Since OCs are largely regulated by RANKL, the fully human anti-RANKL mAb denosumab, FDA approved to treat osteoporosis, could

also be effective treatment to target against MM-related bone lysis. Indeed, denosumab suppressed the bone turnover marker serum C-terminal telopeptide of type I collagen in a phase 2 study of patients with plateau phase or relapsed MM and other solid tumors [31]. In addition, DKK is secreted in high levels in MM patients, thereby inhibiting activity of OB and impairing bone formation. BHQ880, a fully human anti-DKK1 mAb, both inactivated bone integrity and inhibited MM cell growth in the SCID-hu model of human MM. MAbs against BAFF (LY 2127399) and activin A (RAP-011) have also been shown to block OC function and improve bone formation in preclinical studies [33]. Finally, mAbs directed against MM-associated adhesion molecule are under therapeutic development, since they could neutralize the ability of the MM cell to bind to the protective BM micro-environment.

Histone deacetylase inhibition (HDACi)

HDACs have proven to be a promising target for drug intervention, and there are a number of HDAC inhibitors being tested in the pre-clinical and clinical stages [34]. One of the unique opportunities in MM is to target the aggresomal breakdown of protein with either pan HDAC or HDAC6 selective inhibitors [35, 36], either alone or combination with velcade (bortezomib) to concomitantly block Proteasomal protein breakdown. Encouragingly, a phase III clinical trial has suggested that blood type 1,2 HDACi panobinostat may have the ability to overcome velcade resistance despite limited single-agent activity [37], but another type 1, 2 HDACi vorinostat trial showed similar response associated with fatigue, diarrhea, and thrombocytopenia. The more selective HDAC6 inhibitor is currently in clinical trials to enhance activity and tolerability.

Novel targets with new mechanisms of action

Targeting B cell receptor via Bruton's tyrosine kinase (Btk) in hematological malignancies

Btk was first identified in immunodeficient X-linked agammaglobulinemia (XLA) patients, since mutations of this gene cause defective B cell maturation and prevent immunoglobulin secretion. Btk is an essential component of B cell receptor (BCR) signaling pathway and Fcγ Receptor (FcγR) signaling in B cells and myeloid cells, respectively. Upon ligand–receptor binding, Btk, a non-receptor tyrosine kinase, is phosphorylated. Subsequently, phosphorylation of downstream PLCγ, leads to activation of MAPK, NFκB, AKT and STAT3 signaling pathways which regulate growth and survival, as well as cytokine/chemokine secretion. It is a very promising tyrosine kinase inhibitor target in B cell malignancies. The first therapeutic Btk inhibitor ibrutinib (formally PCI-32765), which is orally available and irreversibly binds to Btk with excellent pharmacodyamics, has shown remarkable efficacy with an acceptable safety profile in various B cell malignancies. Phase III clinical

trials in mantle cell lymphoma and chronic lymphocytic leukemia (CLL) are ongoing for FDA approval and it has great promise, either as a single agent or in combination, in other B cell malignancies as well.

In addition, a novel and selective role for Btk has been identified in OC, but not OB, differentiation [38]. Increased expression of Lyn and Syk (upstream of Btk), as well as Src, was found in OC, but not OB. In addition, NFATc1, the major OC transcriptional factor activated following RANKL stimulation, was further upregulated by Btk during OC maturation. Since myeloma is characterized by hyperactive OC and inactive OB, the therapeutic potential of ibrutinib was recently examined in preclinical models of myeloma in its BM micro-environment (Figure 9.5). Ibrutinib potently blocks MM- and OC-related cytokines and chemokines IL-6, MIP-1α, MIP-1β, SDF-1, ARPIL, BAFF, IL-8, activin A and M-CSF at both protein and transcript levels. Importantly, Btk can be activated by SDF-1 in MM cells, and Ibrutinib blocks SDF-1-induced adhesion and migration of MM cells, as in CLL [40]. Excitingly, bone formation activity determined by alkaline phosphatase activity was significantly increased in MM preclinical models. These studies also confirmed *in vivo* anti-MM activity of ibrutinib, which in turn relieved myeloma-suppressed osteoblastogenesis. Thus, Btk activation in the BM milieu not only directly promotes MM cell growth, survival, and interaction with other BM stromal components, but also triggers MM-induced bone lysis. Based upon these data, Btk inhibitors are under clinical evaluation in myeloma.

Waldenstrom's macroglobulinemia (WM) cells express CD19 and B cell receptor (BCR), which mediate growth and survival; and Ibrutinib induces direct cytotoxicity in WM [39]. Moreover, the recently identified MyD88 L265P mutation in 90% WM cells promotes survival of WM cells by activation of Btk [41, 42], further confirming potential clinical benefit of targeting this pathway. Finally, Ibrutinib-inhibited IRF4 activity induced by MyD88 mutation in diffuse large B cell lymphoma [42, 43] further suggest its clinical promise in this setting.

Blocking traffic at the nuclear border via CRM1 inhibition

Mis-localization and disruption of important functions of proteins, especially tumor suppressor proteins (TSP), within the cells, allows cancers to develop, grow

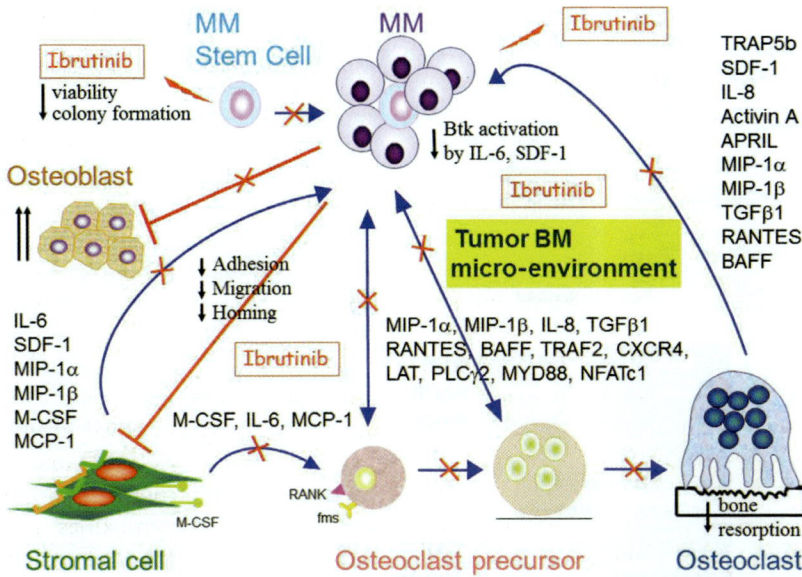

Figure 9.5 Bruton's tyrosine kinase (Btk) inhibition targeting MM cells and the MM BM micro-environment. Treatment with the Btk inhibitor Ibrutinib blocks MM cell growth and survival both by potent blockade of cytokine/chemokine secretion from non-tumor cell components within the BM, and by direct inhibition in tumor cells [39]. Furthermore, Btk inhibition specifically impairs osteoclastogenesis, but not osteoblastogenesis [51]. Drugs targeting Btk, as well as upstream Syk and Lyn, thus represent promising novel therapeutic strategy targeting tumors in the bone marrow (BM) micro-environment in MM and B cell lymphoid malignancies [52].

and survive. CRM1 (XPO1, exportin), the key nuclear chaperon belonging to the karyopherin-β family, transports these TSPs from nucleus into the cytoplasm via binding to the leucine-rich nuclear export signal (NES) in its cargo proteins (Figure 9.6a). An increasingly large number of CRM1-dependent cargo proteins are associated with cancers, since they are important tumor suppressor proteins and transcription factors. For example, CRM1 cargo proteins include p53, p21, topoisomerase II, IκBα/NFκB, NPM, RB, FOXO and BRCA1 [44]. The rationale targeting CRM1 with a new class of cancer drugs is to block the export of these proteins out of the nucleus. Ideally, CRM1 inhibitors can sequester CRM1-target proteins in the nucleus, thereby enhancing cell cycle arrest and apoptosis.

Visual, high-throughput and high-content small molecule screens have identified molecules targeting CRM1. The key contact residues required for the formation of the CRM1-cargo export complex have been resolved [45], and the molecular understanding of the CRM1-cargo binding interface has led to the development of novel small molecule inhibitors of CRM1-cargo interaction with KPT-selective inhibitors of nuclear export (SINE). SINEs are potent, drug-like CRM1 inhibitors that irreversibly inactivate CRM1-directed protein export by covalent modification of essential CRM1-cargo binding residue Cys528. SINEs were recently tested in a broad range of hematological and solid cancers with excellent potency but not apparent toxicity against normal hematopoietic cells [46].

Most recently, a novel role of CRM1 in the pathogenesis of MM was confirmed. Specifically, CRM1 shRNA knockdown leads to MM cell death [47], consistent with a recent report of druggable targets in MM [48]. Importantly, SINE treatment of MM with a variety of genetic alterations and drug sensitivities induced potent and rapid apoptosis [47]. In addition to activating multiple TSPs, SINEs unexpectedly induced a reduction in c-myc and in NFkB activity, known oncogenic drivers in MM and many other tumors. Finally, SINEs showed potent anti-MM activity in an orthotopic *in vivo* model, reducing both tumor burden and osteolytic lesions. This study is also the first to demonstrate a clear and direct effect of SINE on OC formation, at least in part by modulating NFkB activity triggered in OC precursor cells by RANKL stimulation [47]. In contrast, SINEs had no effect on osteoblastogenesis and were not toxic to non-malignant BM accessory cells, i.e. BMSCs, OB. The potent MM cytotoxicity and prolonged host survival demonstrated in our orthotopic MM model, coupled with these beneficial bone effects, provide support for ongoing clinical trials targeting CRM1 with SINE (KPT-330) in MM and other hematologic malignancies.

Conclusions and future directions

During the past two decades, the paradigm for cancer treatment has evolved from relatively nonspecific cytotoxic agents to selective, mechanism-based

(a)

(b)

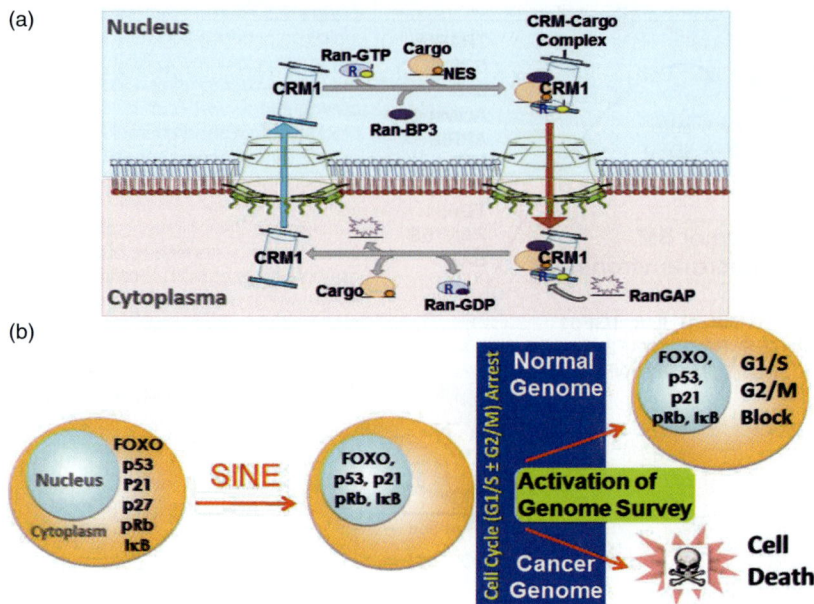

Figure 9.6 Curtailing nuclear transport protein CRM1 in cancer therapies. (a) CRM1 (XPO1, exportin) is the major nuclear export protein which shuttles multiple protein cargoes from the nucleus to the cytoplasm. Specifically, protein cargoes with a canonical leucine-rich nuclear export sequence (NES) require transport through the nuclear pore. CRM1 forms a complex with the protein cargo, RanGTP and RanBP3 for export. Once traversing the nuclear pore, hydrolysis of GTP catalyzed by RanGAP leads to dissociation of the complex, and CRM1 is recycled. (b) Selective inhibitors of nuclear export (SINEs) targeting CRM1 block transport of CRM1-directed client proteins with tumor suppressing activity to the cytoplasm, augmenting their function in the nucleus. These new drugs potently induce growth arrest and preferentially induce tumor cell. For example, these compounds have potent anti-tumor activity in MM, sparing normal hematopoietic cells, bone marrow stromal cells, and osteoblasts. SINEs have shown impressive effects across all cancer types, with ongoing clinial trials cancers including MM to define their efficacy (Clinical Trial NCT01607892).

therapeutics. Novel targeted therapies offer an attractive approach to the future treatment of cancers including MM, with the prospect of individualized therapy based on the genetic expression profiles of individual patient's tumors. However, there are many unanswered questions regarding optimal treatment and long-term management, i.e. MM patients with targeted agents like velcade. Future studies will need to address how best to incorporate targeted agents into existing treatment regimens, to identify those patient subgroups likely to derive most benefit from a given therapy, and to determine when and in which combinations targeted therapy should be administered. For example, MM patients with translocations affecting the MAF family of transcription factors, del17p, or gene-expression profiling-defined high-risk disease have a worse prognosis that is not dramatically improved by current targeted therapies. In this setting, inhibitors targeting Hsp90, HDAC, and most recently, CRM1 have demonstrated potent anti-tumor activities in preclinical models. Therefore, innovative clinical trials with these novel targeted agents should enroll these high-risk patients. Identifying biomarkers predictive will be key, as well as defining combinations based upon blocking multiple signaling pathways. Figuring out when best to test these agents, early or late in the disease course, will also is critical. Finally, mAb based immunotherapeutic approaches are now offering unique treatment opportunities for MM and other cancers.

References

1. Barrett SD, Bridges AJ, Dudley DT, et al. The discovery of the benzhydroxamate MEK inhibitors CI-1040 and PD 0325901. *Bioorg Med Chem Lett.* 2008;**18**:6501–6504.

2. Tai YT, Fulciniti M, Hideshima T, et al. Targeting MEK induces myeloma-cell cytotoxicity and inhibits osteoclastogenesis. *Blood.* 2007;**110**:1656–1663.

3. Kirkwood JM, Bastholt L, Robert C, et al. Phase II, open-label, randomized trial of the MEK1/2 inhibitor selumetinib as monotherapy versus temozolomide in patients with advanced melanoma. *Clin Cancer Res.* 2012;**18**:555–567.

4. Banerji U, Camidge DR, Verheul HM, et al. The first-in-human study of the hydrogen sulfate (Hyd-sulfate) capsule of the MEK1/2 inhibitor AZD6244 (ARRY-142886): a phase I open-label multicenter trial in patients with advanced cancer. *Clin Cancer Res.* 2010;**16**:1613–1623.

5. Yoon J, Koo KH, Choi KY. MEK1/2 inhibitors AS703026 and AZD6244 may be potential therapies for KRAS mutated colorectal cancer that is resistant to EGFR monoclonal

antibody therapy. *Cancer Res.* 2011;**71**:445–453.

6. Gilmartin AG, Bleam MR, Groy A, et al. GSK1120212 (JTP-74057) is an inhibitor of MEK activity and activation with favorable pharmacokinetic properties for sustained in vivo pathway inhibition. *Clin Cancer Res.* 2011;**17**:989–1000.

7. Rinehart J, Adjei AA, Lorusso PM, et al. Multicenter phase II study of the oral MEK inhibitor, CI-1040, in patients with advanced non-small-cell lung, breast, colon, and pancreatic cancer. *J Clin Oncol.* 2004;**22**:4456–4462.

8. Adnane L, Trail PA, Taylor I, Wilhelm SM. Sorafenib (BAY 43-9006, Nexavar), a dual-action inhibitor that targets RAF/MEK/ERK pathway in tumor cells and tyrosine kinases VEGFR/PDGFR in tumor vasculature. *Methods Enzymol.* 2006;**407**:597–612.

9. Wilhelm SM, Adnane L, Newell P, Villanueva A, Llovet JM, Lynch M. Preclinical overview of sorafenib, a multikinase inhibitor that targets both Raf and VEGF and PDGF receptor tyrosine kinase signaling. *Mol Cancer Ther.* 2008;**7**:3129–3140.

10. Messmer D, Fecteau JF, O'Hayre M, Bharati IS, Handel TM, Kipps TJ. Chronic lymphocytic leukemia cells receive RAF-dependent survival signals in response to CXCL12 that are sensitive to inhibition by sorafenib. *Blood.* 2011;**117**:882–889.

11. Widemann BC, Kim A, Fox E, et al. A phase I trial and pharmacokinetic study of the Raf kinase and receptor tyrosine kinase inhibitor sorafenib in children with refractory solid tumors or refractory leukemias. *Clin Cancer Res.* 2012.

12. Flaherty KT, Yasothan U, Kirkpatrick P. Vemurafenib. *Nat Rev Drug Discov.* 2011;**10**:811–812.

13. Kim K, Kong SY, Fulciniti M, et al. Blockade of the MEK/ERK signalling cascade by AS703026, a novel selective MEK1/2 inhibitor, induces pleiotropic anti-myeloma activity in vitro and in vivo. *Br J Haematol.* 2010;**149**:537–549.

14. Chapman MA, Lawrence MS, Keats JJ, et al. Initial genome sequencing and analysis of multiple myeloma. *Nature.* 2011;**471**:467–472.

15. Hideshima T, Mitsiades C, Tonon G, Richardson PG, Anderson KC. Understanding multiple myeloma pathogenesis in the bone marrow to identify new therapeutic targets. *Nat Rev Cancer.* 2007;**7**:585–598.

16. Berns K, Horlings HM, Hennessy BT, et al. A functional genetic approach identifies the PI3K pathway as a major determinant of trastuzumab resistance in breast cancer. *Cancer Cell.* 2007;**12**:395–402.

17. Woyach JA, Johnson AJ, Byrd JC. The B-cell receptor signaling pathway as a therapeutic target in CLL. *Blood.* 2012;**120**:1175–1184.

18. Baumann P, Mandl-Weber S, Oduncu F, Schmidmaier R. The novel orally bioavailable inhibitor of phosphoinositol-3-kinase and mammalian target of rapamycin, NVP-BEZ235, inhibits growth and proliferation in multiple myeloma. *Exp Cell Res.* 2009;**315**:485–497.

19. Leung E, Kim JE, Rewcastle GW, Finlay GJ, Baguley BC. Comparison of the effects of the PI3K/mTOR inhibitors NVP-BEZ235 and GSK2126458 on tamoxifen-resistant breast cancer cells. *Cancer Biol Ther.* 2011;**11**:938–946.

20. Ghobrial IM, Weller E, Vij R, et al. Weekly bortezomib in combination with temsirolimus in relapsed or relapsed and refractory multiple myeloma: a multicentre, phase 1/2, open-label, dose-escalation study. *Lancet Oncol.* 2011;**12**:263–272.

21. Jhaveri K, Taldone T, Modi S, Chiosis G. Advances in the clinical development of heat shock protein 90 (Hsp90) inhibitors in cancers. *Biochim Biophys Acta.* 2012;**1823**:742–755.

22. Erlichman C. Tanespimycin: the opportunities and challenges of targeting heat shock protein 90. *Expert Opin Investig Drugs.* 2009;**18**:861–868.

23. Plesner T, Lokhorst HM, Gimsing P, Nahi H, Lisby S, Richardson P. Daratumumab, a CD38 mab, for the treatment of relapsed/refractory multiple myeloma patients: Preliminary efficacy data from a multicenter phase I/II study. *J Clin Oncol 30, 2012 (suppl; abstr 8019)* 2012.

24. Mitsiades CS, Hideshima T, Chauhan D, et al. Emerging treatments for multiple myeloma: beyond immunomodulatory drugs and bortezomib. *Semin Hematol.* 2009;**46**:166–175.

25. Allegra A, Sant'antonio E, Penna G, et al. Novel therapeutic strategies in multiple myeloma: role of the heat shock protein inhibitors. *Eur J Haematol.* 2011;**86**:93–110.

26. Ellis LM, Hicklin DJ. VEGF-targeted therapy: mechanisms of anti-tumour activity. *Nat Rev Cancer.* 2008;**8**:579–591.

27. Podar K, Tai YT, Hideshima T, Vallet S, Richardson PG, Anderson KC. Emerging therapies for multiple myeloma. *Expert Opin Emerg Drugs.* 2009;**14**:99–127.

28. Anderson KC. The 39th David A. Karnofsky Lecture: bench-to-bedside translation of targeted therapies in multiple myeloma. *J Clin Oncol.* 2012;**30**:445–452.

29. Chauhan D, Tian Z, Nicholson B, et al. A small molecule inhibitor of ubiquitin-specific protease-7 induces apoptosis in multiple myeloma cells and overcomes bortezomib resistance. *Cancer Cell.* 2012;**22**:345–358.

30. McMillin DW, Jacobs HM, Delmore JE, et al. Molecular and cellular effects of NEDD8-activating enzyme inhibition in myeloma. *Mol Cancer Ther.* 2012;**11**:942–951.

31. Tai YT, Anderson KC. Antibody-based therapies in multiple myeloma. *Bone Marrow Res.* 2011;**2011**:924058.

32. Tai YT, Horton HM, Kong SY, et al. Potent in vitro and in vivo activity of an Fc-engineered humanized anti-HM1.24 antibody against multiple myeloma via augmented effector function. *Blood.* 2012;**119**:2074–2082.

33. Raje N, Roodman GD. Advances in the biology and treatment of bone disease in multiple myeloma. *Clin Cancer Res.* 2011;**17**:1278–1286.

34. Hideshima T, Richardson PG, Anderson KC. Mechanism of action of proteasome inhibitors and deacetylase inhibitors and the biological basis of synergy in multiple myeloma. *Mol Cancer Ther.* 2011;**10**:2034–2042.

35. Hideshima T, Bradner JE, Wong J, et al. Small-molecule inhibition of proteasome and aggresome function induces synergistic antitumor activity in multiple myeloma. *Proc Natl Acad Sci U S A.* 2005;**102**:8567–8572.

36. Santo L, Hideshima T, Kung AL, et al. Preclinical activity, pharmacodynamic, and pharmacokinetic properties of a selective HDAC6 inhibitor, ACY-1215, in combination with bortezomib in multiple myeloma. *Blood.* 2012;**119**:2579–2589.

37. Stewart AK. Novel therapeutics in multiple myeloma. *Hematology.* 2012;**17 Suppl 1**:S105–108.

38. Shinohara M, Koga T, Okamoto K, et al. Tyrosine kinases Btk and Tec regulate osteoclast differentiation by linking RANK and ITAM signals. *Cell.* 2008;**132**:794–806.

39. de Rooij MF, Kuil A, Geest CR, et al. The clinically active BTK inhibitor PCI-32765 targets B-cell receptor- and chemokine-controlled adhesion and migration in chronic lymphocytic leukemia. *Blood.* 2012;**119**:2590–2594.

40. Tai YT, Chang BY, Kong SY, et al. Bruton tyrosine kinase inhibition is a novel therapeutic strategy targeting tumor in the bone marrow microenvironment in multiple myeloma. *Blood.* 2012;**120**:1877–1887.

41. Treon SP, Xu L, Yang G, et al. MYD88 L265P somatic mutation in Waldenstrom's macroglobulinemia. *N Engl J Med.* 2012;**367**:826–833.

42. Yang G, Xu L, Zhou Y, et al. Participation of BTK in MYD88 signaling in malignant cells expressing the L265P mutation in Waldenstrom's macroglobulinemia, and effect on tumor cells with BTK-inhibitor PCI-32765 in combination with MYD88 pathway inhibitors. *J Clin Oncol.* 2012 **30**:abstr 8106

43. Yang Y, Shaffer AL, 3rd, Emre NC, et al. Exploiting synthetic lethality for the therapy of ABC diffuse large B cell lymphoma. *Cancer Cell.* 2012;**21**:723–737.

44. Turner JG, Dawson J, Sullivan DM. Nuclear export of proteins and drug resistance in cancer. *Biochem Pharmacol.* 2012;**83**:1021–1032.

45. Xu D, Farmer A, Collett G, Grishin NV, Chook YM. Sequence and structural analyses of nuclear export signals in the NESdb database. *Mol Biol Cell.* 2012;**23**:3677–93.

46. Etchin J, Sun Q, Kentsis A, et al. Anti-leukemic activity of nuclear export inhibitors that spare normal hematopoietic cells. *Leukemia.* 2013;**27**:66–74.

47. Tai YT, Landesman Y, Acharya C, et al. The nuclear export protein CRM1 (exportin 1) regulates multiple myeloma cell growth, osteoclastogenesis, and myeloma-induced osteolysis. *Leukemia* 2013 Apr 16. doi: 10.1038/leu.2013.115. [Epub ahead of print]

48. Tiedemann RE, Zhu YX, Schmidt J, et al. Identification of molecular vulnerabilities in human multiple myeloma cells by RNA interference lethality screening of the druggable genome. *Cancer Res.* 2012;**72**:757–768.

49. Henkin RI. Vismodegib in advanced basal-cell carcinoma. *N Engl J Med.* 2012;**367**:970; author reply 970–971.

50. Lonial S, Vij R, Harousseau JL, et al. Elotuzumab in combination with lenalidomide and low-dose dexamethasone in relapsed or refractory multiple myeloma. *J Clin Oncol.* 2012;**30**:1953–1959.

51. Edwards CM. BTK inhibition in myeloma: targeting the seed and the soil. *Blood.* 2012;**120**:1757–1759.

52. Robak T, Robak E. Tyrosine kinase inhibitors as potential drugs for B-cell lymphoid malignancies and autoimmune disorders. *Expert Opin Investig Drugs.* 2012;**21**:921–947.

Chapter

10

Monoclonal gammopathy of undetermined significance (MGUS) and smoldering multiple myeloma

Efstathios Kastritis and Meletios A. Dimopoulos

The identification of a monoclonal protein in serum protein electrophoresis (SPEP) is a common event requiring medical consultation. A monoclonal protein may be the hallmark of a malignant disease, such as multiple myeloma or Waldenstrom's Macroglobulinemia (and less often of other lymphoproliferative disorders), of diseases associated with a malignant plasma cell clone, such as AL amyloidosis or other plasma cell related disorders, or, quite commonly may have no direct impact and belong to monoclonal gammopathies of undetermined significance (MGUS). Jan Waldenstrom introduced the term "essential hyperglobulinemia" in order to describe patients who had a small serum protein electrophoretic spike but no evidence of overt multiple myeloma (MM), Waldenstrom's macroglobulinemia (WM), primary amyloidosis (AL), or related disorders. The seminal work by Kyle indicated that some patients with this monoclonal gammopathy develop MM, or WM or AL or other lymphoproliferative malignancies, and introduced the term "monoclonal gammopathy of undetermined significance" (MGUS) [1]. Kyle also described patients with histologic and biochemical features of myeloma (bone marrow clonal plasma cells (BMPC) involvement of 10% or higher, presence of a serum M-protein value higher than 3 g/dl) that did not have lytic bone lesions, anemia, renal impairment or other clinical manifestations of myeloma who remained stable, with no need for chemotherapy, for several years [2]. Alexanian also presented data on "indolent myeloma" [3], that included patients who had no clinical features of overt myeloma such as anemia and renal dysfunction and had fewer than three lytic bone lesions. Among these patients, median time to initiation of chemotherapy was two years, but some patients remained stable for

several years. Thus, the term "smoldering" MM or "asymptomatic" or "indolent" MM, entered the clinical practice. The definitions, however, were not strict among different groups. In 2003 a consensus paper defined MGUS and asymptomatic or smoldering myeloma (Table 10.1). MGUS requires that M-protein in serum is <30 g/l and that bone marrow clonal plasma cells are <10% with no evidence of other B cell proliferative disorders and no end organ damage (anemia, renal impairment, hypercalcemia, lytic bone lesions). The diagnosis of asymptomatic MM requires the presence of an M protein in serum ≥30 g/l and/or bone marrow clonal plasma cells ≥10% but no related organ or tissue impairment (no end-organ damage, including bone lesions) or symptoms [5] (Table 10.1). These criteria have remained unchanged since then [4].

The importance of diagnostic definitions and further investigations of these entities lies in their "precursor" nature and their frequency. MGUS is a common "disorder," especially in older patients. These patients do not require therapy, but they have a small (but real) probability of developing a disease, such as MM or WM or AL amyloidosis or other lymphoproliferative disorder that will require treatment. Patients with asymptomatic (smoldering) myeloma do not require immediate therapy but they have a high probability to develop overt (symptomatic) myeloma that requires treatment within a few years of the diagnosis. Furthermore, epidemiological data indicate that MGUS may not be as "innocent" as it was considered but may be associated with an increase in the risk of osteoporosis or thromboembolism. Small plasma cell clones, otherwise considered as an MGUS, are also associated with diverse clinical syndromes varying from peripheral neuropathy to

Myeloma, ed. Stephen A. Schey, Kwee L. Yong, Robert Marcus and Kenneth C. Anderson. Published by Cambridge University Press. © Cambridge University Press 2014.

Table 10.1 Diagnostic criteria for MGUS and SMM

Monoclonal gammopathy of undetermined significance	• Serum monoclonal protein <3.0 g/dl and
	• monoclonal bone marrow plasma cells <10% and
	• no evidence of end-organ damage attributable to the clonal plasma cell disorder:
	    normal serum calcium, hemoglobin level and serum creatinine
	    no bone lesions on full skeletal X-ray survey and/or other imaging if performed
	    no clinical or laboratory features of amyloidosis or light chain deposition disease

Asymptomatic (smoldering) multiple myeloma	• Monoclonal protein present in the serum 3 g per 100 ml or higher or
	• monoclonal plasma cells 10% or greater present in the bone marrow and/or a tissue biopsy
	• no evidence of end-organ damage attributable to the clonal plasma cell disorder:
	    normal serum calcium, hemoglobin level and serum creatinine
	    no bone lesions on full skeletal X-ray survey and/or other imaging if performed
	    no clinical or laboratory features of amyloidosis or light chain deposition disease

more systemic diseases such as POEMS syndrome, Schnitzler's syndrome, and skin mucinosis such as scleromyxedema [6], but these will not be presented in this chapter.

MGUS

MGUS is a common finding and was recognized as such several years ago by Jan Waldenstrom and his group [7,8]: the presence of a monoclonal protein without MM, WM, AL, or a related plasma cell disorder has been reported in approximately 1% of persons older than 50 years of age and in about 3% of those older than 70 years in Sweden [9], Western France [10], and in northern Minnesota [11]. MGUS prevalence increases with age and the age-adjusted prevalence of MGUS in African-Americans was three-fold greater than in Caucasians [12]. Population-based studies have improved our insight into the significance and natural history of MGUS. In a study conducted by Kyle *et al.* in a defined geographic area (Olmsted county, Minessota, USA), serum samples from 21 463 of the 28 038 enumerated residents ≥50 years of age were obtained and a MGUS was identified in 694 (3.2%). Age-adjusted rates were

higher in men than in women (4% vs. 2.7%, P < 0.001) and the prevalence of MGUS was 5.3% among persons ≥70 years of age and 7.5% among those ≥85 years of age. Most persons with MGUS had a monoclonal protein less than 1.0 g /dl (63.5%) while only 4.5% had an M component ≥ 2.0 g/dl. Another significant observation was that uninvolved immunoglobulins were reduced in 27.7% of the persons and that 21.5% of those that were tested had a monoclonal urinary light chain [13]. The Mayo group, led by Dr. Kyle, has also investigated the prognosis of MGUS. In 2002 they reported the results of long term follow up of 1384 MGUS patients who were diagnosed at the Mayo Clinic from 1960 through 1994. During 11 009 person-years of follow-up, MGUS progressed in 115 of the 1384 patients to multiple myeloma, IgM lymphoma, primary amyloidosis, macroglobulinemia, chronic lymphocytic leukemia or plasmacytoma (relative risk of progression, 25, 2.4, 8.4, 46, 0.9 and 8.5, respectively). The overall relative risk of progression was 7.3 in these patients as compared with a similar population of a neighboring state. In 32 additional patients, the monoclonal protein concentration increased to more than 3 g/dl or the percentage of plasma cells in the bone marrow increased to >10% thus these patients were characterized as having a smoldering multiple myeloma, but without progression to overt myeloma or related disorders. The cumulative probability of progression was 12% at 10 years, 25% at 20 years, and 30% at 25 years, averaging a risk of progression to multiple myeloma or related disorders of about 1% per year. The authors identified the initial concentration of serum monoclonal protein as a significant predictor of progression at 20 years [14].

MGUS is not a homogeneous entity. A classification based on the monoclonal Ig type discriminates between IgM MGUS, non-IgM MGUS and light chain MGUS, a recently recognized entity [15]. These distinct types of MGUS differ in their biology and evolution. Non-IgM MGUS and light chain MGUS tend to evolve in to myeloma, while IgM MGUS tends to evolve to Waldenstrom's Macroglobulinemia or other lymphoproliferative disorders and only rarely to IgM myeloma. Immunophenotypic studies have shown that the aberrant cell in non-IgM and light chain MGUS is a plasma cell, while IgM MGUS is characterized by aberrant lymphoid cells with typical lymphoid markers (IgM+, CD5+/−, CD10+/−, CD19+, CD20+ and CD23+).

Two major papers published in 2008 provided solid evidence that an MGUS state almost always precedes multiple myeloma. In the first paper [16], using the database of a large screening program that included 77 469 healthy adults, 71 subjects were identified who developed MM during the course of the study and in whom pre-diagnostic serum samples were available, obtained two to ten years prior to MM diagnosis. A monoclonal immunoglobulin or light chain (by FLC assay) was present in all patients at two years before MM diagnosis and in 90%–98% at three to seven years before MM diagnosis. Furthermore, in half of the study population, the M-protein concentration and the involved FLC-ratio levels showed a yearly increase prior to MM diagnosis. Using a different data base, Weiss et al. [17] identified that a monoclonal immunoglobulin (either intact Ig or a light chain only Ig) was present in 27 out of 30 patients (90%) at least two years before the diagnosis of MM.

These two seminal papers indicate that MGUS always precedes MM as a pre-malignant precursor; however, only a minority will develop an overt malignant condition. Some patients have a relatively rapid evolution while others have a more insidious progression to overt myeloma. Thus, risk stratification, in order to identify MGUS patients at higher risk of development of a malignant disease, is necessary. Identification of those with a higher probability for developing symptomatic disease is based mainly on risk factors associated with tumor burden. The Mayo Clinic group identified the concentration and type of monoclonal protein (non-IgG) as independent predictors of progression while the presence of a monoclonal urinary light chain (kappa or lambda) or a reduction in one or more uninvolved immunoglobulins was not a risk factor for progression [14]. Later, in an attempt to improve prognostication, the Mayo Clinic group proposed a risk stratification system based on the presence of a non-IgG isotype, serum M protein concentration >1.5 g/dl, and abnormal FLC-ratio. Based on these three factors, absolute risk of progression for MGUS patients with zero, one, two and three risk factors was 5%, 21%, 37% and 58%, respectively at 20 years of follow-up [18]. A Italian study analyzed the outcomes of 1283 patients with IgG and IgA MGUS, separately by Ig subtype and in total [19]. In patients with IgG MGUS, serum monoclonal protein >1.5 g/dl, the presence of light chain proteinuria and abnormal (suppressed) serum polyclonal immunoglobulin levels were independent risk factors, with a hazard ratio for ten-year risk of evolution to MM for patients with one or two to three factors of 5.04 and 11.2 times higher compared to those with none. In those subjects with IgA MGUS, hemoglobin levels of <12.5 g/dl and reduced serum polyclonal immunoglobulin correlated with progression. When all patients were included then IgA class, serum monoclonal immunoglobulin levels and light chain proteinuria were the most important variables correlated with disease progression.

In order to refine the prognostic ability of classical clinical and biochemical indices, Perez-Persona et al. used multiparametric flow cytometry as a tool to identify aberrant plasma cell populations [20]. The ratio of aberrant plasma cells to normal bone marrow plasma cells (with a cutoff of 95% of abnormal plasma cells to bone marrow plasma cells) and DNA aneuploidy were identified as risk factors associated with higher risk of progression in a series of 407 subjects with MGUS. By using these independent variables, three risk categories (with none, either or both present) with a progression probability at five years of 2%, 10% and 46%, respectively (P < 0.001) were identified.

123

Insights into the biology

Morphologically plasma cells from MGUS or smoldering MM or symptomatic myeloma are identical, although in some patients with myeloma some immature plasmablasts may be identified by careful examination. However, even at the genetic level, the pre-malignant (such as MGUS) and the malignant condition (MM) share common characteristics, including genetic alterations. MGUS, smoldering MM and symptomatic MM share common cytogenetic features. Hyperdiploidy is found in 42% of MGUS, 63% of SMM, and 57% of MM patients. Similarly, IgH rearrangements were found in 41% of MGUS, 35% of SMM, and 46% of MM patients [21]. Chromosome 13 deletion was higher in MM compared with MGUS (50% vs. 25%). Thus, it seems that the above cytogenetic abnormalities characterize an "initiating" event in the generation of plasma cell neoplasm, while other additional alterations lead to evolution to more aggressive forms, finally leading to myeloma and extramedullary disease. Indeed, cytogenetic abnormalities involving p53 deletions and p18 deletions and mutations, mutations, in N-RAS, K-RAS, MYC up-regulation, and gain or loss of chromosome 1q or 1p, seem to be more prevalent in overt myeloma and correlate with disease progression from MGUS/SMM to myeloma [22].

Using gene-expression profiling (GEP), Zhan *et al.* attempted to identify molecular signatures associated with progression from precursor disease to multiple myeloma. In an initial study published in 2002, hierarchical clustering analysis of normal and MM plasma cells, differentiated four distinct subgroups of MM (MM1, MM2, MM3 and MM4), of which the expression pattern of MM1 was similar to normal PCs and MGUS, whereas MM4 was similar to MM cell lines [23]. In a more recent study, the same investigators identified 52 genes involved in important pathways related to cancer that were differentially expressed in the plasma cells of healthy subjects and patients with stringently defined MGUS/smoldering MM and symptomatic MM. Unsupervised hierarchical clustering created two major cluster branches, one containing 82% of the MGUS patients and the other containing 28% of the MM patients, termed MGUS-like MM (MGUS-L MM). Using the same clustering approach on an independent cohort of 214 patients with MM, 27% were found to be MGUS-L. The MGUS-L signature was also seen in plasma cells from

15 of 20 patients surviving more than ten years after autotransplantation [24]. MicroRNA (miRNA) profiling studies identified that MGUS and multiple myeloma patients seem to up-regulate common miRNAs but also there are differences in the up-regulation of certain other miRNAs [25, 26]. These results provide data supporting the hypothesis of the evolution of MGUS associated plasma cells to symptomatic myeloma associated plasma cells through genomic events and dysregulation of multiple genes and pathways.

However, plasma cell neoplasias are also characterized by alterations in the micro-enviroment of the bone marrow, which supports malignant plasma cell proliferation and survival. An angiogenesis "switch" has been identified by different methods and research groups. The levels of angiogenic cytokines tend to increase as the disease progresses from MGUS to SMM and to symptomatic myeloma [27,28]. The Heidelberg group used imaging techniques (dynamic contrast MRI) to evaluate microcirculatory parameters, which reflects angiogenesis in tumor micro-environment, and a gradual increase in microcirculation was identified when 22 healthy controls were compared to 60 subjects with MGUS, 65 patients with SMM and 75 patients with symptomatic newly diagnosed multiple myeloma [29]. A surplus of expression of proangiogenic over antiangiogenic genes that induces angiogenesis has been proposed as an evolving event in the pathogenesis of myeloma [30].

Pathogenesis

Population based studies provided data that genetic and environmental factors may be associated with an increased prevalence of MGUS. Pesticide exposure was associated with a two-fold increase in the prevalence of MGUS among pesticide applicators [31]. Immune dysregulation due to infections or autoimmune diseases seems to be associated with an increase in the risk of MGUS or MM [32]. MGUS is more prevalent in blacks than in whites; however, there are differences in the isotype of the monoclonal Ig between blacks and whites: IgG is more common in blacks while IgM is more common in whites, serum FLC rations were abnormal more frequently in whites and M protein concentration was higher in whites than in blacks [33]. A familial clustering of MGUS has been observed in small case studies and was confirmed by studies using population-based data: compared with relatives of controls, relatives of

MGUS patients had a 2.8-fold increase in the risk of MGUS, multiple myeloma (relative risk of 2.9), lymphoplasmacytic lymphoma/Waldenstrom Macroglobulinemia (relative risk of 4) and chronic lymphocytic leukemia (relative risk 2) [34]. In another study, serum samples were collected from first-degree relatives of 232 MM and 97 MGUS probands. Age- and sex-adjusted prevalence of MGUS was 8.1% which was associated with an age-adjusted risk ratio of 2.6 compared with the reference population [35]. However, given the low prevalence of MM in the general population and the small risk of disease progression of MGUS to overt malignancy it is not recommended to screen for the identification of monoclonal gammopathy. Family members of patients with MGUS or MM can be informed about an increased relative risk of developing a monoclonal gammopathy but the low absolute risk for development of a plasma cell dyscrasia should be emphasized.

Is MGUS an innocent condition?

Based on the recent findings that an "MGUS" always precedes MM, a monoclonal gammopathy should be considered as a pre-malignant condition. However, MGUS is not only associated with a small risk of development of MM or other lymphoproliferative disease, but also is associated with increased risk for other complications such as bone fractures and thrombosis. In a study based on data from Sweden, the risks of venous and arterial thrombosis in MM and MGUS patients was compared to that of matched controls [36]. As expected, the risk of venous thrombosis for patients with MM was higher compared to controls by a factor of 7.5, 4.6 and 4.1 respectively at one, five, and ten years after MM diagnosis and the corresponding hazards for arterial thrombosis were 1.9, 1.5, and 1.5 at the same time points. However, the respective rates for MGUS patients compared to controls were also increased 3.4, 2.1 and 2.1 times for venous thrombosis and for arterial thrombosis were 1.7, 1.3 and 1.3. The risk of any thromboembolic event was limited in patients with IgG/IgA MGUS. Although patients with IgM MGUS had increased risks for venous and arterial thrombosis, this risk was not correlated with M protein concentration at diagnosis. An older study showed that patients with MGUS had elevated markers of bone resorption compared with healthy controls. However, in contrast to MM patients, this was compensated for by normal

bone formation [27]. In a population-based study using data from Sweden, investigating the risk of skeletal fractures in patients with MGUS, the risks of fractures was assessed in 5326 MGUS patients and compared with 20161 matched controls [37]. MGUS patients had an increased risk of any fracture at 5 years (hazard ratio of 1.74) and 10 (hazard ratio of 1.61). The risk was significantly higher for axial (skull, vertebral/pelvis and sternum/costae) compared with distal (arm and leg) fractures. Risks for fractures did not differ by isotype or M protein concentration at diagnosis. MGUS patients with (vs. without) fractures had no excess risk of MM or Waldenstrom's Macroglobulinemia.

Treatment recommendations

MGUS is an asymptomatic plasma cell disorder with a small risk to transform to overt malignancy. In clinical practice, these patients are followed clinically without treatment until progression. However, MGUS is heterogeneous and still it is very difficult to identify patients at significant risk. Guidelines for the use of bisphosphonates in MGUS are not yet clear except for patients with osteoporosis. In this case, bone density scan (DEXA) should be considered because of the reported increase in skeletal-related events in these patients compared to age-matched controls and if osteoporosis (T score <2) is found then these patients should be treated in a similar manner as patients with osteoporosis. No other treatment recommendation exists for subjects with MGUS.

Smoldering myeloma

The term smoldering myeloma is used interchangeably with the term asymptomatic myeloma or the older term "indolent" myeloma, in analogy with terminology such as indolent lymphoma.

Different diagnostic criteria have been used to define asymptomatic myeloma in the past and thus it is difficult to compare data from different studies. In 2003 the IMWG defined SMM based on an M protein of 3 g/dl or greater and/or a proportion of BMPC of 10% or higher with no symptoms or complications resulting from the monoclonal gammopathy [5] (Table 10.2).

The term asymptomatic myeloma defines a "disease," in contrast with the term MGUS. Thus, the diagnosis of SMM implies that the patient has a

Table 10.2 Differential diagnosis of plasma cell dyscrasias

	M protein	BMPCs	Lytic bone lesions[a]	Anemia[a]	Renal impairment[a]	Hypercalcemia[a]
MGUS	< 3 gr/dl	<10%	No	No	No	No
Smoldering MM	≥ 3 gr/dl[b]	≥10%[b]	No	No	No	No
Symptomatic MM	Any	≥10%[c]	Yes	Yes	Yes	Yes
Solitary plasmacytoma	low	<10%	No	No	No	No

[a] Attributed to the plasma cell dyscrasias.
[b] Either M-protein ≥3 gr/dl or BMPCs ≥10%.
[c] Or presence of a biopsy-proven plasmacytoma with end-organ damage.

substantial risk of progression to a "symptomatic" state, which requires a treatment decision. There is general consensus that patients with SMM should not be treated, but should be followed without therapy [4,38]. This consensus is based on available data from studies conducted in the era before novel agents and in a few studies of thalidomide-based interventions indicating that there is no significant benefit in terms of survival. However, risk stratification is necessary in order to identify those patients at high risk for progression to symptomatic disease in whom, perhaps, alternative strategies should be explored.

In general the rate of progression to MM varies from study to study, according to differences in the definition of SMM and progression to symptomatic disease, but the median time to progression is between two and three years in most cases. Kyle *et al.* have published the outcome of a series of 276 patients with SMM, defined by the standard criteria (i.e. an M component >3 g/dl and/or a BMPCs >10%, without any evidence of end-organ damage) [39]. The cumulative probability of progression was 51% at five years, 66% at ten years and 73% at 15 years. However, the rate of progression was higher in the first five years after diagnosis, 10% per year, while it was reduced at 3% per year for the next five years and thereafter, 1% per year. Several factors were identified as significant predictors of progression to symptomatic MM, including IgA subtype, higher BM infiltration, higher M component, reduction of uninvolved immunoglobulins, pattern of BM involvement. Based on the defining characteristics of SMM, the authors constructed a risk stratification model: patients with both M component >3 g/dl and >10% BMPCs had a 15-year progression rate of 87%, those with a M component <3 g/dl but BMPCs >10% had a 15-year progression rate of 67% and those with

M component >3 g/dl but BMPCs <10% had a rate of progression at 15 years of 39%. It seems that the critical factor is the extent of bone marrow infiltration, rather than the size of the M peak. However, the ratio of free light chains was of prognostic significance when added to the prognostic model. Dispenzieri *et al.* [40] reported that a highly abnormal FLC ratio was an independent prognostic factor and when added to the previous model could discriminate three risk groups (with one, two or three of the risk factors that included an M component >3 g/dl, a BMPCs >10% and a FLC ratio >8 or less than 0.125) with 10-year progression rate of 84%, 64% and 50% if one, two or three risk factors were present.

Rosinol *et al.* [41] identified two types of SMM: evolving SMM, which was characterized by a continued increase in the serum M protein and non-evolving SMM, with long-lasting stable serum or urinary M protein. Interestingly 59% of those with the evolving type of SMM had a previously recognized MGUS as compared with only 4% of those with non-evolving SMM. The median time to progression in the overall series was 3.2 years but the median time to transformation for evolving and non-evolving type was 1.3 vs. 3.9 years respectively (p = 0.007) and the actuarial probability of evolution to symptomatic MM at two and five years for the evolving or non-evolving type was 66% and 88% vs. 12% and 58% respectively. Interestingly in this cohort of patients, only evolving pattern was associated with a shorter time to disease progression while features such as proportion of BMPC as well as the type of heavy and light chain had no impact on disease progression. In a follow up of the above study, by means of comparative genomic hybridization (CGH) analyses, the same group recognized that evolving SMM showed cytogenetic changes consistent with those found in *de novo* symptomatic MM (1q gains, chromosome 13 deletions), while the non-evolving variant showed no 1q gains and deletions were uncommon [42].

Using flow cytometry, Perez-Persona *et al.* studied 93 patients with SMM, and identified that marked predominance of abnormal PCs to BMPC (> 95%) at diagnosis was associated with a significantly higher risk of progression to symptomatic MM(P < 0.001). Immunoparesis was also an independent predictor of progression and three risk categories were identified (according to whether none, one or two factors were present) with probability for progression to symptomatic disease at five years of 4%, 46% and 72% respectively [20].

Imaging studies can provide significant prognostic information in patients with SMM. Moulopoulos *et al.* studied 38 consecutive patients with asymptomatic myeloma with MR imaging of the thoracic and lumbosacral spine [43]. Half of the patients had evidence of marrow involvement at spinal MR imaging (MR patterns of marrow involvement were classified as diffuse, variegated and focal). Patients with abnormal MR imaging required therapy after a median of 16 months, versus 43 months for those with normal MR studies. Recently, a study using whole-body MRI was performed in 149 patients with SMM and focal lesions were identified in 28% of patients [44]. The presence of focal lesions and a number of greater than one focal lesion were the strongest adverse prognostic factors for progression into symptomatic MM. A diffuse infiltration pattern in MRI was also a strong predictor of progression. See Table 10.3 for recommendations for initial assessment and follow up of patients with SMM.

Patterns of progression

According to the IMW criteria progression of SMM to symptomatic MM is defined by the development of one of the following: anemia, lytic bone lesions, renal failure, hypercalcemia (Table 10.4). As mentioned, the rate of progression is higher in the first years after the diagnosis of SMM, while after five years the rate of progression seems to be similar to that of MGUS. Most patients who progress develop anemia or lytic

Table 10.3 Recommendations for initial assessment and follow up of patients with SMM

Initial assessment	Medical history and physical examination
	CBC
	Serum calcium and creatinine
	Protein studies
	• Total serum protein and serum electrophoresis (serum M-protein quantitation)
	• 24-h urine protein electrophoresis (urine M-protein quantitation)
	• Serum and urine immunofixation
	• Serum free light chain measurement (FLC ratio)
	β 2-microglobulin
	Bone marrow aspirate or biopsy
	Skeletal survey
	MRI of thoracic–lumbar spine and pelvis
	DEXA scan
Follow up studies	Medical history and physical examination
	CBC
	Serum calcium and creatinine
	Protein studies
	• Total serum protein and serum electrophoresis (serum M protein quantitation)
	• 24-h urine protein electrophoresis (urine M protein quantitation)
	• Serum free light chain measurement (FLC ratio)
	DEXA scan (yearly?)
	Skeletal survey[a]

[a] For patients at high risk for progression (high levels of M - component, extensive BM infiltration, severely abnormal FLC ratio, abnormal MRI, heavy Bence Jones proteinuria, immunoparesis) follow up studies may be repeated every three to four months.

Table 10.4 Events defining progression to symptomatic MM

Current definition of symptomatic myeloma	Consensus guidelines for diagnostic criteria and indication for treatment and retreatment in plasma cell disorders – IMW Paris 2011
[C] Calcium elevation in the blood (serum calcium >10.5 mg/l or upper limit of normal	[C] Serum calcium >0.25 mmol/l above the upper limit of normal or >2.75 mmol/l, adjusted for serum albumin and ph if available (11.0 mg/dl). Hypercalcemia must be felt related to the underlying clonal plasma cell disorder.
[R] Renal insufficiency (serum creatinine >2 mg/dl)	[R] (1) In a patient with prior estimated glomerular filtration rate (eGFR), a significant drop of eGFR from baseline (>= 35% change over 1 year with no other identifiable cause); OR (2) an eGFR of 50 ml/min with no other identifiable cause; OR (3) evidence of light chain cast nephropathy on renal biopsy.
[A] Anemia (hemoglobin <10 g/dl or 2 g/dl <normal)	[A] Hemoglobin < 2 g/dl the lower limit of normal or baseline or hemoglobin <10 g/dl that is felt related to the underlying clonal plasma cell disorder.
[B] Lytic bone lesions or osteoporosis	[B] Lytic lesion/s are adequate for diagnosis of myeloma. However, if patient has only single lytic lesion then a biopsy confirmation may be required if location accessible. Severe osteopenia with compression fracture will require additional investigation to rule out or confirm myeloma-related bone disease. If skeletal survey is negative for lytic lesion but if MRI performed then three or more hyperintense lesions (focal) or one large macrofocal lesion will be considered as MDE. If PET/CT performed then CT detected lytic lesion > 1 cm OR three or smaller lesions with or without PET positivity should be considered as MDE.
Symptomatic hyperviscosity	If the patient has a symptomatic hyperviscosity that is felt to be related to serum monoclonal protein requiring therapeutic intervention.

bone lesions [3,45], while development of acute renal impairment or hypercalcemia is less common [41]. However, certain patterns of progression may be more frequent in patient presenting at diagnosis with specific features; for example, patients with Bence Jones proteinuria may have a higher probability to progress with renal failure while patients with extensive BM infiltration may present more frequently with anemia or lytic lesions.

Treatment strategies for the management of SMM

Clinical practice guidelines from the IMW or other societies agree that, so far, there are no data to support initiation of therapy in patients with SMM outside the context of a clinical trial. These recommendations were made based on the available data from studies that used alkylating agents and only a few studies that tested novel agents (thalidomide). Currently, ongoing studies explore the role of newer IMiDs (lenalidomide) in the management of patients with SMM and high risk features.

An ideal therapy for SMM should have minimal toxicity, should not limit available options for therapy at progression and should be associated with increased time to disease progression but, most importantly, should prolong survival. Other features of such a therapy should include the mitigation of myeloma complications, for example skeletal events (fractures, need for radiation therapy, etc).

In the past, a few small studies used alkylating agents (melphalan with prednisone, MP) as therapy for patients with SMM and compared to deferred therapy with MP. In all three published studies there was no difference in survival between those who received MP or those who received MP at progression to symptomatic disease. However, none of the studies found any improvement in overall survival [46–48].

Thalidomide is an oral agent with recognized anti-myeloma activity that has direct anti-myeloma effect but also it has been suggested that it has activity on the bone marrow micro-environment that supports the survival and proliferation of malignant plasma cells.

In two small phase II trials, one from the Mayo Clinic, including 29 patients [49], and other from the M. D. Anderson Cancer Center, including 28 patients [50], about one third of the patients showed a partial response (PR). A longer follow up of the Mayo Clinic study indicated a median TTP and PFS of 35 months while response to thalidomide was associated with longer TTP (median TTP was 61 months in those who achieved a PR, 39 months in those achieving MR, and nine months in patients who failed to achieve MR or PR). Median overall survival from diagnosis was 86 months and the median survival measured from onset of symptomatic myeloma was 49 months. In a larger phase II study, Barlogie et al. [51] treated 76 patients with SMM with thalidomide (and pamidronate) at an initial dose of 200 mg/d. At four years from enrollment the PR or better rate was 42% (PR, 25%; near complete response [CR], 12%; CR, 5%) with median times to response of one to two years, while the median time to progression was seven years. Of concern, however, was the observation that achieving a PR was associated with a shorter time to salvage therapy for disease progression (P < 0.001), although OS was similar in the three response categories (70% estimate at six years). Whether this was due to the emergence of resistant clones in patients with high risk disease remains an issue of investigation. A major issue is thalidomide toxicity, especially peripheral neuropathy, but also somnolence, fatigue and constipation. Thus, since data to support a survival benefit are lacking and neurotoxicity is a major concern, thalidomide cannot be considered as an option for patients with SMM.

Bisphosphonates

Another treatment approach is the use of bisphosphonates, which reduce skeletal-related complications in patients with MM and may also prolong survival. Some researchers suggest that bisphosphonates may have a weak anti-tumor effect, but as a monotherapy

this has not been verified. A randomized Italian study showed that pamidronate therapy reduced the number of skeletal events but did not prolong time to progression to symptomatic myeloma or overall survival in patients with early-stage myeloma, after a median follow up of 51 months [52]. A recent update of this study, with a minimum follow up of 5 years for patients still alive, in which 62.9% of patients in the pamidronate-treated group and 62.5% in the control group progressed, confirmed that median time to progression was similar (46 and 48 months, respectively) and that overall survival was also similar. However, skeletal-related events at the time of progression were observed in 72.7% of the controls, but only in 39.2% of pamidronate-treated patients (p = 0.009) [53]. In a similar randomized study, in which 163 patients were randomized to zoledronic acid vs. observation, a significant reduction in the number of skeletal events by the time of progression was observed (55.5% vs. 78.3%, p = 0.04), but again there was no significant prolongation of time to progression to symptomatic myeloma and there was no difference in overall survival [54]. Bisphosphonates may be associated with toxicities such as osteonecrosis of the jaw and renal impairment, thus, long term administration in patients with SMM is not justified, based only on the data that indicate reduction of bone events. However, potential benefits in patients with osteopenia or osteoporosis should be considered and the IMWG has recently proposed that for high-risk SMM and if one cannot differentiate between MM-related versus age-related bone loss, then bisphosphonates at doses and schedule similar to that of symptomatic MM should be considered, especially in patients with abnormal MRIs (http://www.myeloma-paris2011.com/files/files/ConsensusPanel1BoneTheFINAL.pdf).

Lenalidomide

Lenalidomide is a thalidomide derivative that has strong anti-myeloma activity, is orally administered and is not associated with significant neurotoxicity, or other CNS effects. However, in contrast to thalidomide it can cause myelosuppression. Lenalidomide has been approved for patients with relapsed or refractory myeloma and has been shown that it can be administered for prolonged periods with manageable toxicity. In a randomized study from Spain, 124 patients with high-risk SMM (defined by the presence of both bone marrow plasma cells >10% and monoclonal protein

>30g/l or, if only one criterion was present, patients must have had a proportion of aberrant PCs within the total PC BM compartment by immunophenotyping of 95% plus immunoparesis) were randomized to lenalidomide/dexamethasone or observation. Patients who were randomized to the treatment arm received an induction treatment consisting of nine four-week cycles of lenalidomide at a dose of 25 mg daily on days 1–21 plus dexamethasone at a dose of 20 mg daily on days 1–4 and 12–15 (total dose: 160 mg), followed by maintenance until progression of the disease with lenalidomide at dose of 10 mg on days 1–21 every two months, which was later amended into monthly. Among patients treated with len/dex, 81% responded, including a very good PR or better in 25%. In the observation arm, 28 of 60 patients progressed to symptomatic MM in a median of 25 months, while in the treatment group only six patients progressed and the median has not been reached. Interestingly, this is the first study that indicates a possible survival benefit after a median follow up of 22 months, but the data are still immature [55].

Several cytokines have been involved in plasma cell proliferation and survival and have been associated with myeloma progression, especially interleukin-6. Il-1b serum levels have been associated with progression to symptomatic MM, probably reflecting IL-6 activity. In the context of a clinical trial Lust et al. [56] treated 47 patients with SMM with the IL-1R receptor antagonist (anakinra) (which in half of the patients was combined with low dose dexamethasone) in order to interrupt the IL-1/IL-1R/IL-6 stimulatory effect on plasma cells. The investigators followed CRP levels and found a significant increase in time to myeloma progression (>three years) compared to patients who did not had a reduction in CRP levels (six months). Single agent anakinra resulted in minor responses in three patients, while five patients achieved a PR and four patients an MR after addition of dexamethasone. The authors suggested that IL-1R antagonist induced a chronic disease state in certain patients. However, given the non-randomized nature of the study and the toxicity profile of anakinra it is premature to indicate any role for this approach for patients with SMM. However, targeting IL-6 is a reasonable approach and is currently being investigated in clinical trials.

IMW recommendations for patients with SMM

SMM is a condition with a very high probability for progression to symptomatic disease requiring therapy. Also, progression to symptomatic disease is defined by the presence of disease complications, such as lytic bone disease, renal impairment, anemia and hypercalcemia. It is challenging to explain to patients with SMM that they will receive treatment only if they first suffer a complication of their disease. IMW still recommends follow up for patients with SMM, without treatment administration; however there are no formal guidelines concerning follow up for patients with SMM.

Expert recommendations indicate that patients who are diagnosed with SMM should be retested (blood tests, biochemical profile and SPEP) within two to three months to confirm that this is SMM and thereafter, if stable, every three months for the first year to recognize the pattern of evolvement. Thus, for example, in patient with signs of increasing M component or proteinuria or decrease in hemoglobin, additional testing and perhaps consideration for therapy should considered. In patients who remain stable, retesting every four to six months can be scheduled. However, given data regarding risk groups in patients with SMM, perhaps some patients could be considered for closer follow up, for example patients with high M component, high BM infiltration, severely skewed FLC ratio [4,38].

References

1. Kyle, R. A. Monoclonal gammopathy of undetermined significance. Natural history in 241 cases. *Am. J. Med.* 1978; **64**(5):814–26.

2. Kyle, R. A., Greipp, P. R. Smoldering multiple myeloma. *N. Engl. J. Med.* 1980;**302**(24): 1347–9.

3. Alexanian, R. Localized and indolent myeloma. *Blood* 1980;**56** (3):521–5.

4. Kyle, R. A., Durie, B. G., Rajkumar, S. V., *et al.* Monoclonal gammopathy of undetermined significance (MGUS) and smoldering (asymptomatic) multiple myeloma: IMWG consensus perspectives risk factors for progression and guidelines for monitoring and management. *Leukemia* 2010;**24**(6):1121–7.

5. Criteria for the classification of monoclonal gammopathies,

multiple myeloma and related disorders: a report of the International Myeloma Working Group. *Br. J. Haematol.* 2003;**121**(5):749–57.

6. Merlini, G., Stone, M. J. Dangerous small B-cell clones. *Blood* 2006;**108**(8):2520–30.

7. Waldenstrom, J. Studies on conditions associated with disturbed gamma globulin formation (gammopathies). *Harvey Lect.* 1960;**56**:211–31.

8. Dammacco, F., Waldenstrom, J. Bence Jones proteinuria in benign monoclonal gammopathies. Incidence and characteristics. *Acta Med. Scand.* 1968;**184**(5):403–9.

9. Axelsson, U., Bachmann, R., Hallen, J. Frequency of pathological proteins (M-components) on 6,995 sera from an adult population. *Acta Med. Scand.* 1966;**179**(2):235–47.

10. Saleun, J. P., Vicariot, M., Deroff, P., Morin, J. F. Monoclonal gammopathies in the adult population of Finistere, France. *J. Clin. Pathol.* 1982;**35**(1):63–8.

11. Kyle, R. A., Finkelstein, S., Elveback, L. R., Kurland, L. T. Incidence of monoclonal proteins in a Minnesota community with a cluster of multiple myeloma. *Blood* 1972;**40**(5):719–24.

12. Landgren, O., Gridley, G., Turesson, I. *et al.* Risk of monoclonal gammopathy of undetermined significance (MGUS) and subsequent multiple myeloma among African American and white veterans in the United States. *Blood* 2006;**107**(3):904–6.

13. Kyle, R. A., Therneau, T. M., Rajkumar, S. V. *et al.* Prevalence of monoclonal gammopathy of undetermined significance. *N. Engl. J. Med.* 2006;**354**(13):1362–9.

14. Kyle, R. A., Therneau, T. M., Rajkumar, S. V. *et al.* A long-term study of prognosis in monoclonal gammopathy of undetermined

significance. *N. Engl. J. Med.* 2002;**346**(8):564–9.

15. Dispenzieri, A., Katzmann, J. A., Kyle, R. A. *et al.* Prevalence and risk of progression of light-chain monoclonal gammopathy of undetermined significance: a retrospective population-based cohort study. *Lancet* 2010;**375**(9727):1721–8.

16. Landgren, O., Kyle, R. A., Pfeiffer, R. M. *et al.* Monoclonal gammopathy of undetermined significance (MGUS) consistently precedes multiple myeloma: a prospective study. *Blood* 2009;**113**(22):5412–17.

17. Weiss, B. M., Abadie, J., Verma, P., Howard, R. S., Kuehl, W. M. A monoclonal gammopathy precedes multiple myeloma in most patients. *Blood* 2009;**113**(22):5418–22.

18. Rajkumar, S. V., Kyle, R. A., Therneau, T. M. *et al.* Serum free light chain ratio is an independent risk factor for progression in monoclonal gammopathy of undetermined significance. *Blood* 2005;**106**(3):812–17.

19. Rossi, F., Petrucci, M. T., Guffanti, A. *et al.* Proposal and validation of prognostic scoring systems for IgG and IgA monoclonal gammopathies of undetermined significance. *Clin. Cancer Res.* 2009;**15**(13):4439–45.

20. Perez-Persona, E., Vidriales, M. B., Mateo, G. *et al.* New criteria to identify risk of progression in monoclonal gammopathy of uncertain significance and smoldering multiple myeloma based on multiparameter flow cytometry analysis of bone marrow plasma cells. *Blood* 2007;**110**(7):2586–92.

21. Chiecchio, L., Dagrada, G. P., Ibrahim, A. H. *et al.* Timing of acquisition of deletion 13 in plasma cell dyscrasias is dependent on genetic context. *Haematologica* 2009;**94**(12):1708–13.

22. Chiecchio, L., Dagrada, G. P., Protheroe, R. K. *et al.* Loss of 1p and rearrangement of MYC are associated with progression of smouldering myeloma to myeloma: sequential analysis of a single case. *Haematologica* 2009;**94**(7):1024–8.

23. Zhan, F., Hardin, J., Kordsmeier, B. *et al.* Global gene expression profiling of multiple myeloma, monoclonal gammopathy of undetermined significance, and normal bone marrow plasma cells. *Blood* 2002;**99**(5):1745–57.

24. Zhan, F., Barlogie, B., Arzoumanian, V. *et al.* Gene-expression signature of benign monoclonal gammopathy evident in multiple myeloma is linked to good prognosis. *Blood* 2000;**109**(4):1692–700.

25. Pichiorri, F., Suh, S. S., Ladetto, M. *et al.* MicroRNAs regulate critical genes associated with multiple myeloma pathogenesis. *Proc. Natl Acad. Sci. USA* 2008;**105**(35):12 885–90.

26. Pichiorri, F., Suh, S. S., Rocci, A. *et al.* Downregulation of p53-inducible microRNAs 192, 194, and 215 impairs the p53/MDM2 autoregulatory loop in multiple myeloma development. *Cancer Cell* 2010;**18**(4):367–81.

27. Politou, M., Terpos, E., Anagnostopoulos, A. *et al.* Role of receptor activator of nuclear factor-kappa B ligand (RANKL), osteoprotegerin and macrophage protein 1-alpha (MIP-1a) in monoclonal gammopathy of undetermined significance (MGUS). *Br. J. Haematol.* 2004;**126**(5):686–9.

28. Anagnostopoulos, A., Eleftherakis-Papaiakovou, V., Kastritis, E. *et al.* Serum concentrations of angiogenic cytokines in Waldenstrom macroglobulinaemia: the ratio of angiopoietin-1 to angiopoietin-2 and angiogenin correlate with

disease severity. *Br. J. Haematol.* 2007;**137**(6):560–8.

29. Hillengass, J., Zechmann, C., Bauerle, T. *et al.* Dynamic contrast-enhanced magnetic resonance imaging identifies a subgroup of patients with asymptomatic monoclonal plasma cell disease and pathologic microcirculation. *Clin. Cancer Res.* 2009;**15**(9):3118–25.

30. Hose, D., Moreaux, J., Meissner, T. *et al.* Induction of angiogenesis by normal and malignant plasma cells. *Blood* 2009;**114**(1):128–43.

31. Landgren, O., Kyle, R. A., Hoppin, J. A. *et al.* Pesticide exposure and risk of monoclonal gammopathy of undetermined significance in the Agricultural Health Study. *Blood* 2009;**113**(25):6386–91.

32. Brown, L. M., Gridley, G., Check, D., Landgren, O. Risk of multiple myeloma and monoclonal gammopathy of undetermined significance among white and black male United States veterans with prior autoimmune, infectious, inflammatory, and allergic disorders. *Blood* 2008;**111**(7):3388–94.

33. Weiss, B. M., Minter, A., Abadie, J. *et al.* Patterns of monoclonal immunoglobulins and serum free light chains are significantly different in black compared to white monoclonal gammopathy of undetermined significance (MGUS) patients. *Am. J. Hematol.* 2011;**86**(6):475–8.

34. Landgren, O., Linet, M. S., McMaster, M. L. *et al.* Familial characteristics of autoimmune and hematologic disorders in 8,406 multiple myeloma patients: a population-based case-control study. *Int. J. Cancer* 2006;**118**(12):3095–8.

35. Vachon, C. M., Kyle, R. A., Therneau, T. M. *et al.* Increased risk of monoclonal gammopathy in first-degree relatives of patients with multiple myeloma or monoclonal gammopathy of

undetermined significance. *Blood* 2009;**114**(4):785–90.

36. Kristinsson, S. Y., Pfeiffer, R. M., Bjorkholm, M. *et al.* Arterial and venous thrombosis in monoclonal gammopathy of undetermined significance and multiple myeloma: a population-based study. *Blood* 2010;**115**(24):4991–8.

37. Kristinsson, S. Y., Tang, M., Pfeiffer, R. M. *et al.* Monoclonal gammopathy of undetermined significance and risk of skeletal fractures: a population-based study. *Blood* 2010;**116**(15):2651–5.

38. Blade, J., Dimopoulos, M., Rosinol, L., Rajkumar, S. V., Kyle, R. A. Smoldering (asymptomatic) multiple myeloma: current diagnostic criteria, new predictors of outcome, and follow-up recommendations. *J. Clin. Oncol.* 2010;**28**(4):690–7.

39. Kyle, R. A., Remstein, E. D., Therneau, T. M. *et al.* Clinical course and prognosis of smoldering (asymptomatic) multiple myeloma. *N. Engl. J. Med.* 2007;**356**(25):2582–90.

40. Dispenzieri, A., Kyle, R. A., Katzmann, J. A. *et al.* Immunoglobulin free light chain ratio is an independent risk factor for progression of smoldering (asymptomatic) multiple myeloma. *Blood* 2008;**111**(2):785–9.

41. Rosinol, L., Blade, J., Esteve, J. *et al.* Smoldering multiple myeloma: natural history and recognition of an evolving type. *Br. J. Haematol.* 2003;**123**(4):631–6.

42. Rosinol, L., Carrio, A., Blade, J. *et al.* Comparative genomic hybridisation identifies two variants of smoldering multiple myeloma. *Br. J. Haematol.* 2005;**130**(5):729–32.

43. Moulopoulos, L. A., Dimopoulos, M. A., Smith, T. L. *et al.* Prognostic significance of magnetic resonance imaging in patients with asymptomatic

multiple myeloma. *J. Clin. Oncol.* 1995;**13**(1):251–6.

44. Hillengass, J., Fechtner, K., Weber, M. A. *et al.* Prognostic significance of focal lesions in whole-body magnetic resonance imaging in patients with asymptomatic multiple myeloma. *J. Clin. Oncol.* 2010;**28**(9):1606–10.

45. Blade, J., Rosinol, L. Smoldering multiple myeloma and monoclonal gammopathy of undetermined significance. *Curr. Treat. Options Oncol.* 2006;**7**(3):237–45.

46. Hjorth, M., Hellquist, L., Holmberg, E. *et al.* Initial versus deferred melphalan-prednisone therapy for asymptomatic multiple myeloma stage I–a randomized study. Myeloma Group of Western Sweden. *Eur. J. Haematol.* 1993;**50**(2):95–102.

47. Grignani, G., Gobbi, P. G., Formisano, R. *et al.* A prognostic index for multiple myeloma. *Br. J. Cancer* 1996;**73**(9):1101–7.

48. Riccardi, A., Mora, O., Tinelli, C. *et al.* Long-term survival of stage I multiple myeloma given chemotherapy just after diagnosis or at progression of the disease: a multicentre randomized study. Cooperative Group of Study and Treatment of Multiple Myeloma. *Br. J. Cancer* 2000;**82**(7):1254–60.

49. Rajkumar, S. V., Gertz, M. A., Lacy, M. Q. *et al.* Thalidomide as initial therapy for early-stage myeloma. *Leukemia* 2003;**17**(4):775–9.

50. Weber, D., Rankin, K., Gavino, M., Delasalle, K., Alexanian, R. Thalidomide alone or with dexamethasone for previously untreated multiple myeloma. *J. Clin. Oncol.* 2003;**21**(1):16–19.

51. Barlogie, B., van Rhee, F., Shaughnessy, J. D., Jr. *et al.* Seven-year median time to progression with thalidomide for smoldering myeloma: partial response identifies subset requiring earlier

salvage therapy for symptomatic disease. *Blood* 2008;**112**(8): 3122–5.

52. Musto, P., Falcone, A., Sanpaolo, G. *et al.* Pamidronate reduces skeletal events but does not improve progression-free survival in early-stage untreated myeloma: results of a randomized trial. *Leuk. Lymphoma* 2003;**44**(9): 1545–8.

53. D'Arena, G., Gobbi, P. G., Broglia, C. *et al.* Pamidronate versus observation in asymptomatic myeloma: final results with long-term follow-up of a randomized study. *Leuk. Lymphoma* 2011;**52** (5):771–5.

54. Musto, P., Petrucci, M. T., Bringhen, S. *et al.* A multicenter, randomized clinical trial comparing zoledronic acid versus observation in patients with asymptomatic myeloma. *Cancer* 2008;**113**(7):1588–95.

55. Mateos, M.-V., Lopez-Corral, L., Hernandez, M. *et al.* Smoldering multiple myeloma (SMM) at high-risk of progression to symptomatic disease: a phase III, randomized, multicenter trial based on lenalidomide–dexamethasone (len–dex) as induction therapy followed by maintenance therapy with len alone vs no treatment. *ASH Annual Meeting Abstracts* 2010;**116**(21):1935.

56. Lust, J. A., Lacy, M. Q., Zeldenrust, S. R. *et al.* Induction of a chronic disease state in patients with smoldering or indolent multiple myeloma by targeting interleukin 1{beta}-induced interleukin 6 production and the myeloma proliferative component. *Mayo Clin. Proc.* 2009;**84**(2):114–22.

Chapter

11

Multiple myeloma: management of *de novo* disease to include HDT

T. Guglielmelli, P. Sonneveld, A. Broyl and A. Palumbo

Introduction

Treatment strategies of *de novo* symptomatic multiple myeloma (MM) are mainly related to age and comorbidity. Patients <65 years of age without major organ dysfunction (renal, liver, heart and lung) are eligible for intensive chemotherapy and ASCT [1]. The goal of this approach is to obtain a durable complete remission and long-term disease control. A reduced-intensity conditioning regimen followed by ASCT may be also used in patients aged 65–70, or younger patients with pre-existing comorbidities [2]. Patients older than 65 and those who are ineligible for transplantation are candidates for melphalan–prednisone (MP)-based chemotherapy in combination with the new drugs thalidomide, bortezomib and lenalidomide [2].

Risk stratification in multiple myeloma

Multiple myeloma is a heterogeneous disease with variable clinical presentation and prognosis with a survival outcome that ranges from one year in a patient with aggressive disease to ten years in a patient with indolent disease presentation. Evaluation of prognostic factors and risk stratification is important to define appropriate treatment strategies. There is consensus that the current risk stratification is applicable to newly diagnosed patients: a report of the International Myeloma Workshop consensus panel suggested the following parameters: serum beta2 microglobulin and albumin (ISS stage), cytogenetic translocation determined by fluorescent *in situ* hybridization (FISH) analysis [t(4;14), t(14;16), del(17p)], LDH, immunoglobulin type IgA and histology of plasmablastic disease. Additional analyses for risk stratification are conventional cytogenetics, gene expression profiling, labeling index, MRI/PET scan

and DNA copy number alterations by CGH/SNP array [3]. There is a general agreement that risk stratification should be a global stratification and that the risk factors will change in the future with introduction of novel agents and combination therapies. The Mayo Clinic group has recently proposed a risk stratification of multiple myeloma patients based on FISH and GEP (Figure 11.1a). A risk stratification treatment of transplant eligible and ineligible patients has also been suggested (Figure 11.1b) (mSMART: Mayo Stratification for Myeloma and Risk-adapted Therapy, www.msmart.org).

Induction therapies followed by autologous stem cell transplantation

The aim of the induction therapy is the achievement of a rapid and deep response before transplantation. Vincristine–doxorubicin–dexamethasone (VAD) chemotherapy was used as the induction regimen for many years but is no longer recommended following the introduction of novel agents. The two-agent induction regimens most commonly used are dexamethasone in combination with thalidomide (TD), bortezomib (VD) or lenalidomide (RD). TD resulted in nearly complete response (nCR) and in at least very good partial response (VGPR) rates of 8% and 44% respectively [4]. VD demonstrated superior efficacy when compared to VAD with 15% and 38% of patients achieving nCR and very good partial response (VGPR) respectively [5]. RD or lenalidomide plus low-dose dexamethasone (Rd) demonstrated high efficacy in the induction setting, showing 16% nCR and 40% at least VGPR [6]. More recently, three-drug regimens have been introduced with higher response rates and prolongation of PFS. These induction therapies include VD-based regimens in combination

(a)

STANDARD RISK

ANY OTHER THAN THOSE FOR

INTERMEDIATE AND HIGH RISK, INCLUDING:

- hyperdiploid

- t (11;14)

- t (6;14)

INTERMEDIATE RISK

FISH:
- t (4;14)

CYTOGENETIC DEL 13 or HYPERDIPLOIDY

PCLI $\geq$ 3%

HIGH RISK

FISH:
- Del 17p
- t (14;16)
- t (14;20)

GEP:
- high risk signature

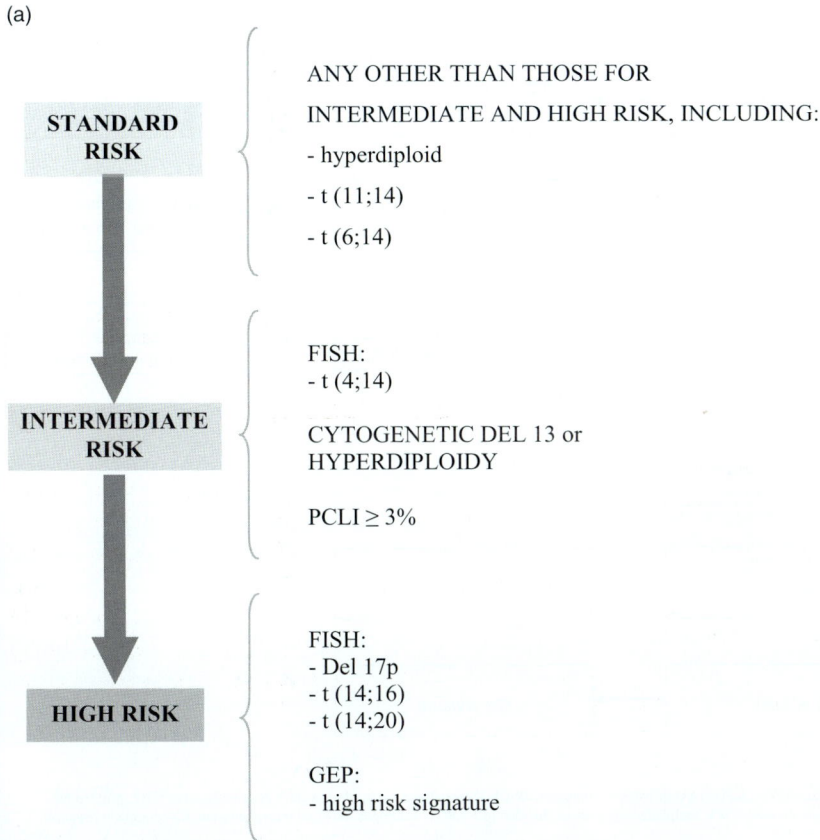

Figure 11.1a mSMART risk classification at diagnosis.

with thalidomide, lenalidomide or chemotherapeutic agents, usually doxorubicin or cyclophosphamide. The first report on triplet therapies focused on the combination of bortezomib–thalidomide–dexamethasone (VTD) [7] and confirmed the significant superiority of VTD over TD, with 32% and 62% of patients achieving nCR and at least VGPR respectively. VD in combination with doxorubicin (PAD) or cyclophosphamide (VCD) showed nCR/VGPR rates of 29/62% [8,9] and 39/61% [10], respectively. More recently, the combination of bortezomib–dexamethasone–lenalidomide (VRD) showed promising results, with 57% and 74% of patients achieving at least nCR and VGPR respectively [11]. These data clearly show that the upfront combination of a proteasome inhibitor (bortezomib) plus an immunomodulatory drug (thalidomide or lenalidomide) is highly effective (see Table 11.1). Four-drug regimens have also been used: the combination of bortezomib–dexamethasone–

thalidomide–cyclophosphamide (VRCD) was equally effective when compared with VRD but was associated with increased toxicity [12]. Longer follow up is needed to evaluate the impact on OS. A randomized trial showed that high-dose melphalan (HDM), namely melphalan 200 mg/m^2, followed by ASCT prolong OS as compared with standard-dose therapy. ASCT remains the gold standard of care in young patients and ongoing trials are evaluating its actual role in the era of novel drugs. The advantage of single- versus double-transplantation is still unclear. Clinical trials demonstrated that only patients who obtain less than a VGPR with the first transplant may benefit from the second transplantation [13,14]. A similar benefit may currently be obtained with consolidation/maintenance therapies based on new drug regimens, thus reserving the second transplant for relapse. Intermediate-dose melphalan (100–140 mg/m^2) followed by ASCT can be used in young patients with pre-existing

(b)

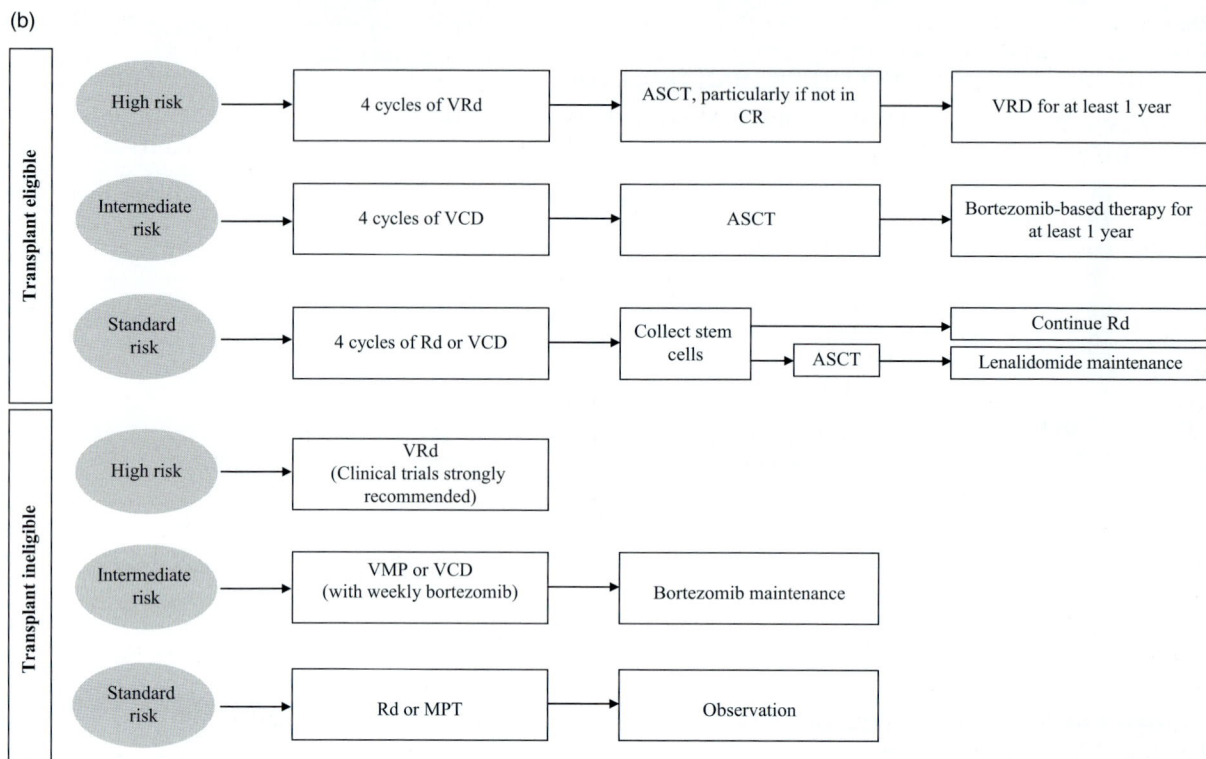

VRD, bortezomib-lenalidomide-dexamethasone; VCD, bortezomib-cyclophosphamide-dexamethasone; VRd, bortezomib-lenalidomide-low dose dexamethasone; VMP, bortezomib-melphalan-prednisone; Rd, lenalidomide plus low dose dexamethasone; MPT, melphalan-prednisone-thalidomide; ASCT, autologus stem cell transplantation; CR, complete response

Figure 11.1b Off-study flow diagram.

Table 11.1 Main induction regimens commonly used in newly diagnosed younger patients with MM

Regimen	Schedule	At least VGPR	PFS	OS
Bortezomib–dexamethsone	Bortezomib 1.3 mg/m^2 intravenous on days 1, 4, 8, 11 every 3 weeks for 4–8 cycles; dexamethasone 40 mg/day on days 1–4 and 9–12 [5].	38%	50% at 36 months	81% at 3 years
Lenalidomide–dexamethasone	Lenalidomide 25 mg/day orally on days 1–21every 4 weeks for 4 cycles; dexamethasone 40 mg/day on days 1, 8, 15, 22 [6].	40%	50% at 25 months	96% at 1 year
Bortezomib–dexamethasone–thalidomide	Bortezomib 1.3 mg/m^2 intravenous on days 1, 4, 8, 11 every 3 weeks for 3 cycles; dexamethasone 320 mg every cycle; thalidomide 200 mg/day orally on days 1–14 every 3 weeks for 3 cycles [7].	63% (CR+nCR)	60% at 3 years	NA
Bortezomib–dexamethasone–cyclophosphamide	Bortezomib 1.3 mg/m^2 intravenous on days 1, 4, 8, 11 every 3 weeks for 4–12 cycles; dexamethasone 40 mg/day on days 1–4, 9–12 and 17–20; cyclophosphamide 300 mg/m^2 orally on days 1, 8, 15, 22 [10].	61%	NA	NA
Bortezomib–dexamethasone–lenalidomide	Bortezomib 1.3 mg/m^2 intravenous on days 1,4,8,11 every 3 weeks for 4–8 cycles; dexamethasone 20 mg/day on days 1, 2, 4, 5, 8, 9, 11, 12; lenalidomide 25 mg/day orally on days 1–14 every 3 weeks for 4–8 cycles [11].	62%	75% at 18 months	97% at 18 months

VGPR, very good partial response; PFS, progression-free survival; OS, overall survival; NA, not available.

comorbidities and in patients aged 65–70 in good clinical condition [2]. Allogeneic transplantation should not be performed outside clinical trials, given the high risk of morbidity and mortality. In very young patients, particularly those with high risk disease at diagnosis, allogeneic transplantation may offer a long-term disease control. Reduced-intensity conditioning (RIC) non-myeloablative allogeneic transplantation reduces transplant-related mortality significantly when compared with myeloablative conditioning, but the relapse/progression rate is higher. Clinical studies comparing ASCT followed by RIC allograft with tandem ASCT have been carried out but the results differ significantly, which may be partially explained by the study design. In the French study including patients with high-risk disease, the outcome of allografting and autografting was similar [15]. The Italian group included all patients, irrespective of the prognostic factors, and demonstrated that allografting confers a long-term survival and disease-free advantage over standard autografting (median OS not reached versus 5.3 years, median event-free survival [EFS] 39 vs. 33 months) [16]. The incorporation of new drugs as induction, consolidation and maintenance therapy along with ASCT or allograft has to be evaluated further in order to select the best therapeutic option for each patient. Randomized trials are needed to directly compare the current best chemotherapeutic approach with best ASCT and allograft strategies and to guide clinical practice for patients.

Induction therapies in patients not eligible for transplantation

Treatment choice should be based on patient's characteristics, in particular age and presence of pre-existing comorbidities. Patients older than 65 are usually not considered eligible for transplant, although a reduced-intensity conditioning regimen (melphalan 100 mg/m^2) followed by ASCT may be used in patients aged 65–70 in good clinical condition. For patients aged 65–75, full-dose chemotherapy is recommended. Patients older than 75 and those who are younger but with pre-existing comorbidities (major organ dysfunction, in particular renal, liver, heart and lung) are suited to the same chemotherapy schedules but with a reduced dose intensity in order to avoid the occurrence of serious adverse events [17]. Combination chemotherapy with melphalan and prednisone (MP) has been used in the treatment of

elderly myeloma patients since the 1960s. Dexamethasone–melphalan combination regimens did not demonstrate an advantage when compared to MP and were associated with more toxic effects. Thalidomide has shown high anti-tumor activity in relapsed/refractory MM patients since the 1990s. More recently, six randomized studies have compared MP with the combination of MP plus thalidomide (MPT) for elderly newly diagnosed MM patients [18]. All these trials demonstrated that MPT improve response rates and prolong PFS when compared with MP while a better OS was only observed in three studies [19–21]. A recent meta-analysis of these studies involving 1685 patients showed that the addition of thalidomide to MP increases PFS by 5.4 months and OS by 6.6 months [25]. Grade 3–4 adverse events occur in around 55% of patients treated with MPT, with a significant risk (20%) of deep venous thrombosis in absence of thromboprophylaxis (see also Table 11.2).

Bortezomib is a new drug that induces reversible inhibition of the proteasome and is the first proteasome inhibitor to be introduced into clinical practice. This novel agent was added to the standard MP (VMP) schedule in elderly, untreated MM patients. A randomized trial comparing VMP with standard MP, reported a significant improvement in the VMP regimen in overall response rates, time to progression (24 months versus 16.6 months) and OS (not reached versus 43 months; three-year OS rates 68.5% versus 54%) [26,27]. This improvement was also confirmed in patients over 75 years old. Neuropathy is a significant risk with VMP therapy as neuropathy occurred in 13% of patients. A recent update of this trial demonstrated that after a median follow-up of 60 months, there was a persistent OS benefit, with 31% reduced risk of death in patients who had received VMP versus MP (median OS 56.4 versus 43.1 months) [28]. A more intense approach, the four-drug combination VMP plus thalidomide (VMPT) led to better overall response rate compared to VMP, but a longer follow-up is needed to assess the effect on survival [29]. Further improvement was achieved by reducing bortezomib schedule from twice- to once-weekly administration. This strategy reduced the incidence of peripheral neuropathy, without negatively affecting efficacy.

MPT and VMP are now considered the standards of care for patients ineligible for transplantation.

Current trials are evaluating the efficacy and safety of the new immunomodulatory drug lenalidomide. Lenalidomide is an oral analog of thalidomide

Table 11.2 Main induction regimens commonly used in newly diagnosed elderly patients with MM

Regimen	Schedule	CR	PFS	OS
Melphalan–prednisone–thalidomide	Melphalan 4 mg/m^2 orally days 1–7; prednisone 40 mg/m^2 days 1–7 for six 4-week cycles; thalidomide 100 mg/day orally until progression [18,19].	13%	50% at 28 months	50% at 52 months
	Melphalan 0.25 mg/kg days 1–4 orally; prednisone 2 mg/kg day 1–4; thalidomide 400 mg/day orally for twelve 6-week cycles [20].	16%	50% at 22 months	50% at 45 months
	Melphalan 0.25 mg/kg; prednisone 1 mg/kg days 1–5; thalidomide 200 mg/day for eight 4-week cycles, followed by 50 mg/day until relapse [21].	23%[a]	50% at 13 months[a]	50% at 44 months
	Melphalan 0.2 mg/kg days 1–4; prednisone 2 mg/kg days 1–4; thalidomide 100 mg/day for twelve 6-week cycles [22].	7%	50% at 24 months	50% at 44 months
	Melphalan 0.25 mg/kg days 1–4; prednisone 100 mg/day days 1–4 for 6-week cycles until plateau; thalidomide 400 mg/day until plateau, reduced to 200 mg/day until progression [23].	13%	50% at 15 months	50% at 32 months
	Melphalan 9 mg/m^2 days 1–4; prednisone 60 mg/m2 days 1–4; thalidomide 100 mg/day for eight 6-week cycles, followed by 100 mg/day until relapse [24].	9%	50% at 21 months[b]	50% at 26 months
Melphalan–prednisone–bortezomib	Melphalan 9 mg/m^2 orally days 1–4 prednisone 60 mg/m^2 days 1–4; bortezomib 1.3 mg/m^2 intravenous days 1, 4, 8, 11, 22, 25, 29, 32 for the first four 6-week cycles and days 1, 8, 15, 22 for the subsequent five 6-week cycles [28].	30	50% at 27 months	50% at 26 months
	Melphalan 9 mg/m^2 orally days 1–4; prednisone 60 mg/m^2 days 1–4; bortezomib 1.3 mg/m^2 intravenous days 1, 8, 15, 22 every 5 weeks for a total of 9 cycles [29].	24%	50% at 22 months	87% at 2 years
Melphalan-prednisone–lenalidomide	Melphalan 0.18 mg/kg orally day 1–4; prednisone 2 mg/kg days 1–4; lenalidomide 10 mg orally days 1–21 for nine 28-day cycles; Lenalidomide 10 mg/day days 1–21 of each 28-day cycle until progression [31].	10%	50% at 31 months	NA

CR, complete response; PFS, progression-free survival; OS, overall survival; NA, not available.
[a] CR plus VGPR (CR alone not available).
[b] Disease-free survival.

designed to have improved efficacy over the parent drug. Lenalidomide has also a different safety profile when compared to thalidomide, with fewer neurological symptoms but more myelosuppression. The combination of melphalan, prednisone and lenalidomide (MPR) has been investigated in a phase I/II study. Patients receiving the standard dose of MP plus lenalidomide 10 mg achieved a PR rate of 81%, including 47% at least VGPR and 24% CR; median PFS was 28.5 months and two-year OS rate was 90%. The major hematologic toxicity was neutropenia (52% of patients experienced grade 3 or 4 neutropenia), and the non-hematologic toxicities included

febrile neutropenia (9.5%), skin rash (9.5%) and thromboembolism (4.8%) [30].

This combination is being assessed in an international randomized trial comparing MPR followed by lenalidomide maintenance (MPR-R) with MPR and MP. MPR-R compared with MP resulted in a higher overall response rate (77% vs. 50%) as well as higher rates of CR (16% vs. 4%) and at least VGPR (32% vs. 12%). MPR-R reduced the risk of disease progression by 66% compared with MP. The PFS benefit associated with MPR-R treatment was evidenced in patients 65 to 75 years of age. Median PFS was 31 months in the MPR-R arm vs. 13 months in the MP arm. Lenalidomide maintenance was well tolerated with no evidence of cumulative toxicity and low rate of adverse events. An increase in the incidence of second primary malignancies (SPMs) was observed in the study of lenalidomide maintenance treatment. The three-year risk of invasive SPMs was 7% with MPR-R and 3% with MP [31]. However, the benefits associated with MPR-R outweigh the increased risk of SPMs, and MPR-R is likely to become another standard therapy for elderly myeloma patients.

Consolidation treatment

The use of consolidation treatment was first introduced in the TT2 regimen [32]. Consolidation chemotherapy consisted of dexamethasone–cyclophosphamide–etoposide–cisplatin (DCEP) versus DCEP alternating with cyclophosphamide–doxorubicin–dexamethasone (CAD). Since similar results arose from these two consolidation arms, the last 90 patients were offered dexamethasone–cisplatin–doxorubicin–cyclophosphamide–etoposide (D-PACE). An alternative consolidation consisting of dexamethasone pulsing was applied monthly when platelet count failed to recover or DCEP was ineffective during induction. Consolidation chemotherapy and dexamethasone consolidation yielded similar post-transplant OS and EFS in TT2. Only a subgroup with cytogenetic abnormalities treated in the control arm of TT2, without thalidomide addition, benefited from consolidation chemotherapy [33,34].

The introduction of novel agents has offered possibilities for improving consolidation treatment.

The Nordic Myeloma Study Group explored the effect of a 21-week consolidation period of single agent bortezomib versus no consolidation, given during months 3–8 after ASCT. Bortezomib consolidation increased CR/nCR rates from 23% at randomization to 54% six months after randomization and from 21% to 35% in the control arm. Twenty percent and 12% in the bortezomib and control groups improved their response from PR to CR/nCR, and a significantly higher percentage of patients in the control group compared to the bortezomib group relapsed during the initial six month observation period, 6% vs. 1% [35].

In addition, lenalidomide consolidation post-ASCT upgraded responses in 15%–20% of patients [36,37].

The Italian study specifically assessed the efficacy and safety of consolidation with VTD and TD; before starting consolidation, CR/nCR rates were not significantly different in the VTD (63%) and TD arms (55%). After consolidation CR/nCR rates were significantly higher for VTD-treated versus TD-treated patients (73% vs. 61%) with an extended three-year progression free survival (60% vs. 48%) [38].

Furthermore, VTD consolidation led to additional shrinkage of residual tumor burden to most patients in CR/VGPR post-ASCT. VTD consolidation was able to induce a molecular response (MR) in almost 20% of patients, measured by qualitative and real-time quantitative polymerase chain reaction (RQ-PCR) of a molecular marker based on the immunoglobulin heavy-chain rearrangement. MRs were stable over time, with no clinical or molecular relapses at a median follow up of 42 months [39].

The study conducted by the Dutch–Belgian cooperative group with the German Multicenter myeloma group strengthens the concept that the ideal therapeutic strategy for transplant-eligible patients with myeloma should be a sequential approach that consists of induction with effective drug combination followed by ASCT and subsequent consolidation/maintenance therapy [9]. In this study, patients who had received PAD induction and bortezomib consolidation/maintenance had superior CR/nCR response rate (31% vs. 15%), better PFS (35 months vs. 28 months) and OS when compared to the VAD group.

Maintenance treatment

Maintenance treatment aims at increasing response duration and prolongation of PFS, without compromising relapse treatment. Several randomized studies have assessed the efficacy of maintenance treatment with thalidomide as single agent or combined with prednisone [33,40–43].

Thalidomide/prednisolone maintenance for 12 months after ASCT improved response, PFS, and OS [43]. The IFM study showed only a survival advantage from single agent thalidomide maintenance in low-risk patients defined by normal β2-microglobulin (β2M) levels, no chromosome 13 abnormalities as determined by FISH, and in patients not achieving VGPR/CR [40]. Two other trials, TT2 and HOVON50/GMMG-HD3, investigated the effect of thalidomide maintenance. Unlike the IFM and Australian trials, thalidomide was given both before and after

HDM [41,44]. In both trials, survival from relapse was significantly shorter after thalidomide maintenance. One of the hypotheses is emergence of tumor-resistant clones in patients with prolonged exposure to thalidomide. Furthermore, patients with cytogenetic abnormalities determined by FISH had no benefit from thalidomide maintenance regarding PFS and a significantly lower OS [42].

More recently, the Mayo Clinic group conducted a randomized controlled trial comparing thalidomide–prednisone (TP) as maintenance therapy versus observation in 332 patients who had undergone ASCT. After a median follow up of 4.1 years, no OS benefit was observed in the TP group versus the observation arm (respective four-year estimates of 68% vs. 60%; P = 0.18); TP improved disease control and was associated with superior PFS (four-year estimates 32% vs. 14%; P <0.0001). TP treatment was associated with a worsening quality of life and a shorter median survival after first disease recurrence (27.7 months vs. 34.1 months in the observation group) [45].

A phase 3, placebo-controlled trial investigated the efficacy of lenalidomide maintenance after transplantation [37]. Lenalidomide maintenance improved PFS to 41 months vs. 23 months from diagnosis in the placebo arm. This benefit was observed across all stratified subgroups of patients including β2M level, chromosome 13 abnormalities, and response after ASCT (CR/VGPR or not). After a follow - up of 45 months, post diagnosis OS remains high and similar in both treatment groups (70%). Recently, a concern about an increased incidence of SPMs following lenalidomide maintenance has been raised. In this trial, the incidence of SPMs was 3.1 per 100 patient-years in the lenalidomide group versus 1.2 per 100 patient-years in the placebo group (P = 0.002); median EFS (taking into account the occurrence of SPMs) was significantly improved with lenalidomide treatment (40 months vs. 27 months with placebo).

Another phase 3 randomized study confirmed the efficacy of lenalidomide maintenance after ASCT in prolonging PFS and OS. After a median follow up of 34 months, 37% of patient who received lenalidomide and 58% of patients with placebo had progressive disease or had died: median time to progression was 46 months in the lenalidomide group versus 27 in the placebo group [46].

The HOVON65/GMMG-HD4 trial assessed the efficacy of bortezomib maintenance following bortezomib-based induction and HDM versus thalidomide maintenance following vincristine-based induction and HDM. Complete response was superior after PAD induction (15% vs. 31%; P < 0.001) and bortezomib maintenance (34% vs. 49%; P < 0.001). After a median follow - up of 41 months, PFS and OS were superior in the PAD arm (median of 28 months vs. 35 months; P = 0.002) [9].

Maintenance treatment in elderly, non-transplant candidates

One of the first trials assessing the efficacy of thalidomide maintenance in elderly patients was the HOVON49. During maintenance, an increase of CR to VGPR from 23% to 28% was observed [21]. Lenalidomide maintenance following MPR induction was compared to maintenance with placebo following MPR or MP induction until progression [31]. Lenalidomide maintenance reduced the risk of disease progression by 66% and improved PFS when compared with placebo (median 31 months vs. 13 months).

Bortezomib maintenance was explored in two trials. Bortezomib, prednisolone (VP) was compared to bortezomib, thalidomide (VT) maintenance after induction treatment with VMP or VTP [47]. The complete response (CR) rate increased from 24% after induction up to 42%, higher for VT versus VP (46% vs. 39%). Median PFS was superior for VT (39 months) compared with VP (32 months) and OS was also longer in VT patients compared with VP (five-year OS of 69% and 50%, respectively) but the differences did not reach statistical significance.

VT maintenance following VMPT (VMPT-VT) was compared to VMP without maintenance treatment. Complete response rates were 38% in the VMPT-VT group and 24% in the VMP group. A significantly higher PFS and OS was observed in the patients treated with VMPT-VT versus VMP [29], thus confirming the role of the four-drug combination followed by maintenance.

Conclusion

Full-dose melphalan followed by ASCT is the treatment of choice in patients younger than 65 years and induction therapy including new drugs seems the most suitable preparatory regimen before transplant. The incorporation of new drugs as induction followed by ASCT appears to lead to VGPR rates slightly superior to those achieved with conventional chemotherapy with new drugs. Randomized trials are needed to directly compare the current best chemotherapeutic approach with best ASCT strategies and to determine the best induction, consolidation, and maintenance therapy.

In elderly patients, randomized phase III studies have shown that MPT, MPV and MPR proved to be more effective than the traditional treatment with MP; hence, they can now be regarded as new standards of care for patients ineligible for ASCT. Maintenance/consolidation therapy showed to improve quality of response and response duration after induction therapy, and the role of novel agents in this setting is now the main focus. Currently there are no guidelines for optimal consolidation or maintenance strategies. Patients should be included in trials to explore the optimal treatment strategy. Outside protocols, comorbidity, previous therapy and prognostic factors such as chromosomal abnormalities could guide the choice of maintenance therapy.

Acknowledgement: the authors thank the editorial assistant Giorgio Schirripa.

References

1. Stewart, A. K., Richardson, P. G., San-Miguel, J. F. How I treat multiple myeloma in younger patients. *Blood* 2009;**114**: 5436–43.

2. Palumbo, A., Sezer, O., Kyle, R. *et al.* International Myeloma Working Group guidelines for the management of multiple myeloma patients ineligible for standard high-dose chemotherapy with autologous stem cell transplantation. *Leukemia* 2009;**23**:1716–30.

3. Munshi, N. C., Anderson, C., Anderson, P. Consensus recommendations for risk stratification in multiple myeloma: report of the international myeloma workshop consensus panel 2. *Blood* 2011:**117**;4696–700.

4. Rajkumar, S. V., Rosiñol, L., Hussein, M. *et al.* Multicenter, randomized, double-blind, placebo-controlled study of thalidomide plus dexamethasone compared with dexamethasone as initial therapy for newly diagnosed multiple myeloma. *J. Clin. Oncol.* 2008;**26**:2171–7.

5. Harousseau, J. L., Attal, M., Avet-Loiseau, H. *et al.* Bortezomib plus dexamethasone is superior to vincristine plus doxorubicin plus dexamethasone as induction treatment prior to autologous stem-cell transplantation in newly diagnosed multiple myeloma: results of the IFM 2005–01 phase III trial. *J. Clin. Oncol.* 2010;**28**:4621–9.

6. Rajkumar, S. V., Jacobus, S., Callander, N. S. *et al.* Lenalidomide plus high-dose dexamethasone versus lenalidomide plus low-dose dexamethasone as initial therapy for newly diagnosed multiple myeloma: an open-label randomised controlled trial. *Lancet Oncol.* 2010;**11**:29–37.

7. Cavo, M., Tacchetti, P., Patriarca, F. *et al.* Bortezomib with thalidomide plus dexamethasone compared with thalidomide plus dexamethasone as induction therapy before, and consolidation therapy after, double autologous stem-cell transplantation in newly diagnosed multiple myeloma: a randomised phase 3 study. *Lancet* 2010;**376**:2075–85.

8. Popat, R., Oakervee, H. E., Hallam, S. *et al.* Bortezomib, doxorubicin and dexamethasone (PAD) front-line treatment of multiple myeloma: updated results after long-term follow-up. *Br. J. Haematol.* 2008;**141**: 512–16.

9. Sonneveld, P., Ingo, G. H., Schmidt-Wolf, I. *et al.* Bortezomib induction and maintenance treatment in patients with newly diagnosed multiple myeloma. Results of the randomized phase III trial HOVON-65/GMMG-HD4. *J. Clin. Oncol.* 2012;**30**:2946–55.

10. Reeder, C. B., Reece, D. E., Kukreti, V. *et al.* Cyclophosphamide, bortezomib and dexamethasone induction for newly diagnosed multiple myeloma: high response rates in a phase II clinical trial. *Leukemia* 2009;**23**:1337–41.

11. Richardson, P. G., Weller, E., Lonial, S. *et al.* Lenalidomide, bortezomib, and dexamethasone combination therapy in patients with newly diagnosed multiple myeloma. *Blood* 2010;**116**: 679–86.

12. Ludwig, H., Viterbo, L., Greil, R. *et al.* Randomized phase II study of bortezomib, thalidomide and dexamethasone with or without cyclophosphamide as induction therapy in previously untreated myeloma. *J. Clin. Oncol.* 2013;**31**:247–55.

13. Attal, M., Harousseau, J. L., Facon, T. *et al.* InterGroupe Francophone du Myélome. Single versus double autologous stem-cell transplantation for multiple myeloma. *N. Engl. J. Med.* 2003;**349**:2495–502.

14. Cavo, M., Tosi, P., Zamagni, E. *et al.* Prospective, randomized study of single compared with double autologous stem-cell transplantation for multiple

myeloma: Bologna 96 clinical study. *J. Clin. Oncol.* 2007;**25**:2434–41.

15. Garban, F., Attal, M., Michallet, M. *et al.* Prospective comparison of autologous stem cell transplantation followed by dose-reduced allograft (IFM99–03 trial) with tandem autologous stem cell transplantation (IFM99–04 trial) in high-risk de novo multiple myeloma. *Blood* 2006;**107**: 3474–80.

16. Giaccone, L., Storer, B., Patriarca, F. *et al.* Long-term follow up of a comparison of non-myeloablative allografting with autografting for newly diagnosed myeloma. *Blood* 2011;**117**:6721–7.

17. Palumbo, A., Mateos, M. V., Bringhen, S. *et al.* Practical management of adverse events in multiple myeloma: can therapy be attenuated in older patients? *Blood Rev.* 2011;**25**:181–91.

18. Palumbo, A., Bringhen, S., Caravita, T. *et al.* Oral melphalan and prednisone chemotherapy plus thalidomide compared with melphalan and prednisone alone in elderly patients with multiple myeloma: randomized controlled trial. *Lancet* 2006;**367**:825–31.

19. Palumbo, A., Bringhen, S., Liberati, A. M. *et al.* Oral melphalan, prednisone, and thalidomide in elderly patients with multiple myeloma: updated results of a randomized controlled trial. *Blood* 2008;**112**:107–14.

20. Facon, T., Mary, J. Y., Hulin, C. *et al.* Melphalan and prednisone plus thalidomide versus melphalan and prednisone alone or reduced-intensity autologous stem cell transplantation in elderly patients with multiple myeloma (IFM 99–06): a randomised trial. *Lancet* 2007;**370**:1209–18.

21. Wijermans, P., Schaafsma, M., Termorshuizen, F. *et al.* Phase III study of the value of thalidomide added to melphalan plus prednisone in elderly patients with

newly diagnosed multiple myeloma: the HOVON 49 Study. *J. Clin. Oncol.* 2010;**28**:3160–6.

22. Hulin, C., Facon, T., Rodon, P. *et al.* Efficacy of melphalan and prednisone plus thalidomide in patients older than 75 years with newly diagnosed multiple myeloma: IFM 01/01 trial. *J. Clin. Oncol.* 2009;**27**:64–70.

23. Waage, A., Gimsing, P., Fayers, P. *et al.* Melphalan and prednisone plus thalidomide or placebo in elderly patients with multiple myeloma. *Blood* 2010;**116**: 1405–12.

24. Beksac, M., Haznedar, R., Firatli-Tuglular, T. *et al.* Addition of thalidomide to oral melphalan/prednisone in patients with multiple myeloma not eligible for transplantation: results of a randomized trial from the Turkish Myeloma Study Group. *Eur. J. Haematol.* 2011;**86**:16–22.

25. Waage, A., Palumbo, A. P., Fayers, P. *et al.* MP versus MPT for previously untreated elderly patients with multiple myeloma: A meta-analysis of 1,682 individual patients data from six randomized clinical trials. *J. Clin. Oncol.* 2010;**28**:605s.

26. San Miguel, I. F., Schlag, R., Khuageva, N. K. *et al.* Bortezomib plus melphalan and prednisone for initial treatment of multiple myeloma. *N. Engl. J. Med.* 2008;**359**:906–17.

27. Mateos, M. V., Richardson, P. G., Schlag, R. *et al.* Bortezomib plus melphalan and prednisone compared with melphalan and prednisone in previously untreated multiple myeloma: updated follow-up and impact of subsequent therapy in the phase III VISTA trial. *J. Clin. Oncol.* 2010;**28**:2259–66.

28. San Miguel, J. F., Schlag, R., Khuageva, N. K. *et al.* Persistent overall survival benefit and no increased risk of second malignancies with bortezomib-

melphalan-prednisone versus melphalan-prednisone in patients with previously untreated myeloma. *J. Clin. Oncol.* 2012 Dec. [epub ahead of print].

29. Palumbo, A., Bringhen, S., Rossi, D. *et al.* Bortezomib-melphalan-prednisone-thalidomide followed by maintenance with bortezomib-thalidomide compared with bortezomib-melphalan-prednisone for initial treatment of multiple myeloma: a randomized controlled trial. *J. Clin. Oncol.* 2010;**28**:5101–9.

30. Palumbo, A., Falco, P., Corradini, P. *et al.* Melphalan, Prednisone and lenalidomide treatment for newly diagnosed myeloma: a report from the GIMEMA-Italian Multiple Myeloma Network. *J. Clin. Oncol.* 2007;**25**:4459–65.

31. Palumbo, A., Hajek, R., Delforge, M. *et al.* Continuous lenalidomide treatment for newly diagnosed multiple myeloma. *N. Engl. J. Med.* 2012;**336**:1759–69.

32. Pineda-Roman, M., Zangari, M., Haessler, J. *et al.* Sustained complete remissions in multiple myeloma linked to bortezomib in total therapy 3: comparison with total therapy 2. *Br. J. Haematol.* 2008;**140**:625–34.

33. Barlogie, B., Tricot, G., Rasmussen, E. *et al.* Total therapy 2 without thalidomide in comparison with total therapy 1: role of intensified induction and post-transplantation consolidation therapies. *Blood* 2006;**107**:2633–8.

34. Zangari, M., van Rhee, F., Anaissie, E. *et al.* Eight-year median survival in multiple myeloma after total therapy 2: roles of thalidomide and consolidation chemotherapy in the context of total therapy 1. *Br. J. Haematol.* 2008;**141**:433–44.

35. Mellqvist, U.-H., Westin, J., Gimsing, P. *et al.* Improved response rate with bortezomib consolidation after high dose

melphalan: first results of a Nordic Myeloma Study Group randomized phase III trial. *Blood.* 2009;**114**:530.

36. Palumbo, A., Gay, F., Falco, P. *et al.* Bortezomib as induction before autologous transplantation, followed by lenalidomide as consolidation-maintenance in untreated multiple myeloma patients. *J. Clin. Oncol.* 2010;**28**:800–7.

37. Attal, M., Lauwers, V., Marit, G. *et al.* Lenalidomide maintenance after stem cell transplantation for multiple myeloma. *N. Eng. J. Med.* 2012:**366**:1782–91.

38. Cavo, M., Pantani, L., Petrucci, M. T. *et al.* Bortezomib-thalidomide-dexamethasone is superior to thalidomide-dexamethasone as consolidation therapy after autologous stem-cell transplantation in patients with newly diagnosed multiple myeloma. *Blood* 2012;**120**:9–19.

39. Ladetto, M., Pagliano, G., Ferrero, S. *et al.* Major tumor shrinking and persistent molecular remissions after consolidation with bortezomib, thalidomide, and dexamethasone in patients with autografted myeloma. *J. Clin. Oncol.* 2010;**28**:2077–84.

40. Attal, M., Harousseau, J. L., Leyvraz, S. *et al.* Maintenance therapy with thalidomide improves survival in patients with multiple myeloma. *Blood* 2006;**108**:3289–94.

41. Lokhorst, H. M., van der Holt, B., Zweegman, S. *et al.* A randomized phase 3 study on the effect of thalidomide combined with adriamycin, dexamethasone, and high-dose melphalan, followed by thalidomide maintenance in patients with multiple myeloma. *Blood* 2010;**115**:1113–20.

42. Morgan, G. J., Gregory, W. M., Davies, F. E. *et al.* The role of maintenence thalidomide therapy in multiple myeloma: MRC myeloma IX results and meta-analysis. *Blood* 2012; **119**:7–15.

43. Spencer, A., Prince, H. M., Roberts, A. W. *et al.* Consolidation therapy with low-dose thalidomide and prednisolone prolongs the survival of multiple myeloma patients undergoing a single autologous stem-cell transplantation procedure. *J. Clin. Oncol.* 2009;**27**:1788–93.

44. Barlogie, B., Tricot, G., Anaissie, E. *et al.* Thalidomide and hematopoietic-cell transplantation for multiple myeloma. *N. Engl. J. Med.* 2006;**354**:1021–30.

45. Stewart, A. K., Trudel, S., Bahlis, N. J. *et al.* A randomized phase III trial of thalidomide and prednisone as maintenance therapy following autologous stem cell transplantation (ASCT) in patients with multiple myeloma (MM) with a quality of life assessment: NCIC CTG MY.10 Trial. *Blood* 2013 Jan. 7 [epub ahead of print].

46. McCarthy, P. L., Owzar, K., Hofmeister, C. C. *et al.* Lenalidomide after stem-cell transplantation for multiple myeloma. *N. Engl. J. Med.* 2012:**336**:1770–81.

47. Mateos, M. V., Oriol, A., Martinez-Lopez, J. *et al.* Maintenance therapy with bortezomib plus thalidomide or bortezomib plus prednisone in elderly multiple myeloma patients included in the GEM2005MAS65 trial *Blood* 2012;**120**:2581–8.

Chapter 12

Treatment of relapsed/refractory myeloma

Matthew J. Streetly, Jacob Laubach, Paul Richardson and Stephen A. Schey

Introduction

Modern treatment of newly diagnosed MM has led to improved responses and markedly improved survival [1,2]. However, despite excellent responses and disease control most patients will eventually relapse and require further therapy. Management of relapsed disease is therefore a critical aspect of overall care. This chapter provides a comprehensive overview of the determinants of and general approaches to therapy as well as a review of specific treatment regimens.

Definition of relapsed and relapsed/refractory MM

The European Group for Blood and Marrow Transplantation (EBMT) [3] criteria and International Myeloma Working Group (IMWG) uniform criteria [4] define progressive disease as $\geq$25% increase (or reappearance from complete response) in the measurable biochemical component (serum monoclonal protein, urine Bence Jones protein or Serum Free Light chain), an increase in bone marrow plasma cells to >10% or the development of new lytic bone lesions/soft tissue plasmacytomas. Clinical relapse is defined as the development of progressive disease and/or myeloma associated end organ dysfunction (CRAB criteria). Primary refractory myeloma refers to disease that fails to achieve at least a minimal response (MR) with initial therapy whilst relapsed and refractory MM is defined as disease that is non-responsive to salvage therapy, or progresses within 60 days of last treatment in patients who previously achieved at least a minimal response (MR).

Determinants of therapy

Disease characteristics, characteristics of prior or ongoing therapy, and patient characteristics are important determinants of therapy in relapsed MM (Figure 12.1).

The cytogenetic signature of the myeloma clone is a major determinant of outcomes and on this basis patients can be identified as high or standard risk on the basis of the detection of high risk cytogenetic/FISH features (e.g. deletion 17p, t(4;14)) [5]. High-risk cytogenetics at diagnosis retains that designation throughout the disease course. The impact of other molecular markers such as gene expression profiles (GEP) and microRNA signatures on response to treatment and outcomes is currently being evaluated.

Clinical manifestations at the time of relapse are also important predictors. An aggressive clinical phenotype characterized by extensive organ dysfunction or extramedullary disease, the presence of

Disease characteristics
- *High versus standard risk cytogenetics*
- *Abnormal versus intact organ function*
- *Presence versus absence of extramedullary disease*

Characteristics of prior or ongoing therapy
- *Short versus prolonged response to prior therapy*
- *Progression on current therapy*
- *Toxicities associated with prior therapy*

Patient characteristics
- *Performance status*
- *Co-morbid medical conditions*
- *Preference regarding mode of chemotherapy administration*
- *Overall goals of care*

Figure 12.1 Determinants of therapy in relapsed multiple myeloma.

Myeloma, ed. Stephen A. Schey, Kwee L. Yong, Robert Marcus and Kenneth C. Anderson. Published by Cambridge University Press.

co-morbidities such as renal impairment, poor bone marrow reserve, peripheral neuropathy, history of previous thromboembolic disease and glucose intolerance guide the choice of therapy. Similarly, the duration of last response and whether the patient relapsed on or off therapy [6] are important considerations when choosing the next treatment. Patient preferences regarding mode of chemotherapy administration, access to health care resources, and goals of care will impact choice of therapy and must be elicited prior to initiation of therapy. Lastly quality of life and costs are becoming increasingly important considerations when deciding therapy.

Risk adapted approach to treatment of relapsed MM

Adverse cytogenetics, aggressive clinical features, short duration of response to prior therapy, or progression on treatment defines high-risk disease whilst the remainder are classified as having standard risk disease. Younger, fitter patients should be assessed for eligibility for autologous stem cell transplantation (ASCT); relapsed patients who have not previously undergone ASCT and those experiencing a prolonged response to their first ASCT are generally considered potential candidates. Response to a particular agent of >18 months suggests re-induction with the same drug alone or in combination with other agents will be effective [7].

High-risk disease is generally treated with three- or four-drug combinations to achieve maximal response. Standard-risk and older less fit patients are generally treated with one- or two-drug regimens that include an agent to which the patient is either naïve or has known sensitivity. Consolidation with ASCT should be considered for patients responding to induction therapy without prior exposure to high-dose therapy and those who sustained a prolonged response to prior transplant.

Specific treatment regimens in relapsed and refractory myeloma
Conventional chemotherapy agents

Conventional therapy refers to chemotherapeutics in use prior to the introduction of the "novel therapies" (thalidomide, lenalidomide, bortezomib) or those with similar modes of action. Few reports of conventional treatments have examined the efficacy of these regimens following treatment with novel therapies. Whilst cross-resistance between the novel therapies and conventional therapies has not been fully established results must be interpreted with caution before applying them to the modern treatment context. The following summarizes key conventional compounds and regimens.

Multiple combination chemotherapy regimens based on the classic VAD (vincristine, adriamycin/doxorubicin, dexamethasone) regimen have been reported for relapsed myeloma (e.g. VAMP, CVAMP, CEVAD, HyperCVAD, VBAP and MOD). Whilst active, they have now been mainly replaced by the introduction of novel targeted therapies because of improved responses with reduced toxicity [8–14]. Similarly, whilst the addition to VAD of drug resistance modifiers such as cyclosporine [15], verapamil [16], interferon [17] and PSC-833 [18] may increase response rates they have not led to longer progression free survival or an improved toxicity profile.

The alkylator-heavy M2 regimen (vincristine, cyclophosphamide, carmustine, melphalan, prednisolone) has a reported overall response rate of 33% [19] with a median response duration of seven months. Oral idarubicin monotherapy [20] was associated with low responses rates (14% MR) but, when used in combination with CCNU and dexamethasone (CIDEX), was associated with 30% PR or greater with acceptable toxicity [21].

Corticosteroids

Steroids have long been known to have activity in relapsed myeloma. Historically, high dose dexamethasone (cumulative dose 480 mg/month) induces responses rates in up to 27% [22]. Consequently, regulatory authorities have required high-dose dexamethasone monotherapy as the comparator arm in advanced relapsed studies [22–25] with PR or better in 18%–24% of patients but PFS is short at 3.5–4.7 months. Steroids, however, are associated with G3/4 fatigue, infection and hyperglycemia in 5%–10% of patients. Less intensive dexamethasone treatment regimens may induce PR or better in 40% but with fewer toxicities [26] whilst single agent methylprednisolone (2 g IV three times weekly) induces response rates in 35% and relapse free and overall survival in responders of 15 months and 19 months respectively [27].

145

Intermediate dose melphalan

A number of studies have examined intermediate dose melphalan (25–50 mg/m^2 IV monthly) in patients relapsing after VAD and/or oral melphalan therapy [28–31]. Overall response rates of 35%–58% are reported with responses lasting 6–16 months. The major toxicities observed were nausea and vomiting as well as prolonged neutropenia.

Fotemustine

Fotemustine is a nitrosourea with significant anti-solid tumor activity and has been reported in two small studies in patients with relapsed myeloma [32,33]. Durable responses have been reported (>PR or better rate of 37%) but the agent is associated with significant G3/4 myelosuppression and mucositis. These encouraging results suggest further evaluation of this as an alternative alkylating agent.

Intensive combination treatment approaches

Approaches using a platinum/etoposide based therapy were pioneered by Barlogie et al. with the EDAP regimen (etoposide, dexamethasone, cytarabine, cisplatin) administered every three to four weeks [34]. In 20 melphalan and/or VAD refractory patients, a 40% response rate was observed, at the cost of 80% neutropenic sepsis admissions and a treatment related mortality of 20%. Patients with better performance status and low tumor burden had a significantly better survival and outcome suggesting a risk adjusted approach should be taken with this more aggressive treatment approach.

The DCEP (dexamethasone, cyclophosphamide, etoposide, cisplatin) regimen has also been studied in a small number of patients, most of whom had received more than two prior lines of therapy. The overall response rate was 58% with a response duration of nine months. A third of patients were able to proceed to consolidation autograft [35].

A third intensive approach using ESHAP (etoposide, methylprednisolone, cytarabine, cisplatin) has been reported in refractory or poor responding patients to first line VAD [36]. A single cycle of treatment was administered and although generally well tolerated 17% of patients were treated for febrile neutropenia and 30% had a decline in renal function not requiring dialysis. Sixty seven percent of patients with VAD refractory or progressive disease had a partial response or better and 76% underwent subsequent

stem cell mobilization which was successful in 84% of those mobilized.

Whilst it is evident that these multi-combination conventional chemotherapies have significant activity in those patients refractory to or relapsing after induction therapy that is based on conventional treatment it must be noted that toxicity is high, the efficacy in post-novel therapy relapsing patients is unknown and they appear to be most appropriately used as a salvage approach prior to a second transplant.

Thalidomide based treatment

Thalidomide monotherapy

The seminal paper by Singhal et al. [37] of thalidomide in relapsed myeloma ushered in a new era in myeloma treatment. Initial observations of thalidomide's anti-angiogenic activity and increased micro-vessel density in bone marrow from myeloma patients suggested a potential anti-myeloma effect. Singhal's initial paper described 84 patients and was updated in 2001 to include 169 previously treated myeloma patients [38]: 30% of patients had a partial response and 14% a complete response which led to a two-year EFS of 26% and OS of 48%. However, responses were not associated with a reduction in marrow micro-vessel density. Treatment was well tolerated with grade 3/4 constipation (16%), neuropathy (9%) and somnolence (25%) the major toxicities.

Numerous thalidomide monotherapy studies followed [39–58]. A systematic review of phase 2 thalidomide monotherapy studies identified 42 clinical trials, reporting on 1674 relapsed myeloma patients [59]. The overall response rate (ORR) was 29.4% and complete response (CR) 1.6%; median time to response was one to two months. The median event free survival (EFS) was 12 months. A dose effect relationship was not detected. Adverse events included somnolence (all grade 54%, G3/4 11%), constipation (all grade 56%, G3/4 16%), peripheral neuropathy (all grade 28%, G3/4 6%), dizziness (22%), rash (15%), neutropenia (15%) and thromboembolism (3%). A significant increase in neuropathy (16% vs. 31%) and somnolence (49% vs. 66%) was observed in trials with a target dose >200mg/d compared with 50–200 mg/day (Table 12.1).

A second systematic review [60] demonstrated comparable responses and outcomes with 28.2% ORRs

Table 12.1 Thalidomide and combinations

Regimen name	Author Year	No. of patients	Details	ORR (CR)	PFS	OS
T	Glasmacher [59] 2006	1674	Metanalysis T: 50 – 800 mg/d	29.4% (1.6%)	3 – 16m (EFS)	5–58m
TD	Von Lilienfeld-Toal [63]	451	Metanalysis T:100 – 400 mg/d D:median 180 mg/month	46% (4%)	3.9 – 12m (EFS)	13–38m
Cyclophosphamide Based						
CT	Hovenga [169] 2004	38	T: 100 – 400 mg/d C: 100 mg/d	53% (11%)	30m	20m
CTD	Kropff [66] 2003	60	T: 100 – 400 mg/d C: iv 300 mg/m^2 bd d1–3 D: 20 mg/m^2 d1–4, 9–12, 17–20 q28	68% (4%)	11m (EFS)	19m
CTD	Garcia-Sanz [65] 2004	71	T: 200–800 mg/d C: 50 mg/d D: 40 mg/d for 4d q21d	53% (2%)	57% at 2y (EFS)	66% at 2 y
CTD	Dimopoulos [64] 2004	53	T: 400 mg od d1–5, 14–18 C: 150 mg/m^2 bd d1–5 D:20 mg/m^2 d1–5, 14–18	55% (5%)	8.2m	17.5m
CTD	Kyriakou [67] 2005	52	T:100 mg/d – 300 mg/d C: 300 mg/m2/week D:40 mg/d d1–4 q28d	61% (17%)	34% at 2y (EFS)	73% at 2 y
CTD	Sidra [69] 2006	62	T: 100 – 200 mg/d C:500mg d1,8,15 D:40 mg d1–4, 15–18	83% (19%)	NR	69% at 2 y
CTD	Roussou [68] 2007	43	T: 400 mg d1–5, 14–18 C:150 mg/m2 bd d1–5 D: 20 mg/m2 d1–5, 14–18 q28 x 3	67% (NR)	10m	NR
CTP	Suvannahsanka [70] 2007	37	T: 200 mg/d C: 50 mg bd d1–21 P: 50 mg alt day q28	57% (20%)	13.2m (DOR 14m)	NR
CTD+E	Moehler [170] 2001	56	T: 400 mg od C: 400 mg/m2 IV d1–4 E:40 mg/m2 d1–4 D:40 mg d1–4 q28	64% (4%)	16m	62% at 1 y
Melphalan Based						
MTD	Srkalovic [73] 2002	21	M: 50 mg iv d1 T: 100–400 mg/d D: 40 mg d1–4	45%	9m	13m
MT	Offidani [71] 2004	27	M:0.2 mg/kg/d d1–4 T: 100–600 mg/d	59%	61% at 2y	61% at 2 y

Table 12.1 (cont.)

Regimen name	Author Year	No. of patients	Details	ORR (CR)	PFS	OS
MPT	Palumbo [72] 2006	24	M: 20 mg/m^2 every 4th cycle T: 50–100 mg/d P: 12.5–50 mg alt day	41%	9m	14m
MPT+Def	Palumbo [171] 2010	24	M: 0.25 mg/kg d1–4 P: 1.5 mg/kg d1–4 T: 50–100 mg/d; De:continuous q35	52%	10m	90% at 1 y
RMPT	Palumbo [117] 2010	44	R:10 mg/d d1–21 M:0.18 mg/kg d1–4 P:2 mg/kgd1–4 T:50–100 mg/d	75%	51% at 1 y	72% at 1 y

T: thalidomide, D: dexamethasone, C: cyclophosphamide, P: prednisolone, E: etoposide, M: melphalan, De: defibrotide, R: lenalidomide (revlimid); ORR: overall response rate; CR: complete response; PFS: progression free survival; OS: overall survival; EFS: event free survival; NR: not reported.

with a 1.6% pooled CR rate. The one-year PFS ranged from 23% to 45% and one-year OS ranged from 49% to 86%. An elevated β-2 microglobulin and advanced age were associated with adverse PFS but other prognostic factors were not consistently identified.

A randomized phase 3 study to define the optimum dose of thalidomide monotherapy (OPTIMUM study [61]) compared 100, 200 and 400 mg/day thalidomide with dexamethasone (480 mg/ cycle) given every 28 days. ORRs between the groups were similar (18%–25%) and no significant prolongation of progression free survival (PFS) with higher doses of thalidomide (6–8.1 months). However, response durations of thalidomide treated patients were significantly prolonged compared with dexamethasone alone but without a clear dose response effect. Adverse events profiles were similar between the thalidomide groups but there was more constipation, neutropenia, peripheral neuropathy and rash compared to dexamethasone.

Thalidomide in combination therapy

Whilst a large number of phase 2 trials and retrospective series with thalidomide combinations with conventional drugs and novel agents such as bortezomib and a corticosteroid have been published there are few reported randomized thalidomide combination trials in relapsed disease (Tables 12.1 and 12.2).

Thalidomide and dexamethasone

Combination studies of thalidomide and dexamethasone have generally been small, phase 2 trials utilizing variable thalidomide and dexamethasone doses. Dimopoulos et al. [62] treated 44 patients at first relapse with thalidomide, starting at 200 mg od and escalating to 400 mg od as tolerated, with dexamethasone (cumulative dose 240 mg/m^2 per cycle). Seventy seven percent of patients were refractory to a prior dexamethasone containing regimen; 55% of patients achieved a partial response and their median progression time exceeded ten months. Toxicities were similar to thalidomide monotherapy with constipation, somnolence and peripheral neuropathy common. Additional adverse events attributable to dexamethasone were also observed such as mood disturbance, headache and edema. Venous thromboembolic events were more prominent (7%) than observed with thalidomide monotherapy.

A systematic review of phase 2 studies of thalidomide/dexamethasone combination treatment identified 12 studies that included over 450 patients [63] treated with a median thalidomide dose of 200 mg/ day (range 100–300 mg/day) and a median cumulative dexamethasone dose of 180 mg/month (range 160–290 mg). Response rates were similar to those previously reported and no dose response was seen for dexamethasone. Responses were rapid (one to

Table 12.2 Thalidomide/bortezomib/intensive combinations

Regimen name	Author (year)	Number of patients	Details	ORR (CR)	PFS	OS
DT-PACE	Lee [113] (2003)	236	D:40 mgd1–4 T: 400 mg/d; cP: 10 mg/m^2/d1–4 A: 10 mg/m^{2}d1–4 C: 400 mg/m^{2}d1–4 E: 40 mg/m^2/dd1–4	32% (7%)		4% TRM
VTD	Ciolli [108] (2006)	18	V: 1 mg/m^2 d1,4,8,11 T: 100 mg/d D: 24 mg d1,2,4,5,8,9,11,12	47% (11%)	NR	NR
ThaLdD	Offidani [172] (2006)	50	T: 100 mg/d; Ld: 40 mg/m^{2}d1 D: 40 mgd1–4, 9–12 q28	76% (26%)	22m	79% at 1y
VMPT	Palumbo [111] (2007)	30	V:1.3–1.6 mg/m^2 d1,4,8,11 M:6 mg/m^2 d1–5 P:60 mg/m^2 d1–5 T:50 mg/d q35	67% (57% CR/VGPR)	61% at 1 y	84% at 1y
ThaLdD v TD (case matched)	Offidani [74] (2007)	47	T: 100 mg/d Ld: 40 mg/m^{2}d1 D: 40 mgd1–4, 9–12 q28	75% vs. 60% (30% vs. 0.5%)	21 vs. 11.5m	33.5 vs. 20m
VTD	Pineda-Roman [112] (2008)	85	V: 1–1.3 mg/m^2 d1,4,8,11 T: 50–200 mg/d D: 20 mg d1,2,4,5,8,9,11,12 q28	64% (6%)		22m
DT-PACE	Srikanth [173] (2008)	26	T: 400 mg/d D:40 mg d1–4 A: 10 mg/m^{2}d1–4 C: 400 mg/m^{2}d1–4 E: 40 mg/m^2/dd1–4 cP: 10 mg/m^2/d1–4	59%	5m	7m
VLdT	Channan-Khan [107] (2009)	23	V: 1.3 mg/m^2 d1,4,15,18 Ld: 20 mg/m2 d1, 15 T: 100–200 mg/d q30	55% (22%)	10.9m	15.7m
VCTD	Kim [109] (2010)	70	V:1.3 d1,4,8,11 C:150 mg/m^2 d1–4 T: 50 mg/d; 20 mg/m^2 d1–4 q28	74% (21%)	14.6m	31.6m
PAD/TD	Lee [174] (2010)	37	V:1.3 d1,4,8,11 A:4 mg/m^2 d1–4 D; 40 mgm^{2}d1–4 6 cycles then T:200 mg/d; D:20 mg/d	81% (32.4%)	18m	35m
ThaLdD-V	Offidani [110] (2011)	46	T:100 mg/d D 20 mg d1,2,4,5,8,9,11,12 Ld:30 mg/m2 d4 V:1.3 mg/m2 d1,4,8,11 q28	76.5% (34.5%)	17.5m	40m

T: thalidomide, D: dexamethasone, C: cyclophosphamide, P: prednisolone, E: etoposide, M: melphalan, De: defibrotide, R: lenalidomide (revlimid), cP: cisplatin, A: Ara-C (cytarabine), V: bortezomib (velcade), Ld: doxil (liposomal doxorubicin); ORR: overall response rate; CR: complete response; PFS: progression free survival; OS: overall survival; EFS: event free survival; NR: not reported.

four months) and median EFS and OS was eight months and 27 months, respectively (Table 12.1). Constipation (37%), somnolence (26%), neuropathy (27%) and depression (10%) were the commonest reported adverse events with 13% of patients discontinuing therapy as a result of toxicity. This review confirmed the higher incidence of VTE with thalidomide/dexamethasone in comparison to thalidomide monotherapy, although no dose relationship was established.

Thalidomide + alkylator +/− corticosteroid

Multiple studies combining variable doses and schedules of cyclophosphamide with thalidomide and a corticosteroid are reported, (CTD) with no obvious significant difference in outcome [64–69]. Treatment has been generally well tolerated with neuropathy, somnolence, constipation and cytopenias, particularly G3/4 neutropenia reported in up to 67% of patients and venous thromboembolic events in up to 11% of patients making thromboprophylaxis important with this combination. Partial response rates of 55%–83% and up to 19% CR rates with PFS of 8–16 months are reported and responses are better for thalidomide naïve patients than those previously exposed to thalidomide (67% vs. 30% $\geq$PR [64]). The substitution of prednisolone for dexamethasone (CTP) [70] induces responses similar to CTD with $\geq$PR 57%, CR 20% and PFS 13.2m with comparable toxicity (G3/4 neutropenia 43%, febrile neutropenia 11%, hyperglycemia 20% and VTE 8%) (Table 12.1).

Thalidomide, combined with melphalan with or without a steroid [71–73] induced 59% PR or better and 5%–12% CR. PFS and OS at two years was 61% for patients achieving a CR.

Thalidomide plus dexamethasone and liposomal doxorubicin

A combination of thalidomide/dexamethasone with liposomal doxorubicin/doxil (ThaDD) was compared to thalidomide/dexamethasone in a case matched analysis [74]. Patients who received ThaDD had superior PR (75% vs. 60%) and CR (30% vs. 10%) and this was associated with a significantly superior PFS (21m vs. 11.5m) and OS (33m vs. 20m) but at the cost of significantly greater G3/4 neutropenia (25% vs. 0%) and G3/4 infections (23% vs. 0%) (Table 12.2).

Lenalidomide based therapy
Lenalidomide monotherapy

Lenalidomide is an orally administered thalidomide analog that exerts anti-tumor effect through various mechanisms, including modulation of the immune response, inhibition of angiogenesis, induction of apoptosis, disruption of interactions between MM cells and the endogenous bone marrow stromal cells, and modulation of cytokines in the bone marrow [75–79].

The first phase 1 study of relapsed myeloma involved 27 patients with a median of three prior regimens utilizing escalating doses of lenalidomide from 5–50 mg/day [80]. The maximum tolerated dose was established as 25 mg daily and a minimal response (MR) or better was reported in 70% of participants.

In a subsequent phase 2 study, 70 patients with relapsed and refractory disease were randomized to either 30 mg once-daily or 15 mg twice-daily lenalidomide for 21 days of every 28-day cycle to better define dose and schedule [81]. The 15 mg twice-daily dose was associated with increased high-grade myelosuppression compared to daily dosing. Non-hematologic toxicity was minimal, with 3% DVT and 2% PN. MR or better was reported in 25%, and median OS was 28 and 27 months in the daily and twice-daily treatment groups, respectively. The addition of dexamethasone for patients with progressive or stable disease after two cycles of therapy was associated with a significant response in 29%.

A large, multi-center phase 2 trial of 30mg of lenalidomide daily in 222 heavily pre-treated patients with relapsed and refractory MM [82] demonstrated 26% PR or better and 44% MR or better. The median TTP, PFS, and OS were 5.2, 4.9 and 23 months respectively. Response rates were similar in patients who previously received thalidomide, and were seen even in those who were thalidomide-refractory, as well as bortezomib-exposed patients. Common grade 3/4 toxicities were primarily related to the marrow-suppressive effects of lenalidomide, and included anemia, thrombocytopenia, and neutropenia.

Lenalidomide plus dexamethasone

Two randomized, double-blind, placebo-controlled studies in patients with relapsed or refractory MM [23,25] used lenalidomide at a dose of 25 mg daily for 21 of a 28 day schedule in combination with dexamethasone. Lenalidomide–dexamethasone produced ORRs of 61% and 60.2% compared to 19.9% and 24% in the placebo–dexamethasone arm. The lenalidomide combination was also associated with a longer median TTP (11.1 months and 11.3 months) compared to placebo–dexamethasone (4.7 months in both studies). VTEs with lenalidomide–dexamethasone (8.5%–15%) were higher than that observed with single-agent lenalidomide studies, and hence VTE-prophylaxis is recommended, with aspirin in low-risk patients and with warfarin or low molecular weight heparin in those at high risk.

The impact of cytogenetics in relapsed MM patients receiving lenalidomide–dexamethasone was evaluated in a cohort of 130 treated at Canadian centers reported by Reece[83]. TTP and OS in patients with t(4;14) and del(13q) were comparable to those without these abnormalities, but patients with del(17p13) had a markedly inferior outcome, with median TTP of just 2.2 months and median OS of 4.7 months.

Lenalidomide in combination therapy

Various lenalidomide-containing combinations have been evaluated in the setting of relapsed MM, building on the distinct and complementary mechanisms of anti-tumor activity of the respective compounds and on that fact that – with a favorable side effect profile overall – lenalidomide represents a suitable partner in such treatment regimens.

Lenalidomide and dexamethasone plus cyclophosphamide

In a phase 1/2 study, 31 patients with a median 3 prior lines of therapy received lenalidomide 25 mg days 1–21 of a 28 day cycle; dexamethasone 20 mg orally days 1–4 and 8–11; and oral cyclophosphamide 300–700 mg/m^2 days 1 and 8 [84]. The MTD was cyclophosphamide 600 mg/m^2 days 1 and 8 in combination with the aforementioned doses and schedule of lenalidomide-dexamethasone. The ORR for the study as a whole (PR or better) was 81%, with a CR rate of 29% and VGPR of 7%. Among ten patients treated at the MTD, the CR rate was 40%. With a median 21 month period of follow-up, the projected two-year PFS was 56% and 30-month OS was 80%. Hematologic toxicities constituted the most frequent grade 3/4 treatment-related adverse events, with neutropenia (41%). Other grade

3/4 non-hematologic toxicities were rare, and included thrombosis in two patients.

Lenalidomide and dexamethasone plus adriamycin

Similar responses are reported when combinations with the anthracycline, adriamycin have been used in this setting but they are generally associated with higher toxicities, primarily myelosuppression, which in the relapsed patient with limited marrow reserve often is a problem requiring G-CSF support.

Bortezomib based therapy

Bortezomib is a boronic acid dipeptide that reversibly inhibits the proteosome, which plays a crucial role in diverse cellular processes. Protein degradation occurs through a two-step process involving ATP-dependent ubiquitination followed by proteolysis within the 20S subunit of the proteosome, which possesses chymotrytic-like, trytpic-like, and post-glutamyl peptide hydrolyzing activity [85]. Bortezomib specifically blocks the chymotryptic-like activity resulting in accumulation of un-degraded proteins that interfere with MM cell survival processes such as tumor–stromal cell adhesion, cytokine production, and angiogenesis leading to tumor cell death [86]. Selected clinical trials involving bortezomib in relapsed MM are summarized in Table 12.3. Its license has recently been amended to allow a change from intravenous to subcutaneous administration given the safer but equally efficacious outcomes [87].

Bortezomib monotherapy

Clinical efficacy for bortezomib was initially demonstrated in a phase 1 trial of patients with refractory hematologic malignancies [88]. The most common high-grade ($\geq$ grade 3) toxicities across all cohorts were thrombocytopenia (37%), anemia (19%), neutropenia (15%), and hyponatremia (15%). The phase 3 APEX study randomized patients to either bortezomib or high-dose dexamethasone [24]. The OR and CR rates in the bortezomib arm were 38% and 6%, respectively. A follow up of this study showed median survival for bortezomib-treated patients to be 29.8 months versus 23.7 months in the dexamethasone group [89].

Table 12.3 Key Bortezomib/Proteosome Inhibitor Studies

Regimen (phase)	Phase	Author (study)	N	ORR%	CR%	TTP mo	OS mo
Btz +/−Dex	2	Richardson [93] (SUMMIT)	202	27	10	7	16
Btz 1.0 (+/−dex)	2	Jagannath [92] (CREST)	28	30 (37)	11 (19)	7	26.7
Btz 1.3(+/−dex)			26	38 (50)	4 (4)	11	60
Btz	3	Richardson [24] (APEX)	333	38	13	6.2	29.8
Dex			336	18	2	3.5	23.7
Btz SC	3	Moreau [175] (MMY-3021)	148	42	20	10.4	1-y 73%
Btz IV			74	42	22	9.4	1-y 77%
Btz + PLD	3	Orlowski [98] (MMY-3001)	324	44	13	9.3	15-mo 76%
Btz			322	41	10	6.5	15-mo 65%
VTD	3	Garderet [176] (MMVAR/IFM 2005–04)	135	86	45	19.5	2-y 71%
TD			134	74	25	13.8	2-y 65%
Btz +Cycl+Pre	1/2	Reece [101] (VCP)	37	88	50	83% at 1y (PFS)	1-y 100%
Btz + Adri + Dex	2	Palumbo [100] (PAD)	64	67	9	34% at 1y (PFS)	1-y 66%
Bendamustine + Btz + Dex	2	Rodon [177] (IFM 2009–01)	83	67	12	67% at 6m (PFS)	6-mo 80%
Btz + Vor	3	Dimopoulos [156] (VANTAGE 088)	637	54	–	7.6	
Btz+ Dex				41		6.8 (PFS)	
Carfilzomib	2	Siegel [161] (PX-171–003-A1)	257	23.7	–	7.8	15.6
Carfilzomib 20 mg/m² 20/27 mg/m²	2	Vij [162] (PX-171–004)	129	42.4	3.4	8.3	–
				52.2	1.5	Not reached	–

Btz: bortezomib; Dex: dexamethasone; PLD: liposomal doxorubicin; VTD: bortezomib (velcade)/thalidomide/dexamethasone; TD: thalidomide/dexamethasone; Cycl: cyclophosphamide; Pre: prednisolone; Adri: adriamcycin (doxorubicin); Vor: vorinostat; ORR: overall response rate; CR: complete response; TTP: time to progression; PFS: progression free survival; OS: overall survival; EFS: event free survival; NR: not reported; SC: subcutaneous; IV: intravenous.

Bortezomib combinations

Pre-clinical evidence of synergy between bortezomib and conventional chemotherapeutic drug classes [90,91] led to the development of a number of combination regimens. Two phase 2 trials looking at the addition of dexamethasone utilized two different bortezomib dosage schedules [92,93] and showed similar OR rates (30% and 38%) and a 10% CR or near complete response (nCR) and a median OS of 16 months. Importantly, a subset analysis demonstrated bortezomib produced comparable response rates and survival among patients with and without del(13) by metaphase cytogenetics [94] supporting other studies demonstrating that response to bortezomib in relapsed/refractory MM is independent of the adverse chromosomal abnormalities del(13) and

t(4;14) [95,96]. The number and type of prior therapies, performance status, beta2-microglobulin, and other adverse prognostic factors were not shown to adversely affect outcomes [97].

Bortezomib plus doxorubicin

Bortezomib alone or in combination with liposomal doxorubicin [98] induces equivalent response rates (39% vs. 40%) in the two arms but the doxorubicin arm yielded superior median TTP (9.3 vs. 6.5 months) and 15-month OS (76% vs. 65%) compared to bortezomib alone. The response rate and median TTP were comparable among patients with and without renal insufficiency (Cr Cl < 60 ml/min), but drug-related toxicities were higher among those with impaired renal function [99]. Bortezomib in combination with doxorubicin and dexamethasone (PAD) [100] is also active producing at least a 67% PR and 25% VGPR or better.

Bortezomib, steroid and an alkylator

Reece *et al.* [101] explored bortezomib with cyclophosphamide and prednisone. The ORR (MR + PR + CR) was 95%, with a CR rate of approximately 50%. The one-year PFS and OS at the highest dose level were 83% and 100%, respectively. Early studies administering bortezomib bi-weekly along with cyclophosphamide and dexamethasone [102–104] produced ORs of 68%–88% with up to 31% CR rates. Treatment was well tolerated with thrombocytopenia, neutropenia, neuropathy and herpes zoster infections reported. Numerous permutations of this schedule have since been published and weekly subcutaneous protocols are now in widespread use producing comparable responses with significantly less toxicity.

A phase 1/2 study [105] has established melphalan 7.5 mg/m^2 as the MTD when used with bortezomib 1.3 mg/m^2 days 1, 4, 8 and 11. ORR was 68%, while CR/nCR rate was 23%. Median PFS was ten months for the study as a whole, and 12 months at the MTD. Grade 3/4 thrombocytopenia occurred in 62% of patients and neutropenia in 57%.

Multiple novel agent combinations

The combination of two novel agents with a steroid or a multi-drug combination with an alkylator or anthracycline has been studied extensively [106–112]. Whilst response rates approaching 100% are seen in *de novo* disease and PFS is improved significantly, there are few randomized comparisons that indicate improved overall survival although there is some increased risk of toxicity, but side effects are generally manageable (Tables 12.3 and 12.4). This, combined with the increased cost of delivering such combinations suggests careful assessment of treatment options is required to balance efficacy with risks. Nonetheless, multidrug novel agent combinations clearly have merit and are especially important for higher risk patients.

DT-PACE

A study published by Lee *et al.* [113] considered two cycles of DT-PACE (Dexamethasone, thalidomide, cisplatin, doxorubicin, cyclophosphamide, etoposide) following VAD or melphalan induction therapy. The response rate was 32%; however, toxicity was very significant, with 12% requiring treatment for

febrile neutropenia; 21% developed nausea and vomiting and 19% developed severe mucositis. Venous thromboembolism (VTE) occurred in 15% of those who did not receive prophylaxis.

Bortezomib plus thalidomide combinations

Pineda-Roman *et al.* [112] explored this combination in a phase 2 study using biweekly bortezomib with thalidomide given starting with cycle two at doses of 50–200 mg/day and dexamethasone 20 mg added on the day of and day after bortezomib during cycle 4 for patients with less than a PR. A minor response (MR) or better occurred in 79% while 63% achieved a PR and 11% CR. The most common grade 3/4 toxicities included thrombocytopenia and neutropenia. Although the cumulative incidence of peripheral neuropathy (PN) is approximately 60%, grade 3/4 PN was infrequent and most cases were reversible. Similar outcomes were observed for patients treated with VTDoxil [107] with 55% PR and 22% CR. These responses were durable with PFS 11.5m but reported neuropathy in this particular study was high (70% G1/2). Interestingly VTE were rarely observed. Garederet *et al.* [114] compared VTD to TD in patients relapsing after ASCT, and demonstrated superior TTP (19.5 vs. 13.8; P = 0.01) and median DOR (17.2 vs. 13.4 months; P = 0.03) with VTD, but no benefit in OS. G3 PN was more frequent with VTD (29% vs. 12%; P = 0.001), as were rates of G3/4 infection and thrombocytopenia.

Thalidomide, bortezomib, alkylator, corticosteroid combinations are reported (VMPT [111], VCTD [109]) with excellent responses (VMPT 67% PR and VCTD 74% PR) that appear sustained (PFS up to 14m) without evidence of significant excess toxicity (Table 12.3).

The combination of bortezomib, thalidomide and dexamethasone with liposomal doxorubicin/doxil (ThaDD-V) [110] also induces excellent responses even when thalidomide or bortezomib has been previously received, with 76% OR rate and 37% CR rate and a median time to progression (TTP) of 18.5 months and OS of 40 months. Peripheral neuropathy was a major adverse event necessitating a reduction in bortezomib and thalidomide dose (G2/3 45%) (Table 12.3).

Bortezomib plus lenalidomide combinations

Preclinical work demonstrates *in vitro* synergistic tumoricidal activity between bortezomib and lenalidomide [79]. A phase 2 study in relapsed/refractory disease of bi-weekly bortezomib and lenalidomide

Table 12.4 Key lenalidomide trials

Study	Phase	Regimen	N	≥PR%	CR/nCR%	TTP mo	PFS mo	OS mo
Weber [25] [MM-009]	3	Len-dex vs dex	177 176	61 19.9	14.1 0.6	11.1 4.7		29.6 20.2
Dimopoulos [23] [MM-010]	3	Len-dex vs dex	176 175	60.2 24.0	15.9 3.4	11.3 4.7		Not reached 20.6
Richardson [178]	2	Lenalidomide, bortezomib, dexamethasone	64	64	25	9.5	9.5	26
Schey [84]	1/2	Cyclophosphamide / len / dex	31	81	29		Not reached 2 yr PFS 56%	Not reached OS at 30 months – 80%
Lentzsch [179]	1/2	Bendamustine/ Len / Dex	36	52	0		4.4	Not reached
Shah [180]	1	Len / Thal / Dex	18	92	15 (nCR)		NA	NA
Niesvizky [181]	1b	Carfilzomib / Len / Dex	32	55	10		NA	NA

PR: partial response; CR: complete response; TTP: time to progression; PFS: progression free survival; OS: overall survival; NA: not available.

days1–14, plus dexamethasone 40 mg (cycles 1–4) or 20 mg (cycles 5–8) [115] demonstrated an MR or better of 86%, with 24% CR/nCR and 67% achieving a PR or better. Response rates were equivalent among patients with standard risk features and those with high-risk disease characterized by advanced ISS stage and cytogenetic abnormalities. Tolerability was favorable, with manageable myelosuppression and limited non-hematologic side effects, including PN.

Lenalidomide plus liposomal doxorubicin, vincristine and dexamethasone

This combination was evaluated by Baz and colleagues [116]. Following induction, maintenance was given with lenalidomide days 1–21 every 28 days along with prednisone 50 mg every other day until progression. The ORR was 75%, with a CR/nCR rate of 29%. Grade 3/4 toxicities occurred in >10% of patients included neutropenia (32%) and thrombocytopenia (13%). Febrile neutropenia occurred in 7% and DVT or PE in 9%. The rate of PN was 35% overall, with 5% of patients developing grade 3/4 PN. The median PFS was 12 months.

Lenalidomide plus melphalan, prednisone and thalidomide

Lenalidomide, melphalan, prednisone and thalidomide has been evaluated by Palumbo [117] in patients who had received one or two prior lines of therapy.

PR or better was seen in 75%, and 34% achieved a VGPR or better. The one-year PFS rate was 51% and one-year OS 72%. G3/4 adverse events included cytopenias, (45% neutropenia; 23% thrombocytopenia) but no G3/4 neuropathy or DVT was observed.

Consolidation following salvage chemotherapy

The availability of novel agents that induce high response rates with much reduced toxicity for the treatment of relapsed myeloma has transformed the transplant landscape in myeloma. However, there continues to be a role for high dose therapy with autologous transplant or allogeneic transplant in selected patients.

Autologous transplant – primary refractory

Stem cell mobilization is usually possible in the context of primary refractory disease and a number of studies have examined outcomes following high dose melphalan autograft despite poor response to initial therapy [118–123]. Although high dose melphalan (200 m/m^2) remains the conditioning of choice a variety of other regimens have been employed. Overall responses are generally good with 69%–92% of patients reported as gaining PR or better and up to 40% having a complete response to autograft. However, the transplant related mortality appears higher in this group (compared with initial responders), reported as 6%–19% at one year and these reports appear durable. A recent study compared stable refractory disease with active progressive disease [122]. It suggested that although responses were equivalent between these two groups (≥PR: 54% vs. 58%) early progression post transplant (< three months) was significantly higher among those with progressing disease pre-transplant (22.5% vs. 2%) and this was associated with a significantly shorter median PFS (0.6 years vs. 2.3 years) and median OS (1.1 years vs. 6 years). Overall these studies suggest that high dose therapy for primary refractory myeloma may not be appropriate in patients with active progressive disease.

Autologous transplant – relapsed disease following a previous autograft

Data for patients receiving a second autograft after relapsing from a first transplant is largely limited to retrospective analyses of single institution data [122,124,125] using a variety of re-induction protocols with conventional chemotherapy. Good prognostic factors identified were albumin > 30 g/l and chemosensitive relapse (OS: 16 months with both factors vs. two months with no factors). A relapse free interval of >18 months post-initial treatment was a significant indicator of event free and overall survival on univariate analysis.

The Royal Marsden Group analyzed 172 patients who had relapsed after a first transplant, 68% of whom received CVAMP as salvage chemotherapy whilst the others received a non-specified salvage approach [126]. Forty eight percent subsequently received a second high dose melphalan autograft based on suitability and patient choice the remainder receiving a variety of other non-high dose treatments. There was no significant difference between these two groups in terms of event free (1.3 vs. 0.9 years) or overall survival (2.9 vs. 1.7 years). A relapse-free interval of >18 months following first transplant was significantly associated with a prolonged overall survival (2.9 vs. 1 years) regardless of whether a second transplant was received although a trend toward superior overall survival for those receiving a second autograft was suggested (4.6 years vs. 2.9 years; p = 0.33). Other studies [127] have suggested that ≥5 prior lines of therapy and poor response to first autograft were poor

prognostic markers for PFS whereas ≥5 prior lines of therapy and time to progression ≤12 months following first autograft were predictive for a poor overall survival.

A case matched analysis comparing outcomes following second autograft with conventional chemotherapy has been carried out [128] showed OR rate following second autograft was 64% (26% CR) with a one-year treatment related mortality of 7% with no treatment related deaths. Second autografts were associated with significantly better four-year overall survival compared with the case matched cohort (32% vs. 22%), attributed to a lower four-year relapse associated mortality (68% vs. 78%) and improved PFS and OS compared with non-transplant treatment. Prognostic factors associated with better outcomes were age <65 years, remission duration of at least 18 months following first transplant and β2M < 2.5 mg/l at diagnosis.

Present available data suggest, therefore, that patients may benefit from consolidation with a second transplant if they have chemosensitive disease and/or have had remission duration of approximately 24 months post first transplant.

Allogeneic transplant

Allogeneic transplant represents an option for a subset of treatment-responsive patients with an available HLA-matched donor, chemotherapy-sensitive disease, and excellent performance status. The potential graft-versus-myeloma effect has stimulated interest in allogeneic ASCT for high-risk patients [129]. The high treatment related mortality (TRM) has been abrogated to some extent by advances in supportive care and utilization of reduced-intensity, non-myeloablative conditioning regimens [130], but transplant related toxicity remains a significant concern and it is generally recommended that allogeneic transplant be performed in the context of a clinical trial whenever possible [131].

New agents on the horizon
Bendamustine

Bendamustine hydrochloride has structural similarities to both alkylating agents and purine analogs with the suggestion of incomplete cross-resistance between bendamustine and other alkylators such as melphalan and cyclophosphamide. When used as a single

155

agent [132], PR or greater is seen in over 50% of patients with a median duration of response of 17 months. Adverse events were generally G1/2 with gastrointestinal upset the major non-hematological G3/4 event occurring in about 4% of patients. G3/4 neutropenia and thrombocytopenia are the most frequent hematological toxicities.

A number of studies have examined single agent bendamustine using a variety of schedules [133–135] in heavily pre-treated populations inducing >30% PR and a median duration of response of approximately ten months. Bendamustine has also been studied in combination with thalidomide and prednisolone, producing 86% PR [136]. The combination is well tolerated with neutropenia and thrombocytopenia being the major G3/4 toxicities.

Pomalidomide

Pomalidomide (CC-4047, Actimid) is an oral immuno-modulatory drug with structural similarities to thalidomide and lenalidomide [137]. It kills myeloma cells by direct toxic action on myeloma cells [138], apoptosis induction via the caspase-8/death receptor pathway [79], reduction of adhesion molecule expression and pro-survival cytokine signaling [139] and augmented natural killer cell activity [76]. But it has more potent *in vitro* anti-tumor necrosis factor alpha and T cell co-stimulatory activity than lenalidomide [140–142].

A first-in-man study of pomalidomide monotherapy in relapsed myeloma [143] identified the MTD in this population as 2 mg/day, and demonstrated G3/4 neutropenia in 58% and G3/4 venous thromboembolism in 16% of patients. The OR rate was 55% and 17% of patients achieved CR. Responses were durable, with a median progression free survival of nine months and OS of 20 months [143]. A second monotherapy study [144] showed an MTD of 5 mg on alternate days; OR was 50% with 10% CR and PFS and OS of 10.5 months and 35.9 months respectively.

Pomalidomide combination therapy with dexamethasone in patients doubly refractory to existing novel therapies, including lenalidomide and bortezomib has shown encouraging results with OR rates exceeding 30% and a 5% CR rate. Significant responses were also observed in patients with poor risk genetic features (Ch 17p PFS was 11.9m and OS 94% at six months [145]. The same group examined the activity of pomalidomide (2 mg od) in combination with dexamethasone in patients refractory to lenalidomide [146] and has also compared two continuous

doses of pomalidomide (2 mg od vs. 4 mg od) in combination with dexamethasone (40 mg weekly) in patients who were refractory to both lenalidomide and bortezomib [147]. Myelosuppression was the main G3/4 toxicity observed, with no major difference between those receiving 2 mg or 4 mg. These studies have collectively demonstrated that pomalidomide has significant anti-myeloma activity even in challenging refractory and heavily pre-treated patients and favorable tolerability (Table 12.5). The pivotal MM-002 study in relapsed and refractory patients has most recently demonstrated an ORR of about 33%, with durable clinical benefit, and expected to result in regulatory approval in 2013 [148].

HDAC inhibitors

Histone acetylation modulates chromatin conformation, and regulates gene expression [149]. Acetylation of histones is controlled by the counter-acting activity of histone deacetylase (HDAC) and histone acetyl transferases [150]. Identification of an imbalance in enzymatic function favoring histone deacetylases in tumor cells sparked interest in inhibitors of this enzyme in cancer therapy [151].

Single agent HDAC inhibition with vorinostat, panobinostat, or romidepsin induces only modest activity [152–154]. However, combination regimens have shown promising results. A phase II study of bortezomib–vorinostat demonstrated 17% ORR among patients refractory to both bortezomib and IMIDs, with a median OS of 11.2 months and two-year OS of 32% [155]. In a study comparing bortezomib–dex versus this plus vorinostat, the addition of vorinostat led to significant improvement in response rate (54% vs. 41%; P < 0.0001) [156]. Unfortunately, the improvement in response translated into only a modest increase in median PFS (7.7 months vs. 6.8 months).

Vorinostat was partnered with lenalidomide and dexamethasone in a phase I study involving patients with rel-refractory MM [157]. The combination was generally well tolerated, with common toxicities including neutropenia, thrombocytopenia, diarrhea, and fatigue. Stable disease was achieved in 87% of patients.

A phase 2 study of the pan-deacetylase inhibitor panobinostat in combination with bortezomib and dexamethasone in relapsed and bortezomib-refractory multiple myeloma (PANORAMA 2 [158]) showed ORR was 29%. Important toxicities included

Table 12.5 Pomalidomide trials

Author (year)	Number of patients	Regimen	Dose	Median prior therapies	Prior Len	Prior BTZ	ORR,% (CR,%)	PFS	OS
Lacy [147] (2011)	35	Pom/Dex	2 mg od d1–28	6	100	100	26 (0)	6.5m;	NR; 78% at 6m
Lacy [147] (2011)	35	Pom/Dex	4 mg od d1–28	6	100	100	28 (3)	3.2m	NR; 67% at 6m
Leleu [182] (2013)	43	Pom/Dex	4 mg od d1–21 q28	5	100	100	35 (2)	5.4m	14.9m
Leleu [182] (2013)	41	Pom/Dex	4 mg od d1–28	5	100	100	34 (5)	4.4m	14.8m
Richardson [183] (2012)	38	Pom+/− Dex	4 mg od d1–21 q28 (MTD)	6	82	74	21 (3)	4.6m	18.3m
Lacy [146] (2010)	34	Pom/Dex	2 mg od d1–28	4	100	59	32 (0)	4.8m	13.9m
Lacy [145] (2009)	60	Pom/Dex	2 mg od d1–28	2	35	33	63 (5)	11.6m	94% at 6m
Streetly [144] (2008)	20	Pom	5 mg ad (MTD)	4	0	85	50 (10)	10.5m	35.9m
Schey [143] (2004)	24	Pom	2 mg od d1–28 (MTD)	3	0	0	55 (17)	39w	90w

Pom: pomalidomide; Dex: dexamethasone; Len: lenalidomide; BTZ: bortezomib; MTD: maximum tolerated dose; ORR: overall response rate; CR: complete response; PFS: progression free survival; OS: overall survival; NR: not reported.

gastrointestinal symptoms and thrombocytopenia. A phase 3 study (PANORAMA 1) comparing bortezomib-dex versus the same plus panobinostat in relapsed and refractory MM is ongoing.

Romidepsin has been evaluated in combination with bortezomib–dexamethasone in a phase 1/2 study in patients with relapsed and refractory MM [159]. A minor response or better was observed in 72% of patients. Important toxicities include neutropenia, thrombocytopenia and gastrointestinal symptoms, but proved manageable.

Second-generation proteosome inhibitors – carfilzomib

Carfilzomib is an irreversible epoxyketone proteosome inhibitor (PI) that is selective for the chymotrypsin-like protease [160]. Two early clinical phase 2 studies have evaluated Carfilzomib in patients with relapsed/refractory myeloma.

In multiply treated and refractory patients single-agent carfilzomib with dexamethasone used as pre-medication [161] induced ORR of 23%, with median DOR of 7.8 months and median OS 15.6 months. Fatigue, nausea, thrombocytopenia, dyspnea, and an increase in serum creatinine were the most common toxicities. When administered to bortezomib-naïve patients [162] a minimal response or better was observed in 59% – 64% of patients. Median overall DOR was 13 months while median TTP was eight months. The rate of PN was low at 17%, which is especially encouraging in this setting, although serious cardiac and pulmonary toxicity was also described, but proved rare.

A number of other proteasome inhibitors are being investigated in early phase clinical trials. These second-generation PIs can be given orally and have been shown to be active in patients who are refractory to or relapse post-bortezomib. Ixazomib (MLN9708) is an orally available reversible proteasome inhibitor that targets the 20S subunit and has been associated with low rates of peripheral neuropathy when given as a single agent. Oprozomib (ONX 0912) is another orally available PI that binds irreversible to the proteasome that shows clinical activity with a low incidence of dose limiting toxicity in early studies.

Signal transduction inhibitors

A number of other agents directed against other targets are in early phase clinical trials such as the kinesin spindle protein inhibitor, ARRY-520. This is well tolerated and produces responses in heavily pretreated patients' refractory to lenalidomide, bortezomib, and dexamethasone. The multi-CDK inhibitor, dinaciclib, similarly has potential anti-myeloma activity as a single agent in patients with relapsed MM.

Monoclonal antibody therapy – elotuzumab

A number of immune strategies utilizing cell based and antibody approaches are under investigation and are discussed elsewhere. Elotuzumab is a humanized monoclonal IgG1 antibody that targets the CS1, a cell surface glycoprotein that is highly expressed on the surface of normal plasma cells and myeloma cells, and at a lower level on the surface of NK cells. It exerts anti-MM activity via direct cytotoxicity and through NK cell-mediated antibody-dependent cellular cytotoxicity [163,164].

In a phase I study, single agent elotuzumab was well tolerated [165], the most common side effects being headache, back pain, cough and fever, but no objective responses were reported.

The combination of elotuzumab plus bortezomib in a phase I study of heavily pre-treated relapsed/refractory disease, 39% of whom had received prior bortezomib [166], did not demonstrate any dose limiting toxicity. The MTD was not reached. Frequent high-grade toxicities included lymphopenia (25%) and fatigue (14%). A partial response or better was observed in 48% of patients, with median TTP of 9.46 months. Another phase I study treated patients with elotuzumab plus lenalidomide and low-dose dex [167]. There were no DLTs although grade 4 anaphylaxis was reported in one patient and grade 4 stridor in another. Partial response or better was observed in 82%, and the median time to progression was not reached after 16.4 months median follow up, which is remarkable in this population. Subsequent phase II studies have confirmed that 10 mg/kg is the preferred dose, and the ORR as well as clinical benefit seen in combination with lenalidomide and dexamethasone has been striking [168].

Other antibodies directed against a number of different targets such as CD38 (daratumumab), anti-BAFF (tabalumab) and DKK1 (BHQ880) are also in early phase studies and demonstrate encouraging results either alone or in combination with other agents.

Conclusions

Relapsed and refractory MM remains an area of enormous clinical challenge and exquisite unmet medical need. Combination therapies targeting clonal heterogeneity and acquired resistance constitute a cornerstone of management, with rational approaches combining novel agents proving key in improving patient outcome.

References

1. Kumar, S. K., Rajkumar, S. V., Dispenzieri, A. *et al*. Improved survival in multiple myeloma and the impact of novel therapies. *Blood* 2008;**111**:2516–20.

2. Venner, C. P., Connors, J. M., Sutherland, H. J. *et al*. Novel agents improve survival of transplant patients with multiple myeloma including those with high-risk disease defined by early relapse (<12 months). *Leuk. Lymphoma* 2011;**52**:34–41.

3. Blade, J., Samson, D., Reece, D. *et al*. Criteria for evaluating disease response and progression in patients with multiple myeloma treated by high-dose therapy and haemopoietic stem cell transplantation. Myeloma Subcommittee of the EBMT. *Br. J. Haematol.* 1998;**102**:1115–23.

4. Durie, B. G., Harousseau, J. L., Miguel, J. S. *et al*. International uniform response criteria for multiple myeloma. *Leukemia* 2006;**20**:1467–73.

5. Rajkumar, S. V., Harousseau, J. L., Durie, B. *et al*. Consensus recommendations for the uniform reporting of clinical trials: report of the International Myeloma Workshop Consensus Panel 1. *Blood*; **117**:4691–5.

6. Avet-Loiseau, H., Soulier, J., Fermand, J. P. *et al*. Impact of high-risk cytogenetics and prior therapy on outcomes in patients with advanced relapsed or refractory multiple myeloma treated with lenalidomide plus dexamethasone. *Leukemia* 2010;**24**:623–8.

7. Conner, T. M., Doan, Q. D., Walters, I. B., LeBlanc, A. L., Beveridge, R. A. An observational, retrospective analysis of

retreatment with bortezomib for multiple myeloma. *Clin. Lymphoma Myeloma* 2008;**8**:140–5.

8. Barlogie, B., Smith, L., Alexanian, R. Effective treatment of advanced multiple myeloma refractory to alkylating agents. *N. Engl. J. Med.* 1984;**310**:1353–6.

9. Bonnet, J., Alexanian, R., Salmon, S. *et al.* Vincristine, BCNU, doxorubicin, and prednisone (VBAP) combination in the treatment of relapsing or resistant multiple myeloma: a Southwest Oncology Group study. *Cancer Treat. Rep.* 1982;**66**:1267–71.

10. Dimopoulos, M. A., Weber, D., Kantarjian, H., Delasalle, K. B., Alexanian, R. HyperCVAD for VAD-resistant multiple myeloma. *Am. J. Hematol.* 1996;**52**:77–81.

11. Forgeson, G. V., Selby, P., Lakhani, S. *et al.* Infused vincristine and adriamycin with high dose methylprednisolone (VAMP) in advanced previously treated multiple myeloma patients. *Br. J. Cancer* 1988;**58**:469–73.

12. Giles, F. J., Wickham, N. R., Rapoport, B. L. *et al.* Cyclophosphamide, etoposide, vincristine, adriamycin, and dexamethasone (CEVAD) regimen in refractory multiple myeloma: an International Oncology Study Group (IOSG) phase II protocol. *Am. J. Hematol.* 2000;**63**:125–30.

13. Lokhorst, H. M., Meuwissen, O. J., Bast, E. J., Dekker, A. W. VAD chemotherapy for refractory multiple myeloma. *Br. J. Haematol.* 1989;**71**:25–30.

14. Phillips, J. K., Sherlaw-Johnson, C., Pearce, R. *et al.* A randomized study of MOD versus VAD in the treatment of relapsed and resistant multiple myeloma. *Leuk. Lymphoma* 1995;**17**:465–72.

15. Sonneveld, P., Schoester, M., de Leeuw, K. Clinical modulation of multidrug resistance in multiple myeloma: effect of cyclosporine on resistant tumor cells. *J. Clin. Oncol.* 1994;**12**:1584–91.

16. Dalton, W. S., Crowley, J. J., Salmon, S. S. *et al.* A phase III randomized study of oral verapamil as a chemosensitizer to reverse drug resistance in patients with refractory myeloma. A Southwest Oncology Group study. *Cancer* 1995;**75**:815–20.

17. Gertz, M. A., Kalish, L. A., Kyle, R. A. *et al.* Phase III study comparing vincristine, doxorubicin (Adriamycin), and dexamethasone (VAD) chemotherapy with VAD plus recombinant interferon alfa-2 in refractory or relapsed multiple myeloma. An Eastern Cooperative Oncology Group study. *Am. J. Clin. Oncol.* 1995;**18**:475–80.

18. Friedenberg, W. R., Rue, M., Blood, E. A. *et al.* Phase III study of PSC-833 (valspodar) in combination with vincristine, doxorubicin, and dexamethasone (valspodar/VAD) versus VAD alone in patients with recurring or refractory multiple myeloma (E1A95): a trial of the Eastern Cooperative Oncology Group. *Cancer* 2006;**106**:830–8.

19. Cavo, M., Galieni, P., Tassi, C., Gobbi, M., Tura, S. M-2 protocol for melphalan-resistant and relapsing multiple myeloma. *Eur. J. Haematol.* 1988;**40**:168–73.

20. Sumpter, K., Powles, R. L., Raje, N. *et al.* Oral idarubicin as a single agent therapy in patients with relapsed or resistant multiple myeloma. *Leuk. Lymphoma* 1999;**35**:593–7.

21. Parameswaran, R., Giles, C., Boots, M. *et al.* CCNU (lomustine), idarubicin and dexamethasone (CIDEX): an effective oral regimen for the treatment of refractory or relapsed myeloma. *Br. J. Haematol.* 2000;**109**:571–5.

22. Alexanian, R., Barlogie, B., Dixon, D. High-dose glucocorticoid treatment of resistant myeloma. *Ann. Intern. Med.* 1986;**105**:8–11.

23. Dimopoulos, M., Spencer, A., Attal, M. *et al.* Lenalidomide plus dexamethasone for relapsed or refractory multiple myeloma. *N. Engl. J. Med.* 2007;**357**:2123–32.

24. Richardson, P. G., Sonneveld, P., Schuster, M. W. *et al.* Bortezomib or high-dose dexamethasone for relapsed multiple myeloma. *N. Engl. J. Med.* 2005;**352**:2487–98.

25. Weber, D. M., Chen, C., Niesvizky, R. *et al.* Lenalidomide plus dexamethasone for relapsed multiple myeloma in North America. *N. Engl. J. Med.* 2007;**357**:2133–42.

26. Tiplady, C. W., Summerfield, G. P. Continuous low-dose dexamethasone in relapsed or refractory multiple myeloma. *Br. J. Haematol.* 2000;**111**:381.

27. Gertz, M. A., Garton, J. P., Greipp, P. R., Witzig, T. E., Kyle, R. A. A phase II study of high-dose methylprednisolone in refractory or relapsed multiple myeloma. *Leukemia* 1995;**9**:2115–18.

28. Back, H., Lindblad, R., Rodjer, S., Westin, J. Single-dose intravenous melphalan in advanced multiple myeloma. *Acta Haematol.* 1990;**83**:183–6.

29. Maniatis, A., Tsakanikas, S., Stamatellou, M., Papanastasiou, K. Intermediate-dose melphalan for refractory myeloma. *Blood* 1989;**74**:1177.

30. Petrucci, M. T., Avvisati, G., Tribalto, M. *et al.* Intermediate-dose (25 mg/m2) intravenous melphalan for patients with multiple myeloma in relapse or refractory to standard treatment. *Eur. J. Haematol.* 1989;**42**:233–7.

31. Tsakanikas, S., Papanastasiou, K., Stamatelou, M., Maniatis, A. Intermediate dose of intravenous melphalan in advanced multiple myeloma. *Oncology* 1991;**48**:369–71.

32. Dumontet, C., Jaubert, J., Sebban, C. *et al.* Clinical and pharmacokinetic phase II study of fotemustine in refractory and relapsing multiple myeloma patients. *Ann. Oncol.* 2003;**14**:615–22.

33. Mangiacavalli, S., Pica, G., Varettoni, M., Lazzarino, M., Corso, A. Efficacy and safety of fotemustine for the treatment of relapsed and refractory multiple myeloma patients. *Eur. J. Haematol.* 2009;**82**:240–1.

34. Barlogie, B., Velasquez, W. S., Alexanian, R., Cabanillas, F. Etoposide, dexamethasone, cytarabine, and cisplatin in vincristine, doxorubicin, and dexamethasone-refractory myeloma. *J. Clin. Oncol.* 1989;**7**:1514–17.

35. Dadacaridou, M., Papanicolaou, X., Maltesas, D. *et al.* Dexamethasone, cyclophosphamide, etoposide and cisplatin (DCEP) for relapsed or refractory multiple myeloma patients. *J. BUON* 2007;**12**:41–4.

36. D'Sa, S., Yong, K., Kyriakou, C. *et al.* Etoposide, methylprednisolone, cytarabine and cisplatin successfully cytoreduces resistant myeloma patients and mobilizes them for transplant without adverse effects. *Br. J. Haematol.* 2004;**125**:756–65.

37. Singhal, S., Mehta, J., Desikan, R. *et al.* Antitumor activity of thalidomide in refractory multiple myeloma. *N. Engl. J. Med.* 1999;**341**:1565–71.

38. Barlogie, B., Desikan, R., Eddlemon, P. *et al.* Extended survival in advanced and refractory multiple myeloma after single-agent thalidomide: identification of prognostic factors in a phase 2 study of 169 patients. *Blood* 2001;**98**:492–4.

39. Cibeira, M. T., Rosinol, L., Ramiro, L. *et al.* Long-term results of thalidomide in refractory and relapsed multiple myeloma with emphasis on response duration. *Eur. J. Haematol.* 2006;**77**:486–92.

40. Fenk, R., Hoyer, B., Steidl, U. *et al.* Single-agent thalidomide for treatment of first relapse following high-dose chemotherapy in patients with multiple myeloma. *Leukemia* 2005;**19**:156–9.

41. Hattori, Y., Okamoto, S., Shimada, N. *et al.* Single-institute phase 2 study of thalidomide treatment for refractory or relapsed multiple myeloma: prognostic factors and unique toxicity profile. *Cancer Sci.* 2008;**99**:1243–50.

42. Huang, S. Y., Tang, J. L., Yao, M. *et al.* Reduction of leukocyte count is associated with thalidomide response in treatment of multiple myeloma. *Ann Hematol.* 2003;**82**:558–64.

43. Hus, I., Dmoszynska, A., Manko, J. *et al.* An evaluation of factors predicting long-term response to thalidomide in 234 patients with relapsed or resistant multiple myeloma. *Br. J. Cancer* 2004;**91**:1873–9.

44. Hus, M., Dmoszynska, A., Soroka-Wojtaszko, M. *et al.* Thalidomide treatment of resistant or relapsed multiple myeloma patients. *Haematologica* 2001;**86**:404–8.

45. Juliusson, G., Celsing, F., Turesson, I. *et al.* Frequent good partial remissions from thalidomide including best response ever in patients with advanced refractory and relapsed myeloma. *Br. J. Haematol.* 2000;**109**:89–96.

46. Kees, M., Dimou, G., Sillaber, C. *et al.* Low dose thalidomide in patients with relapsed or refractory multiple myeloma. *Leuk. Lymphoma* 2003;**44**:1943–6.

47. Kumar, S., Gertz, M. A., Dispenzieri, A. *et al.* Response rate, durability of response, and survival after thalidomide therapy for relapsed multiple myeloma. *Mayo Clin. Proc.* 2003;**78**:34–9.

48. Maisnar, V., Radocha, J., Buchler, T. *et al.* Monotherapy with low-dose thalidomide for relapsed or refractory multiple myeloma: better response rate with earlier treatment. *Eur. J. Haematol.* 2007;**79**:305–9.

49. Mileshkin, L., Biagi, J. J., Mitchell, P. *et al.* Multicenter phase 2 trial of thalidomide in relapsed/refractory multiple myeloma: adverse prognostic impact of advanced age. *Blood* 2003;**102**:69–77.

50. Mohty, M., Attal, M., Marit, G. *et al.* Thalidomide salvage therapy following allogeneic stem cell transplantation for multiple myeloma: a retrospective study from the Intergroupe Francophone du Myelome (IFM) and the Societe Francaise de Greffe de Moelle et Therapie Cellulaire (SFGM-TC). *Bone Marrow Transplant.* 2005;**35**:165–9.

51. Neben, K., Moehler, T., Benner, A. *et al.* Dose-dependent effect of thalidomide on overall survival in relapsed multiple myeloma. *Clin. Cancer Res.* 2002;**8**:3377–82.

52. Richardson, P., Schlossman, R., Jagannath, S. *et al.* Thalidomide for patients with relapsed multiple myeloma after high-dose chemotherapy and stem cell transplantation: results of an open-label multicenter phase 2 study of efficacy, toxicity, and biological activity. *Mayo Clin. Proc.* 2004;**79**:875–82.

53. Rosinol, L., Cibeira, M. T., Blade, J. *et al.* Extramedullary multiple myeloma escapes the effect of thalidomide. *Haematologica* 2004;**89**:832–6.

54. Schey, S. A., Cavenagh, J., Johnson, R. *et al.* A UK myeloma forum phase II study of thalidomide; long term follow-up and recommendations for treatment. *Leuk. Res.* 2003;**27**:909–14.

55. Tosi, P., Zamagni, E., Cellini, C. *et al.* Salvage therapy with thalidomide in patients with advanced relapsed/refractory multiple myeloma. *Haematologica* 2002;**87**:408–14.

56. Waage, A., Gimsing, P., Juliusson, G. *et al.* Early response predicts thalidomide efficiency in patients with advanced multiple myeloma. *Br. J. Haematol.* 2004;**125**:149–55.

57. Wechalekar, A. D., Chen, C. I., Sutton, D. *et al.* Intermediate dose thalidomide (200 mg daily) has comparable efficacy and less toxicity than higher doses in relapsed multiple myeloma. *Leuk. Lymphoma* 2003;**44**:1147–9.

58. Yakoub-Agha, I., Attal, M., Dumontet, C. *et al.* Thalidomide in patients with advanced multiple myeloma: a study of 83 patients–report of the Intergroupe Francophone du Myelome (IFM). *Hematol. J.* 2002;**3**:185–92.

59. Glasmacher, A., Hahn, C., Hoffmann, F. *et al.* A systematic review of phase-II trials of thalidomide monotherapy in patients with relapsed or refractory multiple myeloma. *Br. J. Haematol.* 2006;**132**:584–93.

60. Prince, H. M., Schenkel, B., Mileshkin, L. An analysis of clinical trials assessing the efficacy and safety of single-agent thalidomide in patients with relapsed or refractory multiple myeloma. *Leuk. Lymphoma* 2007;**48**:46–55.

61. Kropff, M., Baylon, H. G., Hillengass, J. *et al.* Thalidomide versus dexamethasone for the treatment of relapsed and/or refractory multiple myeloma: results from OPTIMUM, a randomized trial. *Haematologica* 2012;**97**:784–91.

62. Dimopoulos, M. A., Zervas, K., Kouvatseas, G. *et al.* Thalidomide and dexamethasone combination for refractory multiple myeloma. *Ann. Oncol.* 2001;**12**:991–5.

63. von Lilienfeld-Toal, M., Hahn-Ast, C., Furkert, K. *et al.* A systematic review of phase II trials of thalidomide/dexamethasone combination therapy in patients with relapsed or refractory multiple myeloma. *Eur. J. Haematol.* 2008;**81**:247–52.

64. Dimopoulos, M. A., Hamilos, G., Zomas, A. *et al.* Pulsed cyclophosphamide, thalidomide and dexamethasone: an oral regimen for previously treated patients with multiple myeloma. *Hematol. J.* 2004;**5**:112–17.

65. Garcia-Sanz, R., Gonzalez-Porras, J. R., Hernandez, J. M. *et al.* The oral combination of thalidomide, cyclophosphamide and dexamethasone (ThaCyDex) is effective in relapsed/refractory multiple myeloma. *Leukemia* 2004;**18**:856–63.

66. Kropff, M. H., Lang, N., Bisping, G. *et al.* Hyperfractionated cyclophosphamide in combination with pulsed dexamethasone and thalidomide (HyperCDT) in primary refractory or relapsed multiple myeloma. *Br. J. Haematol.* 2003;**122**:607–16.

67. Kyriakou, C., Thomson, K., D'Sa, S. *et al.* Low-dose thalidomide in combination with oral weekly cyclophosphamide and pulsed dexamethasone is a well tolerated and effective regimen in patients with relapsed and refractory multiple myeloma. *Br. J. Haematol.* 2005;**129**:763–70.

68. Roussou, M., Anagnostopoulos, A., Kastritis, E. *et al.* Pulsed cyclophosphamide, thalidomide and dexamethasone regimen for previously treated patients with multiple myeloma: long term follow up and disease control after subsequent treatments. *Leuk. Lymphoma* 2007;**48**:754–8.

69. Sidra, G., Williams, C. D., Russell, N. H. *et al.* Combination chemotherapy with cyclophosphamide, thalidomide and dexamethasone for patients with refractory, newly diagnosed or relapsed myeloma. *Haematologica* 2006;**91**:862–3.

70. Suvannasankha, A., Fausel, C., Juliar, B. E. *et al.* Final report of toxicity and efficacy of a phase II study of oral cyclophosphamide, thalidomide, and prednisone for patients with relapsed or refractory multiple myeloma: A Hoosier Oncology Group Trial, HEM01–21. *Oncologist* 2007;**12**:99–106.

71. Offidani, M., Corvatta, L., Marconi, M. *et al.* Thalidomide plus oral melphalan compared with thalidomide alone for advanced multiple myeloma. *Hematol. J.* 2004;**5**:312–17.

72. Palumbo, A., Avonto, I., Bruno, B. *et al.* Intravenous melphalan, thalidomide and prednisone in refractory and relapsed multiple myeloma. *Eur. J. Haematol.* 2006;**76**:273–7.

73. Srkalovic, G., Elson, P., Trebisky, B., Karam, M. A., Hussein, M. A. Use of melphalan, thalidomide, and dexamethasone in treatment of refractory and relapsed multiple myeloma. *Med. Oncol.* 2002;**19**:219–26.

74. Offidani, M., Bringhen, S., Corvatta, L. *et al.* Thalidomide-dexamethasone plus pegylated liposomal doxorubicin vs. thalidomide-dexamethasone: a case-matched study in advanced multiple myeloma. *Eur. J. Haematol.* 2007;**78**:297–302.

75. Chang, D. H., Liu, N., Klimek, V. *et al.* Enhancement of ligand-dependent activation of human natural killer T cells by lenalidomide: therapeutic implications. *Blood* 2006;**108**:618–21.

76. Davies, F. E., Raje, N., Hideshima, T. *et al.* Thalidomide and immunomodulatory derivatives augment natural killer cell cytotoxicity in multiple myeloma. *Blood* 2001;**98**:210–16.

77. Dredge, K., Horsfall, R., Robinson, S. P. *et al.* Orally

administered lenalidomide (CC-5013) is anti-angiogenic in vivo and inhibits endothelial cell migration and Akt phosphorylation in vitro. *Microvasc. Res.* 2005;**69**:56–63.

78. LeBlanc, R., Hideshima, T., Catley, L. P. *et al.* Immunomodulatory drug costimulates T cells via the B7-CD28 pathway. *Blood* 2004;**103**:1787–90.

79. Mitsiades, N., Mitsiades, C. S., Poulaki, V. *et al.* Apoptotic signaling induced by immunomodulatory thalidomide analogs in human multiple myeloma cells: therapeutic implications. *Blood* 2002;**99**:4525–30.

80. Richardson, P. G., Schlossman, R. L., Weller, E. *et al.* Immunomodulatory drug CC-5013 overcomes drug resistance and is well tolerated in patients with relapsed multiple myeloma. *Blood* 2002;**100**:3063–7.

81. Richardson, P. G., Blood, E., Mitsiades, C. S. *et al.* A randomized phase 2 study of lenalidomide therapy for patients with relapsed or relapsed and refractory multiple myeloma. *Blood* 2006;**108**:3458–64.

82. Richardson, P., Jagannath, S., Hussein, M. *et al.* Safety and efficacy of single-agent lenalidomide in patients with relapsed and refractory multiple myeloma. *Blood* 2009;**114**:772–8.

83. Reece, D., Song, K. W., Fu, T. *et al.* Influence of cytogenetics in patients with relapsed or refractory multiple myeloma treated with lenalidomide plus dexamethasone: adverse effect of deletion 17p13. *Blood* 2009;**114**:522–5.

84. Schey, S. A., Morgan, G. J., Ramasamy, K. *et al.* The addition of cyclophosphamide to lenalidomide and dexamethasone in multiply relapsed/refractory myeloma patients; a phase I/II

study. *Br. J. Haematol.* 2010;**150**:326–33.

85. Myung, J., Kim, K. B., Crews, C. M. The ubiquitin-proteasome pathway and proteasome inhibitors. *Med. Res. Rev.* 2001;**21**:245–73.

86. Mitsiades, N., Mitsiades, C. S., Poulaki, V. *et al.* Molecular sequelae of proteasome inhibition in human multiple myeloma cells. *Proc. Natl Acad. Sci. USA* 2002;**99**:14 374–9.

87. Moreau, P., Pylypenko, H., Grosicki, S. *et al.* Subcutaneous versus intravenous administration of bortezomib in patients with relapsed multiple myeloma: a randomised, phase 3, non-inferiority study. *Lancet Oncol.*;**12**:431–40.

88. Orlowski, R. Z., Stinchcombe, T. E., Mitchell, B. S. *et al.* Phase I trial of the proteasome inhibitor PS-341 in patients with refractory hematologic malignancies. *J. Clin. Oncol.* 2002;**20**:4420–7.

89. Richardson, P. G., Sonneveld, P., Schuster, M. *et al.* Extended follow-up of a phase 3 trial in relapsed multiple myeloma: final time-to-event results of the APEX trial. *Blood* 2007;**110**:3557–60.

90. Ma, M. H., Yang, H. H., Parker, K. *et al.* The proteasome inhibitor PS-341 markedly enhances sensitivity of multiple myeloma tumor cells to chemotherapeutic agents. *Clin. Cancer Res.* 2003;**9**:1136–44.

91. Mitsiades, N., Mitsiades, C. S., Richardson, P. G. *et al.* The proteasome inhibitor PS-341 potentiates sensitivity of multiple myeloma cells to conventional chemotherapeutic agents: therapeutic applications. *Blood* 2003;**101**:2377–80.

92. Jagannath, S., Barlogie, B., Berenson, J. *et al.* A phase 2 study of two doses of bortezomib in relapsed or refractory myeloma. *Br. J. Haematol.* 2004;**127**:165–72.

93. Richardson, P. G., Barlogie, B., Berenson, J. *et al.* A phase 2 study of bortezomib in relapsed, refractory myeloma. *N. Engl. J. Med.* 2003;**348**:2609–17.

94. Jagannath, S., Richardson, P. G., Sonneveld, P. *et al.* Bortezomib appears to overcome the poor prognosis conferred by chromosome 13 deletion in phase 2 and 3 trials. *Leukemia* 2007;**21**:151–7.

95. Chang, H., Trieu, Y., Qi, X. *et al.* Bortezomib therapy response is independent of cytogenetic abnormalities in relapsed/refractory multiple myeloma. *Leuk. Res.* 2007;**31**:779–82.

96. Sagaster, V., Ludwig, H., Kaufmann, H. *et al.* Bortezomib in relapsed multiple myeloma: response rates and duration of response are independent of a chromosome 13q-deletion. *Leukemia* 2007;**21**:164–8.

97. Richardson, P. G., Barlogie, B., Berenson, J. *et al.* Clinical factors predictive of outcome with bortezomib in patients with relapsed, refractory multiple myeloma. *Blood* 2005;**106**:2977–81.

98. Orlowski, R. Z., Nagler, A., Sonneveld, P. *et al.* Randomized phase III study of pegylated liposomal doxorubicin plus bortezomib compared with bortezomib alone in relapsed or refractory multiple myeloma: combination therapy improves time to progression. *J. Clin. Oncol.* 2007;**25**:3892–901.

99. Blade, J., Sonneveld, P., San Miguel, J. F. *et al.* Pegylated liposomal doxorubicin plus bortezomib in relapsed or refractory multiple myeloma: efficacy and safety in patients with renal function impairment. *Clin. Lymphoma Myeloma* 2008;**8**:352–5.

100. Palumbo, A., Gay, F., Bringhen, S. *et al.* Bortezomib, doxorubicin and dexamethasone in advanced

multiple myeloma. *Ann. Oncol.* 2008;**19**:1160–5.

101. Reece, D. E., Rodriguez, G. P., Chen, C. *et al.* Phase I-II trial of bortezomib plus oral cyclophosphamide and prednisone in relapsed and refractory multiple myeloma. *J. Clin. Oncol.* 2008;**26**:4777–83.

102. Davies, F. E., Wu, P., Jenner, M. *et al.* The combination of cyclophosphamide, velcade and dexamethasone induces high response rates with comparable toxicity to velcade alone and velcade plus dexamethasone. *Haematologica* 2007;**92**:1149–50.

103. Fu, W., Delasalle, K., Wang, J. *et al.* Bortezomib-cyclophosphamide-dexamethasone for relapsing multiple myeloma. *Am. J. Clin. Oncol.* 2012;**35**:562–5.

104. Kropff, M., Bisping, G., Schuck, E. *et al.* Bortezomib in combination with intermediate-dose dexamethasone and continuous low-dose oral cyclophosphamide for relapsed multiple myeloma. *Br. J. Haematol.* 2007;**138**: 330–7.

105. Popat, R., Oakervee, H., Williams, C. *et al.* Bortezomib, low-dose intravenous melphalan, and dexamethasone for patients with relapsed multiple myeloma. *Br. J. Haematol.* 2009;**144**:887–94.

106. Chanan-Khan, A., Miller, K. C. Velcade, Doxil and Thalidomide (VDT) is an effective salvage regimen for patients with relapsed and refractory multiple myeloma. *Leuk. Lymphoma* 2005;**46**:1103–4.

107. Chanan-Khan, A., Miller, K. C., Musial, L. *et al.* Bortezomib in combination with pegylated liposomal doxorubicin and thalidomide is an effective steroid independent salvage regimen for patients with relapsed or refractory multiple myeloma: results of a phase II clinical trial. *Leuk Lymphoma* 2009;**50**: 1096–101.

108. Ciolli, S., Leoni, F., Gigli, F., Rigacci, L., Bosi, A. Low dose velcade, thalidomide and dexamethasone (LD-VTD): an effective regimen for relapsed and refractory multiple myeloma patients. *Leuk. Lymphoma* 2006;**47**:171–3.

109. Kim, Y. K., Sohn, S. K., Lee, J. H. *et al.* Clinical efficacy of a bortezomib, cyclophosphamide, thalidomide, and dexamethasone (Vel-CTD) regimen in patients with relapsed or refractory multiple myeloma: a phase II study. *Ann. Hematol.* 2010;**89**:475–82.

110. Offidani, M., Corvatta, L., Polloni, C. *et al.* Thalidomide, dexamethasone, doxil and velcade (ThaDD-V) followed by consolidation/maintenance therapy in patients with relapsed-refractory multiple myeloma. *Ann. Hematol.* 2011;**90**:1449–56.

111. Palumbo, A., Ambrosini, M. T., Benevolo, G. *et al.* Bortezomib, melphalan, prednisone, and thalidomide for relapsed multiple myeloma. *Blood* 2007;**109**: 2767–72.

112. Pineda-Roman, M., Zangari, M., van Rhee, F. *et al.* VTD combination therapy with bortezomib-thalidomide-dexamethasone is highly effective in advanced and refractory multiple myeloma. *Leukemia* 2008;**22**:1419–27.

113. Lee, C. K., Barlogie, B., Munshi, N. *et al.* DTPACE: an effective, novel combination chemotherapy with thalidomide for previously treated patients with myeloma. *J. Clin. Oncol.* 2003;**21**:2732–9.

114. Garderet, L., Iacobelli, S., Moreau, P. *et al.* Superiority of the triple combination of bortezomib-thalidomide-dexamethasone over the dual combination of thalidomide-dexamethasone in patients with multiple myeloma progressing or relapsing after autologous transplantation: the

MMVAR/IFM 2005–04 Randomized Phase III Trial from the Chronic Leukemia Working Party of the European Group for Blood and Marrow Transplantation. *J. Clin. Oncol.* 2012; **30**:2475–82.

115. Richardson, P. G., Weller, E., Jagannath, S. *et al.* Multicenter, phase I, dose-escalation trial of lenalidomide plus bortezomib for relapsed and relapsed/refractory multiple myeloma. *J. Clin. Oncol.* 2009;**27**:5713–19.

116. Baz, R., Walker, E., Karam, M. A. *et al.* Lenalidomide and pegylated liposomal doxorubicin-based chemotherapy for relapsed or refractory multiple myeloma: safety and efficacy. *Ann. Oncol.* 2006;**17**:1766–71.

117. Palumbo, A., Larocca, A., Falco, P. *et al.* Lenalidomide, melphalan, prednisone and thalidomide (RMPT) for relapsed/refractory multiple myeloma. *Leukemia* 2010;**24**:1037–42.

118. Alexanian, R., Dimopoulos, M. A., Hester, J., Delasalle, K., Champlin, R. Early myeloablative therapy for multiple myeloma. *Blood* 1994;**84**:4278–82.

119. Alexanian, R., Weber, D., Delasalle, K. *et al.* Clinical outcomes with intensive therapy for patients with primary resistant multiple myeloma. *Bone Marrow Transplant* 2004;**34**:229–34.

120. Kumar, S., Lacy, M. Q., Dispenzieri, A. *et al.* High-dose therapy and autologous stem cell transplantation for multiple myeloma poorly responsive to initial therapy. *Bone Marrow Transplant* 2004;**34**:161–7.

121. Rajkumar, S. V., Fonseca, R., Lacy, M. Q. *et al.* Autologous stem cell transplantation for relapsed and primary refractory myeloma. *Bone Marrow Transplant* 1999;**23**:1267–72.

122. Rosinol, L., Garcia-Sanz, R., Lahuerta, J. J. *et al.* Benefit from autologous stem cell

transplantation in primary refractory myeloma? Different outcomes in progressive versus stable disease. *Haematologica* 2012;**97**:616–21.

123. Singhal, S., Powles, R., Sirohi, B. *et al*. Response to induction chemotherapy is not essential to obtain survival benefit from high-dose melphalan and autotransplantation in myeloma. *Bone Marrow Transplant* 2002;**30**:673–9.

124. Lee, C. K., Barlogie, B., Zangari, M. *et al*. Transplantation as salvage therapy for high-risk patients with myeloma in relapse. *Bone Marrow Transplant* 2002;**30**:873–8.

125. Mansi, J. L., Cunningham, D., Viner, C. *et al*. Repeat administration of high dose melphalan in relapsed myeloma. *Br. J. Cancer* 1993;**68**:983–7.

126. Alvares, C. L., Davies, F. E., Horton, C. *et al*. The role of second autografts in the management of myeloma at first relapse. *Haematologica* 2006;**91**:141–2.

127. Olin, R. L., Vogl, D. T., Porter, D. L. *et al*. Second auto-SCT is safe and effective salvage therapy for relapsed multiple myeloma. *Bone Marrow Transplant* 2009;**43**: 417–22.

128. Cook, G., Liakopoulou, E., Pearce, R. *et al*. Factors influencing the outcome of a second autologous stem cell transplant (ASCT) in relapsed multiple myeloma: a study from the British Society of Blood and Marrow Transplantation Registry. *Biol. Blood Marrow Transplant* 2011;**17**:1638–45.

129. Tricot, G., Vesole, D. H., Jagannath, S. *et al*. Graft-versus-myeloma effect: proof of principle. *Blood* 1996;**87**:1196–8.

130. Gahrton, G., Svensson, H., Cavo, M. *et al*. Progress in allogenic bone marrow and peripheral blood stem cell transplantation for

multiple myeloma: a comparison between transplants performed 1983–93 and 1994–8 at European Group for Blood and Marrow Transplantation centres. *Br. J. Haematol.* 2001;**113**:209–16.

131. Lokhorst, H., Einsele, H., Vesole, D. *et al*. International Myeloma Working Group consensus statement regarding the current status of allogeneic stem-cell transplantation for multiple myeloma. *J. Clin. Oncol.* 2010;**28**:4521–30.

132. Bremer, K. High rates of long-lasting remissions after 5-day bendamustine chemotherapy cycles in pre-treated low-grade non-Hodgkin's-lymphomas. *J. Cancer Res. Clin. Oncol.* 2002;**128**:603–9.

133. Damaj, G., Malard, F., Hulin, C. *et al*. Efficacy of bendamustine in relapsed/refractory myeloma patients: results from the French compassionate use program. *Leuk. Lymphoma* 2012;**53**:632–4.

134. Knop, S., Straka, C., Haen, M. *et al*. The efficacy and toxicity of bendamustine in recurrent multiple myeloma after high-dose chemotherapy. *Haematologica* 2005;**90**:1287–8.

135. Michael, M., Bruns, I., Bolke, E. *et al*. Bendamustine in patients with relapsed or refractory multiple myeloma. *Eur. J. Med. Res.* 2010;**15**:13–19.

136. Ponisch, W., Rozanski, M., Goldschmidt, H. *et al*. Combined bendamustine, prednisolone and thalidomide for refractory or relapsed multiple myeloma after autologous stem-cell transplantation or conventional chemotherapy: results of a Phase I clinical trial. *Br. J. Haematol.* 2008;**143**:191–200.

137. Bartlett, J. B., Dredge, K., Dalgleish, A. G. The evolution of thalidomide and its IMiD derivatives as anticancer agents. *Nat. Rev. Cancer* 2004;**4**: 314–22.

138. Hideshima, T., Chauhan, D., Shima, Y. *et al*. Thalidomide and its analogs overcome drug resistance of human multiple myeloma cells to conventional therapy. *Blood* 2000;**96**:2943–50.

139. Gupta, D., Treon, S. P., Shima, Y. *et al*. Adherence of multiple myeloma cells to bone marrow stromal cells upregulates vascular endothelial growth factor secretion: therapeutic applications. *Leukemia* 2001;**15**:1950–61.

140. Corral, L. G., Haslett, P. A., Muller, G. W. *et al*. Differential cytokine modulation and T cell activation by two distinct classes of thalidomide analogues that are potent inhibitors of TNF-alpha. *J. Immunol.* 1999;**163**:380–6.

141. Haslett, P. A., Corral, L. G., Albert, M., Kaplan, G. Thalidomide costimulates primary human T lymphocytes, preferentially inducing proliferation, cytokine production, and cytotoxic responses in the CD8+ subset. *J. Exp. Med.* 1998;**187**:1885–92.

142. Muller, G. W., Chen, R., Huang, S. Y. *et al*. Amino-substituted thalidomide analogs: potent inhibitors of TNF-alpha production. *Bioorg. Med. Chem. Lett.* 1999;**9**:1625–30.

143. Schey, S. A., Fields, P., Bartlett, J. B. *et al*. Phase I study of an immunomodulatory thalidomide analog, CC-4047, in relapsed or refractory multiple myeloma. *J. Clin. Oncol.* 2004;**22**:3269–76.

144. Streetly, M. J., Gyertson, K., Daniel, Y. *et al*. Alternate day pomalidomide retains anti-myeloma effect with reduced adverse events and evidence of in vivo immunomodulation. *Br. J. Haematol.* 2008;**141**:41–51.

145. Lacy, M. Q., Hayman, S. R., Gertz, M. A. *et al*. Pomalidomide (CC4047) plus low-dose dexamethasone as therapy for relapsed multiple myeloma. *J. Clin. Oncol.* 2009;**27**:5008–14.

146. Lacy, M. Q., Hayman, S. R., Gertz, M. A. et al. Pomalidomide (CC4047) plus low dose dexamethasone (Pom/dex) is active and well tolerated in lenalidomide refractory multiple myeloma (MM). Leukemia 2010;24:1934–9.

147. Lacy, M. Q., Allred, J. B., Gertz, M. A. et al. Pomalidomide plus low-dose dexamethasone in myeloma refractory to both bortezomib and lenalidomide: comparison of 2 dosing strategies in dual-refractory disease. Blood 2011;118:2970–5.

148. Richardson, P. G., Siegel, D. S., Vij, R. et al. Randomized, open label phase 1/2 study of pomalidomide (POM) alone or in combination with low-dose dexamethasone (LoDex) in patients (Pts) with relapsed and refractory multiple myeloma who have received prior treatment that includes lenalidomide (LEN) and bortezomib (BORT): phase 2 results. ASH Annual Meeting Abstracts 2011;118:634.

149. Gallinari, P., Di Marco, S., Jones, P., Pallaoro, M., Steinkuhler, C. HDACs, histone deacetylation and gene transcription: from molecular biology to cancer therapeutics. Cell Res. 2007;17:195–211.

150. Roth, S. Y., Denu, J. M., Allis, C. D. Histone acetyltransferases. Ann. Rev. Biochem. 2001;70:81–120.

151. Minucci, S., Pelicci, P. G. Histone deacetylase inhibitors and the promise of epigenetic (and more) treatments for cancer. Nat. Rev. Cancer 2006;6:38–51.

152. Niesvizky, R., Ely, S., Mark, T. et al. Phase 2 trial of the histone deacetylase inhibitor romidepsin for the treatment of refractory multiple myeloma. Cancer 2011;117:336–42.

153. Richardson, P., Mitsiades, C., Colson, K. et al. Phase I trial of oral vorinostat (suberoylanilide hydroxamic acid, SAHA) in patients with advanced multiple myeloma. Leuk. Lymphoma 2008;49:502–7.

154. Wolf, J. L., Siegel, D., Matous, J. et al. A phase II study of oral panobinostat (LBH589) in adult patients with advanced refractory multiple myeloma. ASH Annual Meeting Abstracts 2008;112:2774.

155. Siegel, D. S., Dimopoulos, M. A., Yoon, S.-S. et al. Vantage 095: vorinostat in combination with bortezomib in salvage multiple myeloma patients: final study results of a global phase 2b trial. ASH Annual Meeting Abstracts 2011;118:480.

156. Dimopoulos, M. A., Jagannath, S., Yoon, S.-S. et al. Vantage 088: vorinostat in combination with bortezomib in patients with relapsed/refractory multiple myeloma: results of a global, randomized phase 3 trial. ASH Annual Meeting Abstracts 2011;118:811.

157. Richardson, P., Weber, D., Mitsiades, C. S. et al. A phase I study of vorinostat, lenalidomide, and dexamethasone in patients with relapsed or relapsed and refractory multiple myeloma: excellent tolerability and promising activity in a heavily pretreated population. ASH Annual Meeting Abstracts 2010;116:1951.

158. Richardson, P. G., Alsina, M., Weber, D. M. et al. Phase II study of the pan-deacetylase inhibitor panobinostat in combination with bortezomib and dexamethasone in relapsed and bortezomib-refractory multiple myeloma (PANORAMA 2). ASH Annual Meeting Abstracts 2011;118:814.

159. Harrison, S. J., Quach, H., Link, E. et al. A high rate of durable responses with romidepsin, bortezomib, and dexamethasone in relapsed or refractory multiple myeloma. Blood 2011;118:6274–83.

160. Demo, S. D., Kirk, C. J., Aujay, M. A. et al. Antitumor activity of PR-171, a novel irreversible inhibitor of the proteasome. Cancer Res. 2007;67:6383–91.

161. Siegel, D. S., Martin, T., Wang, M. et al. A phase 2 study of single-agent carfilzomib (PX-171-003-A1) in patients with relapsed and refractory multiple myeloma. Blood 2012;120:2817–25.

162. Vij, R., Wang, M., Kaufman, J. L. et al. An open-label, single-arm, phase 2 (PX-171-004) study of single-agent carfilzomib in bortezomib-naive patients with relapsed and/or refractory multiple myeloma. Blood 2012;119:5661–70.

163. Hsi, E. D., Steinle, R., Balasa, B. et al. CS1, a potential new therapeutic antibody target for the treatment of multiple myeloma. Clin. Cancer Res. 2008;14:2775–84.

164. Tai, Y. T., Dillon, M., Song, W. et al. Anti-CS1 humanized monoclonal antibody HuLuc63 inhibits myeloma cell adhesion and induces antibody-dependent cellular cytotoxicity in the bone marrow milieu. Blood 2008;112:1329–37.

165. Zonder, J. A., Mohrbacher, A. F., Singhal, S. et al. A phase 1, multicenter, open-label, dose escalation study of elotuzumab in patients with advanced multiple myeloma. Blood 2012;120:552–9.

166. Jakubowiak, A. J., Benson, D. M., Bensinger, W. et al. Phase I trial of anti-CS1 monoclonal antibody elotuzumab in combination with bortezomib in the treatment of relapsed/refractory multiple myeloma. J. Clin. Oncol. 2012;30:1960–5.

167. Lonial, S., Vij, R., Harousseau, J. L. et al. Elotuzumab in combination with lenalidomide and low-dose dexamethasone in relapsed or refractory multiple myeloma. J. Clin. Oncol. 2012;30:1953–9.

168. Richardson, P. G., Jagannath, S., Moreau, P. *et al.* A phase 2 study of elotuzumab (Elo) in combination with lenalidomide and low-dose dexamethasone (Ld) in patients (pts) with relapsed/refractory multiple myeloma (R/R MM): updated results. *ASH Annual Meeting Abstracts* 2012;**120**:202.

169. Hovenga, S., Daenen, S. M., de Wolf, J. T. *et al.* Combined thalidomide and cyclophosphamide treatment for refractory or relapsed multiple myeloma patients: a prospective phase II study. *Ann. Hematol.* 2005;**84**:311–16.

170. Moehler, T. M., Neben, K., Benner, A. *et al.* Salvage therapy for multiple myeloma with thalidomide and CED chemotherapy. *Blood* 2001;**98**:3846–8.

171. Palumbo, A., Larocca, A., Genuardi, M. *et al.* Melphalan, prednisone, thalidomide and defibrotide in relapsed/refractory multiple myeloma: results of a multicenter phase I/II trial. *Haematologica* 2010;**95**:1144–9.

172. Offidani, M., Corvatta, L., Marconi, M. *et al.* Low-dose thalidomide with pegylated liposomal doxorubicin and high-dose dexamethasone for relapsed/refractory multiple myeloma: a prospective, multicenter, phase II study. *Haematologica* 2006;**91**:133–6.

173. Srikanth, M., Davies, F. E., Wu, P. *et al.* Survival and outcome of blastoid variant myeloma following treatment with the novel thalidomide containing regime DT-PACE. *Eur. J. Haematol.* 2008;**81**:432–6.

174. Lee, S. S., Suh, C., Kim, B. S. *et al.* Bortezomib, doxorubicin, and dexamethasone combination therapy followed by thalidomide and dexamethasone consolidation as a salvage treatment for relapsed or refractory multiple myeloma: analysis of efficacy and safety. *Ann Hematol* 2010;**89**:905–12.

175. Moreau, P., Pylypenko, H., Grosicki, S. *et al.* Subcutaneous versus intravenous administration of bortezomib in patients with relapsed multiple myeloma: a randomised, phase 3, non-inferiority study. *Lancet Oncol.* 2011;**12**:431–40.

176. Garderet, L., Iacobelli, S., Moreau, P. *et al.* Superiority of the triple combination of bortezomib-thalidomide-dexamethasone over the dual combination of thalidomide-dexamethasone in patients with multiple myeloma progressing or relapsing after autologous transplantation: the MMVAR/IFM 2005–04 randomized phase III trial from the Chronic Leukemia Working Party of the European Group for Blood and Marrow Transplantation. *J. Clin. Oncol.* 2012;**30**:2475–82.

177. Rodon, P., Hulin, C., Pegourie, B. *et al.* Bendamustine, bortezomib and dexamethasone (BVD) in elderly patients with multiple myeloma in first relapse: updated results of the Intergroupe Francophone Du Myelome (IFM) 2009–01 Trial. *ASH Annual Meeting Abstracts* 2012; **120**:4044.

178. Richardson, P. G., Jagannath, S., Jakubowiak, A. J. *et al.* Phase II trial of lenalidomide, bortezomib, and dexamethasone in patients (pts) with relapsed and relapsed/refractory multiple myeloma (MM): updated efficacy and safety data after >2 years of follow-up. *ASH Annual Meeting Abstracts* 2010;**116**:3049.

179. Lentzsch, S., O'Sullivan, A., Kennedy, R. *et al.* Combination of bendamustine, lenalidomide, and dexamethasone (BLD) in patients with refractory or relapsed multiple myeloma is safe and highly effective: results of phase I/II open-label, dose escalation study. *ASH Annual Meeting Abstracts* 2011;**118**:304.

180. Shah, J. J., Orlowski, R. Z., Alexanian, R. *et al.* Phase I trial of the combination of lenalidomide, thalidomide and dexamethasone in relapsed/refractory multiple myeloma. *ASH Annual Meeting Abstracts* 2010;**116**:1948.

181. Niesvizky, R., Wang, L., Orlowski, R. Z. *et al.* Phase Ib multicenter dose escalation study of carfilzomib plus lenalidomide and low dose dexamethasone (CRd) in relapsed and refractory multiple myeloma (MM). *ASH Annual Meeting Abstracts* 2009;**114**:304.

182. Leleu, X., Attal, M., Arnulf, B. *et al.* Pomalidomide plus low dose dexamethasone is active and well tolerated in bortezomib and lenalidomide refractory multiple myeloma: IFM 2009–02. *Blood* 2013 (in press).

183. Richardson, P. G., Siegel, D., Baz, R. *et al.* Phase I study of pomalidomide MTD, safety and efficacy in patients with refractory multiple myeloma who have received lenalidomide and bortezomib. *Blood* 2012 (in press).

Solitary bone and extra-medullary plasmacytoma

Shirley D'Sa and Eve Gallop-Evans

Introduction and epidemiology

Solitary plasmacytoma, which accounts for less than 5% of plasma cell dyscrasias is characterized by a localized proliferation of malignant plasma cells in the absence of evident disease elsewhere. Such a proliferation may arise in a bone (solitary bone plasmacytoma or SBP) or an extra-medullary compartment (extramedullary plasmacytoma or EMP). Plasmacytomas may also arise in a multifocal manner without evidence of malignant plasma cells in the intervening tissues. Extra-medullary plasmacytomas may also arise in the context of multiple myeloma.

Solitary Bone Plasmacytoma

SBP may arise at any age, but the median age of onset at 55 years is 10 years younger than that for myeloma, with a 1.87:1 male to female ratio [1].

Clinical and laboratory features

In two-thirds of cases, SBP arises in the axial skeleton, including the spine (thoracic > lumbar > sacral > cervical spine), skull, ribs and sternum and, in one-third, the appendicular skeleton, including the shoulder girdle, pelvic girdle or the extremities [2]. Localized skeletal pain due to the solitary osteolytic lesion is a typical presentation of SBP. If the spine is affected, spinal cord or nerve root compression may be an important clinical consequence. Other presentations include pathological fracture of the affected bone, a soft tissue mass due to extra-medullary extension of the tumor and in a small proportion, symptoms of peripheral neuropathy.

A monoclonal protein in serum or urine has been reported in 24%–72% of cases, typically less than 5 g/l and 1 g/24 h respectively. In the largest reported series to date, the serum free light chain (SFLC) ratio was noted to be abnormal in 47% and normal in 53% of 116 patients with SBP [3]. Patients with an abnormal SFLC had a higher level of serum paraprotein and higher incidence of monoclonal protein in the urine. Immuneparesis is uncommon in patients with SBP and may be associated with early disease progression if present [4].

Other blood test results including the full blood count, renal function, serum calcium and $\beta_2$microglobulin are normal in patients with SBP; otherwise an alternative explanation for the abnormality should be sought.

Diagnosis and staging

The histological diagnosis is made by biopsy-proven evidence of clonal plasma cells taken from the presenting lesion. Clonality is demonstrated by κ or λ light chain restriction. Monoclonality and/or an aberrant plasma cell phenotype may be demonstrated with useful markers being CD19, CD56, CD27, CD117 and cyclin D1 [5]. International Myeloma Working Group (IMWG) diagnostic criteria [6] for SBP include biopsy-proven plasmacytoma of bone in a single site only, with X-rays and magnetic resonance imaging and/or FDG PET imaging (if performed) negative outside the primary site. The primary lesion may be associated with a low serum and/or urine M component in the absence of monoclonal plasma cells in the bone marrow and myeloma-related organ dysfunction.

MR imaging of the entire spine and pelvis is mandatory in the staging of SBP as occult lesions may be detected by this modality in one-third of patients despite a normal skeletal survey [7]. SBP typically shows low signal intensity on T1-weighted images and high signal intensity on T2-weighted or diffusion-weighted images (Figure 13.1), with homogeneous contrast

Myeloma, ed. Stephen A. Schey, Kwee L. Yong, Robert Marcus and Kenneth C. Anderson. Published by Cambridge University Press. © Cambridge University Press 2014.

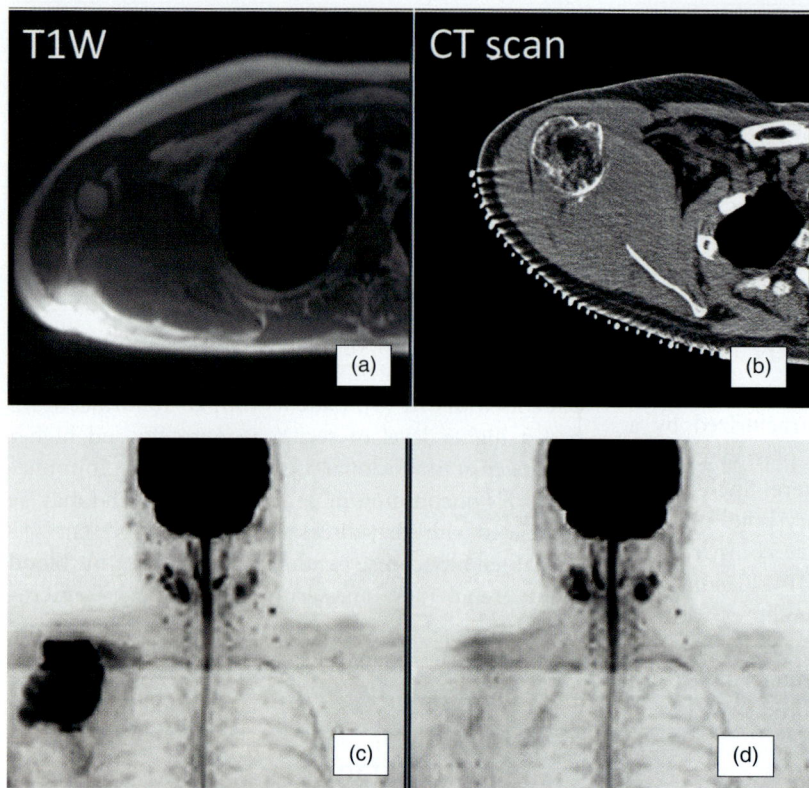

Figure 13.1 A 45 year old male with solitary plasmacytoma of the right scapular bone. Axial images through the proximal right humerus and scapula. The mass is centered on the right scapula glenoid with a large extra-osseous lesion as shown on MR (a) and CT (b). Frontal projection view of a stacked diffusion weighted sequence (b900 s/mm2) presented as a maximum intensity projection (inverted scale). At diagnosis, there is a high signal intensity mass projected over the right scapular bone (c). The high signal intensities of the brain and salivary glands are normal. Following radiotherapy, the signal at the site of disease has disappeared (d).

enhancement of the lesion, but atypical appearances are also possible, so expert review of the imaging is important for an accurate assessment of the condition [8]. There is gathering experience of techniques such as diffusion-weighted whole body MRI, but as yet, evidence for the routine use of this modality is not established. Potential advantages of such a technique include no ionizing radiation, no injections of isotopes or contrast medium, quick to perform and read, potential for quantitative assessments at baseline and following treatment [9].

The role of FDG-PET scanning in plasma cell disorders is also under investigation. PET-CT has also been reported to upstage patients with apparent SBP, by detecting previously unsuspected sites of FDG uptake in eight of 14 patients with SBP [10]. There is evidence for bone marrow SUV max correlation with bone marrow plasma cell percentage in the setting of myeloma and inferior outcome for patients with FDG uptake compared to those without following therapy [11]. Such information may prove to be relevant in the context of plasmacytoma; further studies are warranted. The relative sensitivity and specificity and body coverage of FDG PET and MRI techniques

remains to be clarified; fine-tuning of such imaging techniques will be central to the more accurate primary staging of SBP, so as to permit risk and stage-adapted therapy in the future.

There are emerging flow cytometric data to suggest that the malignant process is active at sites beyond the index lesion from the outset in SBP. Plasma cells with a neoplastic phenotype are detectable in the staging BM of 67% of patients with SBP. In the study by Hill *et al.* [12], they comprised a median of 70% of bone marrow plasma cells and 0.52% of bone marrow leucocytes and their presence was predictive of progression. Further studies of this kind are urgently needed to further the understanding of the pathological nature of SBP and improve the accuracy of staging, so as to apply risk-adapted treatments and hence improve clinical outcome.

Management
Surgery
Surgery may have a role where there is structural instability due to a fracture or rapidly progressive symptoms from cord compression, but is not considered

definitive treatment, even where the diagnostic biopsy appears to have achieved a complete excision.

Radiotherapy

Radical radiotherapy is the treatment of choice for SBP, although there have been no randomized trials. The largest retrospective study included 206 patients with SBP [13]. Treatments included radiotherapy alone (169 patients), RT and chemotherapy (32 patients), and surgery alone (four patients). For patients treated with radiotherapy alone, ten year rates of overall survival, disease-free survival, and local control were 51%, 21% and 78%, with a 71% progression rate to myeloma.

There is little evidence for a dose-response effect over 40 Gy [1,14], even for tumors >5 cm [4,14]. Local control rates of over 85% can be achieved [4,15] but progression to myeloma remains the main problem.

Radiotherapy techniques and beam energies will vary with treatment sites. The clinical target volume should include tumor visible on MRI with a margin of at least 2 cm, or in the case of vertebral involvement, both adjacent vertebrae. If a surgical procedure has been performed, care must be taken to include any areas within the surgical field that may be at risk from tumor contamination. There is no benefit from irradiating the entire medullary cavity of a long bone, or regional lymph nodes.

Chemotherapy

The use of adjuvant chemotherapy for SBP is controversial. Retrospective studies with small numbers of patients have not shown any impact of chemotherapy [16–18]. The only prospective study randomized 53 patients between radiotherapy with or without melphalan and prednisolone given six-weekly for three years [19]. Progression to myeloma occurred in 15 of 28 (54%) patients treated with radiotherapy alone and three of 25 (12%) patients treated with radiotherapy and chemotherapy, and a significant survival benefit seen for the combined treatment group [19]. In a retrospective study of 32 patients with SBP, adjuvant chemotherapy did not affect the incidence of conversion to myeloma, but did appear to delay the median time to progression from 29 to 59 months [20]. Possible consequences of adjuvant cytotoxic therapy in this setting include therapy-induced secondary malignancies and the development of multiresistant subclones, with subsequent compromise of clinical outcome once myeloma has developed [21].

In the era of novel therapies including the immunomodulatory drugs, thalidomide and lenalidomide and the proteasome inhibitor, bortezomib, which have modes of action that are different to conventional cytotoxic drugs, the possibility of adjuvant therapy may warrant reconsideration. These agents have a different side-effect profile compared to cytotoxic agents, and may offer the chance to address the occult neoplastic compartment with limited toxicity. Mateos and colleagues have shown promising results with the use of lenalidomide and dexamethasone therapy in the setting of smoldering myeloma, in which the convention is observation alone [22].

In this phase 3 trial, 119 patients with high-risk smoldering myeloma were randomized to treatment or observation. Patients in the treatment group received an induction regimen (lenalidomide at a dose of 25 mg per day on days 1 to 21, plus dexamethasone at a dose of 20 mg per day on days 1 to 4 and days 12 to 15, at 4-week intervals for nine cycles), followed by a maintenance regimen (lenalidomide at a dose of 10 mg per day on days 1 to 21 of each 28-day cycle for 2 years) until disease progression. The results show, for the first time, that immunomodulatory therapy has significant benefit in terms of progression-free survival in patients with high-risk smoldering myeloma. After a median follow-up of 40 months, the median time to progression was significantly longer in the treatment group than in the observation group (median not reached vs. 21 months; P<0.001). The 3-year survival rate was also higher in the treatment group (94% vs. 80%; P = 0.03). A partial response or better was achieved in 79% of patients in the treatment group after the induction phase and in 90% during the maintenance phase.

This raises the question as to whether a similar outcome could be expected in the setting of SBP, which has parallels with smoldering myeloma in terms of overall disease burden, if novel therapies were employed as part of treatment. Further studies are needed.

Natural history and prognosis

The median overall survival of patients with SBP with current treatment approaches is approximately ten years. The median time to progression to myeloma is two to three years; 15% to 45% of patients remain disease-free at ten years following radiotherapy, but progression can occur as late as 15 years [23]. Relapse rates are higher in older patients [1,13] and in those with an axial rather than appendicular location [2]. The presence of an M protein at the time of diagnosis seems to predict for a higher five-year risk of progression (60% vs. 39%) [24], and persistence of an M protein after radiotherapy also appears to predict for a higher rate of progression to myeloma (91% vs. 29%) [4]. In a study of 116 patients with SBP, a persistent M protein level ≥0.5 g/dl one to two years after diagnosis and an abnormal free light chain ratio at the time of diagnosis were predictive of progression to myeloma at five years. A risk stratification model has been proposed using these two variables, yielding five-year progression rates of 13%, 26% and 62% for those with zero (low risk), one (intermediate risk), or two (high risk) of these risk factors, respectively [3]. Other factors reported to be predictive of progression include plasmacytoma size >5cm, radiotherapy dose, and the presence of neurological symptoms [25]. None of these variables provide a prognostic model that can be used at diagnosis, which is an impediment on the road to risk adapted therapeutic strategies.

Follow up of patients, typically at three to six month intervals should be indefinite, owing to the risk of progression to myeloma, which can occur years later.

Extra-medullary plasmacytoma

Extra-medullary plasmacytomas are plasma cell tumors arising outside the bone marrow, most frequently in the head and neck region (85% of cases), particularly at sites in the upper respiratory tract such as the nasal cavity, sinuses and oropharynx. The next most common site is the gastrointestinal tract, and they can occur less frequently in the bladder, central nervous system, thyroid, breast, testes, lymph nodes and skin. The median age of presentation is 60 years with a 2:1 male to female ratio [25].

Clinical and laboratory features

The clinical presentation depends on the site affected and the local effects of the tumor. Symptoms arising from EMP in the upper respiratory tract include nasal discharge or blockage, epistaxis, hoarseness, hemoptysis and difficulty in breathing; sinus pain and tenderness have also been reported. EMP involving the digestive tract may result in non-specific abdominal pain, gastrointestinal bleeding and weight loss. The stomach and small bowel are more commonly affected than the large bowel [26].

A monoclonal protein is detectable in less than 25% of patients with EMP [25]; immuneparesis is rare, and if present, is regarded by some as an indication of likely occult disease [25]. All other blood tests should be normal. There are few data regarding the utility of the SFLC assay in the setting of EMP.

Diagnosis and staging

The diagnosis of EMP is made by histological confirmation of clonal plasma cells in the index lesion in the absence of evidence for clonal plasmacytosis in the bone marrow. EMP must be distinguished from reactive plasma cell lesions and lymphoma by demonstrating that the infiltrate consists entirely of plasma cells with no B cell component. CD138, MUM1/IRF4, CD20 and PAX5 are the most useful markers although it should be remembered that CD20 and PAX5 are sometimes expressed in plasma cell malignancies. Monoclonality and/or an aberrant plasma cell phenotype should be demonstrated; useful markers include CD19, CD56, CD27, CD117 and cyclin D1 [5]. The importance of histological grade of tumor has been alluded to in previous publications [27], but whether or not higher grade of tumor translates into greater risk of transformation to myeloma and indeed should impact on therapy decisions remains to be ascertained. The extent to which the aerodigestive tract is assessed using endoscopic techniques depends on a careful clinical assessment of the patient's symptoms.

The skeletal survey should be normal and magnetic resonance imaging and/or FDG PET imaging (if performed) must be negative outside the primary site in solitary EMP. FDG uptake on PET-CT may be an important way of identifying regional node involvement, which is present in up to 50% of EMP in the head and neck. This would have potential implications for the radiotherapy field, although the threshold SUV for confirmation of tumor involvement remains contentious [28]. MRI is an important tool for the local assessment of tumor bulk and anatomy; little is known about the role of whole-body MR techniques in the setting of EMP.

Management
Surgery

Surgery can give high rates of local control if complete excision is achieved, particularly if adjuvant radiotherapy is given [29,30], but is usually limited by potential morbidity due to the site of the tumor.

Radiotherapy

Radiotherapy is the primary treatment of choice, giving five year local control rates of 88%–100%, though there is no prospective study data confirming the optimal treatment field and dose.

A retrospective single institution analysis of 67 consecutive patients who received radiotherapy (median dose 50 Gy) for EMP of the head and neck reported five- and ten-year local control rates of 95% and 87%. The five- and ten-year disease free survival rates were 56% and 54% respectively [31]. At a median follow up of 63 months, eight (12%) patients experienced disease progression to multiple myeloma (two patients) and 12 (18%) developed plasmacytoma at another site. A report of 16 patients treated with radiotherapy (median dose 50.4 Gy) found no local relapses, although two patients progressed to MM and four developed plasmacytomas at other sites [32]. Two patients observed following complete surgical excision relapsed at two and 3.3 years respectively, and were successfully treated with salvage radiotherapy.

The optimal dose of radiotherapy is considered to be between 45 Gy and 50 Gy. A report of 17 patients found that doses of 45 Gy or greater were associated with five-year local control rates of 100% compared with 90% for doses of 40 Gy and greater, and 40% for doses below 40 Gy [33].

The primary tumor should be encompassed with a margin of at least 2 cm, and involved nodes included. The role of elective nodal irradiation is unclear. Only one of 51 patients who received radiotherapy to the tumor alone recurred in regional lymph nodes; there were no regional nodal recurrences seen in 16 patients who received radiotherapy to the primary tumor and regional nodes [31].

Adjuvant chemotherapy does not appear to improve relapse rate or increase disease-free survival; however, it is recommended by the UK Myeloma Forum guidelines as a consideration for patients with tumours >5 cm in size and those with high grade tumors. There has been one report, to date, of successful first line treatment of solitary gastric EMP with bortezomib and dexamethasone [34]; bortezomib has also been successfully used to debulk an EMP of the ethmoid and maxillary sinuses prior to 40 Gy radiotherapy [35]. However, the routine use of bortezomib in this setting would be premature, pending further studies.

Natural history and prognosis

Being highly radiosensitive tumors, the local recurrence rate of EMP is less than 10%. Progression to MM at a median of 1.5 to 2.5 years has been reported in 0 to 40% of patients with EMP [36], and as late as 15 years after initial therapy, suggesting that occult disease may be present at diagnosis; indefinite follow up is therefore important for treated EMP patients. Risk factors for progression to myeloma are less well developed than for SBP. Preliminary results of a clinicopathological study of EMP are suggestive of phenotypic and genotypic similarities between myeloma and EMP, including the presence of aberrant phenotype plasma cells in the bone marrow indicating possible occult marrow involvement [37]. Following progression, the clinical course is similar to those with de novo symptomatic myeloma.

Conclusions and future directions

The clinical outcome for patients with SBP and EMP has remained unchanged for many years. Techniques such as immunophenotyping to detect aberrant plasma cells in the bone marrow and imaging techniques that have a functional as well as anatomical capability, such as whole body MRI and FDG-PET CT scanning may improve the sensitivity of detecting occult disease at diagnosis. This could increase the potential for novel, more subtle adjuvant therapies to be applied.

References

1. Ozsahin, M., Tsang, R. W., Poortmans, P. *et al.* Outcomes and patterns of failure in solitary plasmacytoma: a multicenter Rare Cancer Network study of 258 patients. *Int. J. Radiat. Oncol. Biol. Phys.* 2006;**64**(1):210–17.

2. Bataille, R., Sany, J. Solitary myeloma: clinical and prognostic features of a review of 114 cases. *Cancer* 1981;**48**(3):845–51.

3. Dingli, D., Kyle, R. A., Rajkumar, S. V. *et al.* Immunoglobulin free light chains and solitary plasmacytoma of bone. *Blood* 2006;**108**(6):1979–83.

4. Wilder, R. B., Ha, C. S., Cox, J. D. *et al.* Persistence of myeloma protein for more than one year after radiotherapy is an adverse prognostic factor in solitary

plasmacytoma of bone. *Cancer* 2002;**94**(5):1532–7.

5. Rawstron, A. C., Orfao, A., Beksac, M. *et al.* Report of the European Myeloma Network on multiparametric flow cytometry in multiple myeloma and related disorders. *Haematologica* 2008;**93** (3):431–8.

6. Dimopoulos, M., Kyle, R., Fermand, J. P. *et al.* Consensus recommendations for standard investigative workup: report of the International Myeloma Workshop Consensus Panel 3. *Blood* 2011;**117**(18):4701–5.

7. Moulopoulos, L. A., Dimopoulos, M. A., Weber, D. *et al.* Magnetic resonance imaging in the staging of solitary plasmacytoma of bone. *J. Clin. Oncol.* 1993;**11**(7): 1311–15.

8. Chargari, C., Vennarini, S., Servois, V. *et al.* Place of modern imaging modalities for solitary plasmacytoma: Toward improved primary staging and treatment monitoring. *Crit. Rev. Oncol. Hematol.* (in press).

9. Horger, M., Weisel, K., Horger, W. *et al.* Whole-body diffusion-weighted MRI with apparent diffusion coefficient mapping for early response monitoring in multiple myeloma: preliminary results. *AJR Am. J. Roentgenol.* 2011;**196**(6):W790–5.

10. Nanni, C., Rubello, D., Zamagni, E. *et al.* 18F-FDG PET/CT in myeloma with presumed solitary plasmocytoma of bone. *In Vivo* 2008;**22**(4):513–17.

11. Haznedar, R., Aki, S. Z., Akdemir, O. U. *et al.* Value of (18) Fluorodeoxyglucose uptake in positron emission tomography/ computed tomography in predicting survival in multiple myeloma. *Eur. J. Nucl. Med. Mol. Imaging* 2011;**55**:1738–9.

12. Hill, Q., Rawstron, A. C., Child, J. A., De Tute, R., Owen, R. G. Neoplastic plasma cells are demonstrable at bone marrow

sites distant to solitary plasmacytoma of bone and predict for progression to multiple myeloma. *Br. J. Haematol.* 2007;**137**(suppl. 1):18.

13. Knobel, D., Zouhair, A., Tsang, R. W. *et al.* Prognostic factors in solitary plasmacytoma of the bone: a multicenter Rare Cancer Network study. *BMC Cancer* 2006;**6**:118.

14. Tsang, R. W., Gospodarowicz, M. K., Pintilie, M. *et al.* Solitary plasmacytoma treated with radiotherapy: impact of tumor size on outcome. *Int. J. Radiat. Oncol. Biol. Phys.* 2001;**50**(1): 113–20.

15. Dagan, R., Morris, C. G., Kirwan, J., Mendenhall, W. M. Solitary plasmacytoma. *Am. J. Clin. Oncol.* 2009;**32**(6):612–17.

16. Galieni, P., Cavo, M., Avvisati, G. *et al.* Solitary plasmacytoma of bone and extramedullary plasmacytoma: two different entities? *Ann. Oncol.* 1995;**6** (7):687–91.

17. Shih, L. Y., Dunn, P., Leung, W. M., Chen, W. J., Wang, P. N. Localised plasmacytomas in Taiwan: comparison between extramedullary plasmacytoma and solitary plasmacytoma of bone. *Br. J. Cancer* 1995;**71**(1):128–33.

18. Bolek, T. W., Marcus, R. B., Mendenhall, N. P. Solitary plasmacytoma of bone and soft tissue. *Int. J. Radiat. Oncol. Biol. Phys.* 1996;**36**(2):329–33.

19. Aviles, A., Huerta-Guzman, J., Delgado, S., Fernandez, A., Diaz-Maqueo, J. C. Improved outcome in solitary bone plasmacytomata with combined therapy. *Hematol. Oncol.* 1996;**14**(3):111–17.

20. Holland, J., Trenkner, D. A., Wasserman, T. H., Fineberg, B. Plasmacytoma. Treatment results and conversion to myeloma. *Cancer* 1992;**69**(6):1513–17.

21. Delauche-Cavallier, M. C., Laredo, J. D., Wybier, M. *et al.* Solitary

plasmacytoma of the spine. Long-term clinical course. *Cancer* 1988;**61**(8):1707–14.

22. Mateos, M. V., Hernández, M., Giraldo, P. *et al.* Lenalidomide plus dexamethasone for high-risk smoldering multiple myeloma. *N. Engl. J. Med.* 2013;**5**: 1 Aug.

23. Dimopoulos, M. A., Moulopoulos, L. A., Maniatis, A., Alexanian, R. Solitary plasmacytoma of bone and asymptomatic multiple myeloma. *Blood* 2000;**96**(6): 2037–44.

24. Reed, V., Shah, J., Medeiros, L. J. *et al.* Solitary plasmacytomas: outcome and prognostic factors after definitive radiation therapy. *Cancer* (in press).

25. Liebross, R. H., Ha, C. S., Cox, J. D. *et al.* Clinical course of solitary extramedullary plasmacytoma. *Radiother. Oncol.* 1999;**52**(3): 245–9.

26. Dimopoulos, M. A., Hamilos, G. Solitary bone plasmacytoma and extramedullary plasmacytoma. *Curr. Treat. Options Oncol.* 2002;**3** (3):255–9.

27. Bartl, R., Frisch, B., Fateh-Moghadam, A. *et al.* Histologic classification and staging of multiple myeloma. A retrospective and prospective study of 674 cases. *Am. J. Clin. Pathol.* 1987;**87**(3):342–55.

28. Ooi, G. C., Chim, J. C., Au, W. Y., Khong, P. L. Radiologic manifestations of primary solitary extramedullary and multiple solitary plasmacytomas. *Am. J. Roentgenol.* 2006;**186**(3):821–7.

29. Strojan, P., Soba, E., Lamovec, J., Munda, A. Extramedullary plasmacytoma: clinical and histopathologic study. *Int. J. Radiat. Oncol. Biol. Phys.* 2002;**53**(3):692–701.

30. Alexiou, C., Kau, R. J., Dietzfelbinger, H. *et al.* Extramedullary plasmacytoma: tumor occurrence and therapeutic

concepts. *Cancer* 1999;**85**(11):
2305–14.

31. Sasaki, R., Yasuda, K., Abe, E.
    et al. Multi-institutional analysis
    of solitary extramedullary
    plasmacytoma of the head and
    neck treated with curative
    radiotherapy. *Int. J. Radiat. Oncol.
    Biol. Phys.* (in press).

32. Creach, K. M., Foote, R. L.,
    Neben-Wittich, M. A., Kyle, R. A.
    Radiotherapy for extramedullary
    plasmacytoma of the head and
    neck. *Int. J. Radiat. Oncol. Biol.
    Phys.* 2009;**73**(3):789–94.

33. Tournier-Rangeard, L., Lapeyre,
    M., Graff-Caillaud, P. *et al.*

Radiotherapy for solitary
extramedullary plasmacytoma in
the head-and-neck region: A dose
greater than 45 Gy to the target
volume improves the local
control. *Int. J. Radiat. Oncol. Biol.
Phys.* 2006;**64**(4):1013–17.

34. Katodritou, E., Kartsios, C.,
    Gastari, V. *et al.* Successful
    treatment of extramedullary
    gastric plasmacytoma with the
    combination of bortezomib and
    dexamethasone: first reported
    case. *Leuk. Res.* 2008;**32**(2):
    339–41.

35. Varettoni, M., Mangiacavalli, S.,
    Zappasodi, P. *et al.* Efficacy of

Bortezomib followed by local
irradiation in two patients with
extramedullary plasmacytomas.
Leuk. Res. 2008;**32**(5):839–41.

36. Mendenhall, C. M., Thar, T. L.,
    Million, R. R. Solitary
    plasmacytoma of bone and soft
    tissue. *Int. J. Radiat. Oncol. Biol.
    Phys.* 1980;**6**(11):1497–501.

37. Boll, M., Parkins, E., O'Connor, S.
    J., Rawstron, A. C., Owen, R. G.
    Extramedullary plasmacytoma are
    characterized by a 'myeloma-like'
    immunophenotype and genotype
    and occult bone marrow
    involvement. *Br. J. Haematol.*
    2010;**151**(5):525–7.

Amyloidosis

Ashutosh D. Wechalekar, Simon W. Dubrey and Raymond L. Comenzo

Introduction

The common pathophysiologic mechanism in the systemic amyloidoses is proteotoxicity caused by misfolded protein species that are toxic to cells and form interstitial fibrillar deposits of amyloid [1,2]. Organ dysfunction and death, notably from cardiac involvement, remain common occurrences in patients with systemic disease. Systemic immuno-globulin light-chain (AL) amyloidosis, with an incidence of eight to ten cases per million person-years, a median age at diagnosis of 63, and median survival if untreated of 12 months, is the most frequent type encountered in clinical practice [3]. Next most common are the transthyretin (ATTR) types caused by either mutant (hereditary, ATTRm) variants or wild-type ("senile systemic," ATTRwt) transthyretin [4,5]. Secondary amyloidosis (AA), although rare in developed countries, still occurs with autoimmune or inflammatory diseases such as multi-centric Castleman's disease, renal cell cancer, autoimmune disorders and chronic infections due to bronchiectasis or osteomyelitis [6,7]. It is important to note that these non-AL types, as well as other rare hereditary types that cause systemic disease, may confound the diagnosis of AL [8,9]. Critical factors are age and race. Incidence of monoclonal gammopathy increases in the elderly and in blacks; therefore, elderly or black patients with both monoclonal gammopathy and tissue biopsies showing amyloid require direct typing of the amyloid to determine whether it is AL or non-AL in type [9,10]. In this chapter we focus on AL: making the diagnosis, understanding the importance of cardiac involvement and hematologic response to therapy, choosing therapy, and recognizing and managing amyloid-related organ disease.

Making the diagnosis

Clinical presentations are similar for all types of systemic amyloidosis [11]. The pattern of organ involvement, although occasionally suggestive, is not diagnostic of a patient's type of amyloid (Table 14.1). Two potential amyloid-forming precursor proteins can be present in one patient [9]. Elderly men have higher rates of both monoclonal gammopathies and ATTRwt, and blacks also have higher rates of monoclonal gammopathies and a 4% incidence of a mutant gene that can cause ATTRm (Val122Ile) [12]. In these cases, only one type of amyloid usually causes symptomatic disease [13]. If direct tissue typing is not obtained, the risks to the practitioner include failure to diagnose a hereditary disease affecting the patient's kin, treating with chemotherapy inappropriately, or failing to treat at all.

Diagnosis requires tissue biopsy, either of an involved organ or a surrogate site (e.g. abdominal fat), that demonstrates amyloid deposition by classic Congo red staining [14]. Involved-organ biopsies are usually performed based on prior clinical suspicion of disease, particularly renal, gastrointestinal, or cardiac. Congo red-stained biopsy preparations from all sites are subject to error either in sampling or processing. The tissue section can be cut too thin or the mounted section over-stained, giving a false negative or false positive, with the results disputed by pathologists [15,16]. Use of electron microscopy is helpful for confirming the presence of pathognomonic fibrils and, except for renal biopsies, is underutilized due to lack of a priori suspicion of the diagnosis. The first question one may face when the biopsy is read as amyloid is whether the result is reliable, and the second question one does face is what type of amyloid is present. Both questions can be answered by laser

Table 14.1 Types of amyloidosis and possible organ involvement

Type	Heart	Kidneys	Liver/ GI tract	PNS	ST
AL	√	√	√	√	√
ATTRm	√	[√]		√	
ATTRwt	√		[√]		[√]
AFib	[√]	√	√		
AApoA1	√*	√	√		
ALys		√	√		[√]

AL – immunoglobulin light chain; ATTRm – mutant transthyretin; ATTRwt – wild type transthyretin; AFib – fibrinogen A-α; AApoA1 – apolipoprotein A1; ALys – lysozyme; [√] – rare; GI – gastrointestinal tract; PNS – peripheral nerves; ST – soft tissue.

capture mass spectrometry, a technique that employs Congo red-positive areas dissected from slides, digested and analyzed [17]. Amyloid deposits reliably contain the fibrillar amyloid protein (for example, lambda light chains, transthyretin or fibrinogen A α-chain) as well as fellow-passenger proteins such as apo E, serum amyloid P protein and clusterin. A false-positive sample can be clearly identified by this method. Typing by this method is critical if a patient with amyloidosis does not have a monoclonal protein as determined by an evaluation that includes serum and urine immunofixation and the serum free light chain assay, and of course if there are two possible amyloid-forming proteins present in one patient. For typing, immunohistochemical staining is frequently unreliable and inaccurate, and immunogold electron microscopy reliable but limited by serologic dependence [8,18]. Laser capture with mass spectrometry with customized bioinformatic assessment of the constituents of the Congophilic deposits is now the gold standard for amyloid typing, enabling precise identification of type in over 98% of cases. DNA sequencing of genes related to hereditary variants also is a useful tool, particularly for confirming proteomic findings and more pointedly for subsequent screening of kin [9].

Once amyloidosis has been demonstrated by biopsy, subsequent work-up involves identification of the precursor protein and the extent of organ involvement. Testing for a monoclonal gammopathy is performed with serum and urine protein studies and bone marrow biopsy with immunohistochemical staining for CD138, kappa and lambda, and Congo red staining for amyloid [19]. The serum free light chain assay is critical for evaluating and monitoring patients with AL, as many patients lack a circulating intact immunoglobulin and both serum and urine immunofixation have limited sensitivities [20]. The free light chain assay provides a unique scientific and clinical tool in patients with AL since it is a direct measure of the amyloid-forming protein, not simply an indirect measure of clonal plasma cell burden [21]. The use of all three assays can identify a monoclonal protein and/or light chain in 95% of patients [22].

Cytogenetics and fluorescent *in situ* hybridization (FISH) have become routine tests of clonal plasma cells in myeloma patients, enabling the identification of high-risk and standard-risk patients [23]. Patients with abnormalities such as del13 by cytogenetics or t[4;14] or del17p by FISH have shortened overall survival compared to patients with normal cytogenetics and FISH. Therefore, these findings are considered high risk in myeloma [24]. Recently, the t(11:14) and other cytogenetic abnormalities have been identified in the clonal plasma cells of AL patients [25,26]. In one retrospective series, the t [11;14] was associated with shortened survival in AL [26]. We therefore currently recommend that an aspirate marrow sample at baseline in AL patients be sent for cytogenetics and FISH. In addition, high-risk abnormalities have been identified at aggressive plasma cell disease relapse in AL patients, signaling a significant change in the character of the clonal plasma cells [27]. In such instances, repeat cytogenetics and FISH studies are warranted as well.

Rarely, the amyloid-forming light chain is produced by a low-grade lymphoproliferative disorder and therapy then should be tailored to treat the underlying B cell disorder [28,29]. If the monoclonal gammopathy work-up fails to identify a clonal B-cell disorder, then the AL type is highly unlikely and evaluation for other types should commence. Even if the work-up reveals a monoclonal gammopathy, amyloid typing by at least immunohistochemistry should be done in every case in an experienced laboratory. Definitive tissue typing is advised in elderly men and blacks as noted above, in patients diagnosed with dominant peripheral or autonomic neuropathy (a common presentation of hereditary types), and in patients with family histories of amyloidosis.

Imaging of amyloid deposits is difficult but, when possible, may give important information about the

Table 14.2 Organ response and progression criteria in AL

Organ	Response	Progression
Heart	NT-proBNP response (>30% and >300 ng/l decrease in patients with baseline NT-proBNP ≥650 ng/l) OR NYHA class response (≥2 class decrease in subjects with baseline NYHA class 3 or 4)	NT-proBNP progression (>30% and >300 ng/l increase in presence of stable creatinine) OR cTn progression (≥33% increase) OR Ejection fraction progression (≥10% decrease)
Kidney	50% decrease (at least 0.5 g/day) of 24 hour urine protein (urine protein must be >0.5 g/day pretreatment). Creatinine and creatinine clearance must not worsen by 25% over baseline.	50% increase (at least 1 g/day) of 24 hour urine protein to greater than 1 g/day or 25% worsening of serum creatinine or creatinine clearance
Liver	50% decrease in abnormal alkaline phosphatase value Decrease in liver size radiographically at least 2 cm	50% increase of alkaline phosphatase above the lowest value
Peripheral nervous system	Improvement in electromyogram nerve conduction velocity (rare)	Progressive neuropathy by electromyography or nerve conduction velocity

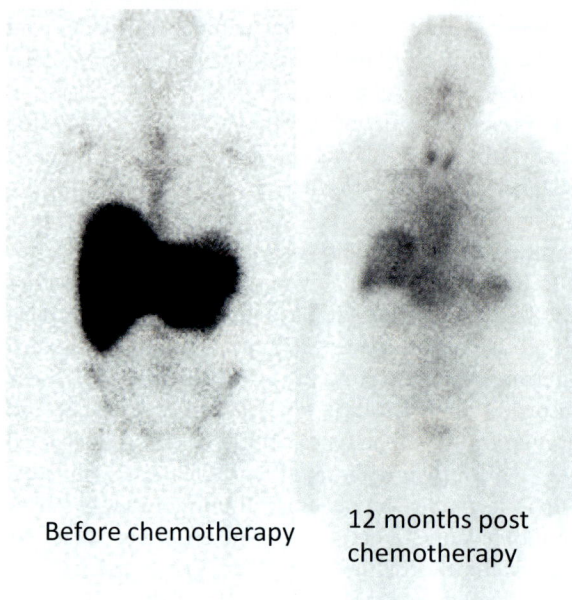

Before chemotherapy   12 months post chemotherapy

Figure 14.1 ^{123}I labeled serum amyloid P component scintigraphy in a patient with AL amyloidosis. There is marked uptake in the liver at presentation in the left-sided panel. Patient had a very good partial response to chemotherapy and the right-sided panel shows complete regression of amyloid from the liver about a year after completion of treatment.

extent of the disease. [123]I labeled serum amyloid P component scintigraphy [30] is used in UK for this purpose and helps to serially monitor changes in the total body amyloid load – and can act as a useful guide to therapy (Figure 14.1). Antibodies to amyloid fibrils also appear to be a useful tracer for positron emission tomographic imaging of amyloid deposits [31].

The importance of cardiac involvement and hematologic response

Criteria for the assessment of organ involvement at baseline have been standardized (Table 14.2) [32,33]. Prognosis in systemic AL amyloidosis remains a function of the extent of cardiac involvement, with median survival of six months for untreated or non-responding patients with symptomatic cardiac AL, and poor hematologic response to therapy [34]. Patients with advanced cardiac involvement and clonal plasma cell disease that fails to respond to initial therapy have short survival [35]. Patients with cardiac involvement can present with progressive dyspnea on exertion, fatigue, findings of diastolic dysfunction and thickening of left ventricular walls in the absence of hypertension, and low voltage on electrocardiogram. Serum troponins (I or T) and B-type natriuretic peptides (either BNP or NT-proBNP) are highly sensitive markers of cardiac involvement, and normal values exclude clinically significant cardiac amyloid [36]. Cardiac MRI is emerging as a useful tool particularly in patients with a thick left ventricular wall and prior hypertension or valvular heart disease, with subendocardial late gadolinium enhancement highly suggestive of amyloid deposition (Figure 14.2) although large studies defining its role or prognostic significance are lacking at this time [37]. ^{99m}Tc-labeled DPD is a bone scanning agent which appears to be specifically taken up by cardiac amyloid deposits and may proven a useful non-invasive tool to differentiate between cardiac AL and ATTR amyloidosis (Figure 14.3).

A cardiac risk assessment or "cardiac staging" system incorporating biomarkers is currently in use, with patients assigned to stage I, II or III based on the presence of 0, 1 or 2 of the biomarkers exceeding threshold levels (NTpro-BNP > 332 ng/l; troponin T > 0.035 µg/l) [38]. Patients in these three stages differ significantly with respect to survival. Patients with stage III cardiac involvement have a median survival of three to four months while those with

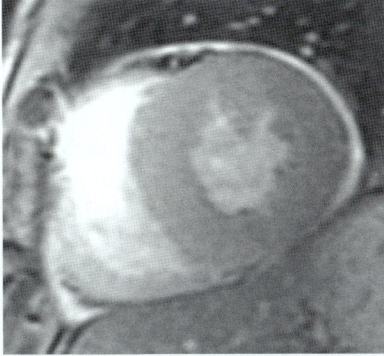

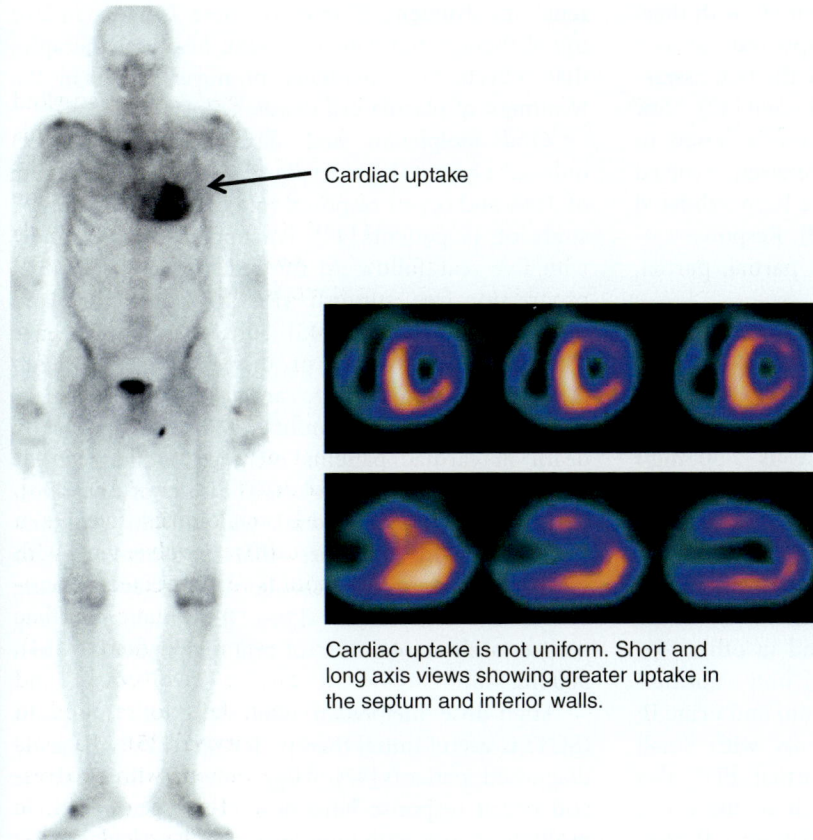

Figure 14.2 Magnetic resonance imaging of the heart in patients with amyloidosis may help to distinguish hypertrophy due to an infiltrative process from that due to hypertension. In this image of the heart of a 49 year old woman with rapidly progressive AL amyloidosis subendocardial enhancement with gadolinium is shown (arrows).

Cardiac uptake

Figure 14.3 ^{99m}Tc-3,3-diphosphono-1,2-propanodicarboxylic acid (DPD) scintigraphy for cardiac amyloidosis. This shows uptake in the heart (normally this should look like a bone scan with no soft tissue uptake) and asymmetric uptake in the myocardium. Patterns and intensity of uptake on DPD scintigraphy may help to differentiate the amyloid type affecting the heart.

Cardiac uptake is not uniform. Short and long axis views showing greater uptake in the septum and inferior walls.

stage I or II disease have much better outcome and could be potential candidates for stem cell transplantation (SCT). In addition, among patients with cardiac involvement, the baseline highly sensitive troponin (hs-Troponin T) is a predictor of survival [39]. Biomarker criteria for clinical cardiac improvement or progression after therapy have been incorporated into the consensus criteria for organ response. Post-therapy, in patients with cardiac involvement, a >30% reduction and a >300 ng/l decrease in the NT-proBNP level from baseline correlate with improved overall survival while increases of that magnitude correlate with progression and worse survival [30].

Staging for cardiac involvement is a critical part of the initial evaluation. In addition to cardiac involvement, the other important prognostic factor is the response to therapy [35,40]. Of note, higher absolute values of the involved free light chain (iFLC), as measured by the serum free light chain assay, are associated with a greater degree of organ involvement and worse overall survival [41]. Post-therapy, achievement of a hematologic response remains the critical variable for predicting organ improvement and prolonged survival [35]. Decreases in the iFLC with therapy are strongly associated with improved survival and serial FLC measurements provide the best assessment of therapeutic efficacy or lack thereof [42]. New criteria for scoring hematologic response based in part on reductions in the difference between involved and uninvolved FLC (the dFLC) have been validated in a large international case series [33]. Response categories include complete, very good partial, partial, and no response.

We hasten to add that 10%–15% of AL patients do not have sufficiently elevated FLC to permit scoring of the dFLC without the iFLC going below the limits of low normal or detectability. Such a scoring algorithm works if the dFLC is >50 mg/l and there is an abnormal kappa to lambda ratio. Patients whose hematologic response cannot be scored in this way, including those with renal insufficiency, remain evaluable based on traditional M protein and marrow biopsy criteria, in some instances for M protein responses and in others for complete hematologic response (CR) only (normalization of the FLC ratio, and/or of serum and urine IF and marrows) [43]. Similarly, patients with small M-proteins (e.g. <0.2 g/dl) and normal FLC also may only be evaluable for CR. In all of these less frequent instances, patients not achieving CR may

be scored as having no hematologic response. Nevertheless, objective measures of organ response and progression will still usually allow reliable clinical assessments and can guide therapy over time and, from the perspective of clinical research, progression-free and overall survival (PFS, OS) still remain key measures of efficacy as well.

Choosing therapy

Therapies for AL are aimed at eliminating the clonal plasma cells producing the toxic precursor protein. Whenever possible, patients should be treated on clinical trials. With current approaches organ improvement can occur in those who achieve at least a partial haematologic response with kidney and liver responses occurring most commonly. Achievement of a >90% reduction in the iFLC or of a CR is associated with organ improvement over 90% of the time [42]. Organ responses can lag six to 12 months after reduction of the iFLC, necessitating best supportive care and collaborative management with other subspecialists, particularly in patients with advanced cardiac or renal involvement. Currently there is no standard initial therapy but rather a menu of initial therapies that reflects the emergence of novel agents in the treatment of plasma cell diseases.

Oral melphalan and dexamethasone (MDex) induced a hematologic response rate of 67%, a CR rate of 33%, and organ response rate of 48% in a phase II study of 45 patients [44]. An update of this cohort with five-year follow-up showed impressive median progression-free survival (PFS) of 3.8 years and median OS of 5.1 years [45]. Subsequent studies have confirmed the activity of this regimen, although outcomes for symptomatic cardiac AL patients remain poor (median OS 10.5 months) [40]. Causes of early death in cardiac patients included sudden cardiac death, infections and strokes. The risks of myelodysplasia and secondary leukemia with monthly oral melphalan remain toxicities that patients need to understand; these risks can be diminished by using cumulative melphalan doses less than 600 mg and certainly a total dose of oral melphalan less than 300 mg [46].

High-dose melphalan with stem cell transplant (SCT) is useful initial therapy for up to 20% of newly diagnosed patients [47]. High rates of hematologic and organ response have now been documented at multiple centers with long-term data reported on over

800 patients and median survivals approaching a decade for SCT patients achieving complete response. Enthusiasm for SCT has been tempered by the high treatment-related mortality (TRM) that remains around 10% even at experienced centers [48]. The use of SCT for AL evolved at a time when no available therapy could reliably produce complete hematologic responses or improve median survival by more than a matter of months [49]. The results with SCT confirmed the direct link of the clonal plasma cell disease to organ damage and survival in AL, showing that elimination of the clonal disease caused reversal of organ damage and prolonged survival [50,51]. Eighty percent of patients achieving a complete hematologic response experience organ responses; half of all patients surviving one year after SCT experience organ responses [47]. The results with SCT propelled development of metrics for organ involvement and response to therapy [32].

We now have numerous therapies that can achieve similar results, including oral melphalan and dexamethasone and bortezomib-based therapies. The sickest AL patients are not candidates for SCT. At best, 20% of newly diagnosed patients are eligible for SCT with effective doses of IV melphalan and with the expectation of a low treatment-related mortality. Indeed, the outcomes reported above with SCT reflect selection bias; that is, choosing the fittest patients for SCT [52–54]. SCT and MDex were compared by the French Myélome Autogreffe Groupe (MAG) in a multi-center randomized phase III trial in newly diagnosed AL patients [55]. There were no significant differences in hematologic or organ responses but median OS was significantly better in the MDex arm (56.9 vs. 22.2 months, $p = 0.04$). However, 22 of the 50 patients assigned to SCT (44%) were not evaluable for response or long-term survival, including 13 who never received SCT due to death or progression and nine who died peri-SCT. Although the up-dated event free survival of patients in both arms continues to show equivalence, confirming the importance of MDex in the treatment of AL, the small number of evaluable SCT patients in the phase III trial, the disparity between outcomes in the SCT arm and SCT results at experienced centers, and the lurking risk of myelodysplasia and secondary leukemia with oral melphalan make it difficult to conclude that equivalence means MDex is best for all.

Over the past decade, with new drugs approved for myeloma, we have witnessed improved survival for many patients. The first novel agent to be investigated in relapsed AL, thalidomide, was poorly tolerated at high doses but in combination with dexamethasone showed efficacy at moderate doses with hematologic responses in 40%–50% of patients post-SCT [56,57]. The combination of oral cyclophosphamide, thalidomide and dexamethsone (CTD) showed promise in the relapsed setting and in a single-center retrospective series of 122 newly diagnosed patients (48% with heart involvement) CTD had high hematologic response rates with a median time to response of two months and 74% survival at three years [58]. CTD is stem-cell sparing, unlike MDex that is stem-cell toxic, and is associated with similar overall response rates. However, due to worries of thalidomide related toxicity, this is not widely used.

In phase II trials, full-dose lenalidomide had significant toxicity requiring dose reductions or discontinuation and was better tolerated at 15 mg/day in combination with weekly dexamethasone (LenDex), with hematologic response rates of 40%–50% [59,60]. Single agent lenalidomide has limited efficacy and is not recommended. In recent reports on over 100 patients with relapsed AL treated with LenDex, there was a 49% hematologic response rate with 16% CR, median OS of about two years and in those achieving CR, a PFS of over three years [61]. In phase I/II studies combining LenDex with oral melphalan or cyclophosphamide, preliminary indications are that dose reductions of the myelosuppressive agents are required and response rates are not substantially different from those seen with MDex or CTD [62]. In a preliminary report on a phase II study of pomalidomide with weekly dexamethasone, over 30% of relapsed AL patients achieved a complete response, highlighting the promise of this potent immunomodulatory (IMiD) therapy [63].

A confounding aspect of IMiD therapy in AL, most applicable to lenaldiomide, is the rise in cardiac biomarker levels that is related to IMiDs [64, 65]. In one trial, asymptomatic increases in NT-proBNP by >30% and >300 ng/l occurred in 67% of patients after cycle 1 [66]. This represents yet another challenge to drug testing in AL – the confounding influence of drug-related side-effects on metrics of organ involvement and response. The pathophysiology of the increase in NT-proBNP due to IMiDs remains uncertain and possible mechanisms may include cardiotoxicity or changes in lean muscle mass.

The safety and preliminary efficacy of bortezomib as a single agent in relapsed AL has been evaluated in a recent phase I/II study of 70 patients [67]. The maximum tolerated dose was not reached, and further evaluation of dosing at both 1.3 mg/m^2 on a twice-weekly (BIW) schedule (i.e. days 1, 4, 8 and 11 every 21 days) and 1.6 mg/m^2 when given weekly (QW) for four out of five weeks, was completed on the phase II level. The most common side-effects were gastrointestinal, neurologic, and fatigue. In the QW cohort (N = 18) there were no instances of >grade 3 peripheral neuropathy (PN), no discontinuations due to PN and only one patient requiring a dose reduction for PN. Overall hematologic and complete response rates were high and as follows: 69% with 38% CR on QW schedule, 67% with 24% CR on BIW schedule, and 39% with 11% CR at lower doses. PFS at one year exceeded 70% and OS 90%. Renal responses have been seen in 14/49 (29%), and objective cardiac responses in 5/39 (13%).

Similar efficacy was seen in a retrospective series of 94 patients (81% previously-treated) receiving bortezomib BIW and dexamethasone. [68] There was a 71% hematologic response rate with 25% CR, a 30% organ response rate, median time to progression of 25 months and one-year survival of 75%. The use of bortezomib and dexamethasone as adjuvant therapy for patients not achieving a CR post-SCT resulted in over 90% of patients improving their hematologic responses, such that at one year post-SCT 65% had achieved a CR and 55% had organ responses [69]. Most striking in the clinical trials and case series in which patients received bortezomib was the rapid time to response, typically one month, a critical variable in AL patients [67]. With weekly and likely subcutaneous dosing, the side effects of bortezomib may be further reduced and dose intensity augmented because of higher weekly doses and fewer interruptions of therapy [70]. The major side effects of bortezomib are gastrointestinal, and range from distension, obstipation, and ileus occasionally requiring conservative in-hospital management, to transient vomiting or diarrhea.

Bortezomib has also been evaluated in combination with MDex (MDB), with a best response rate of over 90% and CR rate over 60% [71]. Of note, in the first 35 patients treated on that trial, 40% required dose reductions of bortezomib for thrombocytopenia or peripheral neuropathy but only one patient was removed from the study for grade 3 PN. These data,

along with the improved survival with bortezomib and oral melphalan and prednisone in myeloma, justify the comparison of MDB with MDex for initial therapy in AL in phase III trials being conducted in the USA by the Eastern Clinic Oncology Group and in the EU by a network of amyloidosis centers. It is not surprising, however, that initial therapy for AL has evolved to include the use of bortezomib, particularly in those with advanced cardiac disease not eligible for phase III trials.

The high response rates, rapidity of response with bortezomib combinations (or even CTD) and being stem cell sparing, makes these regimes attractive in a newly diagnosed AL patient. SCT is becoming a second-line therapy for those who do not respond to initial bortezomib-based therapy and may be as consolidation therapy for those who do. Moreover, because of the risks of myelodysplasia and secondary leukemia, lower and slower responses raise questions about role of MDex in the future for treatment of AL amyloidosis. In patients treated routinely and not on a clinical trial, initial therapy is likely to contain a proteasome inhibitor in combination with other agents such as dexamethasone and an alkylator or may be even an IMiD. Risk-adapted SCT, which tailors the dose of melphalan conditioning to the age and risk status of the patient, may improve early survival with a treatment-related mortality (TRM) of 4% in a recent phase II study [35]. To compensate for the loss of efficacy related to attenuated conditioning, however, adjuvant therapy post-SCT for patients not achieving a CR has been tested and shown to improve hematologic response. Both thalidomide and dexamethasone (TD) and bortezomib and dexamethasone (BD) have been studied as adjuvant therapy post-SCT [35,69]. CR rates at 12 months post-SCT were achieved in 39% and 65% of evaluable patients on these two studies with high rates of organ improvement. However, the high efficacy of novel agent combination regimes in front line treatment, make the role of dose reduced melphalan SCT rather questionable as first line treatment although it may still have a role as consolidation treatment or at relapse.

Every effort should be made to enroll patients in clinical trials. Clinical trials, including multi-center phase I and I/II studies, are required to advance therapy in AL. Ideally such trials should be widely available at multiple centers. Single-center phase II trials make limited contributions to advances in therapy, particularly if both newly diagnosed and relapsed patients are eligible for the trial and time-to-event endpoints are not reported. There are several study populations among AL patients in addition to newly diagnosed untreated patients. AL patients with advanced cardiac disease, who are often excluded from clinical trials, provide a unique and unfortunate opportunity to conduct novel phase II and III trials employing overall survival as a primary endpoint because survival in this study population can be determined in a limited timeframe. Such trials could significantly change practice. There is also a previously treated population of patients with relapsing disease surviving three or more years from diagnosis, a population which no longer contains those with advanced cardiac disease. Relapsed patients are excellent candidates for multi-center trials of novel agents in all phases. A phase I clinical trial with the novel oral proteasome inhibitor MLN9708 in AL is under way for them, and trials with other proteasome inhibitors are planned. Currently there is no standard therapy for patients with relapsed AL but the use of second-line SCT or MDex will likely become more routine as initial therapy with bortezomib-based regimens becomes more prevalent. Patients treated initially with non-bortezomib based therapies should receive bortezomib-based regimens as second-line therapy.

Recognizing and managing amyloid related organ disease

Cardiac amyloid causes a restrictive cardiomyopathy with reduced cardiac output and, when combined with autonomic dysfunction and the hypoalbuminemia of nephrosis, can lead to severe cardiovascular compromise [37]. One must use vasoactive medications in such patients with caution since their hearts are "stiff" and under-filled. Diuretics such as furosemide or bumetanide are standard therapy but they may compromise cardiac output and cause chronic nausea and vomiting due to hypovolemia [72]. Close clinical monitoring with frequent adjustments of dose are mandatory. Patients must be taught to limit their salt intake and weigh themselves daily. Lower extremity edema can be problematic and result in complications of venous stasis; although support stockings may help, their use is difficult for many patients. For those with chronic autonomic insufficiency and orthostasis, midodrine is useful. Fludrocortisone has to be used with caution in

patients with cardiac disease and clearly has no role in any patient on diuretics. In order to minimize the risk of syncope and the trauma of falls, patients must be taught to rise slowly and carefully from the lying to sitting to standing position, and men must be advised to urinate in the seated position.

Among the agents used to treat cardiac failure, low doses of beta blockers may be of limited use to manage arrhythmic tendencies. Cardiac amyloid patients poorly tolerate angiotensin converting enzyme inhibitors, angiotensin receptor blockers, calcium channel blockers and digoxin [19]. These drugs generally must be avoided. Bi-ventricular pacing has not been studied in these patients but may be of benefit, although pacemakers for AV block and AICDS have not prevented dysrhythmias or death [73,74]. Sudden death in cardiac amyloidosis is usually caused by electro-mechanical dissociation. In a report on 53 patients with amyloid cardiomyopathy (33 with AL, the rest with other types) with AICD implantation, a high rate of appropriate AICD shocks were delivered to the AL group with no overall survival benefit [75]. Young patients with advanced cardiac amyloidosis and limited other organ involvement should be evaluated for cardiac transplant. There have been numerous patients who have successfully undergone cardiac allograft and then SCT; the feasibility of this approach is established [76,77]. Hematologic response to treatment with normalization of the iFLC in cardiac patients is associated with reductions in the cardiac biomarker levels (Figure 14.4a) [78]. Moreover, reductions in diuretic requirements are also a common feature of hematologic response and organ improvement.

Over 60% of patients with AL amyloidosis have renal involvement and the most common presentation is proteinuria [79]. Nearly 70% of patients with renal involvement have nephrotic range proteinuria/albuminuria [80] and most have minimal free light chains in the urine [81], [82]. Amyloidosis is present in 3% of renal biopsies [83]. The level of urine protein excretion per day has no impact on survival but patients with higher levels of proteinuria have greater morbidity associated with stem cell mobilization including increased fluid retention and transient acute renal failure [84] in addition to having a higher risk of progressing to end-stage renal failure. The major consequences of renal amyloid are severe serum hypoalbuminemia and eventual renal failure [85]. The loss of albumin results in reduced

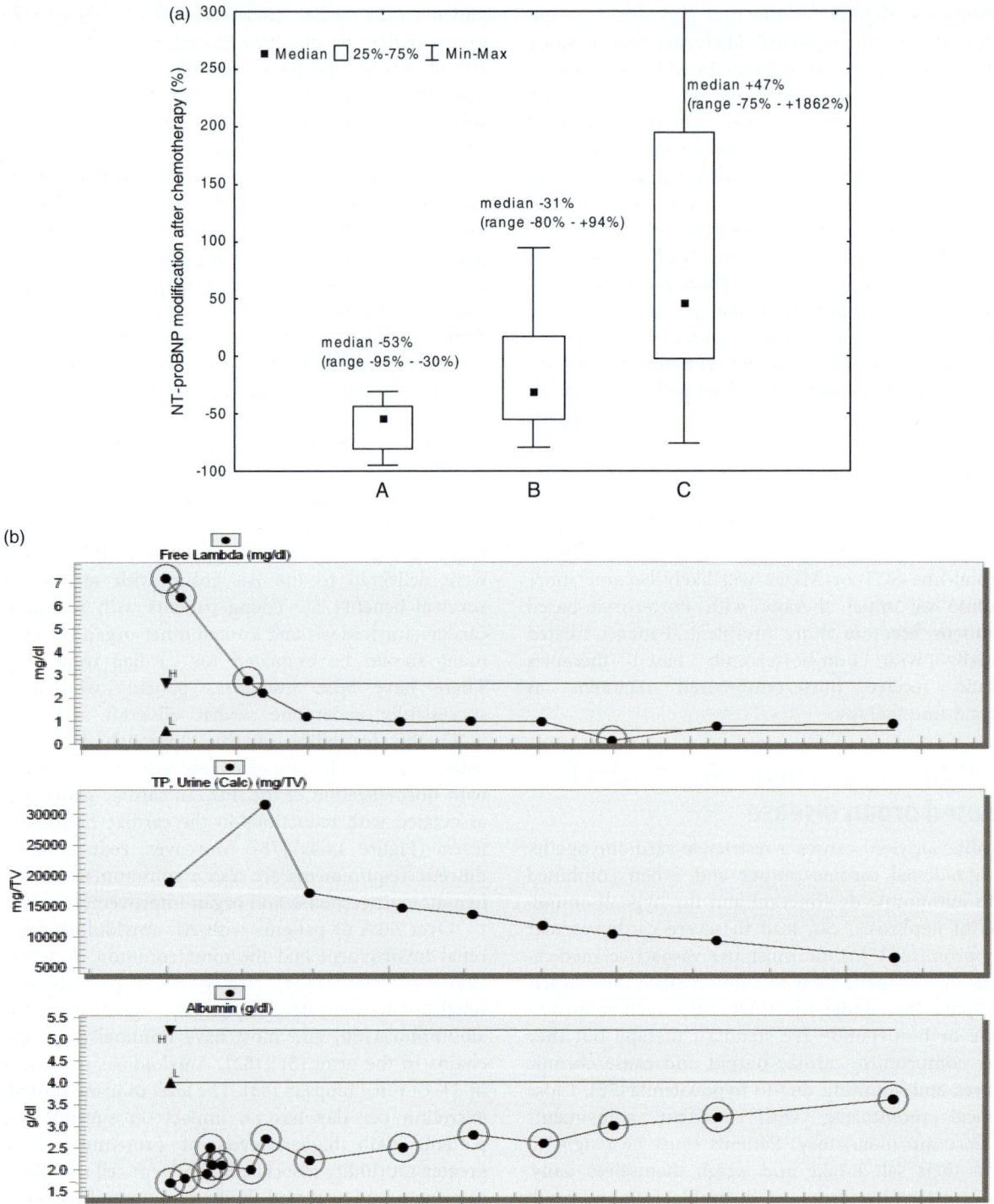

Figure 14.4 In (a), the box-and-whiskers plots depict the changes in NT-proBNP levels in patients who had complete (group A), partial (>50% reduction, group B) or no response to treatment (group C), demonstrating how the organ responses follow hematologic responses (reprinted from reference [76]. Hematologic responses were light-chain based and NT-proBNP measurements were obtained at baseline and at three months after therapy [78]. In (b), the response of a patient with renal involvement is shown. In the top panel the reductions in the involved free light chains with each cycle of MDex are shown and in the lower panels the changes in total daily urine protein and serum albumin are depicted. The incremental improvements in proteinuria and serum albumin occur in time after normalization of the involved free light chain level.

intravascular oncotic pressure and edema of the lower extremities and presacral area. In severe cases it can lead to anasarca, ascites and pleural effusions. The edema generally requires diuretics for control but diuresis may aggravate intravascular volume contraction and exacerbate hypotension. Intravenous salt poor albumin infusion given once or twice times weekly are often very useful, especially during chemotherapy, to allow adequate diuresis. Over a quarter of all patients presenting with renal amyloidosis will develop end-stage renal failure [80] and this figure is likely to increase with longer survival in patients who do not achieve near complete responses to chemotherapy. Renal transplantation has been performed in patients with AL but recurrence is common without effective therapy. Hematologic response to treatment with normalization of the iFLC in renal patients is associated with reductions in proteinuria (Figure 14.4b).

Hepatomegaly is found by physical examination in one-fourth of patients with AL and is associated with an elevated serum alkaline phosphatase level and early satiety [86]. Hepatomegaly may be due to heart failure or direct infiltration of the liver; most patients are asymptomatic and will have alkaline phosphatase elevation with normal transaminases. When two organs are involved with amyloid, the most common presentation is combined hepatic and renal. Half of the patients with hepatic amyloid have >1 g of daily proteinuria. Hepatomegaly is usually out of proportion to the degree of abnormal liver function tests [86]. Elevation of the bilirubin level is generally a preterminal finding. Rarely, a patient can present with splenic or hepatic rupture – this is a common presenting feature of the rare hereditary amyloidosis syndrome due to lysozyme mutations and should be ruled out if organ rupture is a presenting feature. Portal hypertension with varices and bleeding has been reported but is rare [87]. Ascites is usually due to associated nephrotic syndrome, hypoalbuminemia, and congestive heart failure, not to portal hypertension. The diagnosis is easily confirmed with liver biopsy with a low complication rate but can also be appreciated by scintigraphy. The presence of Howell–Jolly bodies on the peripheral blood film is specific for splenic amyloid and, like the abnormal liver function tests and hepatomegaly, is reversible with hematologic response to therapy [50].

Most patients with amyloidosis will have deposits seen in GI tract biopsies [88]. Usually these are vascular deposits only and do not produce symptoms – such patients should not be classed as having GI amyloidosis. Fewer than 5% of patients with AL will present with symptoms referable to the GI tract [89]. GI symptoms in amyloidosis may either be due to direct amyloid infiltration (rare) or due to autonomic involvement (commoner) but can be very difficult to differentiate on clinical grounds alone. The presence of anorexia and weight loss does not correlate with the presence of GI amyloid deposits. Malabsorption with steatorrhea is seen in <5% of patients. When symptoms are present, they can include pseudo-obstruction [90], and advanced GI tract involvement can lead to long-term dependence on total parenteral nutrition [91]. Patients can have intractable nausea and vomiting and often do not respond to enteral feeding or pharmacologic interventions.

The most common presenting symptoms of small bowel involvement are diarrhea, anorexia and dizziness [92]. The median weight loss is 30 pounds, and 50% of patients have orthostatic hypotension – latter suggesting associated autonomic neuropathy [89,93]. Small bowel dilatation can be seen as thickening, nodularity and delayed transit. There is usually a significant delay from the onset of symptoms to the recognition of amyloid. The diarrhea of amyloid is difficult to treat [94]. Loperamide, diphenoxylate, octreotide and tincture of opium have all been tried with limited success. Somastatin analogs (octreotide or lanreotide) are helpful when opioids fail to control diarrhea. Amyloidosis can present as ischemic colitis with deposits obstructing the vessels of the lamina propria and muscularis mucosa; it can lead to chronic mucosal sloughing and hemorrhage [95]. There is a risk for GI bleeding in patients who undergo SCT [96]. GI bleeding has been associated with an inferior outcome in SCT [97].

Peripheral neuropathy due to AL is present in one patient in five [89]. Isolated peripheral neuropathy is a relatively rare presentation of amyloidosis. When patients present with dominant neuropathy, consideration needs to be given to the possibility of hereditary amyloidosis as noted above. The most common symptoms are paresthesias, muscle weakness, numbness, pain, orthostasis, urinary retention and impotence [98]. Syncope is seen in 12% of patients, and dysesthesias and distal burning sensations in one-quarter [98]. The lower extremities are involved before the upper extremities in 90% of patients and two-thirds of patients have autonomic symptoms. Cranial nerve involvement is rare. Carpal tunnel syndrome is seen in half of patients with amyloid peripheral neuropathy and a third have significant weight loss [98]. Peripheral nervous system involvement is reversible with hematologic response to therapy [50,91].

Significant delays in diagnosis are common in patients with amyloid-related peripheral neuropathy. Sural nerve biopsy may demonstrate deposits in endoneurial capillaries [98] but, no matter the biopsy result, patients with peripheral neuropathy should have serum FLC and serum and urine immunofixation studies performed because the discovery of a monoclonal paraprotein limits the differential diagnosis to gammopathy-related neuropathy, POEMS syndrome (polyneuropathy, organomegaly, endocrinopathy, M protein, skin changes), cryoglobulinemia and AL. Since amyloidosis preferentially causes loss of small unmyelinated fibers, an electromyogram can be normal early in the disease course. Amyloid is often deposited proximally at the level of the nerve root causing distal demyelination and therefore the sural nerve biopsy is often negative.

Involvement of the respiratory tract is usually asymptomatic [99]. Almost 40% of patients with amyloid deposits in the lungs have localized forms and do not have systemic amyloidosis [100,101]. In patients who have systemic amyloidosis and lung involvement, the symptoms of concurrent cardiac involvement may dominate. Gas exchange in the lungs is preserved until late in the disease [102]. Pulmonary amyloidosis presents radiographically as an interstitial or reticulonodular infiltrate with or without pleural effusion. Bronchoscopic lung biopsy is safe and is not associated with an increased bleeding risk. The chest X-ray is not specific, demonstrating an interstitial process that can be misinterpreted as fibrosis. In patients who have dyspnea due to interstitial lung disease, low doses of prednisone may produce symptomatic benefit. Pleural infiltration with amyloid can result in pleural effusions.

Bleeding can be a serious complication of amyloidosis [103]. Periorbital purpura is a presenting feature and, in absence of trauma or a known bleeding diathesis, is almost pathognomonic of AL amyloidosis. The most common manifestations of bleeding are skin and oral mucosal purpura. Deficiency of factor X is seen in <5% of patients and is associated with hepatosplenic involvement.

Bleeding associated with factor X deficiency is generally seen only when the level falls below 25%. Normalization of factor X levels following SCT has been reported but severe factor X deficiency is associated with increased mortality with SCT [104]. The management of factor X deficiency prior to SCT has included splenectomy and the use of recombinant human factor VIIa [35]. Highly purified factor X concentrate is now available and may have a role in these cases. Recurrent abdominal pain in such cases may be due to recurrent pericapsular hematomata – which can be a cause of morbidity or mortality if it leads to organ rupture [105]. Acquired von Willebrand's disease or abnormal glycosylation of other coagulation factors has been described and may result in intractable bleeding [106].

Paradoxically, patients with AL amyloidosis may also be significantly prothrombotic especially in the presence of marked nephrosis, worsened by therapy with IMiDs. The same patients may also have vascular amyloid deposits leading to increased vascular fragility and higher bleeding risk – treatment of thrombosis becomes very complex. True thromboembolic disease rarely complicates AL but in patients with advanced cardiac involvement it can be a cause of early death [40,107]. In one series of 40 patients with AL and documented thromboembolic disease, thromboembolism was seen more than one month following the diagnosis of AL; 29 of the 40 events were venous and 11 arterial [108]. Risk factors for thrombosis included nephrotic syndrome, immobilization, tobacco use, heart failure and disseminated intravascular coagulation. Five of the 40 patients had activated protein C resistance. The mortality associated with thromboembolism was 20%, with 45% of patients dying within a year of the thrombotic event.

Conclusions

Over the past 20 years, the development of SCT and then the use of novel agents to treat the clonal plasma cell disease that underlies systemic AL amyloidosis have had a profound impact on patient survival. We now know that AL-related organ damage can be reversed in many cases with effective control of the AL light chain protein. But at diagnosis about 15% of patients are too sick to benefit from any therapy because their cardiac amyloid is too advanced; early death remains a major part of the profile of AL. Newer therapies are on the horizon which offer hope to such patients. Immunotherapy appears to be one such promising approach. Anti-serum amyloid P component antibodies (SAP is a part of all amyloid deposits) lead to rapid amyloid regression in a mouse model and human trials will start in the near future. Late in the course of disease patients still develop renal failure requiring dialysis; this is despite long-term control of the iFLC and because of persistent nephrotic-range proteinuria and progression of glomerular and tubular scarring. Although the metrics for assessing AL organ damage have improved and have found their place in clinical care, we do not have agents to mitigate the damage caused to hearts or kidneys by amyloid disease, as we have for myeloma bone disease in the form of bisphosphonates. Indeed, much has improved for newly diagnosed AL patients but much remains to be done.

References

1. Pepys, M. B. Amyloidosis. *Annu. Rev. Med.* 2006;**57**:223–41.

2. Bellotti, V., Nuvolone, M., Giorgetti, S. *et al.* The workings of the amyloid diseases. *Ann. Med.* 2007;**39**(3):200–7.

3. Gertz, M. A. How to manage primary amyloidosis. *Leukemia* Aug 26 2011.

4. Benson, M. D. The hereditary amyloidoses. *Best Pract. Res. Clin. Rheumatol.* 2003;**17**(6):909–27.

5. Ng, B., Connors, L. H., Davidoff, R., Skinner, M., Falk, R. H. Senile systemic amyloidosis presenting with heart failure: a comparison with light chain-associated amyloidosis. *Arch. Intern. Med.* 2005;**165**(12):1425–9.

6. Leung, K. T., Wong, K. M., Choi, K. S., Chau, K. F., Li, C. S. Multicentric Castleman's disease complicated by secondary renal amyloidosis. *Nephrology (Carlton)* 2004;**9**(6):392–3.

7. Tanaka, F., Migita, K., Honda, S. *et al.* Clinical outcome and survival of secondary (AA) amyloidosis. *Clin. Exp. Rheumatol.* 2003;**21**(3):343–6.

8. Lachmann, H. J., Booth, D. R., Booth, S. E. *et al.* Misdiagnosis of hereditary amyloidosis as AL (primary) amyloidosis. *N. Engl. J. Med.* 2002;**346**(23):1786–91.

9. Comenzo, R. L., Zhou, P., Fleisher, M., Clark, B., Teruya-Feldstein, J. Seeking confidence in the diagnosis of systemic AL (Ig light-chain) amyloidosis: patients can have both monoclonal gammopathies and hereditary amyloid proteins. *Blood* 2006; **107**(9):3489–91.

10. Landgren, O., Weiss, B. M. Patterns of monoclonal gammopathy of undetermined significance and multiple myeloma in various ethnic/racial groups: support for genetic factors in pathogenesis. *Leukemia* 2009;**23**(10):1691–7.

11. Merlini, G., Westermark, P. The systemic amyloidoses: clearer understanding of the molecular mechanisms offers hope for more effective therapies. *J. Intern. Med.* 2004;**255**(2):159–78.

12. Jacobson, D. R., Pastore, R. D., Yaghoubian, R. *et al.* Variant-sequence transthyretin (isoleucine 122) in late-onset cardiac amyloidosis in black Americans. *N. Engl. J. Med.* 1997;**336**(7):466–73.

13. Wechalekar, A. D., Offer, M., Gillmore, J. D., Hawkins, P. N., Lachmann, H. J. Cardiac amyloidosis, a monoclonal gammopathy and a potentially misleading mutation. *Nature Clin. Pract.* 2009;**6**(2):128–33.

14. Falk, R. H., Comenzo, R. L., Skinner, M. The systemic amyloidoses. *N. Engl. J. Med.* 1997;**337**(13):898–909.

15. Bely, M., Makovitzky, J. Sensitivity and specificity of Congo red staining according to Romhanyi. Comparison with Puchtler's or Bennhold's methods. *Acta Histochem.* 2006;**108**(3):175–80.

16. Giorgadze, T. A., Shiina, N., Baloch, Z. W., Tomaszewski, J. E., Gupta, P. K. Improved detection of amyloid in fat pad aspiration: an evaluation of Congo red stain by fluorescent microscopy. *Diagn. Cytopathol.* 2004; **31**(5):300–6.

17. Vrana, J. A., Gamez, J. D., Madden, B. J. *et al.* Classification of amyloidosis by laser microdissection and mass spectrometry-based proteomic analysis in clinical biopsy specimens. *Blood* 2009; **114**(24):4957–9.

18. Solomon, A., Murphy, C. L., Westermark, P. Unreliability of immunohistochemistry for typing amyloid deposits. *Arch. Pathol. Lab. Med.* 2008;**132**(1):14; author reply -5.

19. Palladini, G., Perfetti, V., Merlini, G. Therapy and management of systemic AL (primary) amyloidosis. *Swiss Med. Wkly* 2006;**136**(45–46):715–20.

20. Dispenzieri, A., Kyle, R., Merlini, G. *et al.* International Myeloma Working Group guidelines for serum-free light chain analysis in multiple myeloma and related disorders. *Leukemia* 2009; **23**(2):215–24.

21. Bochtler, T., Hegenbart, U., Heiss, C. *et al.* Evaluation of the serum-free light chain test in untreated patients with AL amyloidosis. *Haematologica* 2008;**93**(3):459–62.

22. Obici, L., Perfetti, V., Palladini, G., Moratti, R., Merlini, G. Clinical aspects of systemic

amyloid diseases. *Biochim. Biophys. Acta* 2005;**1753**(1):11–22.

23. Avet-Loiseau, H., Attal, M., Moreau, P. *et al.* Genetic abnormalities and survival in multiple myeloma: the experience of the Intergroupe Francophone du Myelome. *Blood* 2007; **109**(8):3489–95.

24. Fonseca, R., Bergsagel, P. L., Drach, J. *et al.* International Myeloma Working Group molecular classification of multiple myeloma: spotlight review. *Leukemia* 2009; **23**(12):2210–21.

25. Bochtler, T., Hegenbart, U., Cremer, F. W. *et al.* Evaluation of the cytogenetic aberration pattern in amyloid light chain amyloidosis as compared with monoclonal gammopathy of undetermined significance reveals common pathways of karyotypic instability. *Blood* 2008;**111**(9):4700–5.

26. Bryce, A. H., Ketterling, R. P., Gertz, M. A. *et al.* Translocation t(11;14) and survival of patients with light chain (AL) amyloidosis. *Haematologica* 2009;**94**(3):380–6.

27. Hoffman, J., Jhanwar, S., Comenzo, R. L. AL amyloidosis and progression to multiple myeloma with gain(1q). *Br. J. Haematol.* 2009;**144**(6):963–4.

28. Cohen, A. D., Zhou, P., Xiao, Q. *et al.* Systemic AL amyloidosis due to non-Hodgkin's lymphoma: an unusual clinicopathologic association. *Br. J. Haematol.* 2004;**124**(3):309–14.

29. Palladini, G., Foli, A., Russo, P. *et al.* Treatment of IgM-associated AL amyloidosis with the combination of rituximab, bortezomib, and dexamethasone. *Clin. Lymphoma Myeloma Leuk.* 2011;**11**(1):143–5.

30. Hawkins, P. N., Lavender, J. P., Pepys, M. B. Evaluation of systemic amyloidosis by scintigraphy with 123I-labeled serum amyloid P component. *N. Engl. J. Med.* 1990;**323**:508–13.

31. Wall, J. S., Kennel, S. J., Stuckey, A. C. *et al.* Radioimmunodetection of amyloid deposits in patients with AL amyloidosis. *Blood* 2010; **116**(13):2241–4.

32. Gertz, M. A., Comenzo, R., Falk, R. H. *et al.* Definition of organ involvement and treatment response in immunoglobulin light chain amyloidosis (AL): a consensus opinion from the 10th International Symposium on Amyloid and Amyloidosis, Tours, France, 18–22 April 2004. *Am. J. Hematol.* 2005;**79**(4):319–28.

33. Palladini, G., Dispenzieri, A., Gertz, M. A. *et al.* New criteria for response to treatment in immunoglobulin light chain amyloidosis based on free light chain measurement and cardiac biomarkers: impact on survival outcomes. *J. Clin. Oncol.* 2012;**30**(36):454–9.

34. Palladini, G., Kyle, R. A., Larson, D. R. *et al.* Multicentre versus single centre approach to rare diseases: the model of systemic light chain amyloidosis. *Amyloid* 2005;**12**(2):120–6.

35. Cohen, A. D., Zhou, P., Chou, J. *et al.* Risk-adapted autologous stem cell transplantation with adjuvant dexamethasone +/− thalidomide for systemic light-chain amyloidosis: results of a phase II trial. *Br. J. Haematol.* 2007;**139**(2):224–33.

36. Dispenzieri, A., Kyle, R. A., Gertz, M. A. *et al.* Survival in patients with primary systemic amyloidosis and raised serum cardiac troponins. *Lancet* 2003;**361**(9371):1787–9.

37. Falk, R. H. Cardiac amyloidosis: a treatable disease, often overlooked. *Circulation* 2011; **124**(9):1079–85.

38. Dispenzieri, A., Gertz, M. A., Kyle, R. A. *et al.* Prognostication of survival using cardiac troponins and N-terminal pro-brain natriuretic peptide in patients with primary systemic amyloidosis undergoing peripheral blood stem

cell transplantation. *Blood* 2004; **104**(6):1881–7.

39. Palladini, G., Barassi, A., Klersy, C. *et al.* The combination of high-sensitivity cardiac troponin T (hs-cTnT) at presentation and changes in N-terminal natriuretic peptide type B (NT-proBNP) after chemotherapy best predicts survival in AL amyloidosis. *Blood* 2010;**116**(18):3426–30.

40. Lebovic, D., Hoffman, J., Levine, B. M. *et al.* Predictors of survival in patients with systemic light-chain amyloidosis and cardiac involvement initially ineligible for stem cell transplantation and treated with oral melphalan and dexamethasone. *Br. J. Haematol.* 2008;**143**(3):369–73.

41. Dispenzieri, A., Lacy, M. Q., Katzmann, J. A. *et al.* Absolute values of immunoglobulin free light chains are prognostic in patients with primary systemic amyloidosis undergoing peripheral blood stem cell transplantation. *Blood* 2006; **107**(8):3378–83.

42. Sanchorawala, V., Seldin, D. C., Magnani, B., Skinner, M., Wright, D. G. Serum free light-chain responses after high-dose intravenous melphalan and autologous stem cell transplantation for AL (primary) amyloidosis. *Bone Marrow Transplant* 2005;**36**(7):597–600.

43. Durie, B. G., Harousseau, J. L., Miguel, J. S. *et al.* International uniform response criteria for multiple myeloma. *Leukemia* 2006;**20**(9):1467–73.

44. Palladini, G., Perfetti, V., Obici, L. *et al.* Association of melphalan and high-dose dexamethasone is effective and well tolerated in patients with AL (primary) amyloidosis who are ineligible for stem cell transplantation. *Blood* 2004;**103**(8):2936–8.

45. Palladini, G., Russo, P., Nuvolone, M. *et al.* Treatment with oral melphalan plus dexamethasone

produces long-term remissions in AL amyloidosis. *Blood* 2007; **110**(2):787–8.

46. Gertz, M. A., Lacy, M. Q., Lust, J. A. *et al.* Long-term risk of myelodysplasia in melphalan-treated patients with immunoglobulin light-chain amyloidosis. *Haematologica* 2008;**93**(9):1402–6.

47. Cibeira, M. T., Sanchorawala, V., Seldin, D. C. *et al.* Outcome of AL amyloidosis after high-dose melphalan and autologous stem cell transplantation: long-term results in a series of 421 patients. *Blood* 2011 Aug 9.

48. Gertz, M. A., Blood, E., Vesole, D. H. *et al.* A multicenter phase 2 trial of stem cell transplantation for immunoglobulin light-chain amyloidosis (E4A97): an Eastern Cooperative Oncology Group Study. *Bone Marrow Transplant* 2004;**34**(2):149–54.

49. Comenzo, R. L., Vosburgh, E., Simms, R. W. *et al.* Dose-intensive melphalan with blood stem cell support for the treatment of AL amyloidosis: one-year follow-up in five patients. *Blood* 1996; **88**(7):2801–6.

50. Comenzo, R. L., Vosburgh, E., Falk, R. H. *et al.* Dose-intensive melphalan with blood stem-cell support for the treatment of AL (amyloid light-chain) amyloidosis: survival and responses in 25 patients. *Blood* 1998;**91**(10): 3662–70.

51. Comenzo, R. L., Sanchorawala, V., Fisher, C. *et al.* Intermediate-dose intravenous melphalan and blood stem cells mobilized with sequential GM+G-CSF or G-CSF alone to treat AL (amyloid light chain) amyloidosis. *Br. J. Haematol.* 1999;**104**(3): 553–9.

52. Mollee, P. N., Wechalekar, A. D., Pereira, D. L. *et al.* Autologous stem cell transplantation in primary systemic amyloidosis: the impact of selection criteria on outcome. *Bone Marrow Transplant* 2004;**33**(3):271–7.

53. Wechalekar, A. D., Hawkins, P. N., Gillmore, J. D. Perspectives in treatment of AL amyloidosis. *Br. J. Haematol.* 2008;**140**(4): 365–77.

54. Goodman, H. J., Gillmore, J. D., Lachmann, H. J. *et al.* Outcome of autologous stem cell transplantation for AL amyloidosis in the UK. *Br. J. Haematol.* 2006;**134**(4):417–25.

55. Jaccard, A., Moreau, P., Leblond, V. *et al.* High-dose melphalan versus melphalan plus dexamethasone for AL amyloidosis. *N. Engl. J. Med.* 2007;**357**(11):1083–93.

56. Dispenzieri, A., Lacy, M. Q., Rajkumar, S. V. *et al.* Poor tolerance to high doses of thalidomide in patients with primary systemic amyloidosis. *Amyloid* 2003;**10**(4):257–61.

57. Seldin, D. C., Choufani, E. B., Dember, L. M. *et al.* Tolerability and efficacy of thalidomide for the treatment of patients with light chain-associated (AL) amyloidosis. *Clin. Lymphoma* 2003;**3**(4):241–6.

58. Wechalekar, A. D., Goodman, H. J., Lachmann, H. J. *et al.* Safety and efficacy of risk-adapted cyclophosphamide, thalidomide, and dexamethasone in systemic AL amyloidosis. *Blood* 2007; **109**(2):457–64.

59. Sanchorawala, V., Wright, D. G., Rosenzweig, M. *et al.* Lenalidomide and dexamethasone in the treatment of AL amyloidosis: results of a phase 2 trial. *Blood* 2007;**109**(2):492–6.

60. Dispenzieri, A., Lacy, M. Q., Zeldenrust, S. R. *et al.* The activity of lenalidomide with or without dexamethasone in patients with primary systemic amyloidosis. *Blood* 2007;**109**(2):465–70.

61. Sanchorawala, V., Finn, K. T., Fennessey, S. *et al.* Durable hematologic complete responses can be achieved with lenalidomide in AL amyloidosis. *Blood* 2010;**116**(11):1990–1.

62. Moreau, P., Jaccard, A., Benboubker, L. *et al.* Lenalidomide in combination with melphalan and dexamethasone in patients with newly diagnosed AL amyloidosis: a multicenter phase 1/2 dose-escalation study. *Blood* 2010; **116**(23):4777–82.

63. Dispenzieri, A., Hayman, S. R., Buadi, F. *et al.* Pomalidomide and dexamethasone for previously treated AL: a phase 2 study. *Amyloid* 2010;**17**:87a.

64. Tapan, U., Seldin, D. C., Finn, K. T. *et al.* Increases in B-type natriuretic peptide (BNP) during treatment with lenalidomide in AL amyloidosis. *Blood* 2011; **116**(23):5071–2.

65. Dispenzieri, A., Dingli, D., Kumar, S. K. *et al.* Discordance between serum cardiac biomarker and immunoglobulin-free light-chain response in patients with immunoglobulin light-chain amyloidosis treated with immune modulatory drugs. *Am. J. Hematol.* 2010;**85**(10):757–9.

66. Russo, P., Zenone Bragotti, L., Musca, F. *et al.* A phase II trial of cyclophosphamide, lenalidomide and dexamethasone (CLD) in previously treated patients with AL amyloidosis. *Amyloid* 2010;**17**:169a.

67. Reece, D. E., Hegenbart, U., Sanchorawala, V. *et al.* Efficacy and safety of once-weekly and twice-weekly bortezomib in patients with relapsed systemic AL amyloidosis: results of a phase 1/2 study. *Blood* 2011;**118**(4):865–73.

68. Kastritis, E., Anagnostopoulos, A., Roussou, M. *et al.* Treatment of light chain (AL) amyloidosis with the combination of bortezomib and dexamethasone. *Haematologica* 2007;**92**(10): 1351–8.

69. Landau, H., Bello, C., Hoover, E. et al. Adjuvant bortezomib and dexamethasone following risk-adapted melphalan and stem cell transplant in systemic AL amyloidosis. *Amyloid* 2010;**17**:80a.

70. Moreau, P., Pylypenko, H., Grosicki, S. et al. Subcutaneous versus intravenous administration of bortezomib in patients with relapsed multiple myeloma: a randomised, phase 3, non-inferiority study. *Lancet Oncol.* 2011;**12**(5):431–40.

71. Zonder, J., Snyder, R., Matous, J. et al. Rapid haematologic and organ responses in patients with AL amyloid treated with bortezomib plus melphalan and dexamethasone. *Amyloid* 2010;**17**:86a.

72. Sack, F. U., Kristen, A., Goldschmidt, H. et al. Treatment options for severe cardiac amyloidosis: heart transplantation combined with chemotherapy and stem cell transplantation for patients with AL-amyloidosis and heart and liver transplantation for patients with ATTR-amyloidosis. *Eur. J. Cardiothorac Surg.* 2008; **33**(2):257–62.

73. Mathew, V., Olson, L. J., Gertz, M. A., Hayes, D. L. Symptomatic conduction system disease in cardiac amyloidosis. *Am. J. Cardiol.* 1997;**80**(11):1491–2.

74. Kristen, A. V., Dengler, T. J., Hegenbart, U. et al. Prophylactic implantation of cardioverter-defibrillator in patients with severe cardiac amyloidosis and high risk for sudden cardiac death. *Heart Rhythm* 2008;**5**(2):235–40.

75. Lin, G. D. A., Grogan, M., Kyle, R., Brady, P. A. Outcomes of implantable defibrillators in patients with cardiac amyloidosis. *Amyloid* 2010;**17**:166a.

76. Maurer, M. S., Raina, A., Hesdorffer, C. et al. Cardiac transplantation using extended-donor criteria organs for systemic amyloidosis complicated by heart failure. *Transplantation* 2007; **83**(5):539–45.

77. Gillmore, J. D., Goodman, H. J., Lachmann, H. J. et al. Sequential heart and autologous stem cell transplantation for systemic AL amyloidosis. *Blood* 2006; **107**(3):1227–9.

78. Palladini, G., Lavatelli, F., Russo, P. et al. Circulating amyloidogenic free light chains and serum N-terminal natriuretic peptide type B decrease simultaneously in association with improvement of survival in AL. *Blood* 2006; **107**(10):3854–8.

79. Leung, N., Rajkumar, S. V. Renal manifestations of plasma cell disorders. *Am. J. Kidney Dis.* 2007;**50**(1):155–65.

80. Pinney, J. H., Lachmann, H. J., Bansi, L. et al. Outcome in renal Al amyloidosis after chemotherapy. *J. Clin. Oncol.* 2011;**29**(6):674–81.

81. Leung, N., Dispenzieri, A., Lacy, M. Q. et al. Severity of baseline proteinuria predicts renal response in immunoglobulin light chain-associated amyloidosis after autologous stem cell transplantation. *Clin. J. Am. Soc. Nephrol.* 2007;**2**(3):440–4.

82. Gertz, M. A., Lacy, M. Q., Dispenzieri, A., Hayman, S. R. Amyloidosis: diagnosis and management. *Clin. Lymphoma Myeloma* 2005;**6**(3):208–19.

83. Gertz, M. A., Lacy, M. Q., Dispenzieri, A. Immunoglobulin light chain amyloidosis and the kidney. *Kidney Int.* 2002; **61**(1):1–9.

84. Leung, N., Leung, T. R., Cha, S. S. et al. Excessive fluid accumulation during stem cell mobilization: a novel prognostic factor of first-year survival after stem cell transplantation in AL amyloidosis patients. *Blood* 2005; **106**(10):3353–7.

85. Dember, L. M. Amyloidosis-associated kidney disease. *J. Am. Soc. Nephrol.* 2006;**17**(12): 3458–71.

86. Park, M. A., Mueller, P. S., Kyle, R. A. et al. Primary (AL) hepatic amyloidosis: clinical features and natural history in 98 patients. *Medicine (Baltimore)* 2003; **82**(5):291–8.

87. Culafic, D., Perisic, M., Boricic, I., Culafic-Vojinovic, V., Vukcevic, M. Primary amyloidosis presenting with cholestasis and hyperkinetic portal hypertension. *J. Gastrointestin. Liver Dis.* 2007;**16**(2):201–4.

88. James, D. G., Zuckerman, G. R., Sayuk, G. S., Wang, H. L., Prakash, C. Clinical recognition of Al type amyloidosis of the luminal gastrointestinal tract. *Clin. Gastroenterol. Hepatol.* 2007; **5**(5):582–8.

89. Kyle, R. A., Gertz, M. A. Primary systemic amyloidosis: clinical and laboratory features in 474 cases. *Semin. Hematol.* 1995;**32**(1): 45–59.

90. Lau, C. F., Fok, K. O., Hui, P. K. et al. Intestinal obstruction and gastrointestinal bleeding due to systemic amyloidosis in a woman with occult plasma cell dyscrasia. *Eur. J. Gastroenterol Hepatol.* 1999;**11**(6):681–5.

91. Comenzo, R. L. Advances in the treatment of plasma cell diseases. *Hosp. Pract. (Minneap).* 1996; **31**(8):67–70, 3–4, 9–84 passim.

92. Hurlstone, D. P. Iron-deficiency anemia complicating AL amyloidosis with recurrent small bowel pseudo-obstruction and hindgut sparing. *J. Gastroenterol. Hepatol.* 2002;**17**(5):623–4.

93. Ebert, E. C., Nagar, M. Gastrointestinal manifestations of amyloidosis. *Am. J. Gastroenterol.* 2008;**103**(3):776–87.

94. Guirl, M. J., Hogenauer, C., Santa Ana, C. A. et al. Rapid intestinal transit as a primary cause of severe chronic diarrhea in patients with amyloidosis.

Am. J. Gastroenterol. 2003;
98(10):2219–25.

95. Trinh, T. D., Jones, B., Fishman, E. K. Amyloidosis of the colon presenting as ischemic colitis: a case report and review of the literature. *Gastrointest. Radiol.* 1991;**16**(2):133–6.

96. Kumar, S., Dispenzieri, A., Lacy, M. Q., Litzow, M. R., Gertz, M. A. High incidence of gastrointestinal tract bleeding after autologous stem cell transplant for primary systemic amyloidosis. *Bone Marrow Transplant* 2001; **28**(4):381–5.

97. Gertz, M. A., Lacy, M. Q., Gastineau, D. A. *et al.* Blood stem cell transplantation as therapy for primary systemic amyloidosis (AL). *Bone Marrow Transplant* 2000;**26**(9):963–9.

98. Rajkumar, S. V., Gertz, M. A., Kyle, R. A. Prognosis of patients with primary systemic amyloidosis who present with dominant neuropathy. *Am. J. Med.* 1998;**104**(3):232–7.

99. Lachmann, H. J., Hawkins, P. N. Amyloidosis and the lung. *Chron. Respir. Dis.* 2006;**3**(4):203–14.

100. Kumaran, R., Saleh, A., Amin, B., Raoof, S. A 73-year-old woman with mild shortness of breath and multiple central calcified pulmonary nodules. *Chest* 2008;**134**(2):460–4.

101. Pitz, M. W., Gibson, I. W., Johnston, J. B. Isolated pulmonary amyloidosis: case report and review of the literature. *Am. J. Hematol.* 2006;**81**(3): 212–13.

102. Cordier, J. F. Pulmonary amyloidosis in hematological disorders. *Semin. Respir. Crit. Care Med.* 2005;**26**(5):502–13.

103. Mumford, A. D., O'Donnell, J., Gillmore, J. D. *et al.* Bleeding symptoms and coagulation abnormalities in 337 patients with AL-amyloidosis. *Br. J. Haematol.* 2000;**110**(2):454–60.

104. Choufani, E. B., Sanchorawala, V., Ernst, T. *et al.* Acquired factor X deficiency in patients with amyloid light-chain amyloidosis: incidence, bleeding manifestations, and response to high-dose chemotherapy. *Blood* 2001;**97**(6):1885–7.

105. Kyle, R. A., Gertz, M. A., Greipp, P. R. *et al.* A trial of three regimens for primary amyloidosis: colchicine alone, melphalan and prednisone, and melphalan, prednisone, and colchicine. *N. Engl. J. Med.* 1997; **336**(17):1202–7.

106. Kos, C. A., Ward, J. E., Malek, K. *et al.* Association of acquired von Willebrand syndrome with AL amyloidosis. *Am. J. Hematol.* 2007;**82**(5):363–7.

107. Feng, D., Edwards, W. D., Oh, J. K. *et al.* Intracardiac thrombosis and embolism in patients with cardiac amyloidosis. *Circulation* 2007;**116**(21):2420–6.

108. Halligan, C. S., Lacy, M. Q., Vincent Rajkumar, S. *et al.* Natural history of thromboembolism in AL amyloidosis. *Amyloid* 2006; **13**(1):31–6.

Table 15.1 Clinical and laboratory findings for 149 consecutive newly diagnosed patients with the consensus panel diagnosis of WM presenting to the Dana Farber Cancer Institute

	Median	Range	Institutional normal reference range
Age (years)	59	34–84	NA
Gender (male/female)	85/64		NA
Bone marrow involvement	30%	5%–95%	NA
Adenopathy	16%		NA
Splenomegaly	10%		NA
IgM (mg/dl)	2870	267–12 400	40–230
IgG (mg/dl)	587	47–2770	700–1600
IgA (mg/dl)	47	8–509	70–400
Serum viscosity (cp)	2.0	1.4–6.6	1.4–1.9
Hct (%)	35.0%	17.2%–45.4%	34.8–43.6
Plt ($\times 10^9$/l)	253	24–649	155–410
Wbc ($\times 10^9$/l)	6.0	0.3–13	3.8–9.2
B$_2$M (mg/dl)	3.0	1.3–13.7	0–2.7
LDH	395	122–1131	313–618

NA (not applicable).

Table 15.2 Physicochemical and immunological properties of the monoclonal IgM protein in Waldenstrom's macroglobulinemia

Properties of IgM monoclonal protein	Diagnostic condition	Clinical manifestations
Pentameric structure	Hyperviscosity	Headaches, blurred vision, epistaxis, retinal hemorrhages, leg cramps, impaired mentation, intracranial hemorrhage
Precipitation on cooling	Cryoglobulinemia (Type I)	Raynaud's phenomenom, acrocyanosis, ulcers, purpura, cold urticaria
Auto-antibody activity to myelin associated glycoprotein (MAG), ganglioside M1 (GM1), sulfatide moieties on peripheral nerve sheaths	Peripheral neuropathies	Sensorimotor neuropathies, painful neuropathies, ataxic gait, bilateral foot drop
Auto-antibody activity to IgG	Cryoglobulinemia (Type II)	Purpura, arthralgias, renal failure, sensorimotor neuropathies
Auto-antibody activity to red blood cell antigens	Cold agglutinins	Hemolytic anemia, Raynaud's phenomenom, acrocyanosis, livedo reticularis
Tissue deposition as amorphous aggregates	Organ dysfunction	Skin: bullous skin disease, papules, Schnitzler's syndrome GI: diarrhea, malabsorption, bleeding Kidney: proteinuria, renal failure (light chain component)
Tissue deposition as amyloid fibrils (light chain component most commonly)	Organ dysfunction	Fatigue, weight loss, edema, hepatomegaly, macroglossia, organ dysfunction of involved organs: heart, kidney, liver, peripheral sensory and autonomic nerves

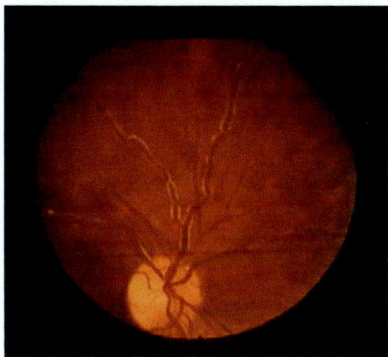

Figure 15.2
Funduscopic examination of a patient with Waldenstrom's macroglobulinemia demonstrating hyperviscosity related changes including dilated retinal vessels, peripheral hemorrhages and "venous sausaging" (courtesy of Marvin Stone M.D.).

increase in the resistance to blood flow and the resulting impaired transit through the microcirculatory system are rather complex [38–40]. The main determinants are: (1) a high concentration of monoclonal IgMs, which may form aggregates and may bind water through their carbohydrate component; and (2) their interaction with blood cells. Monoclonal IgMs increase red cell aggregation (*rouleaux* formation) and red cell internal viscosity while also reducing deformability. The possible presence of cryoglobulins can contribute to increasing blood viscosity as well as to the tendency to induce erythrocyte aggregation. Serum viscosity is proportional to IgM concentration up to 30 g/l, then increases sharply at higher levels. Plasma viscosity and hematocrit are directly regulated by the body. Increased plasma viscosity may also contribute to inappropriately low erythropoietin production, which is the major reason for anemia in these patients [41]. Clinical manifestations are related to circulatory disturbances that can be best appreciated by ophthalmoscopy, which shows distended and tortuous retinal veins, hemorrhages and papilledema [42] (Figure 15.2). Symptoms usually occur when the monoclonal IgM concentration exceeds 50 g/l or when serum viscosity is >4.0 centipoises (cp), but there is a great individual variability, with some patients showing no evidence of hyperviscosity even at 10 cp [38]. The most common symptoms are oronasal bleeding, visual disturbances due to retinal bleeding, and dizziness that may rarely lead to coma. Heart failure can be aggravated, particularly in the elderly, owing to increased blood viscosity, expanded plasma volume, and anemia. Inappropriate transfusion can exacerbate hyperviscosity and may precipitate cardiac failure.

Cryoglobulinemia

In up to 20% of WM patients, the monoclonal IgM can behave as a cryoglobulin (type I), but it is symptomatic in 5% or less of the cases [43]. Cryoprecipitation is mainly dependent on the concentration of monoclonal IgM; for this reason plasmapheresis or plasma exchange are commonly effective in this condition. Symptoms result from impaired blood flow in small vessels and include Raynaud's phenomenon, acrocyanosis and necrosis of the regions most exposed to cold, such as the tip of the nose, ears, fingers and toes (Figure 15.3), malleolar ulcers, purpura and cold urticaria. Renal manifestations may occur but are infrequent.

Auto-antibody activity

Monoclonal IgM may exert its pathogenic effects through specific recognition of autologous antigens, the most notable being nerve constituents, immunoglobulin determinants and red blood cell antigens.

IgM related neuropathy

The presence of peripheral neuropathy has been estimated to range from 5% to 38% in WM patients [44–48]. The nerve damage is mediated by diverse pathogenetic mechanisms: IgM antibody activity toward nerve constituents causing demyelinating polyneuropathies; endoneurial granulofibrillar deposits of IgM without antibody activity, associated with axonal polyneuropathy; occasionally by tubular deposits in the endoneurium associated with IgM cryoglobulin and, rarely, by amyloid deposits or by neoplastic cell infiltration of nerve structures [49]. Half of the patients with IgM neuropathy have a distinctive clinical syndrome that is associated with antibodies against a minor 100-kDa glycoprotein component of nerve, myelin-associated glycoprotein (MAG). Anti-MAG antibodies are generally monoclonal IgMκ, and usually also exhibit reactivity with other glycoproteins or glycolipids that share antigenic determinants with MAG [50–52]. The anti-MAG-related neuropathy is typically distal and symmetrical, affecting both motor and sensory functions; it is slowly progressive with a long period of stability [45,53]. Most patients present with sensory complaints (paresthesias, aching discomfort, dysesthesias, or lancinating pains), imbalance and gait ataxia, owing to lack of proprioception, and leg muscles atrophy in advanced stage. Patients with predominantly demyelinating sensory neuropathy in association with

193

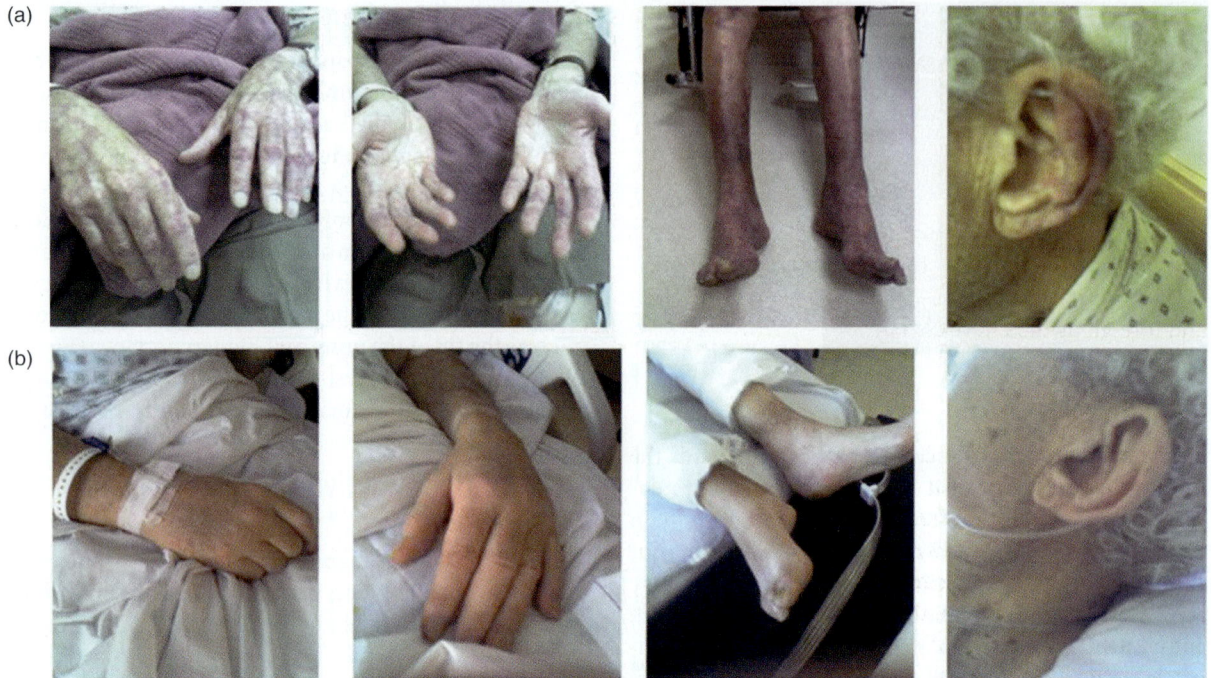

Figure 15.3 Cryoglobulinemia manifesting with severe acrocyanosis in a patient with Waldenstrom's macroglobulinemia before (a) and following warming and plasmapheresis (b).

monoclonal IgM to gangliosides with disialosyl moieties, such as GD1b, GD3, GD2, GT1b, and GQ1b, have also been reported [54,55]. Anti-GD1b and anti-GQ1b antibodies were significantly associated with predominantly sensory ataxic neuropathy [59]. These antiganglioside monoclonal IgMs present core clinical features of chronic ataxic neuropathy with variably present ophthalmoplegia and/or red blood cell cold agglutinating activity. The disialosyl epitope is also present on red blood cell glycophorins, thereby accounting for the red cell cold agglutinin activity of anti-Pr2 specificity [56,57]. Monoclonal IgM proteins that bind to gangliosides with a terminal trisaccharide moiety, including GM2 and GalNac-GD1A, are associated with chronic demyelinating neuropathy and severe sensory ataxia, unresponsive to corticosteroids [58,60]. Antiganglioside IgM proteins may also cross-react with lipopolysaccharides of *Campylobacter jejuni*, whose infection is known to precipitate the Miller Fisher syndrome, a variant of the Guillain–Barré syndrome [59]. This finding indicates that molecular mimicry may play a role in this condition. Antisulfatide monoclonal IgM proteins, associated with sensory/sensorimotor neuropathy, have been detected in 5% of patients with IgM monoclonal

gammopathy and neuropathy [60]. Motor neuron disease has been reported in patients with WM, and monoclonal IgM with anti-GM1 and sulfoglucuronyl paragloboside activity [61]. POEMS (polyneuropathy, organomegaly, endocrinopathy, M protein, and skin changes) syndrome is rarely associated with WM [62].

Cold agglutinin hemolytic anemia

Monoclonal IgM may present with cold agglutinin activity, i.e. it can recognize specific red cell antigens at temperatures below physiological, producing chronic hemolytic anemia. This disorder occurs in <10% of WM patients [63] and is associated with cold agglutinin titers >1:1000 in most cases. The monoclonal component is usually an IgMκ and reacts most commonly with I/i antigens, with complement fixation and activation [64,65]. Mild chronic hemolytic anemia can be exacerbated after cold exposure but rarely does hemoglobin drop below 70 g/l. The hemolysis is usually extravascular (removal of C3b opsonized cells by the reticuloendotelial system, primarily in the liver) and rarely intravascular from complement destruction of red blood cell (RBC) membrane. The agglutination of RBCs in the cooler peripheral circulation also causes Raynaud's syndrome, acrocyanosis and livedo reticularis. Macroglobulins with the properties of both cryoglobulins and cold agglutinins with anti-Pr specificity have been reported. These properties may have as a common basis the immune binding of the sialic acid-containing carbohydrate present on red blood cell glycophorins and on Ig molecules. Several other macroglobulins with various antibody activity toward autologous antigens (i.e. phospholipids, tissue and plasma proteins, etc.) and foreign ligands have also been reported.

Tissue deposition

The monoclonal protein can deposit in several tissues as amorphous aggregates. Linear deposition of monoclonal IgM along the skin basement membrane is associated with bullous skin disease [66]. Amorphous IgM deposits in the dermis determine the so-called IgM storage papules on the extensor surface of the extremities – macroglobulinemia cutis [67]. Deposition of monoclonal IgM in the lamina propria and/or submucosa of the intestine may be associated with diarrhea, malabsorption and gastrointestinal bleeding [68,69]. It is well known that kidney involvement is less common and less severe in WM than in multiple myeloma, probably because the amount of light chain excreted in the urine is generally lower in WM than in myeloma and because of the absence of contributing factors, such as hypercalcemia, although cast nephropathy has also been described in WM [70]. On the other hand, the IgM macromolecule is more susceptible to being trapped in the glomerular loops where ultra-filtration presumably contributes to its precipitation, forming subendothelial deposits of aggregated IgM proteins that occlude the glomerular capillaries. [71] Mild and reversible proteinuria may result and most patients are asymptomatic. The deposition of monoclonal light chain as fibrillar amyloid deposits (AL amyloidosis) is uncommon in patients with WM [72]. Clinical expression and prognosis are similar to those of other AL patients with involvement of heart (44%), kidneys (32%), liver (14%), lungs (10%), peripheral/autonomic nerves (38%) and soft tissues (18%). However, the incidence of cardiac and pulmonary involvement is higher in patients with monoclonal IgM than with other immunoglobulin isotypes. The association of WM with reactive amyloidosis (AA) has been documented rarely [73,74]. Simultaneous occurrence of fibrillary glomerulopathy, characterized by glomerular deposits of wide non-congophilic fibrils and amyloid deposits, has been reported in WM [75].

Manifestations related to tissue infiltration by neoplastic cells

Tissue infiltration by neoplastic cells is rare and can involve various organs and tissues, from the bone marrow (described later) to the liver, spleen, lymph nodes, and possibly the lungs, gastrointestinal tract, kidneys, skin, eyes and central nervous system. Pulmonary involvement in the form of masses, nodules, diffuse infiltrate, or pleural effusions is relatively rare, since the overall incidence of pulmonary and pleural findings reported for WM is only 3%–5% [76–78]. Cough is the most common presenting symptom, followed by dyspnea and chest pain. Chest radiographic findings include parenchymal infiltrates, confluent masses, and effusions. Malabsorption, diarrhea, bleeding or obstruction may indicate involvement of the gastrointestinal tract at the level of the stomach, duodenum or small intestine [79–82]. In contrast to multiple myeloma, infiltration of the kidney interstitium with lymphoplasmacytoid cell has been reported in WM [83], while renal or perirenal masses are not uncommon [84]. The skin can be the site of dense lymphoplasmacytic infiltrates, similar to that seen in the liver, spleen, and lymph nodes, forming cutaneous plaques and, rarely, nodules [85]. Chronic urticaria and IgM gammopathy are the two cardinal features of the Schnitzler syndrome, which is not usually associated initially with clinical features of WM [86], although evolution to WM is not uncommon. Thus, close follow up of these patients is warranted. Invasion of articular and periarticular structures by WM malignant cells is rarely reported [87]. The neoplastic cells can infiltrate the periorbital structures, lacrimal gland, and retro-orbital lymphoid tissues, resulting in ocular nerve palsies [88,89]. Direct infiltration of the central nervous system by monoclonal lymphoplasmacytic cells as infiltrates or as tumors constitutes the rarely observed Bing–Neel syndrome, characterized clinically by confusion, memory loss, disorientation, and motor dysfunction (reviewed in Civit *et al.* [90]).

Laboratory investigations and findings
Hematological abnormalities

Anemia is the most common finding in patients with symptomatic WM and is caused by a combination of factors: mild decrease in red cell survival, impaired erythropoiesis, hemolysis, moderate plasma volume expansion, and blood loss from the gastrointestinal tract. Blood smears are usually normocytic and normochromic, and rouleaux formation is often pronounced. Electronically measured mean corpuscular volume may be elevated spuriously owing to erythrocyte aggregation. In addition, the hemoglobin estimate can be inaccurate, i.e. falsely high, because of interaction between the monoclonal protein and the diluent used in some automated analyzers [91]. Leukocyte and platelet counts are usually within the reference range at presentation, although patients may occasionally present with severe thrombocytopenia. As reported above, monoclonal B lymphocytes expressing surface IgM and late-differentiation B cell markers are uncommonly detected in blood by flow cytometry. A raised erythrocyte sedimentation rate is almost constantly observed in WM and may be the first clue to the presence of the macroglobulin. The clotting abnormality detected most frequently is prolongation of thrombin time. AL amyloidosis should be suspected in all patients with nephrotic syndrome, cardiomyopathy, hepatomegaly or peripheral neuropathy. Diagnosis requires the demonstration of green birefringence under polarized light of amyloid deposits stained with Congo red.

Biochemical investigations

High-resolution electrophoresis combined with immunofixation of serum and urine are recommended for identification and characterization of the IgM monoclonal protein. The light chain of the monoclonal IgM is κ in 75%–80% of patients. A few WM patients have more than one M component. The concentration of the serum monoclonal protein is very variable but in most cases lies within the range of 15–45 g/l. Densitometry should be adopted to determine IgM levels for serial evaluations because nephelometry is unreliable and shows large intralaboratory as well as interlaboratory variation. The presence of cold agglutinins or cryoglobulins may affect determination of IgM levels and, therefore, testing for cold agglutinins and cryoglobulins should be performed at diagnosis. If present, subsequent serum samples should be analyzed under warm conditions for determination of serum monoclonal IgM level. Although Bence Jones proteinuria is frequently present, it exceeds 1 g per 24 h in only 3% of cases. While IgM levels are elevated in WM patients, IgA and IgG levels

are most often depressed and do not demonstrate recovery even after successful treatment suggesting that patients with WM harbor a defect which prevents normal plasma cell development and/or Ig heavy chain rearrangements [92,93].

Serum viscosity

Because of its large size (almost 1 000 000 Da), most IgM molecules are retained within the intravascular compartment and can exert an undue effect on serum viscosity. Therefore, serum viscosity should be measured if the patient has signs or symptoms of hyperviscosity syndrome. Fundoscopy remains an excellent indicator of clinically relevant hyperviscosity. Among the first clinical signs of hyperviscosity, the appearance of peripheral and mid-peripheral dot and blot-like hemorrhages in the retina, which are best appreciated with indirect ophthalmoscopy and scleral depression [42]. In more severe cases of hyperviscosity, dot, blot and flame shaped hemorrhages can appear in the macular area along with markedly dilated and tortuous veins with focal constrictions resulting in "venous sausaging," as well as papilledema.

Bone marrow findings

The bone marrow is always involved in WM. Central to the diagnosis of WM is the demonstration, by trephine biopsy, of *bone marrow infiltration by a lymphoplasmacytic cell population* constituted by small lymphocytes with evidence of plasmacytoid/plasma cell differentiation (Figure 15.1). The pattern of bone marrow infiltration may be diffuse, interstitial, or nodular, showing usually an intertrabecular pattern of infiltration. A solely paratrabecular pattern of infiltration is unusual and should raise the possibility of follicular lymphoma [1]. The bone marrow infiltration should routinely be confirmed by *immunophenotypic studies* (flow cytometry and/or immunohistochemistry) showing the following profile: sIgM$^+$CD19$^+$CD20$^+$CD22$^+$CD79$^+$ [23–25]. Up to 20% of cases may express either CD5, CD10 or CD23 [26]. In these cases, care should be taken to satisfactorily exclude chronic lymphocytic leukemia and mantle cell lymphoma [1]. "Intranuclear" periodic acid-Schiff (PAS)-positive inclusions (Dutcher–Fahey bodies) [94] consisting of IgM deposits in the perinuclear space, and sometimes in intranuclear vacuoles, may be seen occasionally in lymphoid cells in WM.

An increased number of mast cells, usually in association with the lymphoid aggregates is commonly found in WM, and their presence may help in differentiating WM from other B cell lymphomas [1,2].

Other investigations

Magnetic resonance imaging (MRI) of the spine in conjunction with computed tomography (CT) of the abdomen and pelvis are useful in evaluating the disease status in WM [95]. Bone marrow involvement can be documented by MRI studies of the spine in over 90% of patients, while CT of the abdomen and pelvis demonstrated enlarged nodes in 43% of WM patients [95]. Lymph node biopsy may show preserved architecture or replacement by infiltration of neoplastic cells with lymphoplasmacytoid, lymphoplasmacytic or polymorphous cytological patterns. The residual disease after high-dose chemotherapy with allogeneic or autologous stem cell rescue can be monitored by polymerase chain reaction (PCR)-based methods using primers specific for the monoclonal Ig variable regions.

Prognosis

Waldenström's macroglobulinemia typically presents as an indolent disease though considerable variability in prognosis can be seen. The median survival reported in several large series has ranged from five to ten years [96–102], although in a recent study of 436 consecutive patients with WM, the median overall survival from time of diagnosis was in excess of ten years [103]. The presence of 6q deletions as a prognostic marker remains controversial [14,16]. Age is consistently an important prognostic factor (>60–70 years) [96,97,99,102], but this factor is often impacted by unrelated morbidities. Anemia which reflects both marrow involvement and the serum level of the IgM monoclonal protein (due to the impact of IgM on intravascular fluid retention) has emerged as a strong adverse prognostic factor with hemoglobin levels of <9–12 g/dl associated with decreased survival in several series [96–99,102]. Cytopenias have also been regularly identified as a significant predictor of survival [97]. However, the precise level of cytopenias with prognostic significance remains to be determined [99]. Some series have identified a platelet count of <100–150×10^9/l and a granulocyte count of $<1.5 \times 10^9$/l as independent prognostic factors [96,97,99,102]. The number of cytopenias

in a given patient has been proposed as a strong prognostic factor [97]. Serum albumin levels have also correlated with survival in WM patients in certain but not all studies using multivariate analyses [97,99,100]. High beta-2 microglobulin levels (>3–3.5 g/dl) were shown in several studies [98–102], a high serum IgM M protein (>7 g/dl) [102] as well as a low serum IgM M protein (<4 g/dl) [100] and the presence of cryoglobulins [96] as adverse factors. A few scoring systems have been proposed based on these analyses (Table 15.3).

Treatment of Waldenström's macroglobulinemia: treatment indications

Consensus guidelines on indications for treatment initiation were formulated as part of the 2nd International Workshop on Waldenström's Macroglobulinemia [99]. Initiation of therapy should not be based on the IgM levels since this may not correlate with either disease burden or symptomatic status [103]. Initiation of therapy is appropriate for patients with constitutional symptoms, such as recurrent fever, night sweats, fatigue due to anemia, or weight loss. The presence of progressive, symptomatic lymphadenopathy or splenomegaly provides additional reasons to begin therapy. The presence of anemia with a hemoglobin value of ≤10 g/dl or a platelet count ≤100 × 10^9/l on this basis of disease is also a reasonable indication for treatment initiation. Certain complications of WM, such as hyperviscosity syndrome, symptomatic sensorimotor peripheral neuropathy, systemic amyloidosis, renal insufficiency, or symptomatic cryoglobulinemia are also indications for therapy.

Treatment options

A precise therapeutic algorithm for therapy of WM remains to be defined given the paucity of randomized clinical trials. Active agents include alkylators (chlorambucil, cyclophosphamide), nucleoside analogs (cladribine, fludarabine), monoclonal antibodies (rituximab, ofatumumab, alemtuzumab), bortezomib, thalidomide, everolimus and bendamustine [103,104]. Combination therapy particularly with rituximab has been associated with improved clinical outcomes. Individual patient considerations, including the presence of cytopenias, need for more rapid disease control, age and candidacy

Table 15.3 Prognostic scoring systems in Waldenstrom's macroglobulinemia

Study	Adverse prognostic factors	Number of groups	Survival
Gobbi et al. [96]	Hb < 9 g/dl Age >70 years Weight loss Cryoglobulinemia	prognostic factors 2–4 prognostic factors	Median: 48 months Median: 80 months
Morel et al. [97]	Age ≥ 65 years Albumin <4 g/dl Number of cytopenias: Hb <12 g/dl Platelets <150 × 10^9/l Wbc <4 × 10^9/l	prognostic factors 2 prognostic factors 3–4 prognostic factors	5 years: 87% 5 years: 62% 5 years: 25%
Dhodapkar et al. [98]	β_2M ≥3 g/dl Hb <12 g/dl IgM <4 g/dl	β_2M < 3 mg/dl + Hb ≥ 12 g/dl β_2M < 3 mg/dl + Hb < 12 g/dl β_2M ≥ 3 mg/dl + IgM ≥ 4 g/dl β_2M ≥ 3 mg/dl + IgM < 4 g/dl	5 years: 87% 5 years: 63% 5 years: 53% 5 years: 21%
Application of international staging system criteria for myeloma to WM Dimopoulos et al. [100]	Albumin ≤3.5 g/dl β_2M ≥3.5 mg/l	Albumin ≥ 3.5 g/dl + β_2M < 3.5 mg/dl Albumin ≤ 3.5 g/dl + β_2M < 3.5 or β_2M 3.5–5.5 mg/dl β_2M > 5.5 mg/dl	Median: NR Median: 116 months Median: 54 months
International prognostic scoring system for WM Morel et al. [102]	Age > 65 years Hb <11.5 g/dl Platelets <100 × 10^9/l β_2M >3 mg/l IgM >7 g/dl	prognostic factors[a] 2 prognostic factors[b] 3–5 prognostic factors	5 years: 87% 5 years: 68% 5 years: 36%

[a] Excluding age.
[b] Or age >65.

for autologous transplant therapy, should be taken into account in making the choice of a first-line agent. For patients who are candidates for autologous transplant therapy, exposure to continuous chlorambucil or nucleoside analog therapy should be limited given potential for stem cell damage. The use of nucleoside analogs may also increase risk for histological transformation to diffuse large B cell lymphoma, as well as myelodysplasia and acute myelogenous leukemia [105].

Chlorambucil

Oral alkylating drugs, alone and in combination therapy with steroids, have been extensively evaluated in the upfront treatment of WM. The greatest experience with oral alkylator therapy has been with chlorambucil, which has been administered on both a continuous (i.e. daily dose schedule) as well as an intermittent schedule. Patients receiving chlorambucil on a continuous schedule typically receive 0.1 mg/kg per day, whilst on the intermittent schedule patients will typically receive 0.3 mg/kg for seven days, every six weeks. In a prospective randomized study, Kyle et al. [106] reported no significant difference in the overall response rate between these schedules, although interestingly the median response duration was greater for patients receiving intermittent versus continuously dosed chlorambucil (46 months vs. 26 months). Despite the favorable median response duration in this study for use of the intermittent schedule, no difference in the median overall survival was observed. Moreover, an increased incidence for development of myelodysplasia and acute myelogenous leukemia with the intermittent (three of 22 patients) versus the continuous (0 of 24 patients) chlorambucil schedule prompted the authors of this study to express preference for use of continuous chlorambucil dosing. The use of steroids in combination with alkylator therapy has also been explored. Dimopoulos and Alexanian [107] evaluated chlorambucil (8 mg/m^2) along with prednisone (40 mg/m^2) given orally for ten days, every six weeks, and reported a major response (i.e. reduction of IgM by greater than 50%) in 72% of patients. Non-chlorambucil-based alkylator regimens employing melphalan and cyclophosphamide in combination with steroids have also been examined by Petrucci et al. [108] and Case et al. [109] producing slightly higher overall response rates and response durations, although the benefit of these more complex regimens over chlorambucil remains to be demonstrated. Facon et al. [110] have evaluated parameters predicting for response to alkylator therapy. Their studies in patients receiving single-agent chlorambucil demonstrated that age 60, male sex, symptomatic status and cytopenias (but, interestingly, not high tumor burden and serum IgM levels) were associated with poor response to alkylator therapy. Additional factors to be taken into account in considering alkylator therapy for patients with WM include necessity for more rapid disease control given the slow nature of response to alkylator therapy, as well as consideration for preserving stem cells in patients who are candidates for autologous transplant therapy.

Nucleoside analogs

Both cladribine and fludarabine have been extensively evaluated in untreated as well as previously treated WM patients. Cladribine administered as a single agent by continuous intravenous infusion, by two-hour daily infusion, or by subcutaneous bolus injections for five to seven days has resulted in major responses in 40%–90% of patients who received primary therapy, whilst in the salvage setting responses have ranged from 38% to 54% [110–117]. Median time to achievement of response in responding patients following cladribine ranged from 1.2 to five months. The overall response rate with daily infusional fludarabine therapy administered mainly on five-day schedules in previously untreated and treated WM patients has ranged from 38 to 100% and 30%–40%, respectively [118–123], which are on par with the response data for cladribine. Median time to achievement of response for fludarabine was also on par with cladribine at three to six months.

In general, response rates and durations of responses have been greater for patients receiving nucleoside analogs as first-line agents, although in several of the above studies wherein both untreated and previously treated patients were enrolled, no substantial difference in the overall response rate was reported. Myelosuppression commonly occurred following prolonged exposure to either of the nucleoside analogs, as did lymphopenia with sustained depletion of both CD4$^+$ and CD8+ T-lymphocytes observed in WM patients one year following initiation of therapy [110,112]. Treatment-related mortality due to myelosuppression and/or opportunistic infections attributable to immunosuppression occurred in up to 5% of all treated patients in some series with either nucleoside analog. Factors predicting for response to nucleoside analogs in WM included age at start of treatment (<70 years), pre-treatment hemoglobin >95 g/l, platelets >75 000/mm^3, disease relapsing off therapy, patients with resistant disease within the first year of diagnosis, and a long interval between first-line therapy and initiation of a nucleoside analog in relapsing patients [110,116,122]. There are limited data on the use of an alternate nucleoside analog to salvage patients whose disease relapsed or demonstrated resistance off cladribine or fludarabine therapy [124,125]. Three of four (75%) patients responded to cladribine to salvage patients who progressed following an unmaintained remission to fludarabine, whereas only one of ten (10%) with disease resistant to fludarabine responded to cladribine [126]. However, Lewandowski et al. [125] reported a response in two of six patients (33%) and disease stabilization in the remaining patients to fludarabine, in spite of an inadequate response or progressive disease following cladribine therapy. The combination of nucleoside analogs with cyclophosphamide and/or rituximab has been investigated and discussed below.

The safety of nucleoside analogs has been the subject of investigation in several recent studies. Thomas et al. recently reported their experiences in harvesting stem cells in 21 patients with symptomatic WM in whom autologous peripheral blood stem cell collection was attempted. Autologous stem cell collection succeeded on the first attempt in 14/15 patients who received non-nucleoside analog based therapy versus 2/6 patients who received a nucleoside analog [127]. The long term safety of nucleoside analogs in WM was recently examined by Leleu et al. [105] in a large series of WM patients.

A seven-fold increase in transformation to an aggressive lymphoma, and a three-fold increase in the development of acute myelogenous leukemia/myelodysplasia were observed amongst patients who received a nucleoside analog versus other therapies for their WM. A recent meta-analysis by Leleu et al.[126] of several trials utilizing nucleoside analogs in WM patients, which included patients who had previously received an alkylator agent showed a crude incidence of 6.6%–10% for development of disease transformation, and 1.4%–8.9% for development of myelodysplasia or acute myelogenous leukemia. None of the studied risk factors, i.e. gender, age, family history of WM or B cell malignancies, typical markers of tumor burden and prognosis, type of nucleoside analog therapy (cladribine versus fludarabine), time from diagnosis to nucleoside analog use, nucleoside analog treatment as primary or salvage therapy, as well as treatment with an oral alkylator (i.e. chlorambucil), predicted for the occurrence of transformation or development of myelodysplasia/acute myelogenous leukemia for WM patients treated with a nucleoside analog [126].

Monoclonal antibodies

Rituximab is a chimeric monoclonal antibody which targets CD20, a widely expressed antigen on lymphoplasmacytic cells in WM [128]. Several retrospective and prospective studies have indicated that rituximab, when used at standard dosimetry (i.e. four weekly infusions at 375 mg/m^2) induced major responses in approximately 27%–35% of previously treated and untreated patients [129–135]. Furthermore, it was shown in some of these studies, that patients who achieved minor responses or even stable disease benefited from rituximab as evidenced by improved hemoglobin and platelet counts, and reduction of lymphadenopathy and/or splenomegaly. The median time to treatment failure in these studies was found to range from eight to 27+ months. Studies evaluating an extended rituximab schedule consisting of four weekly courses at 375 mg/m^2 per week, repeated three months later by another four-week course have demonstrated major response rates of 44%–48%, with time to progression estimates of 16+ to 29+ months [135,136].

In many WM patients, a transient increase of serum IgM (IgM flare) may be noted immediately following initiation of rituximab treatment [135,137–139]. The IgM flare may be related to release of interleukin-6 by bystander immune in response to binding of rituximab to FcγRIIA receptors, and also occurs in response to intravenous immunoglobulin administration in WM patients [140]. The IgM flare in response to rituximab does not herald treatment failure, and while most patients will return to their baseline serum IgM level by 12 weeks, some patients may flare for months despite having tumor responses in their bone marrow. Patients with baseline serum IgM levels of >50 g/dl or serum viscosity of >3.5 cp may be particularly at risk for a hyperviscosity related event and in such patients plasmapheresis should be considered or rituximab omitted for the first few cycles of therapy until IgM levels decline to safer levels [103]. Because of the decreased likelihood of response in patients with higher IgM levels, as well as the possibility that serum IgM and viscosity levels may abruptly rise, rituximab monotherapy should not be used as sole therapy for the treatment of patients at risk for hyperviscosity symptoms.

Time to response after rituximab is slow and exceeds three months on the average. The time to best response in one study was 18 months [136]. Patients with baseline serum IgM levels of <60g/dl are more likely to respond, irrespective of the underlying bone marrow involvement by tumor cells [135,136]. A recent analysis of 52 patients who were treated with single agent rituximab has indicated that the objective response rate was significantly lower in patients who had either low serum albumin (<35 g/l) or elevated serum monoclonal protein (>40 g/l M spike). Furthermore, the presence of both adverse prognostic factors was related with a short time to progression (3.6 months). Moreover, patients who had normal serum albumin and relatively low serum monoclonal protein levels derived a substantial benefit from rituximab with a time to progression exceeding 40 months [141].

The genetic background of patients may also be important for determining response to rituximab. In particular, a correlation between polymorphisms at position 158 in the Fc gamma RIIIa receptor (CD16), an activating Fc receptor on important effector cells that mediate antibody-dependent cell-mediated cytotoxicity (ADCC), and rituximab response was observed in WM patients. Individuals may encode either the amino acid valine or phenylalanine at position 158 in the FcγRIIIa receptor. WM patients who carried the valine amino acid (either in a homozygous or heterozygous pattern) had a four-fold higher major response rate to rituximab versus those patients who expressed phenylalanine in a homozygous pattern [142]. The attainment of better categorical responses, i.e. very good partial response or complete resonse following rituximab based therapy appears also dependent on the presence of at least one valine amino acid at FcγRIIIa-158 [143].

Ofatumumab is a fully humanized CD20-directed monoclonal antibody that targets the small loop of CD20, a target which is different than that of rituximab. A 43% overall response rate was observed in a small series of symptomatic WM patients following ofatumumab administration, which included untreated and previously treated patients [144]. An IgM flare with symptomatic hyperviscosity was also observed in this series necessitating plasmapheresis. Additionally, ofatumumab has been successfully administered to WM patients who demonstrated intolerance to rituximab [144,145].

The activity of alemtuzumab has also been investigated in WM patients given the broad expression of CD52 [129]. The WMCTG recently reported a multi-center study in symptomatic WM patients, whose median prior therapies was 2 (range 0–5), and 43% had refractory disease [146]. Patients received alemtuzumab intravenously at 30 mg three times weekly for up to 12 weeks, after test dosing, and received hydrocortisone, acyclovir and bactrim or equivalent prophylaxis. The overall response rate in this series was 75%, and included major responses in 36% of patients. With a median follow up of 64 months, the median time to progression was 14.5 months. Hematological and infectious complications, including CMV reactivation were more common in previously treated patients and indirectly associated with three deaths. Long term follow up revealed late-onset idiopathic thrombocytopenia in four patients at a median of 13.6 months following therapy, and contributed to one death. High rates of response with the use of alemtuzumab were also observed by Owen et al. [147] who reported their preliminary experience in a small series of heavily pretreated WM patients. The median number of prior therapies in this series was 4, and similar to this study patients received up to 12 weeks of therapy (at 30 mg IV three times weekly) following initial dose

escalation. Among the seven patients treated with alemtuzumab, five achieved a partial response and one a complete response. Disseminated aspergillus and mycobacterial infections contributed to two deaths in this series.

Bortezomib

Bortezomib is a proteasome inhibitor which has been extensively investigated in WM. In a multi-center study of the WMCTG, 27 patients received up to eight cycles of bortezomib at 1.3 mg/m^2 on days 1, 4, 8 and 11 [148]. All but one patient had relapsed/or refractory disease. Following therapy, median serum IgM levels declined from 4660 mg/dl to 2092 mg/dl (p < 0.0001). The overall response rate was 85%, with 10 and 13 patients achieving a minor (<25% decrease in IgM) and major (<50% decrease in IgM) response. Responses were prompt, and occurred at median of 1.4 months. The median time to progression for all responding patients in this study was 7.9 (range 3–21.4+) months, and the most common grade III/IV toxicities occurring in ≥5% of patients were sensory neuropathies (22.2%); leukopenia (18.5%); neutropenia (14.8%); dizziness (11.1%); and thrombocytopenia (7.4%). Importantly, sensory neuropathies resolved or improved in nearly all patients following cessation of therapy. As part of an NCI-Canada study, Chen et al. [149] treated 27 patients with both untreated (44%) and previously treated (56%) disease. Patients in this study received bortezomib utilizing the standard schedule until they either demonstrated progressive disease, or two cycles beyond a complete response or stable disease. The overall response rate in this study was 78%, with major responses observed in 44% of patients. Sensory neuropathy occurred in 20 patients, five with grade >3, and occurred following two to four cycles of therapy. Among the 20 patients developing a neuropathy, 14 patients resolved and one patient demonstrated a one-grade improvement at 2–13 months. In addition to the above experiences with bortezomib monotherapy in WM, Dimopoulos et al. [150] observed major responses in six of ten (60%) previously treated WM patients, while Goy et al. [151] observed a major response in one of two WM patients who were included in a series of relapsed or refractory patients with non-Hodgkin's lymphoma (NHL). The combination of bortezomib with steroids and/or rituximab has also been investigated and is discussed below.

Immunomodulatory agents

Thalidomide as monotherapy, and in combination with dexamethasone and/or clarithromycin has been examined in WM. Dimopoulos et al. [152] demonstrated a major response in five of 20 (25%) previously untreated and treated patients who received single-agent thalidomide. Dose escalation from the thalidomide start dose of 200 mg daily was hindered by development of side effects, including the development of peripheral neuropathy in five patients obligating discontinuation or dose reduction. Low doses of thalidomide (50 mg orally daily) in combination with dexamethasone (40 mg orally once a week) and clarithromycin (250 mg orally twice a day) have also been examined, with 10 of 12 (83%) previously treated patients demonstrating at least a major response [153]. However, in a follow-up study by Dimopoulos et al. [154] using a higher thalidomide dose (200 mg orally daily) along with dexamathasone (40 g orally once a week) and clarithromycin (500 mg orally twice a day), only two of ten (20%) previously treated patients responded. Thalidomide, as well as lenalidomide has been investigated in combination with rituximab and these studies are discussed below.

Bendamustine

Bendamustine is a recently approved agent for the treatment of relapsed/refractory indolent non-Hodgkin's lymphoma (NHL). Bendamustine has structural similarities to both alkylating agents and purine analogs [155]. Bendamustine in combination with rituximab has been investigated in both previously untreated, as well as relapsed/refractory WM patients and is discussed below.

Everolimus

Everolimus is an oral inhibitor of the mTOR pathway, which is approved for the treatment of renal cell carcinoma. The Akt-mTOR-p70 pathway is active in WM, and inhibition of this pathway leads to apoptosis of primary WM cells, and WM cell lines [156,157]. Fifty patients with a median of three prior therapies were treated with everolimus in a joint Dana Farber/Mayo Clinic study [158]. The overall response rate was 70%, with 42% of patients attaining a major response. The progression free survival at 12 months was estimated to be 62%. Grade 3 or higher related toxicities were observed in 56% of patients with cytopenias

constituting the most common toxicity. Pulmonary toxicity occurred in 10% of patients. Dose reductions due to toxicity occurred in 52% of patients. A clinical trial examining the activity of everolimus in previously untreated patients with WM has been initiated by the WMCTG. IgM discordance to bone marrow tumor burden was common in this upfront study, and therefore serial bone marrow biopsies are important in assessing disease response to everolimus.

Combination strategies

Because rituximab is an active and a non-myelosuppressive agent, its combination with various chemotherapeutic agents has been extensively explored in WM. The combination of CHOP (cyclophosphamide, doxorubicin, vincristine, prednisone) with rituximab (CHOP-R) was investigated in a randomized frontline study by the German Low Grade Lymphoma Study Group (GLSG) involving 69 patients, most of whom had WM [159]. The addition of rituximab to CHOP resulted in a higher overall response rate (94% vs. 67%) and median time to progression (63 months vs. 22 months) in comparison to patients treated with CHOP alone. Dimopoulos et al. [160] investigated the combination of rituximab, dexamethasone and oral cyclophosphamide (RCD) as primary therapy in 72 patients with WM. At least a major response was observed in 74% of patients in this study, and the two-year progression free survival was 67%. Therapy was well tolerated, though one patient died of interstitial pneumonia. In the salvage setting, the use of CHOP-R has been investigated in relapsed/refractory WM patients [161]. Among 13 evaluable patients, ten patients achieved a major response (77%) including three CR and seven PR, and two patients achieved a minor response. In a retrospective study, Ioakimidis et al. [162] examined the outcomes of symptomatic WM patients who received CHOP-R, CVP-R, or CP-R. Baseline characteristics for all three cohorts were similar for age, prior therapies, bone marrow involvement, hematocrit, platelet count and serum beta-2 microglobulin, though serum IgM levels were higher in patients treated with CHOP-R. The overall response rates to therapy were comparable among all three treatment groups: CHOP-R (96%); CVP-R (88%) and CP-R (95%), though more CR were observed among patients treated with either CVP-R or CHOP-R. Comparison of adverse events for these regimens showed a higher incidence for neutropenic fever as well as treatment related neuropathy in patients receiving CHOP-R and CVP-R versus CPR. These results suggest that in WM, the use of doxorubicin and vincristine may be omitted in order to minimize treatment related complications.

Combination therapy with nucleoside analogs has been investigated as both firstline and salvage therapy in WM. Weber et al. [163] administered rituximab along with cladribine and cyclophosphamide to 17 previously untreated patients with WM. At least a partial response was documented in 94% of WM patients including a complete response in 18%. With a median follow up of 21 months no patient has relapsed. Laszlo et al. [164] recently evaluated the combination of subcutaneous cladribine with rituximab in 29 WM patients with either untreated or previously treated disease. Intended therapy consisted of rituximab on day 1 followed by subcutaneous cladribine 0.1 mg/kg for five consecutive days, administered monthly for four cycles. With a median follow-up of 43 months, the overall response rate observed was 89.6%, with seven complete responses (CR), 16 partial responses, and three minor responses. Response activity was similar between untreated and previously treated patients. No major infections were observed despite the lack of antimicrobial prophylaxis. In a study by the WMCTG, the combination of rituximab and fludarabine was administered to 43 WM patients, 32 (75%) of whom were previously untreated [165]. The overall response rate was 95.3%, and 83% of patients achieved a major response. The median time to progression was 51.2 months in this series, and was longer for those patients who were previously untreated and for those achieving at least a very good partial response. Hematological toxicity was common, particularly neutropenia and thrombocytopenia. Two deaths occurred in this study due to non-pneumocystis carinii pneumonia. Secondary malignanices including transformation to aggressive lymphoma and development of myelodysplasia or AML were observed in six patients in this series. The addition of rituximab to fludarabine and cyclophosphamide has also been explored in the salvage setting by Tam et al., wherein four of five patients demonstrated a response [166]. Hensel et al. [167] administered rituximab along with pentostatin and cyclophosphamide to 13 patients with untreated and previously treated WM or lymphoplasmacytic lymphoma. A major response was observed in 77% or patients. The addition of alkylating agents to

nucleoside analogs has also been explored in WM. Weber et al. [163] administered two cycles of oral cyclophosphamide along with subcutaneous cladribine to 37 patients with previously untreated WM. At least a partial response was observed in 84% of patients and the median duration of response was 36 months. Dimopoulos et al. [168] examined fludarabine in combination with intravenous cyclophosphamide and observed partial responses in six of 11 (55%) patients with either primary refractory disease, or who relapsed on treatment. The combination of fludarabine plus cyclosphosphamide (FC) was also evaluated in a recent study by Tamburini et al. [169] involving 49 patients, 35 of whom were previously treated. Seventy-eight percent of the patients in this study achieved a response, and median time to treatment failure was 27 months. Hematological toxicity was commonly observed and three patients died of treatment related toxicities. Two interesting findings in this study was the development of acute leukemia in two patients, histologic transformation to diffuse large cell lymphoma in one patient, and two cases of solid malignancies (prostate and melanoma), as well as failure to mobilize stem cells in four of six patients. Tedeschi et al. [170] recently completed a multicenter study on with fludarabine, cyclophosphamide and rituximab (FCR) in symptomatic WM patients with untreated or relapsed/refractory disease to one line of chemotherapy. Treatment consisted of rituximab at 375 mg/m^2 on day 1, fludarabine at 25 mg/m^2 and cyclophosphamide at 250 mg/m^2 by intravenous administration on days two to four every four weeks. Forty-three patients were accrued to this study. The overall response rate was 89%, with 83% of patients attaining a major remission, and 14% a complete response. Prolonged neutropenia was observed in up to a third of patients. With a median follow up of 15 months, the median progression free survival for this study has not been reached.

The combination of bortezomib, dexamethasone and rituximab (BDR) has been investigated as primary therapy in patients with WM by the WMCTG. An overall response rate of 96%, major response rate of 83%, and complete attainment in 22% was observed with BDR [171]. The updated median progression free survival in this study was >56.1 months. The incidence of grade 3 neuropathy was 30% in this study which utilized a twice a week schedule for bortezomib administration at 1.3 mg/m^2. Peripheral neuropathy from bortezomib was reversible in most patients in this study following discontinuation of therapy, and patients benefitted with pregabalin. An increased incidence of herpes zoster was also observed with BDR prompting the use of prophylactic antiviral therapy. An alternative schedule for bortezomib administration (i.e. weekly at 1.6 mg/m^2) in combination with rituximab and/or dexamethasone has been investigated in several studies with overall response rates of 80%–90% [172–174]. A lower incidence of peripheral neuropathy was observed in two studies using once a week bortezomib [172,174]. The impact of once versus twice a week bortezomib administration on progression free survival remains to be clarified.

The combination of immunomodulator agents (thalidomide, lenalidomide) with rituximab was investigated by the WMCTG. Thalidomide was administered at 200 mg daily for two weeks, followed by 400 mg daily and thereafter for one year. Patients received four weekly infusions of rituximab at 375 mg/m^2 beginning one week after initiation of thalidomide, followed by four additional weekly infusions of rituximab at 375 mg/m^2 beginning at week 13. The overall and major response rate was 72% and 64%, respectively, and the median time to progression was 38 months in this series [175]. Dose reduction and/or discontinuation of thalidomide was common, and mainly attributed to treatment related neuropathy. The investigators concluded in this study that lower doses of thalidomide (i.e. 50–100 mg/day) should be considered in this patient population. The combination of lenalidomide with rituximab was investigated by the WMCTG using lenalidomide at 25 mg daily on a syncopated schedule wherein therapy was administered for three weeks, followed by a one week pause for an intended duration of 48 weeks [176]. Patients received one week of therapy with lenalidomide, after which rituximab (375 mg/m^2) was administered weekly on weeks two to five, then 13 to 16. The overall and a major response rates in this study were 50% and 25%, respectively, and a median TTP for responders was 18.9 months. In two patients with bulky disease, significant reduction in extramedullary disease was observed. However, an acute decrease in hematocrit were observed during first two weeks of lenalidomide therapy in 13/16 (81%) patients with a median absolute decrease in hematocrit of 4.8%, resulting in anemia related complications and hospitalizations in four patients. Despite dose reduction, most patients in this study continued to demonstrate aggravated anemia with lenalidomide. There was no evidence of hemolysis or more general myelosuppression with lenalidomide in this study. Therefore, the mechanism for lenalidomide related anemia in WM patients remains to be determined, and the use of this agent among WM patients should be avoided.

The use of bendamustine in combination with rituximab was explored by Rummel et al. [177] in the frontline therapy of WM. As part of a randomized study, patients received six cycles of bendamustine plus rituximab (Benda-R) or CHOP-R. A total of 546 patients were enrolled in this study for indolent NHL patients, and included 40 patients with WM [8]. For patients receiving Benda-R, bendamustine was administered at 90 mg/m^2 on days 1 and 2, and rituximab at 375 mg/m^2 on day 1. The overall response rate was 96% for Benda-R, and 94% for CHOP-R treated patients. With a median observation period of 26 months, 20/23 (87%) Benda-R versus 9/17 (53%) CHOP-R treated WM patients remain free of progression. Importantly, Benda-R was associated with a lower incidence of grade 3 or 4 neutropenia, infectious complications, and alopecia. In the salvage setting, the outcome of 30 WM patients with relapsed/refractory disease who received bendamustine alone, or with with a CD20-directed antibody was reported by Treon et al. [145] An overall response rate of 83.3% was reported [145]. The median estimated progression free survival for all patients was 13.2 months. Overall therapy was well tolerated. Prolonged myelosuppression was more common in patients who received prior nucleoside analogs.

Maintenance therapy

A role for maintenance rituximab in WM patients following response to a rituximab containing regimen was raised in a study examining the outcome of 248 WM rituximab naïve patients who were either observed or received maintenance rituximab [178]. In this retrospective study, categorical responses improved in 16/162 (10%) of observed patients, and in 36/86 (41.8%) of patients who received maintenance rituximab following induction therapy. Both progression free (56.3 months vs. 28.6 months) and overall survival (>120 months vs. 116 months) were longer in patients who received maintenance rituximab. Improved progression free survival was evident despite previous treatment status, induction with rituximab alone or in combination therapy. Best serum IgM response was lower, and hematocrit higher in those patients receiving maintenance rituximab. Among patients receiving maintenance rituximab, an increased number of infectious events, predominantly sinusitis and bronchitis were observed, though were mainly grade 1 or 2.

High-dose therapy and stem cell transplantation

The use of stem cell transplantation (SCT) therapy has also been explored in WM patients. Desikan et al. [179] reported their initial experience of high-dose chemotherapy and autologous stem cell transplant, which has more recently been updated by Munshi and Barlogi [180]. Their studies involved eight previously treated WM patients between the ages of 45 and 69 years, who received either melphalan at 200 mg/m^2 ($n = 7$) or melphalan at 140 mg/m^2 along with total body irradiation. Stem cells were successfully collected in all eight patients, although a second collection procedure was required for two patients who had extensive previous nucleoside analog exposure. There were no transplant related mortalities and toxicities were manageable. All eight patients responded, with seven of eight patients achieving a major response, and one patient achieving a complete response with durations of response raging from 5+ to 77+ months. Dreger et al. [181] investigated the use of the DEXA-BEAM (dexamethasone, BCNU, etoposide, cytarabine, melphalan) regimen followed by myeloablative therapy with cyclophosphamide, and total body irradiation and autologous stem cell transplantation in seven WM patients, which included four untreated patients. Serum IgM levels declined by >50% following DEXA-BEAM and myeloablative therapy for six of seven patients, with progression-free survival ranging from 4+ to 30+ months. All three evaluable patients, who were previously treated, also attained a major response in a study by Anagnostopoulos et al. [182] in which WM patients received various preparative regimens and showed event-free survivals of 26+, 31 and 108+ months. Tournilhac et al. [183] recently reported the outcome of 18 WM patients in France who received high-dose chemotherapy followed by autologous stem cell transplantation. All patients were previously treated with a median of three (range 1–5) prior regimens. Therapy was well tolerated with an improvement in response status observed for seven patients (six PR to CR; one SD to PR), while only one patient demonstrated progressive disease. The median event-free survival for all non-progressing patients

was 12 months. Tournilhac et al. [183] have also reported the outcome of allogeneic transplantation in ten previously treated WM patients (ages 35–46) who received a median of three prior therapies, including three patients with progressive disease despite therapy. Two of three patients with progressive disease responded, and an improvement in response status was observed in five patients. The median event-free survival for non-progressing, evaluable patients was 31 months. Concerning in this series was the death of three patients owing to transplantation related toxicity. Anagnostopoulos et al. [184] have also reported on a retrospective review of WM patients who underwent either autologous or allogeneic transplantation, and whose outcomes were reported to the International Blood and Marrow Transplant Registry. Seventy-eight percent of patients in this cohort had two or more previous therapies, and 58% of them were resistant to their previous therapy. The relapse rate at three years was 29% in the allogeneic group, and 24% in the autologous group. Non-relapse mortality however was 40% in the allogeneic group, and 11% in the autologous group in this series.

Kyriakou et al. [185] reported on the outcome of WM patients in the European Bone Marrow Transplant (EBMT) registry who received either an autologous or allogeneic SCT. Among 158 patients receiving an autologous SCT, which included primarily relapsed or refractory patients, the five-year progression free and overall survival rates were 39.7% and 68.5%, respectively. Non-relapse mortality at one year was 3.8%. Chemorefractory disease, and the number of prior lines of therapy at time of the autologous SCT were the most important prognostic factor for progression free and overall survival. The achievement of a negative immunofixation after autologous SCT had a positive impact on progression free survival. When used as consolidation at first response, autologous transplantation provided a progression-free survival of 44% at five years. In the allogeneic SCT experience from the EBMT, the long-term outcome of 86 WM patients was reported by Kyriakou et al. [186] A total of 86 patients received allograft by either myeloablative ($n = 37$) or reduced-intensity ($n = 49$) conditioning. The median age of patients in this series was 49 years, and 47 patients had three or more previous lines of therapy. Eight patients failed prior autologous SCT. Fifty-nine patients (68.6%) had chemotherapy-sensitive disease at the time of allogeneic SCT. Non-relapse mortality at three

205

Table 15.4 Summary of updated response criteria adopted at the Sixth International Workshop on Waldenstrom's macroglobulinemia [189]

Complete response	CR	IgM in normal range, and disappearance of monoclonal protein by immunofixation; no histological evidence of bone marrow involvement, and resolution of any adenopathy/organomegaly (if present at baseline), along with no signs or symptoms attributable to WM. Reconfirmation of the CR status is required by repeat immunofixation studies
Very good partial response	VGPR	A ≥90% reduction of serum IgM and decrease in adenopathy/organomegaly (if present at baseline) on physical examination or on CT scan. No new symptoms or signs of active disease
Partial response	PR	A ≥50% reduction of serum IgM and decrease in adenopathy/organomegaly (if present at baseline) on physical examination or on CT scan. No new symptoms or signs of active disease
Minor response	MR	A ≥25% but <50% reduction of serum IgM. No new symptoms or signs of active disease
Stable disease	SD	A <25% reduction and <25% increase of serum IgM without progression of adenopathy/organomegaly, cytopenias or clinically significant symptoms due to disease and/or signs of WM
Progressive disease	PD	A ≥25% increase in serum IgM by protein confirmed by a second measurement or progression of clinically significant findings due to disease (i.e. anemia, thrombocytopenia, leukopenia, bulky adenopathy/organomegaly) or symptoms (unexplained recurrent fever ≥ 38.4 °C, drenching night sweats, ≥10% body weight loss, or hyperviscosity, neuropathy, symptomatic cryoglobulinemia or amyloidosis) attributable to WM

years was 33% for patients receiving a myeloablative transplant, and 23% for those who received reduced-intensity conditioning. The overall response rate was 75.6%. The relapse rates at three years were 11% for myeloablative, and 25% for reduced-intensity conditioning recipients. Five-year progression-free and overall survival for WM patients who received a myeloablative allogeneic SCT were 56% and 62%, and for patients who received reduced intensity conditioning were 49% and 64%, respectively. The occurrence of chronic graft-versus-host disease was associated with improved progression free survival, and suggested the existence of a clinically relevant graft-versus-WM effect in this study.

Response criteria in Waldenstrom's macroglobulinemia

As part of the Second and Third International Workshops on WM, consensus panels developed guidelines for uniform response criteria in WM [187,188]. The category of minor response was adopted at the Third International Workshop of WM, given that clinically meaningful responses were observed with newer biological agents and is based on ≥25% to < 50% decrease in serum IgM level, which is used as a surrogate marker of disease in WM. At the Sixth International Workshop on WM, the categorical response of very good partial response (VGPR), i.e. 90% reduction in IgM levels was adopted given reports of improved clinical outcome associated with VGPR or better response achievement [143,189]. In distinction, the term major response is used to denote a response of ≥ 50% in serum IgM levels, and includes partial or better responses [188]. Response categories and criteria for progressive disease in WM based on consensus recommendations are summarized in Table 15.4.

An important concern with the use of IgM as a surrogate marker of disease is that it can fluctuate, independent of tumor cell killing, particularly with newer biologically targeted agents such as rituximab, bortezomib and everolimus [136–138,148,189]. Rituximab induces a spike or flare in serum IgM levels which can occur when used as monotherapy and in combination with other agents including cyclophosphamide, nucleoside analogs, thalidomide and lenalidomide, and last for several weeks to months [162,175,176,190], whereas bortezomib and everolimus can suppress IgM levels independent of tumor cell killing in certain patients [148,189,191]. Moreover, Vargnese et al [192] showed that in patients treated with selective B cell depleting agents such as rituximab and alemtuzumab, residual IgM producing plasma cells are spared and continue to persist, thus potentially skewing the relative response and assessment to treatment. Therefore, in circumstances where the serum IgM levels appear out of context with the clinical progress of the patient, a bone marrow biopsy should be considered in order to clarify the patient's underlying disease burden. Soluble CD27 may serve as an alternative surrogate marker in WM, and remains a faithful marker of disease in patients experiencing a rituximab related IgM flare, as well as plasmapheresis [33,193].

References

1. Owen, R. G., Treon, S. P., Al-Katib, A. et al. Clinicopathological definition of Waldenström's macroglobulinemia: Consensus Panel Recommendations from the Second International Workshop on Waldenström's macroglobulinemia. *Semin. Oncol.* 2003;**30**:110–15.

2. World Health Organization Classification of Tumours of Haematopoietic and Lymphoid Tissues. Swerdlow, S. H., Campo, E., Harris, N. L. et al., editions, IARC Press, Lyon 2008.

3. Groves, F. D., Travis, L. B., Devesa, S. S., Ries, L. A., Fraumeni, J. F., Jr. Waldenström's macroglobulinemia: incidence patterns in the United States, 1988–1994. *Cancer* 1998;**82**:1078–81.

4. Varettoni, M., Tedesci, A., Arcaini, L. et al. Risk of second cancers in Waldenstrom Macroglobulinemia. *Ann. Oncol.* 2011; Apr 27. Epb ahead of print.

5. Hanzis, C., Ojha, R. P., Hunter, Z. et al. Associated malignancies in patients with Waldenström's Macroglobulinemia and their kin. *Clin. Lymphoma Myeloma Leuk.* 2011;**11**:88–92.

6. Renier, G., Ifrah, N., Chevailler, A. et al. Four brothers with Waldenstrom's Macroglobulinemia. *Cancer* 1989;**64**:1554–9.

7. Treon, S. P., Hunter, Z. R., Aggarwal, A. et al. Characterization of familial Waldenstrom's macroglobulinemia. *Ann. Oncol.* 2006;**17**:488–94.

8. Kristinsson, S. Y., Bjorkholm, M., Goldin, L. R. et al. Risk of lymphoproliferative disorders among first-degree relatives of lymphoplasmacytic lymphoma/Waldenstrom's macroglobulinemia patients: a population-based study in Sweden. *Blood* 2008;**112**:3052–6.

9. McMaster, M. L., Csako, G., Giambarresi, T. R. et al. Long-term evaluation of three multiple-case Waldenstrom's macroglobulinemia families. *Clin. Cancer Res.* 2007;**13**:5063–9.

10. Ogmundsdottir, H. M., Sveinsdottir, S., Sigfusson, A. et al. Enhanced B cell survival in familial macroglobulinaemia is associated with increased expression of Bcl-2. *Clin. Exp. Immunol.* 1999;**117**:252–60.

11. Ogmundsdottir, H. M., Steingrimsdottir, H., Haraldsdottir, V. Familial paraproteinemia: hyper-responsive B-cells as endophenotype. *Clin. Lymphoma Myeloma Leuke.* 2011;**11**:82–4.

12. Silvestri, F., Barillari, G., Fanin, R. et al. Risk of hepatitis C virus infection, Waldenström's macroglobulinemia, and monoclonal gammopathies. *Blood* 1996;**88**:1125–6.

13. Leleu, X., O'Connor, K., Ho, A. et al. Hepatitis C Viral Infection Is Not Associated with Waldenström's Macroglobulinemia. *Am. J. Hematol.* 2007;**82**:83–4.

14. Schop, R. F., Kuehl, W. M., Van Wier, S. A. et al. Waldenström macroglobulinemia neoplastic cells lack immunoglobulin heavy chain locus translocations but have frequent 6q deletions. *Blood* 2002;**100**:2996–3001.

15. Ocio, E. M., Schop, R. F., Gonzalez, B. et al. 6q deletion in Waldenstrom's macroglobulinemia is associated with features of adverse prognosis. *Br. J. Haematol.* 2007;**136**:80–6.

16. Chang, H., Qi, C., Trieu, Y. et al. Prognostic relevance of 6q deletion in Waldenstrom's macroglobulinemia. *Clin. Lymph. Myeloma* 2009;**9**:36–8.

17. Nguyen-Khac, F., Lejeune, J., Chapiro, E. et al. Cytogenetic abnormalities In a cohort of 171 patients with Waldenström Macroglobulinemia before treatment: clinical and biological correlations. *Blood* 2010;**116**: Abstract 801.

18. Rivera, A. I., Li, M. M., Beltran, G., Krause, J. R. Trisomy 4 as the sole cytogenetic abnormality in a Waldenstrom macroglobulinemia. *Cancer Genet. Cytogenet.* 2002;**133**:172–3.

19. Avet-Loiseau, H., Garand, R., Lode, L., Robillard, N., Bataille, R. 14q32 translocations discriminate IgM multiple myeloma from Waldenstrom's macroglobulinemia. *Semin. Oncol.* 2003;**30**:153–5.

20. Preud'homme, J. L., Seligmann, M. Immunoglobulins on the surface of lymphoid cells in Waldenström's macroglobulinemia. *J. Clin. Invest.* 1972;**51**:701–5.

21. Smith, B. R., Robert, N. J., Ault, K. A. In Waldenstrom's macroglobulinemia the quantity of detectable circulating monoclonal B lymphocytes correlates with clinical course. *Blood* 1983;**61**:911–14.

22. Levy, Y., Fermand, J. P., Navarro, S. et al. Interleukin 6 dependence

of spontaneous in vitro differentiation of B cells from patients with IgM gammopathy. *Proc. Natl Acad. Sci. USA* 1990;**87**:3309–13.

23. Owen, R. G., Barrans, S. L., Richards, S. J. *et al.* Waldenström macroglobulinemia. Development of diagnostic criteria and identification of prognostic factors. *Am. J. Clin. Pathol.* 2001;**116**:420–8.

24. Feiner, H. D., Rizk, C. C., Finfer, M. D. *et al.* IgM monoclonal gammopathy/Waldenström's macroglobulinemia: a morphological and immunophenotypic study of the bone marrow. *Mod. Pathol.* 1990;**3**:348–56.

25. San Miguel, J. F., Vidriales, M. B., Ocio, E. *et al.* Immunophenotypic analysis of Waldenstrom's macroglobulinemia. *Semin. Oncol.* 2003;**30**:187–95.

26. Hunter, Z. R., Branagan, A. R., Manning, R. *et al.* CD5, CD10, CD23 expression in Waldenstrom's Macroglobulinemia. *Clin. Lymph.* 2005;**5**:246–9.

27. Wagner, S. D., Martinelli, V., Luzzatto, L. Similar patterns of V kappa gene usage but different degrees of somatic mutation in hairy cell leukemia, prolymphocytic leukemia, Waldenström's macroglobulinemia, and myeloma. *Blood* 1994;**83**:3647–53.

28. Aoki, H., Takishita, M., Kosaka, M., Saito, S. Frequent somatic mutations in D and/or JH segments of Ig gene in Waldenström's macroglobulinemia and chronic lymphocytic leukemia (CLL) with Richter's syndrome but not in common CLL. *Blood* 1995;**85**:1913–19.

29. Shiokawa, S., Suehiro, Y., Uike, N., Muta, K., Nishimura, J. Sequence and expression analyses of mu and delta transcripts in patients with Waldenström's macroglobulinemia. *Am. J. Hematol.* 2001;**68**:139–43.

30. Sahota, S. S., Forconi, F., Ottensmeier, C. H. *et al.* Typical Waldenström macroglobulinemia is derived from a B-cell arrested after cessation of somatic mutation but prior to isotype switch events. *Blood* 2002;**100**:1505–7.

31. Paramithiotis, E., Cooper, M. D. Memory B lymphocytes migrate to bone marrow in humans. *Proc. Natl Acad. Sci. USA* 1997;**94**:208–12.

32. Tournilhac, O., Santos, D. D., Xu, L. *et al.* Mast cells in Waldenstrom's Macroglobulinemia support lymphoplasmacytic cell growth through CD154/CD40 signaling. *Ann. Oncol.* 2006;**17**:1275–82.

33. Ho, A., Leleu, X., Hatjiharissi, E. *et al.* CD27-CD70 interactions in the pathogenesis of Waldenstrom's Macroglobulinemia. *Blood* 2008;**112**:4683–9.

34. Ngo, H. T., Leleu, X., Lee, J., Jia, X. *et al.* SDF-1/CXCR4 and VLA-4 interaction regulates homing in Waldenstrom macroglobulinemia. *Blood* 2008;**112**:150–8.

35. Merlini, G., Farhangi, M., Osserman, E. F. Monoclonal immunoglobulins with antibody activity in myeloma, macroglobulinemia and related plasma cell dyscrasias. *Semin. Oncol.* 1986;**13**:350–65.

36. Farhangi, M., Merlini, G. The clinical implications of monoclonal immunoglobulins. *Semin. Oncol.* 1986;**13**:366–79.

37. Marmont, A. M., Merlini, G. Monoclonal autoimmunity in hematology. *Haematologica* 1991;**76**:449–59.

38. Mackenzie, M. R., Babcock, J. Studies of the hyperviscosity syndrome. II. Macroglobulinemia. *J. Lab. Clin. Med.* 1975;**85**:227–34.

39. Gertz, M. A., Kyle, R. A. Hyperviscosity syndrome. *J. Intens. Care. Med.* 1995;**10**:128–41.

40. Kwaan, H. C., Bongu, A. The hyperviscosity syndromes. *Semin. Thromb. Hemost.* 1999;**25**:199–208.

41. Singh, A., Eckardt, K. U., Zimmermann, A. *et al.* Increased plasma viscosity as a reason for inappropriate erythropoietin formation. *J. Clin. Invest.* 1993;**91**:251–6.

42. Menke, M. N., Feke, G. T., McMeel, J. W. *et al.* Hyperviscosity-related retinopathy in Waldenstrom's Macroglobulinemia. *Arch. Opthalmol.* 2006;**124**:1601–6.

43. Merlini, G., Baldini, L., Broglia, C. *et al.* Prognostic factors in symptomatic Waldenström's macroglobulinemia. *Semin. Oncol.* 2003;**30**:211–15.

44. Dellagi, K., Dupouey, P., Brouet, J. C. *et al.* Waldenström's macroglobulinemia and peripheral neuropathy:a clinical and immunologic study of 25 patients. *Blood* 1983;**62**:280–5.

45. Nobile-Orazio, E., Marmiroli, P., Baldini, L. *et al.* Peripheral neuropathy in macroglobulinemia:incidence and antigen-specificity of M proteins. *Neurology* 1987;**37**:1506–14.

46. Nemni, R., Gerosa, E., Piccolo, G., Merlini, G. Neuropathies associated with monoclonal gammapathies. *Haematologica* 1994;**79**:557–66.

47. Ropper, A. H., Gorson, K. C. Neuropathies associated with paraproteinemia. *N. Engl. J. Med.* 1998;**338**:1601–7.

48. Treon, S. P., Hanzis, C. A., Ioakimidis, L. I. *et al.* Clinical characteristics and treatment outcome of disease-related peripheral neuropathy in Waldenstrom's macroglobulinemia. *Proc. Am. Soc. Clin. Oncol.* 2010;**28**:abstract 8114.

49. Vital, A. Paraproteinemic neuropathies. *Brain. Pathol.* 2001;**11**:399–407.

50. Latov, N., Braun, P. E., Gross, R. B. *et al.* Plasma cell dyscrasia and peripheral neuropathy: identification of the myelin antigens that react with human paraproteins. *Proc. Natl Acad. Sci. USA* 1981;**78**:7139–42.

51. Chassande, B., Leger, J. M., Younes-Chennoufi, A. B. *et al.* Peripheral neuropathy associated with IgM monoclonal gammopathy: correlations between M-protein antibody activity and clinical/electrophysiological features in 40 cases. *Muscle Nerve* 1998;**21**:55–62.

52. Weiss, M. D., Dalakas, M. C., Lauter, C. J., Willison, H. J., Quarles, R. H. Variability in the binding of anti-MAG and anti-SGPG antibodies to target antigens in demyelinating neuropathy and IgM paraproteinemia. *J. Neuroimmunol.* 1999;**95**:174–84.

53. Latov, N., Hays, A. P., Sherman, W. H. Peripheral neuropathy and anti-MAG antibodies. *Crit. Rev. Neurobiol.* 1988;**3**:301–32.

54. Dalakas, M. C., Quarles, R. H. Autoimmune ataxic neuropathies (sensory ganglionopathies): are glycolipids the responsible autoantigens? *Ann. Neurol.* 1996;**39**:419–22.

55. Eurelings, M., Ang, C. W., Notermans, N. C. *et al.* Antiganglioside antibodies in polyneuropathy associated with monoclonal gammopathy. *Neurology* 2001;**57**:1909–12.

56. Ilyas, A. A., Quarles, R. H., Dalakas, M. C., Fishman, P. H., Brady, R. O. Monoclonal IgM in a patient with paraproteinemic polyneuropathy binds to gangliosides containing disialosyl groups. *Ann. Neurol.* 1985;**18**:655–9.

57. Willison, H. J., O'Leary, C. P., Veitch, J. *et al.* The clinical and laboratory features of chronic sensory ataxic neuropathy with anti-disialosyl IgM antibodies. *Brain* 2001;**124**:1968–77.

58. Lopate, G., Choksi, R., Pestronk, A. Severe sensory ataxia and demyelinating polyneuropathy with IgM anti-GM2 and GalNAc-GD1A antibodies. *Muscle Nerve* 2002;**25**:828–36.

59. Jacobs, B. C., O'Hanlon, G. M., Breedland, E. G. *et al.* Human IgM paraproteins demonstrate shared reactivity between Campylobacter jejuni lipopolysaccharides and human peripheral nerve disialylated gangliosides. *J. Neuroimmunol.* 1997;**80**:23–30.

60. Nobile-Orazio, E., Manfredini, E., Carpo, M. *et al.* Frequency and clinical correlates of antineural IgM antibodies in neuropathy associated with IgM monoclonal gammopathy. *Ann. Neurol.* 1994;**36**:416–24.

61. Gordon, P. H., Rowland, L. P., Younger, D. S. *et al.* Lymphoproliferative disorders and motor neuron disease:an update. *Neurology* 1997;**48**: 1671–8.

62. Pavord, S. R., Murphy, P. T., Mitchell, V. E. POEMS syndrome and Waldenström's macroglobulinaemia. *J. Clin. Pathol.* 1996;**49**:181–2.

63. Crisp, D., Pruzanski, W. B-cell neoplasms with homogeneous cold-reacting antibodies (cold agglutinins). *Am. J. Med.* 1982;**72**:915–22.

64. Pruzanski, W., Shumak, K. H. Biologic activity of cold-reacting autoantibodies (first of two parts). *N. Engl. J. Med.* 1977;**297**:538–42.

65. Pruzanski, W., Shumak, K. H. Biologic activity of cold-reacting autoantibodies (second of two parts). *N. Engl. J. Med.* 1977;**297**:583–9.

66. Whittaker, S. J., Bhogal, B. S., Black, M. M. Acquired immunobullous disease:a cutaneous manifestation of IgM macroglobulinaemia. *Br. J. Dermatol.* 1996;**135**:283–6.

67. Daoud, M. S., Lust, J. A., Kyle, R. A., Pittelkow, M. R. Monoclonal gammopathies and associated skin disorders. *J. Am. Acad. Dermatol.* 1999;**40**:507–35.

68. Gad, A., Willen, R., Carlen, B., Gyland, F., Wickander, M. Duodenal involvement in Waldenström's macroglobulinemia. *J. Clin. Gastroenterol.* 1995;**20**:174–6.

69. Case records of the Massachusetts General Hospital. Weekly clinicopathological exercises. Case 3–1990. A 66-year-old woman with Waldenström's macroglobulinemia, diarrhea, anemia, and persistent gastrointestinal bleeding. *N. Engl. J. Med.* 1990;**322**:183–92.

70. Isaac, J., Herrera, G. A. Cast nephropathy in a case of Waldenström's macroglobulinemia. *Nephron* 2002;**91**:512–15.

71. Morel-Maroger, L., Basch, A., Danon, F., Verroust, P., Richet, G. Pathology of the kidney in Waldenström's macroglobulinemia. Study of sixteen cases. *N. Engl. J. Med.* 1970;**283**:123–9.

72. Gertz, M. A., Kyle, R. A., Noel, P. Primary systemic amyloidosis: a rare complication of immunoglobulin M monoclonal gammopathies and Waldenström's macroglobulinemia. *J. Clin. Oncol.* 1993;**11**:914–20.

73. Moyner, K., Sletten, K., Husby, G., Natvig, J. B. An unusually large (83 amino acid residues) amyloid fibril protein AA from a patient with Waldenström's macroglobulinaemia and amyloidosis. *Scand. J. Immunol.* 1980;**11**:549–54.

74. Gardyn, J., Schwartz, A., Gal, R. *et al.* Waldenström's

macroglobulinemia associated with AA amyloidosis. *Int. J. Hematol.* 2001;**74**:76–8.

75. Dussol, B., Kaplanski, G., Daniel, L. *et al.* Simultaneous occurrence of fibrillary glomerulopathy and AL amyloid. *Nephrol. Dial. Transplant* 1998;**13**:2630–2.

76. Rausch, P. G., Herion, J. C. Pulmonary manifestations of Waldenström macroglobulinemia. *Am. J. Hematol.* 1980;**9**:201–9.

77. Fadil, A., Taylor, D. E. The lung and Waldenström's macroglobulinemia. *South Med. J.* 1998;**91**:681–5.

78. Kyrtsonis, M. C., Angelopoulou, M. K., Kontopidou, F. N. *et al.* Primary lung involvement in Waldenström's macroglobulinaemia:report of two cases and review of the literature. *Acta Haematol.* 2001;**105**:92–6.

79. Kaila, V. L., el Newihi, H. M., Dreiling, B. J., Lynch, C. A., Mihas, A. A. Waldenström's macroglobulinemia of the stomach presenting with upper gastrointestinal hemorrhage. *Gastrointest. Endosc.* 1996;**44**:73–5.

80. Yasui, O., Tukamoto, F., Sasaki, N. *et al.* Malignant lymphoma of the transverse colon associated with macroglobulinemia. *Am. J. Gastroenterol.* 1997;**92**:2299–301.

81. Rosenthal, J. A., Curran, W. J., Jr, Schuster, S. J. Waldenström's macroglobulinemia resulting from localized gastric lymphoplasmacytoid lymphoma. *Am. J. Hematol.* 1998;**58**:244–5.

82. Recine, M. A., Perez, M. T., Cabello-Inchausti, B., Lilenbaum, R. C., Robinson, M. J. Extranodal lymphoplasmacytoid lymphoma (immunocytoma) presenting as small intestinal obstruction. *Arch. Pathol. Lab. Med.* 2001;**125**:677–9.

83. Veltman, G. A., van Veen, S., Kluin-Nelemans, J. C., Bruijn, J. A., van Es, L. A. Renal disease in Waldenström's macroglobulinaemia. *Nephrol. Dial. Transplant* 1997;**12**:1256–9.

84. Moore, D. F., Jr, Moulopoulos, L. A., Dimopoulos, M. A. Waldenström macroglobulinemia presenting as a renal or perirenal mass:clinical and radiographic features. *Leuk. Lymphoma* 1995;**17**:331–4.

85. Mascaro, J. M., Montserrat, E., Estrach, T. *et al.* Specific cutaneous manifestations of Waldenström's macroglobulinaemia. A report of two cases. *Br. J. Dermatol.* 1982;**106**:17–22.

86. Schnitzler, L., Schubert, B., Boasson, M., Gardais, J., Tourmen, A. Urticaire chronique, lésions osseuses, macroglobulinémie IgM:Maladie de Waldenström? *Bull. Soc. Fr. Dermatol. Syphiligr.* 1974;**81**: 363–8.

87. Roux, S., Fermand, J. P., Brechignac, S. *et al.* Tumoral joint involvement in multiple myeloma and Waldenström's macroglobulinemia – report of 4 cases. *J. Rheumatol.* 1996;**23**:2175–8.

88. Orellana, J., Friedman A. H. Ocular manifestations of multiple myeloma, Waldenström's macroglobulinemia and benign monoclonal gammopathy. *Surv. Ophthalmol.* 1981;**26**:157–69.

89. Ettl, A. R., Birbamer, G. G., Philipp, W. Orbital involvement in Waldenström's macroglobulinemia:ultrasound, computed tomography and magnetic resonance findings. *Ophthalmologica* 1992;**205**:40–5.

90. Civit, T., Coulbois, S., Baylac, F., Taillandier, L., Auque, J. [Waldenström's macroglobulinemia and cerebral lymphoplasmocytic proliferation: Bing and Neel syndrome. Apropos of a new case.] *Neurochirurgie* 1997;**43**:245–9.

91. McMullin, M. F., Wilkin, H. J., Elder, E. Inaccurate haemoglobin estimation in Waldenström's macroglobulinaemia. *J. Clin. Pathol.* 1995;**48**:787.

92. Treon, S. P., Branagan, A. R., Hunter, Z. *et al.* IgA and IgG hypogammaglobulinemia persists in most patients with Waldenstrom's macroglobulinemia despite therapeutic responses, including complete remissions. *Blood* 2004;**104**:306b.

93. Treon, S. P., Hunter, Z., Ciccarelli, B. T. *et al.* IgA and IgG Hypogammaglobulinemia is a constitutive feature in most Waldenstrom's Macroglobulinemia patients and may be related to mutations associated with common variable immunodeficiency disorder (CVID). *Blood* 2008;**112**:3749.

94. Dutcher, T. F., Fahey, J. L. The histopathology of macroglobulinemia of Waldenström. *J. Natl Cancer Inst.* 1959;**22**:887–917.

95. Moulopoulos, L. A., Dimopoulos, M. A., Varma, D. G. *et al.* Waldenström macroglobulinemia: MR imaging of the spine and CT of the abdomen and pelvis. *Radiology* 1993;**188**:669–73.

96. Gobbi, P. G., Bettini, R., Montecucco, C. *et al.* Study of prognosis in Waldenström's macroglobulinemia:a proposal for a simple binary classification with clinical and investigational utility. *Blood* 1994;**83**:2939–45.

97. Morel, P., Monconduit, M., Jacomy, D. *et al.* Prognostic factors in Waldenström macroglobulinemia:a report on 232 patients with the description of a new scoring system and its validation on 253 other patients. *Blood* 2000;**96**:852–8.

98. Dhodapkar, M. V., Jacobson, J. L., Gertz, M. A. *et al.* Prognostic factors and response to fludarabine therapy in patients

with Waldenström macroglobulinemia:results of United States intergroup trial (Southwest Oncology Group S9003). *Blood* 2001; **98**:41–8.

99. Kyle, R. A., Treon, S. P., Alexanian, R. *et al.* Prognostic markers and criteria to initiate therapy in Waldenström's macroglobulinemia: Consensus Panel Recommendations from the Second International Workshop on Waldenström's macroglobulinemia. *Semin. Oncol.* 2003;**30**:116–20.

100. Dimopoulos, M., Gika, D., Zervas, K. *et al.* The international staging system for multiple myeloma is applicable in symptomatic Waldenstrom's macroglobulinemia. *Leuk. Lymph.* 2004;**45**:1809–13.

101. Anagnostopoulos, A., Zervas, K., Kyrtsonis, M. *et al.* Prognostic value of serum beta 2-microglobulin in patients with Waldenstrom's macroglobulinemia requiring therapy. *Clin. Lymph. Myeloma* 2006;**7**:205–9.

102. Morel, P., Duhamel, A., Gobbi, P. *et al.* International prognostic scoring system for Waldenstrom Macroglobulinemia. *Blood* 2009;**113**:4163–70.

103. Treon, S. P. How I treat Waldenstrom's macroglobulinemia. *Blood* 2009;**114**:419–31.

104. Dimopoulos, M. A., Gertz, M. A., Kastritis, E. *et al.* Update on treatment recommendations from the Fourth International Workshop on Waldenström's Macroglobulinemia. *J. Clin. Oncol.* 2009;**27**:120–6.

105. Leleu, X. P., Manning, R., Soumerai, J. D. *et al.* Increased incidence of transformation and myelodysplasia/acute leukemia in patients with Waldenström macroglobulinemia treated with nucleoside analogs. *J. Clin. Oncol.* 2009;**27**:250–5.

106. Kyle, R. A., Greipp, P. R., Gertz, M. A. *et al.* Waldenström's macroglobulinaemia:a prospective study comparing daily with intermittent oral chlorambucil. *Br. J. Haematol.* 2000;**108**:737–42.

107. Dimopoulos, M. A., Alexanian, R. Waldenström's macroglobulinemia. *Blood* 1994;**83**:1452–9.

108. Petrucci, M. T., Avvisati, G., Tribalto, M., Giovangrossi, P., Mandelli, F. Waldenström's macroglobulinaemia:results of a combined oral treatment in 34 newly diagnosed patients. *J. Intern. Med.* 1989;**226**:443–7.

109. Case, D. C., Jr, Ervin, T. J., Boyd, M. A., Redfield, D. L. Waldenström's macroglobulinemia: long-term results with the M-2 protocol. *Cancer Invest.* 1991;**9**:1–7.

110. Facon, T., Brouillard, M., Duhamel, A. *et al.* Prognostic factors in Waldenström's macroglobulinemia: a report of 167 cases. *J. Clin. Oncol.* 1993;**11**:1553–8.

111. Dimopoulos, M. A., Kantarjian, H., Weber, D. *et al.* Primary therapy of Waldenström's macroglobulinemia with 2-chlorodeoxyadenosine. *J. Clin. Oncol.* 1994;**12**:2694–8.

112. Delannoy, A., Ferrant, A., Martiat, P. *et al.* 2-Chlorodeoxyadenosine therapy in Waldenström's macroglobulinaemia. *Nouv. Rev. Fr. Hematol.* 1994;**36**:317–20.

113. Fridrik, M. A., Jager, G., Baldinger, C. *et al.* First-line treatment of Waldenström's disease with cladribine. Arbeitsgemeinschaft Medikamentose Tumortherapie. *Ann. Hematol.* 1997;**74**:7–10.

114. Liu, E. S., Burian, C., Miller, W. E., Saven, A. Bolus administration of cladribine in the treatment of Waldenström macroglobulinaemia. *Br. J. Haematol.* 1998;**103**:690–5.

115. Hellmann, A., Lewandowski, K., Zaucha, J. M. *et al.* Effect of a 2-hour infusion of 2-chlorodeoxyadenosine in the treatment of refractory or previously untreated Waldenström's macroglobulinemia. *Eur. J. Haematol.* 1999;**63**:35–41.

116. Betticher, D. C., Hsu Schmitz, S. F., Ratschiller, D. *et al.* Cladribine (2-CDA) given as subcutaneous bolus injections is active in pretreated Waldenström's macroglobulinaemia. Swiss Group for Clinical Cancer Research (SAKK). *Br. J. Haematol.* 1997;**99**:358–63.

117. Dimopoulos, M. A., Weber, D., Delasalle, K. B., Keating, M., Alexanian, R. Treatment of Waldenström's macroglobulinemia resistant to standard therapy with 2-chlorodeoxyadenosine: identification of prognostic factors. *Ann. Oncol.* 1995;**6**:49–52.

118. Dimopoulos, M. A., O'Brien, S., Kantarjian, H. *et al.* Fludarabine therapy in Waldenström's macroglobulinemia. *Am. J. Med.* 1993;**95**:49–52.

119. Foran, J. M., Rohatiner, A. Z., Coiffier, B. *et al.* Multicenter phase II study of fludarabine phosphate for patients with newly diagnosed lymphoplasmacytoid lymphoma, Waldenström's macroglobulinemia, and mantle-cell lymphoma. *J. Clin. Oncol.* 1999;**17**:546–53.

120. Thalhammer-Scherrer, R., Geissler, K., Schwarzinger, I. *et al.* Fludarabine therapy in Waldenström's macroglobulinemia. *Ann. Hematol.* 2000;**79**:556–9.

121. Dhodapkar, M. V., Jacobson, J. L., Gertz, M. A. *et al.* Prognostic factors and response to fludarabine therapy in patients with Waldenström macroglobulinemia:results of

United States intergroup trial (Southwest Oncology Group S9003). *Blood* 2001;**98**:41–8.

122. Zinzani, P. L., Gherlinzoni, F., Bendandi, M. *et al.* Fludarabine treatment in resistant Waldenström's macroglobulinemia. *Eur. J. Haematol.* 1995;**54**:120–3.

123. Leblond, V., Ben Othman, T., Deconinck, E. *et al.* Activity of fludarabine in previously treated Waldenström's macroglobulinemia: a report of 71 cases. Groupe Cooperatif Macroglobulinemie. *J. Clin. Oncol.* 1998;**16**:2060–4.

124. Dimopoulos, M. A., Weber, D. M., Kantarjian, H., Keating, M., Alexanian, R. 2-Chlorodeoxyadenosine therapy of patients with Waldenström macroglobulinemia previously treated with fludarabine. *Ann. Oncol.* 1994;**5**:288–9.

125. Lewandowski, K., Halaburda, K., Hellmann, A. Fludarabine therapy in Waldenström's macroglobulinemia patients treated previously with 2-chlorodeoxyadenosine. *Leuk. Lymphoma* 2002;**43**:361–3.

126. Leleu, X., Tamburini, J., Roccaro, A. *et al.* Balancing risk versus benefit in the treatment of Waldenstrom's macroglobulinemia patients with nucleoside analogue based therapy. *Clin. Lymph. Myeloma* 2009; **9**(1): 71–3.

127. Thomas, S., Hosing, C., Delasalle, K. B. *et al.* Success rates of autologous stem cell collection in patients with Waldenstrom's macroglobulinemia. *Proc. 5th International Workshop on Waldenstrom's Macroglobulinemia* 2008 (Supplemental Abstract).

128. Treon, S. P., Kelliher, A., Keele, B. *et al.* Expression of serotherapy target antigens in Waldenstrom's macroglobulinemia:Therapeutic applications and considerations. *Semin. Oncol.* 2003;**30**:248–52.

129. Treon, S. P., Shima, Y., Preffer, F. I. *et al.* Treatment of plasma cell dyscrasias with antibody-mediated immunotherapy. *Semin. Oncol.* 1999;**26** (Suppl 14): 97–106.

130. Byrd, J. C., White, C. A., Link, B. *et al.* Rituximab therapy in Waldenstrom's macroglobulinemia:preliminary evidence of clinical activity. *Ann. Oncol.* 1999;**10**:1525–7.

131. Weber, D. M., Gavino, M., Huh, Y. *et al.* Phenotypic and clinical evidence supports rituximab for Waldenstrom's macroglobulinemia. *Blood* 1999;**94**:125a.

132. Foran, J. M., Rohatiner, A. Z., Cunningham, D. *et al.* European phase II study of rituximab (chimeric anti-CD20 monoclonal antibody) for patients with newly diagnosed mantle-cell lymphoma and previously treated mantle-cell lymphoma, immunocytoma, and small B-cell lymphocytic lymphoma. *J. Clin. Oncol.* 2000;**18**:317–24.

133. Treon, S. P., Agus, D. B., Link, B. *et al.* CD20-Directed antibody-mediated immunotherapy induces responses and facilitates hematologic recovery in patients with Waldenstrom's macroglobulinemia. *J. Immunother.* 2001;**24**:272–9.

134. Gertz, M. A., Rue, M., Blood, E. *et al.* Multicenter phase 2 trial of rituximab for Waldenstrom macroglobulinemia (WM): an Eastern Cooperative Oncology Group Study (E3A98). *Leuk. Lymphoma* 2004;**45**:2047–55.

135. Dimopoulos, M. A., Zervas, C., Zomas, A. *et al.* Treatment of Waldenstrom's macroglobulinemia with rituximab. *J. Clin. Oncol.* 2002;**20**:2327–33.

136. Treon, S. P., Emmanouilides, C., Kimby, E. *et al.* Extended rituximab therapy in Waldenström's Macroglobulinemia. *Ann. Oncol.* 2005;**16**:132–8.

137. Donnelly, G. B., Bober-Sorcinelli, K., Jacobson, R., Portlock, C. S. Abrupt IgM rise following treatment with rituximab in patients with Waldenstrom's macroglobulinemia. *Blood* 2001;**98**:240b.

138. Treon, S. P., Branagan, A. R., Anderson, K. C. Paradoxical increases in serum IgM levels and serum viscosity following rituximab therapy in patients with Waldenstrom's macroglobulinemia. *Blood* 2003;**102**:690a.

139. Ghobrial, I. M., Fonseca, R., Greipp, P. R. *et al.* The initial "flare" of IgM level after rituximab therapy in patients diagnosed with Waldenstrom Macroglobulinemia:An Eastern Cooperative Oncology Group Study. *Blood* 2003; **102**:448α.

140. Yang, G., Xu, L., Hunter, Z. R. *et al.* The Rituximab and IVIG Related IgM Flare In Waldenstrom's Macroglobulinemia Is Associated with Monocytic Activation of FCGR2A Signaling, and Triggering of IL-6 Release by the PI3K/AKT and MAPK Pathways. *Proc. Am. Blood* 2010;**116**:2870.

141. Dimopoulos, M. A., Anagnostopoulos, A., Zervas, C. *et al.* Predictive factors for response to rituximab in Waldenstrom's macroglobulinemia. *Clin. Lymphoma* 2005;**5**:270–2.

142. Treon, S. P., Hansen, M., Branagan, A. R. *et al.* Polymorphisms in FcγRIIIA (CD16) receptor expression are associated with clinical responses to Rituximab in Waldenstrom's Macroglobulinemia. *J. Clin. Oncol.* 2005;**23**:474–81.

143. Treon, S. P., Yang, G., Hanzis, C. *et al.* Attainment of complete/very

good partial response following rituximab-based therapy is an important determinant to progression-free survival, and is impacted by polymorphisms in FCGR3A in Waldenstrom macroglobulinaemia. *Br. J. Haematol.* 2011; May 12 [Epub ahead of print].

144. Furman, R. R., Eradat, H., Switzky, J. C. *et al.* A phase II trial of ofatumumab in subjects with Waldenstrom's Macroglobulinemia. *Blood* 2010; **116**:Abstract 1795.

145. Treon, S. P., Hanzis, C., Tripsas, C. *et al.* Bendamustine therapy in patients with relapsed or refractory Waldenström's Macroglobulinemia. *Clin. Lymphoma Myeloma Leuk.* 2011;**11**:133–5.

146. Treon, S. P., Soumerai, J. D., Hunter, Z. R. *et al.* Long-term follow-up of symptomatic patients with lymphoplasmacytic lymphoma/Waldenstrom's macroglobulinemia treated with the anti-CD52 monoclonal antibody alemtuzumab. *Blood* 2011; May 12 [Epub ahead of print].

147. Owen, R. G., Rawstron, A. C., Osterborg, A. *et al.* Activity of alemtuzumab in relapsed/ refractory Waldenstrom's macroglobulinemia. *Blood* 2003;**102**:644a.

148. Treon, S. P., Hunter, Z. R., Matous, J., *et al.* Multicenter clinical trial of bortezomib in relapsed/refractory Waldenstrom's macroglobulinemia: results of WMCTG trial 03–248. *Clin. Cancer Res.* 2007;**13**: 3320–5.

149. Chen, C. I., Kouroukis, C. T., White, D. *et al.* Bortezomib is active in patients with untreated or relapsed Waldenstrom's macroglobulinemia: a phase II study of the National Cancer Institute of Canada Clinical Trials

Group. *J. Clin. Oncol.* 2007;**25**:1570–5.

150. Dimopoulos, M. A., Anagnostopoulos, A., Kyrtsonis, M. C. *et al.* Treatment of relapsed or refractory Waldenstrom's macroglobulinemia with bortezomib. *Haematologica* 2005;**90**:1655–7.

151. Goy, A., Younes, A., McLaughlin, P. *et al.* Phase II study of proteasome inhibitor bortezomib in relapsed or refractory B-cell non-Hodgkin's lymphoma. *J. Clin.* 2005;**23**:657–8.

152. Dimopoulos, M. A., Zomas, A., Viniou, N. A. *et al.* Treatment of Waldenström's macroglobulinemia with thalidomide. *J. Clin. Oncol.* 2001;**19**:3596–601.

153. Coleman, C., Leonard, J., Lyons, L., Szelenyi, H., Niesvizky, R. Treatment of Waldenström's macroglobulinemia with clarithromycin, low-dose thalidomide and dexamethasone. *Semin. Oncol.* 2003;**30**:270–4.

154. Dimopoulos, M. A., Zomas, K., Tsatalas, K. *et al.* Treatment of Waldenström's macroglobulinemia with single agent thalidomide or with combination of clarithromycin, thalidomide and dexamethasone. *Semin. Oncol.* 2003;**30**:265–9.

155. Cheson, B. D., Rummel, M. J. Bendamustine: rebirth of an old drug. *J. Clin. Oncol.* 2009;**27**:1492–501.

156. Hatjiharissi, E., Mitsiades, C. S., Ciccarelli, B. *et al.* Comprehensive molecular characterization of malignant and microenvironmental cells in Waldenstrom's Macroglobulinemia by gene expression profiling. *Blood* 2007;**110**:abstract 3174.

157. Leleu, X., Jia, X., Runnels, J. *et al.* The Akt pathway regulates survival and homing in Waldenstrom

macroglobulinemia. *Blood* 2007;**110**:4417–26.

158. Ghobrial, I., Gertz, M., LaPlant, B. *et al.* Phase II trial of the oral mammalian target of rapamycin inhibitor everolimus in relapsed or refractory Waldenström macroglobulinemia. *J. Clin. Oncol.* 2010;**28**:1408–14.

159. Buske, C., Hoster, E., Dreyling, M. H. *et al.* The addition of rituximab to front-line therapy with CHOP (R-CHOP) results in a higher response rate and longer time to treatment failure in patients with lymphoplasmacytic lymphoma:results of a randomized trial of the German Low-Grade Lymphoma Study Group (GLSG). *Leukemia* 2009;**23**:153–61.

160. Dimopoulos, M. A., Anagnostopoulos, A., Kyrtsonis, M. C. *et al.* Primary treatment of Waldenstrom's macroglobulinemia with dexamethasone, rituximab and cyclophosphamide. *J. Clin. Oncol.* 2007;**25**:3344–9.

161. Treon, S. P., Hunter, Z., Branagan, A. CHOP plus rituximab therapy in Waldenström's macroglobulinemia. *Clin. Lymphoma Myeloma* 2005;**5**: 273–7.

162. Ioakimidis, L., Patterson, C. J., Hunter, Z. R. *et al.* Comparative outcomes following CP-R, CVP-R and CHOP-R in Waldenstrom's Macroglobulinemia. *Clin. Lymphoma Myeloma* 2009;**9**:62–6.

163. Weber, D. M., Dimopoulos, M. A., Delasalle, K. *et al.* 2-chlorodeoxyadenosine alone and in combination for previously untreated Waldenstrom's macroglobulinemia. *Semin. Oncol.* 2003;**30**:243–7.

164. Laszlo, D., Andreola, G., Rigacci, L. *et al.* Rituximab and subcutaneous 2-chloro-2'-deoxyadenosine combination treatment for patients with Waldenstrom

macroglobulinemia:clinical and biologic results of a phase II multicenter study. *J. Clin. Oncol.* 2010;**28**:2233–8.

165. Treon, S. P., Branagan, A. R., Ioakimidis, L. *et al.* Long term outcomes to fludarabine and rituximab in Waldenstrom's macroglobulinemia. *Blood* 2009 [Epub ahead of print].

166. Tam, C. S., Wolf, M. M., Westerman, D. *et al.* Fludarabine combination therapy is highly effective in first-line and salvage treatment of patients with Waldenstrom's macroglobulinemia. *Clin. Lymphoma Myeloma* 2005;**6**: 136–9.

167. Hensel, M., Villalobos, M., Kornacker, M. *et al.* Pentostatin/ cyclophosphamide with or without rituximab:an effective regimen for patients with Waldenstrom's macroglobulinemia/ lymphoplasmacytic lymphoma. *Clin. Lymphoma Myeloma* 2005;**6**:131–5.

168. Dimopoulos, M. A., Hamilos, G., Efstathiou, E. *et al.* Treatment of Waldenstrom's macroglobulinemia with the combination of fludarabine and cyclophosphamide. *Leuk. Lymphoma* 2003;**44**: 993–6.

169. Tamburini, J., Levy, V., Chateilex, C. *et al.* Fludarabine plus cyclophosphamide in Waldenstrom's macroglobulinemia: results in 49 patients. *Leukemia* 2005; **19**:1831–4.

170. Tedeschi, A., Benevolo, G., Varettoni, M. *et al.* Results of a phase II multicenter study of immunochemotherapy with fludarabine, cyclophosphamide and rituximab (FCR) for symptomatic Waldenstrom's Macroglobulinemia. *Blood* 2008;**112**: abstract 3692.

171. Treon, S. P., Ioakimidis, L., Soumerai, J. D. *et al.* Primary therapy of Waldenstrom's Macroglobulinemia with bortezomib, dexamethasone and rituximab: results of WMCTG clinical trial 05–180. *J. Clin. Oncol.* 2009;**27**:3830–5.

172. Ghobrial, I. M., Xie, W., Padmanabhan, S. *et al.* Phase II trial of weekly bortezomib in combination with rituximab in untreated patients with Waldenström Macroglobulinemia. *Am. J. Hematol.* 2010;**85**:670–4.

173. Agathocleous, A., Rule, S., Johson, P. Preliminary results of a phase I/II study of weekly or twice weekly bortezomib in combination with rituximab in patients with follicular lymphoma, mantle cell lymphoma, and Waldenstrom's macroglobulinemia. *Blood* 2007;**110**:abstract 2559.

174. Dimopoulos, M. A., García-Sanz, R., Gavriatopoulou, M. *et al.* Primary therapy of Waldenstrom's Macroglobulinemia (WM) with weekly bortezomib, low-dose dexamethasone and rituximab (BDR): a phase II study of the European Myeloma Network. *Blood* 2010;**116**: abstract 1941.

175. Treon, S. P., Soumerai, J. D., Branagan, A. R. *et al.* Thalidomide and rituximab in Waldenstrom's Macroglobulinemia. *Blood* 2008;**112**:4452–7.

176. Treon, S. P., Soumerai, J. D., Branagan, A. R. *et al.* Lenalidomide and rituximab in Waldenstrom's Macroglobulinemia. *Clin. Cancer Res.* 2008;**15**:355–60.

177. Rummel, M. J., von Gruenhagen, U., Niederle, N. *et al.* Bendamustine plus rituximab versus CHOP plus rituximab in the firstline treatment of patients with follicular, indolent and mantle cell lymphomas: results of a randomized phase III study of the Study Group Indolent Lymphomas (StiL). *Blood* 2008;**112**:abstract 2596.

178. Treon, S. P., Hanzis, C., Manning, R. J. *et al.* Maintenance rituximab is associated with improved clinical outcome in rituximab naïve patients with Waldenstrom's Macroglobulinemia who respond to a rituximab containing regimen. *Br. J. Haematol.* 2011, May [Epub ahead of print].

179. Desikan, R., Dhodapkar, M., Siegel, D. *et al.* High-dose therapy with autologous haemopoietic stem cell support for Waldenström's macroglobulinaemia. *Br. J. Haematol.* 1999;**105**:993–6.

180. Munshi, N. C., Barlogie, B. Role for high dose therapy with autologous hematopoietic stem cell support in Waldenström's macroglobulinemia. *Semin. Oncol.* 2003;**30**:282–5.

181. Dreger, P., Glass, B., Kuse, R. *et al.* Myeloablative radiochemotherapy followed by reinfusion of purged autologous stem cells for Waldenström's macroglobulinaemia. *Br. J. Haematol.* 1999;**106**:115–18.

182. Anagnostopoulos, A., Dimopoulos, M. A., Aleman, A. *et al.* High-dose chemotherapy followed by stem cell transplantation in patients with resistant Waldenström's macroglobulinemia. *Bone Marrow Transplant* 2001;**27**:1027–9.

183. Tournilhac, O., Leblond, V., Tabrizi, R. *et al.* Transplantation in Waldenström's macroglobulinemia – the french experience. *Semin. Oncol.* 2003;**30**:291–6.

184. Anagnostopoulos, A., Hari, P. N., Perez, W. S. *et al.* Autologous or allogeneic stem cell transplantation in patients with Waldenstrom's macroglobulinemia. *Biol. Blood Marrow Transplant* 2006;**12**: 845–54.

185. Kyriakou, C., Canals, C., Sibon, D. et al. High-dose therapy and autologous stem-cell transplantation in Waldenstrom macroglobulinemia: the Lymphoma Working Party of the European Group for Blood and Marrow Transplantation. *J. Clin. Oncol.* 2010;**28**:2227–32.

186. Kyriakou, C., Canals, C., Cornelissen, J. J. et al. Allogeneic stem-cell transplantation in patients with Waldenström macroglobulinemia: report from the Lymphoma Working Party of the European Group for Blood and Marrow Transplantation. *J. Clin. Oncol.* 2010;**28**:4926–34.

187. Weber, D., Treon, S. P., Emmanouilides, C. et al. Uniform response criteria in Waldenstrom's macroglobulinemia: consensus panel recommendations from the Second International Workshop on Waldenstrom's Macroglobulinemia. *Semin. Oncol.* 2003;**30**:127–31.

188. Kimby, E., Treon, S. P., Anagnostopoulos, A. et al. Update on recommendations for assessing response from the Third International Workshop on Waldenstrom's Macroglobulinemia. *Clin. Lymph. Myeloma* 2006;**6**:380–3.

189. Treon, S. P., Merlini, G., Morra, E. et al. Report from the Sixth International Workshop on Waldenstrom's Macroglobulinemia. *Clin. Lymph. Myeloma Leukemia* 2011;**11**:69–73.

190. Nichols, G. L., Savage, D. G. Timing of rituximab/fludarabine in Waldenstrom's macroglobulinemia may avert hyperviscosity. *Blood* 2004;**104**:237b.

191. Strauss, S. J., Maharaj, L., Hoare, S. et al. Bortezomib therapy in patients with relapsed or refractory lymphoma: Potential correlation of in vitro sensitivity and tumor necrosis factor alpha response with clinical activity. *J. Clin. Oncol.* 2006;**24**:2105–12.

192. Varghese, A. M., Rawstron, A. C., Ashcroft, A. J. et al. Assessment of bone marrow response in Waldenström's macroglobulinemia. *Clin. Lymph. Myeloma* 2009;**9**:53–5.

193. Ciccarelli, B. T., Yang, G., Hatjiharissi, E. et al. Soluble CD27 is a faithful marker of disease burden and is unaffected by the rituximab induced IgM flare, as well as plasmapheresis in patients with Waldenstrom's macroglobulinemia. *Clin. Lymph. Myeloma* 2009;**9**:56–8.

Chapter

16

Castleman's disease

Karthik Ramasamy

Introduction

Castleman's disease was first described in a case report by Dr. Benjamin Castleman and Towne in 1954 [1]. Following this initial description, a case series of mediastinal lymph node hyperplasia which was subsequently coined as Castleman's disease was published [2]. Castleman's disease is a non-clonal lymphoproliferative disorder characterized by angiofollicular lymph node hyperplasia, widespread lymphadenopathy and marked constitutional symptoms in affected patients. Castleman's disease is frequently associated with both human immunodeficiency virus (HIV) and human herpes virus 8 (HHV8) infections. Castleman's disease not infrequently presents with either polyneuropathy, organomegaly, endocrinopathy, M protein and skin changes (POEMS syndrome), Hodgkin's disease, non-Hodgkin's lymphoma, or Kaposi's sarcoma. Clinical presentation can be more localized, with absence of systemic symptoms termed as unicentric presentation. Patients with multi-centric Castleman's disease present with constitutional symptoms and multiple lymph node areas or organs are involved. Although unicentric presentation is frequent and curable in most patients with surgical resection and/or radiotherapy, management of Multicentric Castleman's disease is challenging. There are two main histological subtypes described in Castleman's disease: hyaline vascular subtype and plasma cell variant. Occasionally mixed patterns can occur. In HIV positive patients, lymph nodes are ubiquitously positive for HHV8 infection. There is significant clinical heterogeneity, and the factors guiding therapy are clinical features, HIV status, performance status, localized or multi-centric presentation and in some cases the type of hematological neoplasm associated with. Castleman's disease is a rare condition and no official incidence or prevalence figures are available. The National Cancer Institute in the USA has assigned an orphan status to Castleman's disease.

Castleman's disease is characterized by enlarged lymph nodes demonstrating globally altered nodal architecture involving the germinal center, mantle zone and interfollicular areas. There are key differences in the histopathological changes observed in these regions, between the hyaline vascular subtype and plasma cell variant [3]. In this chapter we describe the pathophysiology, clinical presentation investigations, and report on treatments available for patients with both HIV positive and HIV negative patients with Castleman's disease.

Pathophysiology

Castleman's disease (CD) displays a wide variation in presenting symptoms and signs, which are determined by extent of the disease, lymph node histology, HIV status, IL6 levels, associated autoimmune phenomena and overlap with other hematological or non-hematological disorders. Diagnosis of Castleman's disease is based on clinical features and pathologic findings from lymph node biopsy. Classification of Castleman's disease has been based on clinical presentation, either unicentric disease or multi-centric disease and histopathologic subtype hyaline vascular disease or plasma cell variant. However, significant overlap of these disease features is noted with a diagnosis of a mixed pathologic type in 10%–15% of patients. Unicentric and multi-centric disease are hence part of a continuous spectrum ranging from unifocal disease involving a single lymph node region or organ, and unicentric disease defined as unifocal disease plus a group of satellites. In multi- centric disease, multiple groups of lymph nodes in different areas are involved.

Myeloma, ed. Stephen A. Schey, Kwee L. Yong, Robert Marcus and Kenneth C. Anderson. Published by Cambridge University Press. © Cambridge University Press 2014.

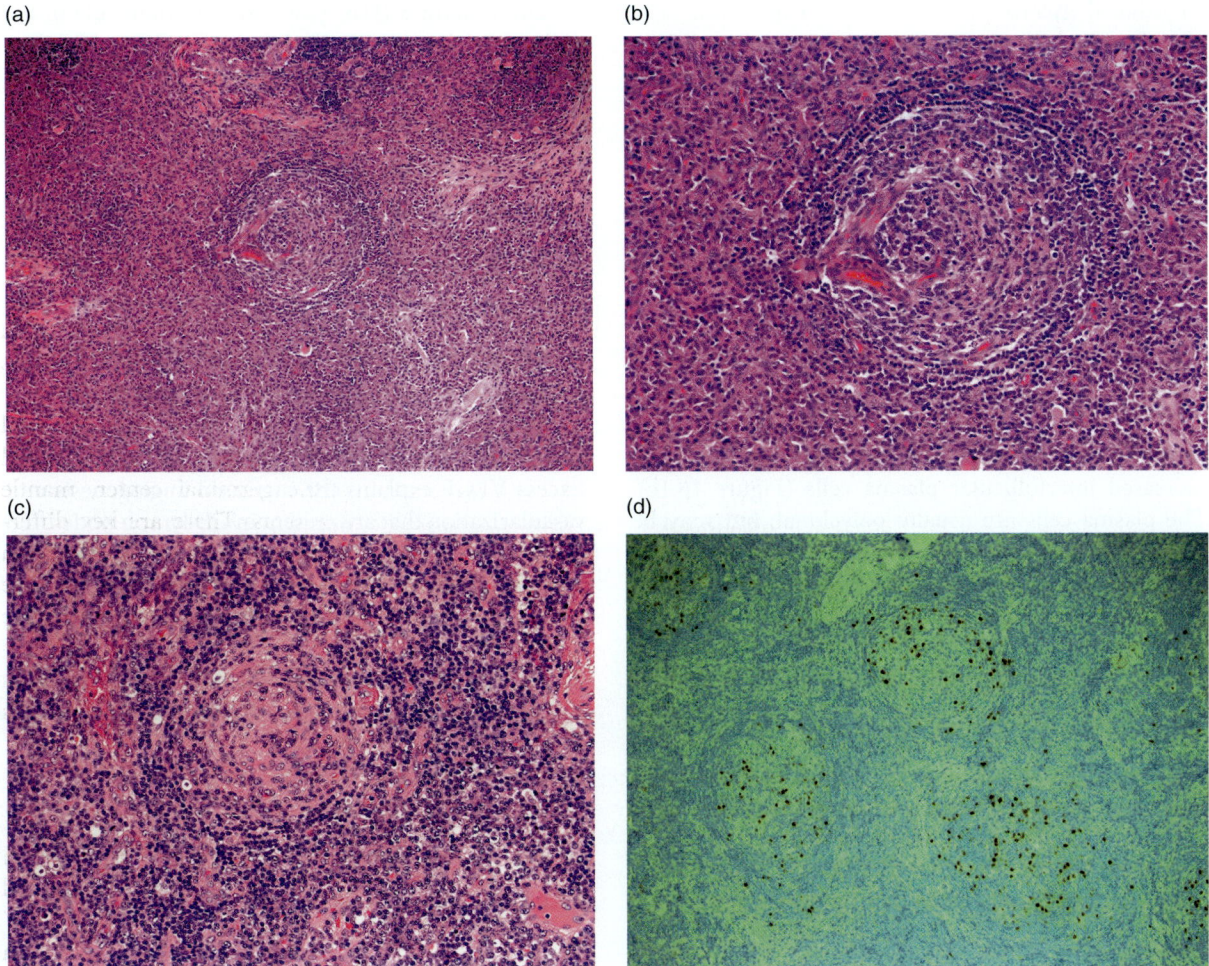

Figure 16.1 Histological changes in Castleman's disease. (a) Hyaline vascular variant of Castleman's disease. (b) Onion-skin histological pattern in Hyaline vascular variant of Castleman's disease. (c) Plasma cell variant of Castleman's disease. (d) HHV8 DNA positivity demonstrated in plasma cell variant Castleman's disease.

Pathologic diagnosis of CD requires an adequate sample and considerable expertise in morphological interpretation of lymphoproliferative disorders [3]. There is a global architectural change observed in lymph nodes excised from patients with CD. A diagnosis of Castleman's disease is reliably made only by studying the whole lymph node architecture from a surgical biopsy, and fine needle aspirates can be unhelpful and potentially misleading.

Hyaline vascular variant is characterized by lymphoid proliferation wherein the follicles are regressing with atrophic germinal centers, and have expanded mantle zones with small lymphocytes arranged concentrically in an onion-skin fashion (Figure 16.1a). The interfollicular region is variably expanded with prominent hyalinized vascular proliferation; expanded, often dysplastic follicular dendritic cell networks [4]. High endothelial venules are present in the paracortical region. Plasma cells are not abundant. The appearance of the hyalinized blood vessel penetrating the follicle together with the concentric rimming by mantle zone lymphocytes is often described as resembling a lollipop. Aggregates of plasmacytoid dendritic cells are frequently noted in the interfollicular region. There is a prominent loss or rarification of sinusoids. Interfollicular area is expanded with fibroblastic reticulum cells and mature small T lymphocytes (Figure 16.1b).

The vascular proliferation in hyaline vascular histology is believed to be driven by increased vascular

217

endothelial growth factor (VEGF) expression. The vascular thickening and hyalinization observed in CD is most likely due to a VEGF-induced increase in vascular permeability and leakage of protein-rich plasma in the subendothelium [5]. Lymphocytes are polyclonal on molecular analysis. Follicular dendritic cells (FDCs) in CD demonstrate moderate to strong expression of epidermal growth factor receptor (EGFR) [6]. Increased VEGF expression is believed to contribute to the development of vascular neoplasms in CD.

In plasma cell variant Castleman's disease, the lymph nodes in contrast show preserved architecture with hyperplastic follicles and a normal follicular dendritic cell network. The most striking feature is increased interfollicular plasma cells (Figure 16.1c). The plasma cells are usually polyclonal, but may be monotypic and usually lambda light chain restricted, especially in cases associated with osteosclerotic myeloma or POEMS syndrome. Monoclonality is rare and may herald development of a lymphoma. Notable difference between hyaline vascular disease and plasma cell variant relates to the follicular dendritic cell network. The FDC network is normal in plasma cell disease, while it is expanded or disrupted in hyaline vascular disease with multiple tight collections of follicular dendritic cells [7]. Morphological findings in hyaline vascular disease are diagnostic of Castleman's disease. However, it is difficult to differentiate the plasma cell variant from other conditions such as reactive changes in autoimmune disease, Castleman's disease-like changes associated with HIV infection, collagen vascular and mixed connective tissue disease, plasmacytic lymphoma, marginal zone lymphoma with plasmacytoid differentiation, plasmacytoma and plasmablastic lymphoma. Exclusion of these reactive states is essential to make a diagnosis of plasma cell variant Castleman's disease.

Multi-centric CD can be associated with the presence of HHV8. This is considered a separate entity because of this distinct association, the presence of immunodeficiency, and certain unique histologic features. The lymph nodes in HHV8-associated CD have increased numbers of plasmablasts, present in the outer mantle zones of some follicles (Figure 16.1d). These plasmablasts are lambda-light chain restricted, uniformly express cytoplasmic IgM, and may colonize the germinal centers. They are polyclonal and have heterogeneous, weak expression of CD20[8].

Interleukin 6 (IL6) plays an important role in the pathophysiology of CD. IL6 heterodimerizes with either soluble IL6 receptor alpha (IL6Rα), or IL6 receptor bound to gp130 signaling complex at the cell surface, resulting in activation of the JAK/STAT signaling pathway [9]. IL6 also activates the mitogen activated protein kinase (MAPK) cascade. IL6 production has a triple role in Castleman's disease: it induces B-cell proliferation, mediates inflammatory clinical symptoms, and induces VEGF and angiogenesis [10]. Serum IL6 levels observed in CD is much higher than seen in other hematological malignancies such as Hodgkin's disease, NHL, rheumatoid syndromes and myeloma. Excess IL6 induces a proinflammatory syndrome that leads to constitutional symptoms, with elevation of acute phase reactants. Excess VEGF explains the increased angiogenesis and vascularization that are present in CD lymph nodes. IL6 is a potent growth and survival factor for B-lymphocytes and plasma cells. Autoimmune phenomena, such as cytopenias, are thought to arise due to IL6-induced immune dysregulation. Excess IL6 may cause immune dysregulation by impairing dendritic cell maturation and promoting a Th2 type skewed pattern. It has been suggested that IL6-induced expansion of autoantibody-producing CD5-positive B-lymphocytes may be responsible for autoimmune phenomena [11]. Autoimmune hemolytic anemia and thrombocytopenia, Evan's syndrome, pure red cell aplasia, acquired factor VIII deficiency, systemic lupus erythematosus and myasthenia gravis have all been described The key role of IL6 is exemplified by the improvement in symptoms correlating with lowered IL6 levels [10]. Also therapeutic intervention by interrupting IL6 signaling with antibodies directed either at IL6 or IL6 receptor leads to disease response in CD [12]. Human-IL6 transgenic mice develop a CD-like syndrome with plasmacytosis, splenomegaly, enlarged lymph nodes, fever, cachexia and anemia, which responds to administration of anti-IL6R monoclonal antibodies [13]. The HHV8-genome encodes a number of homologs of human cellular genes, including viral IL6 (vIL6), which induces proliferation of HHV8-infected cells. However, HHV8-infected cells secrete vIL6 at low levels [14], and vIL6 has a low affinity for the human IL6R. Human IL6 secretion, likely to be stimulated both in autocrine and/or paracrine fashion, remains the most important mediator in the pathogenesis of CD. Although host mRNA is degraded via viral shutoff exonuclease in HHV8 lytic infection, IL6 mRNA is up regulated, resulting in increased transcription and secretion of human IL6 from HHV8-infected cells [15]. Reasons underlying excess IL6 production in HIV-negative CD is poorly understood. HHV8-derived DNA, mRNA, and proteins have been detected in the peripheral blood mononuclear cells and lymph nodes of a variable percentage of HIV-negative CD patients [16]. Detection rates are dependent on the type of material and the sensitivity of the techniques used.

HHV8 was found to be causally related to Kaposi sarcoma (KS) in HIV-positive and HIV-negative patients in the mid 1990s [17]. The target of HHV8 infection in Kaposi sarcoma is vascular endothelial cells, which are subsequently transformed into the abundant spindle cells embedded in fibrovascular stroma typically containing hyalinized granules [18]. HHV8 infection is mostly latent and viral replication occurs at a low level [19]. The important role of HHV8 in the pathogenesis of Castleman's disease is well recognized [20]. HHV8 infection is ubiquitous in HIV-positive CD, and present in the majority of HIV-negative patients with multicentric disease. HHV8 infection is also associated with B cell derived primary effusion lymphomas or body-cavity-based lymphomas [19].

Kaposi sarcoma and Castleman's disease have a number of clinicopathologic features in common. These conditions are inflammatory, related to HHV8 infection, associated with hyalinizing processes, produce a fibrovascular stroma, and are often associated with HIV infection. In HIV positive patients with Castleman's disease, the lymph nodes are often also involved by Kaposi sarcoma [21], which usually affects endothelial cells [18]. It has been hypothesized that the association of Castleman's disease and Kaposi sarcoma (KS) in a single lymph node is due to lytic HHV8 infection of B-lymphoid cells. This exposes susceptible endothelial cells to extreme HHV8 viral loads resulting in the formation of KS changes in multicentric Castleman's disease-related lymph nodes. Expression of viral IL6 (vIL6) is induced by the lytic program of viral replication [22]. Lytic cycle of HHV8 in lymphovascular cells leads to destruction of these cells resulting in a hyaline scar. Production of vIL6 triggers new vessel formation with formation of penetrating vessels via basic fibroblast growth factor and VEGF [23]. This results in expansion of the lymphovascular epithelial cell reservoir of HHV8- infected cells. In addition, the chemotactic effect of human IL6 leads to cluster formation of plasmablasts around small vessels. In patients

with HHV8 positive Castleman's disease, response to therapy correlates with falling HHV8 DNA levels by PCR in peripheral blood of treated patients [24].

Clinical features and Investigations

Patients with CD have varying initial clinical presentations due to the nature of the disease localization, HIV status, associated disease and the presentation is driven by the underlying pathological subtype. It is not uncommon for patients to be diagnosed with CD from lymph node biopsy done to exclude lymphoma. But patients do present with more serious clinical features secondary to compression of neurovascular structures or other organs. This is usually observed in patients presenting with mediastinal mass or intra-abdominal mass [25]. Occasionally non lymph-node sites such as lungs, orbits, mouth, or nasopharynx are involved. Patients with unicentric disease are likely to be HIV negative and a hyaline vascular variant histology. Systemic symptoms do not dominate their presenting feature. Patients with multi-centric CD present with systemic B symptoms due to cytokine activation with fever, weight loss, night sweats, weakness and fatigue. Fluid retention in individuals with multi-centric disease may be pronounced with edema, ascites, pleural or pericardial effusions. These features are due to extensive nature of the disease and high levels of pro-inflammatory cytokine IL6 secretion. Rarely patients present with multiorgan dysfunction [26]. Investigations as listed on Table 16.1 should be performed in all patients with a suspected diagnosis of Castleman's disease.

In some patients, disease can sometimes behave more indolently, and therapy is reserved until when patients are symptomatic. Clinical features which necessitate institution of therapy are listed in Table 16.2. These clinical features have been coined as MCD attack indicating a need for therapy [28]. There is a subset of patients where disease is more aggressive and patients need urgent therapy. Some patients with CD may become systemically ill from unusual pulmonary complications, such as acute reticulonodular interstitial pneumonitis, and development of acute respiratory distress syndrome [29]. Infiltration of the skin with Kaposi's-like lesions and other non-specific skin rashes can occur. Sensory neuropathy is noted in up to 20% of patients. Proinflammatory states induce anemia and vascular permeability and a prothrombotic state. Immune

Table 16.1 Clinical investigations in patients with suspected Castleman's disease

Investigation	Details
Blood profile	Full blood count, ESR, liver profile, renal profile, bone profile
Markers of disease activity	CRP, IL6 levels, VEGF levels and HHV8 DNA PCR (in positive patients). HIV testing where status is unknown
HIV positive patients	CD4 count, HIV viral copy numbers
Biopsy	Lymph node biopsy reviewed by experienced pathologist. Exclude concomitant Kaposi sarcoma. Staining for HHV8 DNA, EBER
Staging	CT chest/abdomen/pelvis. CT/PET scan if appropriate [27]
Bone marrow examination	To exclude plasma cell dyscrasias and NHL
Other tests	Endocrine screen, serum electrophoresis with paraprotein analysis, hemolysis screen

Table 16.2 Clinical features consistent with MCD attack

Fever
At least three of the following other MCD-related symptoms:
    Peripheral lymphadenopathy
    Enlarged spleen
    Edema
    Pleural effusion
    Ascites
    Cough
    Nasal obstruction
    Xerostomia
    Rash
    Central neurologic symptoms
    Jaundice
    Autoimmune hemolytic anemia

Increased serum C-reactive protein level >20 mg/l in the absence of any other etiology

Adapted from Gerard et al. [28]

reconstitution inflammatory syndrome might explain the observation that some HIV positive patients develop CD within weeks of starting highly active antiretroviral therapy [30]. A degree of immune competence is necessary to establish the signs and symptoms of CD. This coincides with the observation that CD4 counts and HIV viral titers are inversely correlated with the development of CD.

Treatment

To date there are no randomized studies to guide the management of patients with CD but an approach based largely on whether the disease is unicentric or multicentric, the HIV status and associated co-morbidities can guide treatment. A pragmatic algorithm is provided (Figure 16.2)

Unicentric disease is managed with local therapy. It is important to determine whether the tumor is surgically resectable and the fitness of the patient. If a surgical option is feasible, this approach is preferred, as up to 95% of patients are cured and this results in resolution of symptoms and involution of satellite lymph nodes [3,25]. In patients with unresectable disease or those unfit for surgery, radiotherapy

should be considered. Local radiotherapy can lead to either a complete or partial responses with good symptom resolution [31]. Long term follow up is essential as local relapses have been reported following surgery and radiotherapy [31,32].

Multi-centric Castleman's disease in HIV negative patients

Patients with multi-centric CD are symptomatic and therapy is indicated to alleviate symptoms and improve outcome. In HIV negative patients therapy is directed to reduce HHV8 proliferation, reduce IL6 levels and debulk proliferating B cell tumor mass. Steroids delivered at high doses will improve symptoms and even induce disease response with reduction in lymph node mass. Although significant remissions with steroid therapy alone have been reported, the risk of infections is significantly high [33]. Addition of chemotherapy to steroids has been reported to induce complete remissions in this group of patients. Lymphoma-based chemotherapeutic regimens CHOP (cyclophosphamide, doxorubicin, vincristine and prednisone) or fractionated cyclophosphamide, vincristine, doxorubicin, and dexamethasone (CVAD) induces complete responses in approximately 50% of patients, but relapses occur with a median survival of 19 months [25]. Rituximab therapy with or without steroids induces responses in HIV negative CD

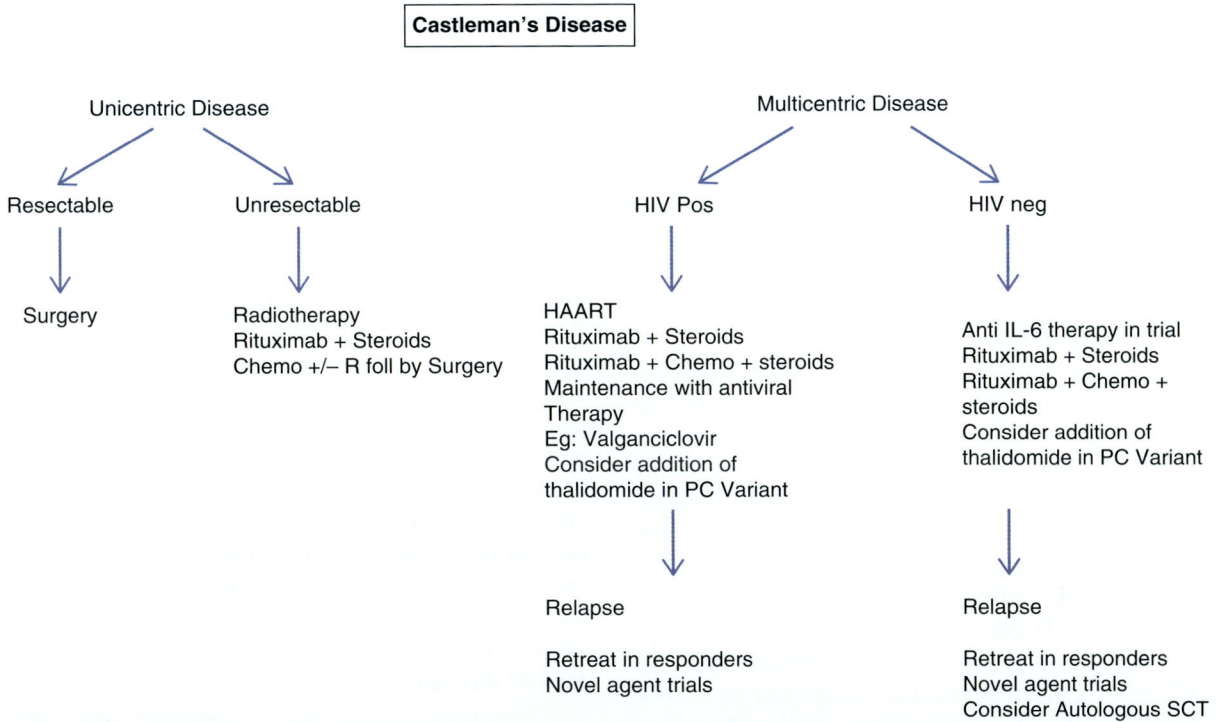

Figure 16.2 A pragmatic treatment algorithm for management of Castleman's disease.

patients with some near complete responses [34,35]. There are reports of thalidomide in combination with rituximab inducing significant responses in HIV negative CD without significant toxicity [36]. Reports of single agent activity have been demonstrated in CD with thalidomide, bortezomib [37] and alpha interferon [38] therapy. Although patients with HIV negative multicentric CD do not frequently express HHV8 DNA, antiviral therapy has been explored in this group of patients. Therapies considered include ganciclovir, valganciclovir (oral pro drug), or foscarnet. Efficacy of valganciclovir in suppressing HHV8 replication was tested in a randomized trial [39] with patients randomized to the valganciclovir arm having a significant reduction in oral HHV8 shedding in comparison to patients in the placebo arm.

IL6 levels are significantly elevated in these patients and interruption of this pathway with a biologic, without use of chemotherapy has been an active area of research over the years. The first drug to be tested (suramin, polysulfated naphthylurea) was originally developed as an anti-parasitic drug. Suramin use induced, complete remission in two patients with multi-centric CD [40]. Suramin inhibits proliferation in lymphoid cell lines by interfering with the IL6 signaling pathway. Unfortunately similar success with this drug has not been replicated. Two other agents have been tested in patients with CD. Tocilizumab is a monoclonal antibody which blocks the human IL6 receptor and blocks the crucial role of IL6 in CD progression. This drug has now been approved for use in patients with HIV negative CD in Japan [41]. In a phase II single agent study, 35 patients were treated with twice-weekly infusion of tocilizumab for 16 weeks. Rapid normalization of inflammatory markers and hemoglobin was observed with concomitant resolution of constitutional symptoms, an increase in body mass index, and reduction in lymphadenopathy [12]. Thirty patients continued to receive tocilizumab for five years, and the remissions were durable. The key issue with this agent is that continued therapy with tocilizumab is required as relapses were observed upon stopping therapy. Tocilizumab also decreases hepcidin secretion by downregulating the IL6 pathway. This results in an improvement in anemia of inflammation observed in patients with CD [42]. Siltuximab is a new anti-IL6, chimeric monoclonal antibody with potential therapeutic benefit under investigation in patients with CD. In the open label dose finding study, 18 (78%)

of 23 patients achieved clinical benefit response (CBR), and 12 patients (52%) demonstrated objective tumor response. All 11 patients treated with the highest dose of 12 mg/kg demonstrated clinical benefit, and eight patients (73%) achieved objective tumor response. Both tocilizumab and siltuximab were well tolerated with few adverse events in studies. Both agents can induce hyperlipidemia, and monitoring of cholesterol and triglycerides is recommended.

HIV positive Castleman's Disease

Treatment of patients with HIV positive CD is particularly challenging. This is partly due to a 15-fold increased risk of developing HHV8-asssociated non-Hodgkin lymphoma as compared with the general HIV positive population [43]. There is also a substantially increased frequency of Kaposi sarcoma in HIV positive CD patients [44]. Historically prognosis has been poor with probably some improvement more recently [44]. Highly active anti-retroviral therapy (HAART) does not prevent the development of CD in HIV positive patients, and it is not effective on its own in inducing remissions. In fact, exacerbations have been reported after initiation of anti-retroviral therapy, perhaps as part of an immune reconstitution syndrome [30]. A recent detailed review suggests that HAART improves CD4-positive counts, reduces viral load, and prevents progression to lymphoma and development of Kaposi sarcoma in CD patients, thus reducing the mortality rate and possibly improving overall outcome [45]. Use of chemotherapy has been explored with single agent etoposide and vinblastine [45]. Etoposide given at a single intravenous dose (120–150 mg/m2) followed by weekly oral maintenance therapy (100–120 mg/m2) provides good disease control [46]. More recently rituximab therapy as a single agent has been investigated in multiple studies. Rituximab monotherapy achieves high response rates in HIV positive patients with CD. A phase 2 trial using rituximab in 21 patients achieved two-year overall survival and disease free survival rates of 95% and 79%, respectively [47]. In the prospective open label ANRS117

Castleman's trial, rituximab as monotherapy was investigated in 24 chemotherapy-dependent patients [28]. Sustained remission was observed in more than 90% of patients at two months and the overall survival rate was 92%, and patients tolerated rituximab well. However, there were reports of rituximab induced exacerbations of Kaposi sarcoma and rituximab monotherapy may not be optimal due to early disease progression [48]. Ideal therapy for HIV positive CD patients is a combinatorial approach. Owing to early deaths observed in patients with rituximab monotherapy, use of chemotherapy should be considered in the acute setting. Combination of chemotherapy, rituximab and HAART could potentially improve response rates and salvage patients with high disease burden. This could be followed by a maintenance approach with either antiviral therapy +/− rituximab to reduce risk or relapse or disease progression. As thalidomide induces additional responses in patients with plasmacytic variant CD [36], maintenance thalidomide remains a reasonable option for this group of patients who can tolerate this therapy.

Conclusion

Considerable progress has been made in the understanding of Castleman's disease over the last couple of decades. Expert multidisciplinary input is required at diagnosis to understand the biology and stage of the disease. Distinct clinical categories of unicentric and multi-centric disease are recognized with a goal of cure for patients with unicentric disease. Survival in patients with HIV positive Castleman's disease has improved with addition of rituximab therapy and further clinical studies are underway to further improve the outcome in this group with a combinatorial approach with chemoimmunotherapy and antiviral approach. Use of anti-IL6 therapies has been exciting in patients with HIV negative CD. This has paved a way of treating CD with a non-chemotherapeutic approach and therefore limiting toxicity. Drugs currently used in management of myeloma will be explored in patients with plasma cell variant CD in the near future.

References

1. Castleman, B., Towne, V. W. Case records of the Massachusetts General Hospital; weekly clinicopathological exercises; founded by Richard C. Cabot. *N. Engl. J. Med.* 1954; **251**(10):396–400.

2. Castleman, B., Iverson, L., Menendez, V. P. Localized mediastinal lymph node hyperplasia resembling thymoma. *Cancer* 1956;**9**(4): 822–30.

3. Keller, A. R., Hochholzer, L., Castleman, B. Hyaline-vascular and plasma-cell types of giant lymph node hyperplasia of the

mediastinum and other locations. *Cancer* 1972;**29**(3):670–83.

4. Cronin, D. M., Warnke, R. A. Castleman disease: an update on classification and the spectrum of associated lesions. *Adv. Anat. Pathol.* 2009;**16**(4):236–46.

5. Bates, D. O., Harper, S. J. Regulation of vascular permeability by vascular endothelial growth factors. *Vascul. Pharmacol.* 2002;**39**(4–5): 225–37.

6. Lee, J., Ban, J. Y., Won, K. Y. *et al.* Expression of EGFR and follicular dendritic markers in lymphoid follicles from patients with Castleman's disease. *Oncol. Rep.* 2008;**20**(4):851–6.

7. McClain, K. L., Natkunam, Y., Swerdlow, S. H. Atypical cellular disorders. *Hematology. Am. Soc. Hematol. Educ. Program* 2004:283–96.

8. Du, M. Q., Liu, H., Diss, T. C. *et al.* Kaposi sarcoma-associated herpesvirus infects monotypic (IgM lambda) but polyclonal naive B cells in Castleman disease and associated lymphoproliferative disorders. *Blood* 2001;**97**(7):2130–6.

9. Heinrich, P. C., Behrmann, I., Haan, S. *et al.* Principles of interleukin (IL)-6-type cytokine signalling and its regulation. *Biochem. J.* 2003;**374**(Pt 1):1–20.

10. Yoshizaki, K., Matsuda, T., Nishimoto, N. *et al.* Pathogenic significance of interleukin-6 (IL-6/BSF-2) in Castleman's disease. *Blood* 1989;**74**(4):1360–7.

11. Hall, P. A., Donaghy, M., Cotter, F. E., Stansfield, A. G., Levison, D. A. An immunohistological and genotypic study of the plasma cell form of Castleman's disease. *Histopathology* 1989;**14**(4): 333–46; discussion 429–32.

12. Nishimoto, N., Kanakura, Y., Aozasa, K. *et al.* Humanized anti-interleukin-6 receptor antibody treatment of multicentric

Castleman disease. *Blood* 2005;**106**(8):2627–32.

13. Katsume, A., Saito, H., Yamada, Y. *et al.* Anti-interleukin 6 (IL-6) receptor antibody suppresses Castleman's disease like symptoms emerged in IL-6 transgenic mice. *Cytokine* 2002; **20**(6):304–11.

14. Chen, D., Choi, Y. B., Sandford, G., Nicholas, J. Determinants of secretion and intracellular localization of human herpesvirus 8 interleukin-6. *J. Virol.* 2009; **83**(13):6874–82.

15. Glaunsinger, B., Ganem, D. Highly selective escape from KSHV-mediated host mRNA shutoff and its implications for viral pathogenesis. *J. Exp. Med.* 2004;**200**(3):391–8.

16. Yamasaki, S., Iino, T., Nakamura, M. *et al.* Detection of human herpesvirus-8 in peripheral blood mononuclear cells from adult Japanese patients with multicentric Castleman's disease. *Br. J. Haematol.* 2003; **120**(3):471–7.

17. Chang, Y., Cesarman, E., Pessin, M. S. *et al.* Identification of herpesvirus-like DNA sequences in AIDS-associated Kaposi's sarcoma. *Science* 1994; **266**(5192):1865–9.

18. Pyakurel, P., Pak, F., Mwakigonja, A. R. *et al.* Lymphatic and vascular origin of Kaposi's sarcoma spindle cells during tumor development. *Int. J. Cancer* 2006;**119**(6):1262–7.

19. Ablashi, D. V., Chatlynne, L. G., Whitman, J. E., Jr., Cesarman, E. Spectrum of Kaposi's sarcoma-associated herpesvirus, or human herpesvirus 8, diseases. *Clin. Microbiol. Rev.* 2002;**15**(3): 439–64.

20. Hengge, U. R., Ruzicka, T., Tyring, S. K. *et al.* Update on Kaposi's sarcoma and other HHV8 associated diseases. Part 2: pathogenesis, Castleman's disease, and pleural effusion lymphoma.

Lancet. Infect. Dis. 2002;**2**(6): 344–52.

21. Naresh, K. N., Rice, A. J., Bower, M. Lymph nodes involved by multicentric Castleman disease among HIV-positive individuals are often involved by Kaposi sarcoma. *Am. J. Surg. Pathol.* 2008;**32**(7):1006–12.

22. Parravicini, C., Corbellino, M., Paulli, M. *et al.* Expression of a virus-derived cytokine, KSHV vIL-6, in HIV-seronegative Castleman's disease. *Am. J. Pathol.* 1997;**151**(6):1517–22.

23. Foss, H. D., Araujo, I., Demel, G. *et al.* Expression of vascular endothelial growth factor in lymphomas and Castleman's disease. *J. Pathol.* 1997;**183**(1): 44–50.

24. Casper, C., Nichols, W. G., Huang, M. L., Corey, L., Wald, A. Remission of HHV-8 and HIV-associated multicentric Castleman disease with ganciclovir treatment. *Blood* 2004;**103**(5):1632–4.

25. Herrada, J., Cabanillas, F., Rice, L., Manning, J., Pugh, W. The clinical behavior of localized and multicentric Castleman disease. *Ann. Intern. Med.* 1998;**128** (8):657–62.

26. Weisenburger, D. D., Nathwani, B. N., Winberg, C. D., Rappaport, H. Multicentric angiofollicular lymph node hyperplasia: a clinicopathologic study of 16 cases. *Hum. Pathol.* 1985; **16**(2):162–72.

27. Barker, R., Kazmi, F., Stebbing, J. *et al.* FDG-PET/CT imaging in the management of HIV-associated multicentric Castleman's disease. *Eur. J. Nucl. Med. Mol. Imaging* 2009;**36**(4):648–52.

28. Gerard, L., Berezne, A., Galicier, L. *et al.* Prospective study of rituximab in chemotherapy-dependent human immunodeficiency virus associated multicentric Castleman's disease: ANRS 117

CastlemaB Trial. *J. Clin. Oncol.* 2007;**25**(22):3350–6.

29. Guihot, A., Couderc, L. J., Rivaud, E. *et al.* Thoracic radiographic and CT findings of multicentric Castleman disease in HIV-infected patients. *J. Thorac. Imaging* 2007;**22**(2):207–11.

30. Zietz, C., Bogner, J. R., Goebel, F. D., Lohrs, U. An unusual cluster of cases of Castleman's disease during highly active antiretroviral therapy for AIDS. *N. Engl. J. Med.* 1999;**340**(24):1923–4.

31. Chronowski, G. M., Ha, C. S., Wilder, R. B. *et al.* Treatment of unicentric and multicentric Castleman disease and the role of radiotherapy. *Cancer* 2001;**92**(3): 670–6.

32. Olscamp, G., Weisbrod, G., Sanders, D., Delarue, N., Mustard, R. Castleman disease: unusual manifestations of an unusual disorder. *Radiology* 1980;**135**(1): 43–8.

33. Frizzera, G., Peterson, B. A., Bayrd, E. D., Goldman, A. A systemic lymphoproliferative disorder with morphologic features of Castleman's disease: clinical findings and clinicopathologic correlations in 15 patients. *J. Clin. Oncol.* 1985; **3**(9):1202–16.

34. Ide, M., Kawachi, Y., Izumi, Y., Kasagi, K., Ogino, T. Long-term remission in HIV-negative patients with multicentric Castleman's disease using rituximab. *Eur. J. Haematol.* 2006;**76**(2):119–23.

35. Ocio, E. M., Sanchez-Guijo, F. M., Diez-Campelo, M. *et al.* Efficacy of rituximab in an aggressive form of multicentric Castleman disease associated with immune phenomena. *Am. J. Hematol.* 2005;**78**(4):302–5.

36. Ramasamy, K., Gandhi, S., Tenant-Flowers, M. *et al.* Rituximab and thalidomide combination therapy for Castleman disease. *Br. J. Haematol.* 2012;**158**(3):421–3.

37. Hess, G., Wagner, V., Kreft, A., Heussel, C. P., Huber, C. Effects of bortezomib on pro-inflammatory cytokine levels and transfusion dependency in a patient with multicentric Castleman disease. *Br. J. Haematol.* 2006;**134**(5): 544–5.

38. Tamayo, M., Gonzalez, C., Majado, M. J., Candel, R., Ramos, J. Long-term complete remission after interferon treatment in a case of multicentric Castelman's disease. *Am. J. Hematol.* 1995; **49**(4):359–60.

39. Casper, C., Krantz, E. M., Corey, L. *et al.* Valganciclovir for suppression of human herpesvirus-8 replication: a randomized, double-blind, placebo-controlled, crossover trial. *J. Infect. Dis.* 2008; **198**(1):23–30.

40. Stein, C. A., LaRocca, R. V., Thomas, R., McAtee, N., Myers, C. E. Suramin: an anticancer drug with a unique mechanism of action. *J. Clin. Oncol.* 1989; **7**(4):499–508.

41. Matsuyama, M., Suzuki, T., Tsuboi, H. *et al.* Anti-interleukin-6 receptor antibody (tocilizumab) treatment of multicentric Castleman's disease. *Intern. Med.* 2007;**46**(11):771–4.

42. Song, S. N., Tomosugi, N., Kawabata, H. *et al.* Down-regulation of hepcidin resulting from long-term treatment with an anti-IL-6 receptor antibody (tocilizumab) improves anemia of inflammation in multicentric Castleman disease. *Blood* 2010;**116**(18):3627–34.

43. Oksenhendler, E., Boulanger, E., Galicier, L. *et al.* High incidence of Kaposi sarcoma-associated herpesvirus-related non-Hodgkin lymphoma in patients with HIV infection and multicentric Castleman disease. *Blood* 2002; **99**(7):2331–6.

44. Oksenhendler, E., Duarte, M., Soulier, J. *et al.* Multicentric Castleman's disease in HIV infection: a clinical and pathological study of 20 patients. *Aids* 1996;**10**(1):61–7.

45. Oksenhendler, E. HIV-associated multicentric Castleman disease. *Curr. Opin. HIV. AIDS* 2009; **4**(1):16–21.

46. Scott, D., Cabral, L., Harrington, W. J., Jr. Treatment of HIV-associated multicentric Castleman's disease with oral etoposide. *Am. J. Hematol.* 2001;**66**(2):148–50.

47. Bower, M., Powles, T., Williams, S. *et al.* Brief communication: rituximab in HIV-associated multicentric Castleman disease. *Ann. Intern. Med.* 2007; **147**(12):836–9.

48. Bower, M., Newsom-Davis, T., Naresh, K. *et al.* Clinical features and outcome in HIV-associated multicentric Castleman's disease. *J. Clin. Oncol.* 2011;**29**(18): 2481–6.

Chapter

17

POEMS syndrome and paraproteinemic syndromes: management and follow-up

Angela Dispenzieri and Suzanne R. Hayman

Introduction

POEMS syndrome is an atypical plasma cell disorders, composed of a diverse group of diseases that often share little other than an underlying plasma cell clone. The pathophysiologic relationship between the plasma cell dyscrasia is often cryptic in many of these disorders. However, understanding that there may be relationships between bone marrow and distant organ systems is important to arrive at a diagnosis and management plan. A convenient means of characterizing these disorders is by their dominant clinical feature: neuropathy, dermopathy and nephropathy (Figure 17.1). Some atypical plasma cell disorders will have phenotypes that cross many systems, as will be specified in the following pages. The most common atypical plasma cell disorder, light chain (AL) amyloidosis, may affect almost any organ system but will be discussed in a separate chapter.

Atypical PCD with peripheral neuropathy as dominant phenotype

Chemotherapy-induced peripheral neuropathy, Waldenstrom's macroglobulinemia, multiple myeloma, and light chain amyloid are important etiologies for plasma cell disorder (PCD)-associated neuropathy, but these are beyond the scope of this review. In this section the focus will be upon POEMS (polyneuropathy, organomegaly, endocrinopathy, M protein and skin changes) syndrome and MGUS (monoclonal gammopathy of undetermined significance) associated peripheral neuropathy.

POEMS syndrome

POEMS syndrome is a rare paraneoplastic syndrome due to an underlying plasma cell disorder. This acronym refers to several, but not all, of the features of the syndrome: polyradiculoneuropathy, organomegaly, endocrinopathy, monoclonal plasma cell disorder and skin changes [1]. There are two important points about this acronym: (1) not all of the features within the acronym are required to a diagnosis of POEMS syndrome; and (2) there are other important features not included in the POEMS acronym, including papilledema, extravascular volume overload, sclerotic bone lesions, thrombocytosis/erythrocytosis (P.E.S.T.), elevated VEGF levels, abnormal pulmonary function tests and a predisposition towards thrombosis. There is a Castleman disease variant of POEMS syndrome, which may not be associated with a clonal plasma cell disorder. Other names of the POEMS syndrome that are less frequently used are osteosclerotic myeloma, Takatsuki syndrome or Crow–Fukase syndrome [2,3]. The disease was initially thought to be more common in patients of Japanese descent given the largest initial reports from Japan [2,3]. However, over the years, large series have also been reported from France, the United States, China and India [4–8].

The pathogenesis of the syndrome is not well understood. There are several characteristics that differentiate POEMS syndrome from standard multiple myeloma (MM). First, the dominant symptoms in POEMS syndrome have little to do with bone pain, extremes of bone marrow infiltration by plasma cells, or renal failure. Instead the dominant symptoms of the syndrome are typically neuropathy, endocrine dysfunction and volume overload. Second, vascular

Myeloma, ed. Stephen A. Schey, Kwee L. Yong, Robert Marcus and Kenneth C. Anderson. Published by Cambridge University Press. © Cambridge University Press 2014.

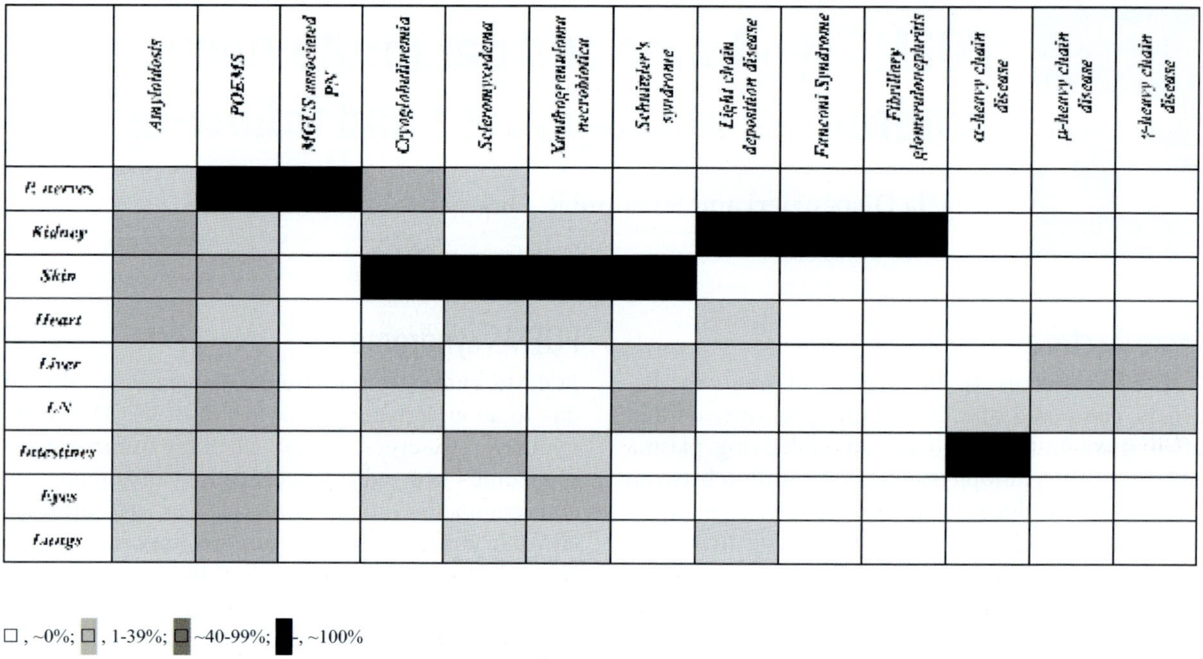

	Amyloidosis	POEMS	MGUS associated PN	Cryoglobulinemia	Scleromyxedema	Xanthogranuloma necrobiotica	Schnitzler's syndrome	Light chain deposition disease	Fanconi Syndrome	Fibrillary glomerulonephritis	α-heavy chain disease	μ-heavy chain disease	γ-heavy chain disease
P. nerves	░	■	■	░	░								
Kidney	░			░				■	■	■			
Skin	░	░		■	■	■	■	░					
Heart	░	░			░			░					
Liver	░	░						░				░	░
LN	░	░					░				░	░	
Intestines	░				░							■	░
Eyes	░	░					░						
Lungs	░	░			░				░				

□, ~0%; ░, 1–39%; ▒, ~40–99%; ■, ~100%

Figure 17.1 System involvement by various atypical plasma cell disorders.

endothelial growth factor (VEGF) levels are high in POEMS. Third, sclerotic bone lesions (rather than pure lytic lesions) are present in the majority of cases. Fourth, the overall survival is typically superior amongst patients with POEMS syndrome. Lastly, lambda clones predominate in POEMS syndrome [9].

VEGF is the cytokine that correlates best with disease activity, although it may not be the driving force of the disease based on the mixed results seen with anti-VEGF therapy. VEGF is known to target endothelial cells, induce a rapid and reversible increase in vascular permeability, and be important in angiogenesis. It is expressed by osteoblasts, in bone tissue, macrophages, tumor cells (including plasma cells) and megakaryocytes/platelets. Both IL-1β and IL-6 have been shown to stimulate VEGF production.

Diagnosis

The diagnosis is made based on a composite of clinical and laboratory features (Table 17.1). The constellation of neuropathy and any of the following should elicit an in depth search for POEMS syndrome: a lambda restricted monoclonal protein; thrombocytosis; anasarca; or papilledema. Making the diagnosis can be a challenge, but a good history and physical examination followed by appropriate testing – most notably

radiographic assessment of bones, measurement of VEGF, and careful analysis of a bone marrow biopsy [10] – can differentiate this syndrome from other conditions like chronic inflammatory polyradiculoneuropathy (CIDP), monoclonal gammopathy of undetermined significance (MGUS) neuropathy and immunoglobulin light chain amyloid neuropathy. As will be discussed, there is a Castleman's variant of POEMS syndrome that does not have a clonal plasma cell proliferative disorder underlying, but have many of the other paraneoplastic features [11].

A thorough review of systems and physical examination are required. The neuropathy is the dominant complaint. The quality and extent of the neuropathy, which tends to be peripheral, ascending, symmetrical, and affecting both sensation and motor function, should be elicited [12]; pain may be a dominant feature in about 10%–15% of patients, and in one report as many as 50% of patients had hyperesthesia [13]. Papilledema is present in at least one-third of patients.

Skin manifestations include hyperpigmentation, a recent out-cropping of hemangioma, hypertrichosis, dependent rubor and acrocyanosis, white nails, sclerodermoid changes, flushing or clubbing. Respiratory complaints are usually limited given patients'

Table 17.1 Criteria for the diagnosis of POEMS syndrome[a]

Mandatory major criteria	1. Polyneuropathy (typically demyelinating)
	2. Monoclonal plasma cell-proliferative disorder (almost always λ)
Other major criteria **(one required)**	3. Castleman disease[b]
	4. Sclerotic bone lesions
	5. Vascular endothelial growth factor elevation
Minor criteria	6. Organomegaly (splenomegaly, hepatomegaly, or lymphadenopathy)
	7. Extravascular volume overload (edema, pleural effusion, or ascites)
	8. Endocrinopathy (adrenal, thyroid,[c] pituitary, gonadal, parathyroid, pancreatic[c])
	9. Skin changes (hyperpigmentation, hypertrichosis, glomeruloid hemangiomata, plethora, acrocyanosis, flushing, white nails)
	10. Papilledema
	11. Thrombocytosis/polycythemia[d]
Other symptoms and signs	Clubbing, weight loss, hyperhidrosis, pulmonary hypertension/restrictive lung disease, thrombotic diatheses, diarrhea, low vitamin B_{12} values

[a] POEMS: polyneuropathy, organomegaly, endocrinopathy, M protein, skin changes. The diagnosis of POEMS syndrome is confirmed when both of the mandatory major criteria, one of the three other major criteria, and one of the six minor criteria are present.
[b] There is a Castleman disease variant of POEMS syndrome that occurs *without* evidence of a clonal plasma cell disorder that is not accounted for in this table. This entity should be considered separately.
[c] Because of the high prevalence of diabetes mellitus and thyroid abnormalities, this diagnosis alone is not sufficient to meet this minor criterion.
[d] Approximately 50% of patients will have bone marrow changes that distinguish it from a typical MGUS or myeloma bone marrow. Anemia and/or thrombocytopenia are distinctively unusual in this syndrome unless Castleman disease is present.
Reprinted with permission from reference [30].

neurologic status impairing their ability to induce cardiovascular challenges. In a series of 137 POEMS syndrome patients seen at our institution between 1975 and 2003, at presentation the frequency with which patients reported dyspnea, chest pain, cough and orthopnea, were 20%, 10%, 8% and 7%, respectively [14].

Patients are at increased risk for arterial and/or venous thromboses during their course, with nearly 20% of patients experiencing one of these complications [9,15]. Ten percent of patients present with a cerebrovascular event, most commonly embolic or vessel dissection with resulting stenosis [16].

On physical examination, objective evidence of the symptoms described above can be found in addition to non-bulky adenopathy, gynecomastia, darkened areolae, diminished breath sounds, hepatosplenomegaly, areflexia and a steppage gait, commonly with a positive Romberg sign. In our experience, finger-nail clubbing is seen in about 4% of cases, but others have reported rates as high as 49%.

Laboratory findings are notable for an absence of cytopenias. In fact, nearly half of patients will have thrombocytosis or erythrocytosis [17]. In the series of Li and colleagues, 26% of patients had anemia, which the authors attributed to impaired renal function [7]. Their series was enriched with Castleman disease patients (25%), which may have also contributed to this unprecedentedly high rate of anemia.

Serum creatinine levels are normal in most cases, but serum cystatin C, which is a surrogate marker for renal function, is high in 71% of patients [18]. In our experience, at presentation, fewer than 10% of patients have proteinuria exceeding 0.5 g/24 h, and only 6% have a serum creatinine greater than or equal to 1.5 mg/dl. Four percent of patients developed renal failure as preterminal events [17]. In a recent series from China, 37% of patients had a CrCl of less than 60 ml/min, and 9% had a CrCl of less than 30 ml/min. In our experience, renal disease is more likely to occur in patients who have co-existing Castleman disease.

Endocrinopathy is a central but poorly understood feature of POEMS. In a recent series [19], approximately 84% of patients had a recognized endocrinopathy, with hypogonadism as the most common endocrine abnormality, followed by thyroid mortality can be minimized by recognizing and treating an engraftment syndrome characterized by fevers, rash, diarrhea, weight gain, and respiratory symptoms and signs that occurs anytime between days 7 to 15 post-stem cell infusion.

Other promising treatments include lenalidomide, thalidomide and bortezomib, all of which are drugs that can have anti-VEGF and anti-TNF effects. Enthusiasm for the latter two therapies should be tempered by the high rate of peripheral neuropathy induced by these drugs. Dramatic improvements have been reported with lenalidomide and dexamethasone with good effect. One patient relapsed five months after discontinuing therapy, but responded to reintroduction of the drug. Although an anti-VEGF strategy is appealing, the results with bevacizumab have been mixed [30]. Only one of the reports in which bevacizumab was reported to be of benefit was the drug used as monotherapy. Three patients receiving it died. Single agent IV IG or plasmapheresis is not helpful. Other treatments like interferon-alpha, tamoxifen, trans-retinoic acid, ticlopidine, argatroban, and strontium-89 have been reported as having activity mostly as single case reports [9].

Attention to supportive care is imperative. Orthotics, physical therapy and CPAP all play an important role in patients' recovery. Ankle foot orthotics can increase mobility and reduce falls. Physical therapy reduces the risk for permanent contractures and leads to improved function both in the long and short term. For those with severe neuromuscular weakness, CPAP and/or biBAP provides better oxygenation and potentially reduces the risk complications associated with hypoventilation like pulmonary infection and pulmonary hypertension.

Patients must be followed carefully on a quarterly basis tracking the status of deficits comparing these to baseline. VEGF responses may occur as soon as three months, but they can be delayed. VEGF is an imperfect marker since discordance between disease activity and response has been reported, so trends rather than absolute values should direct therapeutic decisions. Serum M protein responses by protein electrophoresis, immunofixation electrophoresis, or serum immunoglobulin free light chains also pose a challenge. The size of the M protein is typically small making standard multiple myeloma response criteria inapplicable in most cases. In addition, patients can derive significant clinical benefit in the absence of and M protein response. Finally, despite the fact that the immunoglobulin free light chains are elevated in 90% of POEMS patients, the ratio is normal in all but 18%, making the test of limited value for patients with POEMS syndrome.

MGUS associated peripheral neuropathy

MGUS associated peripheral neuropathy is a diagnosis of exclusion. There is no assay to prove that the MGUS is driving the neuropathy for any given patient. The pathogenesis of MGUS neuropathy (especially IgM) is sometimes related to the reactivity of the monoclonal immunoglobulins to specific antigens expressed on peripheral nerves such as myelin associated glycoprotein (MAG) [34], gangliosides, chondroitin sulfate and sulfatide. There is still some debate regarding the sensitivity and specificity of the MAG assays. IgM with complement can be found within the myelin and extending throughout the compact myelin in both large and small myelinated fibers. There is no correlation between the size of the M protein and the anti-MAG titers. Quarles and Weiss provide a comprehensive review of autoantibodies associated with PN [35]

Typically MGUS associated neuropathy has the following features: (1) an M protein in the serum, most commonly IgM, followed in frequency by IgG and then IgA; (2) a symmetric sensorimotor polyradiculopathy or neuropathy which begins insidiously and is usually slowly progressive; (3) no cranial nerves involvement; (4) occurrence most common in sixth to the seventh decade of life; and (5) a predisposition for males. Paresthesias, ataxia and pain may be predominant features. Symptoms usually begin with paresthesias and numbness distally in the feet or hands, and early motor symptoms are rare or minor. The neuropathy then progresses proximally in stocking/glove distribution and may involve motor as well as sensory functions. There is no correlation between the size of the monoclonal protein and the severity of the neuropathy. Roughly 50% of MGUS neuropathies are associated with IgM gammopathy; about one-half to two-thirds of these monoclonal proteins will have anti-MAG activity [36,37].

Treatment and prognosis

Initiation of treatment is largely based on comparing the potential risk of therapy to its potential benefit. Nobile-Orazio et al. analyzed the long-term outcome of 25 of the 26 patients with neuropathy and high anti-MAG IgM [38]. After a mean follow-up of

Table 17.3 Randomized trials to treat MGUS associated peripheral neuropathy

Reference	N	Treatment	
[39]	39	Double blind plasma exchange vs. sham	Improvement in NDS with PE; especially in IgA and IgG patients
[42]	24	Chlorambucil vs. chlorambucil and plasma exchange	Sensory component of NDS improved slightly in both arms. No difference between treatments
[104]	20	Open randomized IFN-α vs. IV IG	8/10 vs 1/10 improved NDS at 6 months; persistent at 12 months. Sensory improvement only. Decreased IgM in 2 IFN-α patients. MAG Ab persist
[43]	22	IV Ig vs. placebo	Improved handgrip, 10 m walking time, and sensory symptom score in IV Ig group as compared to baseline. Only difference at 4 weeks was hand grip.
[41]	24	Double blind randomized IFN-α vs. placebo	3/12 patients in each arm improved clinically. No benefit to IFN-α

NDS, neuropathy disability score.
Modified from Dispenzieri and Kyle [105].

8.5 years and a mean duration of neuropathy symptoms of 11.8 years (range 3–18, >10 years in 16), 17 patients (68%) were alive. The eight (32%) who died did so 3–15 years after neuropathy onset; in none of them was death caused by the neuropathy, although in three it was possibly related to the therapy for the neuropathy. At last follow-up or prior to death, 11 patients (44%) were disabled by severe hand tremor, gait ataxia or both, with disability rates at 5, 10 and 15 years from neuropathy onset of 16%, 24% and 50%, respectively. Of the 19 patients treated during the follow-up, only five (26%) reported a consistent and four a slight improvement in the neuropathy after one treatment or more; only one patient had persistent improvement throughout the follow-up period. Severe adverse events, possibly related to therapy, occurred during treatment in half [38].

Treatment strategies are directed toward reducing the IgM paraprotein level either by removing the antibody or targeting the presumed monoclonal B cell clone, or toward interfering with the presumed effector mechanisms such as complement activation or macrophage recruitment. There are limited published data regarding efficacy of the various immunosuppressive regimes in IgM paraproteinemic neuropathies and only six randomized controlled trials (Table 17.3) [39–43]. Most case series are small, include diverse groups of patients and measurements of efficacy differ between trials.

Plasma exchange was superior to sham exchange, especially for non-IgM patients [39]. In another randomized trial in IgM MGUS patients, comparing chlorambucil orally or chlorambucil plus 15 courses of plasma exchange demonstrated no difference in the two treatment groups [42]. Alkylators may be used, with the knowledge that secondary myelodysplastic syndrome or acute leukemia are possible complications. Small studies indicate response rates of ~33%. Corticosteroids are not usually effective in patients with neuropathy and IgM MGUS. Based on the results of a small open label randomized study in which patients were randomized to either IFN-α or IV Ig, it was thought that IFN-α was an effective therapy in patients with IgM MAG associated PN. A successor study, which was a blinded comparison of IFN-α and placebo, however, was negative [41].

Intravenous gammaglobulin produces may be used for patients with sensorimotor peripheral neuropathy and MGUS. Intravenous immunoglobulin is beneficial in 25%–50% of patients. Dalakas et al. randomized 11 patients with IgM MAG associated PN to either intravenous gammaglobulin or placebo; at three months, patients crossed over to the other therapy. There was improvement in 27% [40]. Comi et al. treated 22 patients with IgM MAG associated PN with either intravenous gammaglobulin or placebo, and found short-term intrapatient improvement [43].

Response rates of 66%–100% have been observed with anti-CD20 antibodies. Pestronk et al. treated 21 patients with IgM-associated neuropathy with rituximab, with an option to retreat, followed by a maintenance course of a dose every ten weeks

231

for two years. Eighty-one percent had improvement in the functional scores over baseline at the conclusion of the study [44].

Atypical PCD with dermopathy as dominant phenotype

Cryoglobulinemia

Cryoglobulins are immunoglobulins that precipitate in the cold. A distinct syndrome of purpura, arthralgias, asthenia, renal disease and neuropathy – often occurring with immune complex deposition or vasculitis, or both – is termed cryoglobulinemia. The Brouet classification system is as follows: type I, isolated monoclonal immunoglobulins; type II, a monoclonal component, usually IgM, possessing activity toward polyclonal immunoglobulins, usually IgG; and type III, polyclonal immunoglobulins of more than one isotype [45]. This classification provided a framework by which clinical correlations could be made. Associated conditions, such as lymphoproliferative disorders, connective tissue disorders, infection, and liver disease were observed in some patients [46,47]. In several large series, 34% to 71% of cryoglobulinemia cases were not associated with other specific disease states and were termed "essential" or primary cryoglobulinemia [46,48]. In 1990, hepatitis C virus (HCV) was recognized as an etiologic factor for the majority of these cases [49,50].

Cryoglobulinemia is driven primarily by four classes of disease: liver disease (predominantly HCV), infection (again, predominantly HCV), connective tissue disease and lymphoproliferative disease. These diseases induce a seemingly non-specific stimulation of B cells, frequently resulting in polyclonal hypergammaglobulinemia. When these various antibodies are produced, antibodies to autoantigens may also result. In animal models, a strong B cell stimulus disrupts the sequential order of idiotype–anti-idiotype interactions, resulting in both immunosuppression and idiotype–anti-idiotype immune complexes [51]. Furthermore, poorly regulated production and clearance of IgM rheumatoid factor contribute to immune complex formation and pathologic conditions, which include vasculitis, nephritis and vascular occlusion.

The prevalence of cryoglobulinemia is difficult to estimate both because of its clinical polymorphism and because of the necessity of separating the laboratory finding of cryoglobulins from the symptomatic disease state. Although only a minority of patients with serum cryoglobulins has symptoms referable to them, cryoglobulins may be found in patients with cirrhosis (up to 45%), alcoholic hepatitis (32%), autoimmune hepatitis (40%), subacute bacterial endocarditis (90%), rheumatoid arthritis (47%), IgG myeloma (10%) and Waldenström macroglobulinemia (19%).

Results of most studies show that the median age at diagnosis is the early to mid 50s. In some studies, the female predominance for cryoglobulinemia is greater than 2:1. Involvement of the skin, peripheral nerves, kidneys and liver is common. Lymphadenopathy is present in approximately 17% of patients [46,52]. On autopsy, widespread vasculitis involving small and medium vessels in the heart, gastrointestinal tract, central nervous system, muscles, lungs, and adrenal glands may also be seen [46,53]. Type I cryoglobulinemia is usually asymptomatic. When symptomatic, it most commonly causes occlusive symptoms rather than the vasculitis of types II and III [46,52,54]. Symptoms of hyperviscosity may occur. Type II cryoglobulinemia is more frequently symptomatic (61% of patients) than type III (21% of patients) [55].

Purpura is present in 55%–100% of patients with mixed cryoglobulinemia. The incidence varies from 15% to 33% in type I, from 60% to 93% in type II, and from 70% to 83% in type III [56]. Petechiae and palpable purpura are the most common lesions, although ecchymoses, erythematous spots and dermal nodules occur in as many as 20% of patients. Bullous or vesicular lesions are distinctly uncommon [54]. Successive purpuric rashes, which may be preceded by a burning or itching sensation, occur most commonly on the lower extremities, gradually extending to the thighs and lower abdomen. Occasionally the arms are involved, but the face and trunk are generally spared [54]. Head and mucosal involvement, livedoid vasculitis and cold-induced acrocyanosis of the helices of the ears are more frequently observed in type I; infarction, hemorrhagic crusts or ulcers occur in 10%–25% of all patients with mixed cryoglobulinemia [57]. Showers of purpura last for one to two weeks and occur once or twice a month. Cold precipitates these types of lesions in only 10%–30% of the patients [54,57]. Raynaud phenomenon occurs in about 19%–50% of patients; in a quarter of these, the symptoms may be severe, including necrosis of fingertips [54]. Skin necrosis, urticaria and livedo, which are all rare, are more commonly associated with exposure to cold.

Peripheral neuropathy is much more common than central nervous system involvement. Peripheral nerve involvement is described in 12%–56% of patients. The presentation may be an acute or subacute distal symmetric polyneuropathy or a mononeuritis multiplex with a chronic or chronic-relapsing evolution [58]. The neuropathy is most often characterized by axonal degeneration. Epineurial vasculitis is a common finding on sural nerve biopsy. Even when other manifestations of mixed cryoglobulinemia are stable over time, there may be worsening of the peripheral neuropathy [59].

Approximately 21%–39% of patients with mixed cryoglobulinemia have renal involvement. The incidence of renal injury is highest in patients with type II cryoglobulins [48,60]. Proteinuria greater than 0.5 g/d and hematuria are the most common features of renal disease at diagnosis; nephrotic syndrome affects approximately 20% of patients and acute nephritic syndrome affects approximately 25% of patients. Although cryopathic membranoproliferative glomerulonephritis portends a poor prognosis, progression to end-stage renal failure due to sclerosing nephritis is uncommon [61]. Among patients with mixed cryoglobulinemia-associated membranoproliferative glomerulonephritis followed up for a median of 11 years, 15% had disease progression to end-stage renal failure, and 43% died of cardiovascular, hepatic or infectious causes.

Hepatomegaly is present in up to 70% of patients, and splenomegaly is present in up to 52% of patients. Among patients with symptomatic cryoglobulinemia, liver failure is the cause of death in 2.5%–7.6% of patients and in 5.6%–29% of all reported deaths. Histologic findings include portal fibrosis, chronic persistent hepatitis, chronic active hepatitis, chronic active hepatitis with cirrhosis and post-necrotic cirrhosis. Most specimens are characterized by a diffuse lymphocytic infiltrate ranging from minimal periportal to extensive infiltration with nodule formation. These changes correlate with the severity of other pathologic findings. The lymphoid population in the liver may show the histologic and immunophenotypic findings of lymphoplasmacytoid lymphoma/immunocytoma, and frequently the lymphoid elements arrange in pseudo-follicular structures in the liver with morphologic features similar to those previously reported in chronic HCV without cryoglobulinemia [62].

Treatment and prognosis

Cryoglobulinemia has a fluctuating course with spontaneous exacerbation and remission, making randomized controlled clinical trials essential in evaluating the response to therapy. Unfortunately, such studies are rare. Overall, the prognosis is reasonably good with a median overall survival of more than ten years. The most common causes of death include renal failure, infection, lymphoproliferative disorders, liver failure, cardiovascular complications and hemorrhage. For 15% of individuals the disease was complicated by malignancy [63].

For mildly symptomatic patients (purpura, asthenia, arthralgia and mild sensory neuropathy), conservative management may be most appropriate: bed rest, analgesics, low-dose corticosteroid therapy, low-antigen content diet and protective measures against cold. For severe disease (glomerulonephritis, motor neuropathy and systemic vasculitis) plasmapheresis, high-dose corticosteroid therapy and cytotoxic therapy may be indicated. In HCV driven mixed cryoglobulinemia, interferon-alpha (FN)-based therapy is generally considered to be first-line [64–69]. For patients with symptomatic type I cryoglobulinemia, anti-CD20 therapy and/or cytotoxic therapy appropriate for the lymphoproliferative disorder remains the therapy of choice. Similarly, treatment of underlying connective tissue disease or infection would be first-line therapy in appropriate situations. The importance of not over treating patients must be emphasized. Clinical trials are needed to clarify these issues (Table 17.4).

Once the acute exacerbation has been mitigated, those patients who are HCV positive antiviral strategies are implemented in HCV positive patients to consolidate and maintain response. The ribavirin and IFN-α combination can be effective in the setting of renal disease [70,71]. See recent consensus recommendations [72]. One should be cognoscente of reports of peripheral neuropathy and, nephritis, vasculitis and ischemic events.

Anti-CD20 therapy with rituximab has been shown to produce responses in patients with all types of cryoglobulinemia; however, those patients with HCV are at risk for increased HCV replication [73,74]. The initial increase in the cryoglobulin level after rituximab therapy for type II cryoglobulinemia secondary to Waldenstrom macroglobulinemia does not indicate failure of response [75].

Although not formally studied, high-dose therapy with autologous stem cell transplantation may be considered for patients with symptomatic, refractory cryoglobulinemia that results from a plasmaproliferative disorder. There is an increased risk of lethal

Table 17.5 Diagnostic criteria of the Schnitzler syndrome [89,90]

Major
  Chronic urticarial rash
  Monoclonal **IgM** (or IgG: variant type)

Minor
  Intermittent fever
  Arthragia or arthritis
  Bone pain
  Lymphadenopathy
  Hepato- and/or splenomegaly
  Elevated ESR and/or leukocytosis
  Bone abnormalities (radiologic or histologic)

To meet criteria, patient must have both major criteria, and at least two minor criteria after exclusion of other causes.

monoclonal protein has also been described [90]. The mean age is early fifties. The pathophysiology of this disorder is not well understood. It has been postulated that the monoclonal protein serves as an autoantibody that, when deposited, triggers a local inflammatory response that could induce the skin lesions. Cytokine aberrations have been implicated including elevations in interleukin-6 and antibodies against interleukin-1. The demonstrated clinical efficacy of the interleukin-1β inhibitor anakinra against this disorder would suggest that interleukin-1β plays an important role in the pathophysiology [90–93].

The typical histologic appearance of a skin lesion is that of neutrophilic urticaria [94]. There is edema and a perivascular infiltrate of neutrophils and eosinophils in the papillary dermis. Fibrinoid deposits may be seen around dilated superficial blood vessels. However, fibrinoid necrosis, the hallmark of fully developed leukocytoclastic vasculitis, is not seen and immunofluorescence studies are usually negative, although IgM has been seen along the dermal–epidermal junction [95].

Diagnostic criteria by Lipsker *et al.* are shown in Table 17.5. The rash is pale rose, slightly elevated papules and plaques. Individual lesions measure 0.5–3 cm in diameter. New lesions appear daily and disappear in 12–24 h. The course may be chronic and unrelenting, but patients can go one to two weeks without eruptions. Head and neck are usually spared, and the trunk and extremities are most commonly affected. Approximately 45% of patients experience pruritus, but this tends to be a later finding. Angioedema is rare.

Extra-dermatological manifestations include: fever (88%), arthralgia/arthritis (82%), bone pain (72%), weight loss (64%), lymphadenopathy (44%), hepatomegaly (29%) and splenomegaly (12%) [90]. Typical laboratory findings include a moderately increased erythrocyte sedimentation rate, leukocytosis, mild anemia and an elevated C reactive protein. On immunofixation, an IgM monoclonal protein will be found. Since the monoclonal protein is typically small, it can be missed by merely measuring quantitative immunoglobulins by nephelometry or by screening with a serum protein electrophoresis. Occasionally, there will be a monoclonal IgG monoclonal protein instead. Complement levels are normal. The bone marrow biopsy may be "negative" and lymph nodes tend to show only reactive hyperplasia. Bone radiographs are most commonly normal, but increased bone density, lytic lesions, and periosteal apposition have been described [89,90].

Treatment and prognosis

Treatments that have provided varying degrees of relief include anakinra (an interleukin-receptor antagonist), oral glucocorticoids, thalidomide, PUVA (psoralen and ultraviolet irradiation), anti-histamines, non-steroidal anti-inflammatory drugs, interferon, rituximab, intravenous gammaglobulin, colchicine, dapsone, cyclosporin, alkylating agents purine nucleoside analogs, methotrexate and plasma exchange [89, 90]. Patients are at risk for both progression to Waldenstrom macroglobulinemia and AA amyloidosis. AL amyloidosis has not been reported. In a recent study of 94 patients, the 15 year survival rate was 91% [90]. In this same series, 11 patients developed Waldenstrom macroglobulinemia.

Atypical PCD with Nephropathy as Dominant Phenotype

The most common atypical plasma cell disorder with nephropathy as the dominant phenotype is light chain (AL) amyloidosis, but this topic is discussed in another chapter. The other disorders are listed in Table 17.1 and described in greater detail below.

Non-amyloidogenic light chain deposition disease (LCDD)

LCDD is a systemic disorder first described by Randall in 1976 [96] The light chains are produced by clonal plasma cells, which are most typically few in number; however, this disorder can also occur in the context of active multiple myeloma. LCDD is due to pathologic protein deposition in various tissues and organs. Even less commonly, the immunoglobulin heavy chain can deposit either alone or in combination with light chains. These conditions are referred to as heavy chain deposition disease and light and heavy chain deposition disease, respectively [97,98].

The organ most commonly involved is the kidney. Nodular glomerulosclerosis is commonly seen. The light chains most frequently found within these deposits are κ 1 and κ IV. It has been suggested that somatic mutations of specific amino acid sequences in the light chains affecting the three-dimensional confirmation of the protein. Unlike the light chain deposits observed in patients with primary systemic amyloidosis, these infiltrates are not congophilic by light microscopy. On electron microscopy, amorphous nodular deposits are seen in the glomeruli, the interstitium, along the tubular basement membranes, and in blood vessel walls.

The most common area of involvement is the kidney, but other organs like the heart, liver and lung have been described. Patients may be asymptomatic and have an incidental finding of renal insufficiency or proteinuria. In one series of 63 cases of LCDD, the median age was 52 years with approximately two-thirds of patients male [99] Ninety-six percent presented with renal insufficiency and 84% with proteinuria greater than 1 g/day. Approximately two-thirds of patients will have monoclonal kappa deposition, with the other third being lambda. The size of the serum and/or urine monoclonal protein is often small with approximately one-third of patients meeting criteria for MGUS rather than multiple myeloma. Not uncommonly, the clinical phenotype of these patients is more akin to AL amyloidosis than multiple myeloma.

Treatment and prognosis

The prognosis of patients who have this disorder depends on whether there is underlying multiple myeloma. In two retrospective studies of patients with LCDD, five-year actuarial patient survival and survival free of end-stage renal disease were 40%–70% and 37%, respectively [99,100]. Renal prognosis was linked to age and presenting creatinine, while overall survival was tied to age and extrarenal sites of involvement.

There is no standard therapy. For those who meet criteria for active multiple myeloma, chemotherapy is appropriate. During the era in which low-dose alkylators were the only therapies available, a common strategy was to avoid therapy with the understanding that renal failure would ensue; this risk was felt to be preferable over the risk alkylator induced myelodysplasia. Salvage renal allografting is feasible, but allograft survival is short if measures to significantly reduce light chain production have not been employed. High-dose chemotherapy and peripheral blood stem cell transplant, however, offers a treatment option for these patients with a lower risk of secondary myelodysplasia, but with a risk of precipitating renal failure [101,102]. It is not known what role novel agents like thalidomide and bortezomib may play in the care of these patients. The use of lenalidomide may be curtailed by the extent of renal failure in these patients.

Acquired Fanconi syndrome

Fanconi syndrome is a rare complication of plasma cell dyscrasias characterized by diffuse failure in reabsorption at the level of the proximal renal tubule and resulting in glycosuria, generalized aminoaciduria and hypophosphatemia [103]. Fanconi first described the syndrome in children. Subsequently, acquired forms were described in adults. The syndrome is usually associated with MGUS. Overt hematologic malignancies like multiple myeloma, Waldenstrom macroglobulinemia, or other lymphoproliferative disorders may be present at diagnosis or with further follow up. The crystals that deposit in the proximal renal tubules are composed of a portion of the variable region of the monoclonal light chain. The κ-variable domains from patients with this syndrome have been shown to be highly resistant to protease degradation and to have unusual self-reactivity to form crystals. It is thought that these light chains do not undergo complete proteolysis and therefore accumulate in the lysosomal compartment of the cells in the renal tubules.

In the Mayo series of 32 patients with Fanconi's syndrome, nearly 50% of patients presented with bone pain as their main complaint [103]. Approximately one-third had asymptomatic renal insufficiency, proteinuria or glycosuria, while the remainder presented with fatigue. Hypokalemia, hypophosphatemia and hypouricemia were present in 44%, 50% and 66%,

237

respectively. All patients tested had aminoaciduria and glucosuria. Bence Jones proteinuria is usually present and is almost always of the κ type.

Treatment and prognosis

Treatment consists of supplementation with phosphorus, calcium and vitamin D. The prognosis is good in the absence of overt malignant disease. The median time from diagnosis to end-stage renal failure was 196 months in one series [103]. Chemotherapy may benefit patients with rapidly progressive renal failure or symptomatic malignancy, but patients treated with alkylators are at risk for secondary myelodysplastic syndrome or acute leukemia.

Fibrillary glomerulonephritis

Fibrillary glomerulonephritis may occur in association with monoclonal gammopathy. The causal relationship is not always iron-clad. The clinical presentation includes hematuria, proteinuira and renal insufficiency. Extrarenal manifestations have been reported. On electron microcroscopy is found randomly arranged extracellular Congo red fibrils with diameter ranging from 13 mm to 29 mm. Common histologies include membranoproliferative glomerulonephritis, diffuse proliferative GN and crescents. The deposits more commonly contain IgG1 and IgG4. Immunotactoid glomerulonephritis is probably a subgroup of fibrillary GN. The size range of fibrils for this disorder tends to be larger (20–55 nm) and have a hollow center. These deposits often stain positive for monoclonal immunoglobulins.

Other atypical plasma cell disorders

The heavy chain diseases are a rare group of disorders with diverse clinical presentations [45]. The three conditions (α-, γ-, and μ-HCD) are discussed together because they are lymphoproliferative or plasmaproliferative disorders that share the generation and secretion of an isolated heavy chain fragment. α-HCD (Mediterranean lymphoma or immunoproliferative small intestinal disease) is the most common and has the most uniform presentation; γ- and μ-HCD have variable clinical presentations and histopathologic features. In the majority of cases, the heavy chain fragment is not secreted in large quantities, and immunofixation or immunoelectrophoresis is required to detect the abnormality. Screening the serum and urine

of patients with lymphoplasmacytoid NHL would most likely identify more patients with γ- or μ-HCD.

α-Heavy chain disease

Mediterranean lymphoma is a primary small intestinal lymphoma coupled with intestinal malabsorption. An isolated IgA immunoglobulin heavy chain fragment was recognized in association with this condition. Because some patients had benign-appearing lymphocytes in their small bowel, the term "α-HCD" was preferred over "Mediterranean lymphoma" by some authors. A consensus panel in 1976 concluded that α-HCD and Mediterranean lymphoma represented a spectrum of disease with benign, intermediate, and overtly malignant stages, and the term "immunoproliferative small intestinal disease" came into use.

Histologic features of IPSID range from early lymphoplasmacytic intestinal infiltration to overt malignant diffuse large B cell lymphoma. This entity shares morphologic features of mucosa-associated lymphoid tissue (MALT) in that there are lymphoepithelial lesions, centroyte-like cells, and plasma–cell differentiation. The hypothesis that chronic antigenic stimulation by intestinal organisms is the cause of this disorder is credible and can be modeled after the MALT lymphoma paradigm. C jejuni is now considered to be a possible offending organism, but this will need to be confirmed.

The standard accepted treatment for the early stage is broad-spectrum antibiotics, with or without corticosteroids. In the absence of a documented parasite or an intestinal bacterial overgrowth, therapy with tetracycline or metronidazole and ampicillin is appropriate. Lecuit et al. demonstrated response of IPSID after clearance of C jejuni. Response to antibiotics usually occurs promptly; however, a minimum six-month trial of tetracycline (1–2 g/d) is recommended for establishing responsiveness of the lesion. In patients with more advanced stages, or unresponsive early stages, total abdominal radiation or combination chemotherapy, or both, have been used (remission rate, 64%). Overall five-year survival rates are 60%–70%.

γ-Heavy chain disease

γ-HCD has a diverse clinical phenotype. Although most patients present with weakness, fatigue, fever, lymphadenopathy (62%), hepatomegaly (58%), splenomegaly (59%) and lymphoma, other features, such as autoimmune hemolytic anemia and idiopathic thrombocytopenic purpura, may also be seen. Cutaneous and subcutaneous involvement is not uncommon. Several cases have arisen in patients with long-standing connective tissue disorders such as rheumatoid arthritis, lupus, keratoconjunctivitis sicca, vasculitis and myasthenia gravis. A normochromic anemia is a presenting feature in about 79% of patients. About 10% have either a Coombs-positive or Coombs-negative autoimmune hemolytic anemia. Thrombocytopenia may be present in as many as 22% of patients. Proteinuria can range from none to 20 g/d. Bone marrow most commonly demonstrates an increase of plasma cells, lymphocytes, or plasmacytoid lymphocytes; occasionally eosinophilia is seen. The lymphoproliferative disorders range from benign lymphoplasma cell proliferative disorder to plasmacytoma, to chronic lymphocytic leukemia, to angioimmunoblastic lymphoma to diffuse large cell lymphoma. Lytic bone disease occurs rarely. Amyloid deposits may be present.

Treatment and prognosis

The median survival is 7.4 years, with a range of one month to more than 25 years. Single-agent therapy with prednisone and combination chemotherapy with cyclophosphamide, vincristine and prednisone has been used with benefit. Wahner-Roedler *et al.* reported a rituximab response in one patient. Patients with aggressive lymphomas should receive a regimen containing anthracycline.

μ-Heavy chain disease

μ-HCD is a rare poorly understood condition. Common clinical presentations include splenomegaly and hepatomegaly. Lymphadenopathy is less common. About one-third of patients have chronic lymphocytic leukemia. Some patients with μ-HCD have features resembling those of lymphoma or multiple myeloma with amyloid arthropathy.

Hypogammaglobulinemia is present in about one-half of the patients and a free monoclonal IgM fragment is found in the serum of all patients [104, 105]. Lytic bone lesions or osteoporosis occur in a minority of patients. Bone marrow plasma cells tend to be vacuolated. Survival ranges from less than one month to 11 years (median, 24 months).

Treatment and prognosis

There is no standard treatment for this disorder, but it is generally treated as a low-grade lymphoproliferative disease with observation alone for asymptomatic patients and low-intensity chemotherapy for symptomatic patients.

A. D. and this work are support in part by NIH grants CA125614, CA62242, CA107476, and CA111345 and the Predolin Foundation and the JABBS Foundation.

Conflict of interest

Research dollars from Celgene, Travel compensation from Binding Site and Celgene, and unpaid advisory board to Onyx and Millenium.

References

1. Bardwick, P. A., Zvaifler, N. J., Gill, G. N. *et al.* Plasma cell dyscrasia with polyneuropathy, organomegaly, endocrinopathy, M protein, and skin changes: the POEMS syndrome. Report on two cases and a review of the literature. *Medicine* 1980; **59**(4):311–22.

2. Takatsuki, K., Sanada, I. Plasma cell dyscrasia with polyneuropathy and endocrine disorder: clinical and laboratory features of 109 reported cases. *Jpn. J. Clin. Oncol.* 1983;**13**(3):543–55.

3. Nakanishi, T., Sobue, I., Toyokura, Y. *et al.* The Crow-Fukase syndrome: a study of 102 cases in Japan. *Neurology* 1984; **34**(6):712–20.

4. Singh, D., Wadhwa, J., Kumar, L. *et al.* POEMS syndrome: experience with fourteen cases. *Leuk. Lymphoma* 2003;**44**(10): 1749–52.

5. Soubrier, M. J., Dubost, J. J., Sauvezie, B. J. POEMS syndrome: a study of 25 cases and a review of the literature. French Study Group on POEMS Syndrome. *Am. J. Med.* 1994;**97**(6):543–53.

6. Zhang, B., Song, X., Liang, B. *et al.* The clinical study of POEMS syndrome in China. *Neuro. Endocrin. Lett.* 2010;**31**(2):229–37.

7. Li, J., Zhou, D. B., Huang, Z. *et al.* Clinical characteristics and long-term outcome of patients with POEMS syndrome in China. *Annals. Hematol.* 2011;**90**(7): 819–26.

8. Kulkarni, G. B., Mahadevan, A., Taly, A. B. *et al.* Clinicopathological profile of polyneuropathy, organomegaly, endocrinopathy, M protein and skin changes (POEMS) syndrome. *J. Clin. Neurosci.* 2011;**18**(3):356–60.

9. Dispenzieri, A. POEMS Syndrome. *Blood. Reviews* 2007; **21**(6):285–99.

10. Dao, L. N., Hanson, C. A., Dispenzieri, A. *et al.* Bone marrow

histopathology in POEMS syndrome: a distinctive combination of plasma cell, lymphoid and myeloid findings in 87 patients. *Blood* 2011;**117** (24):6438–44.

11. Dispenzieri, A. Castleman disease. *Cancer Treatment Res.* 2008;**142**:293–330.

12. Kelly, J. J., Jr., Kyle, R. A., Miles, J. M., Dyck, P. J. Osteosclerotic myeloma and peripheral neuropathy. *Neurology* 1983;**33** (2):202–10.

13. Koike, H., Iijima, M., Mori, K. *et al.* Neuropathic pain correlates with myelinated fibre loss and cytokine profile in POEMS syndrome. *J. Neurol. Neurosurg. Psych.* 2008;**79**(10):1171–9.

14. Allam, J. S., Kennedy, C. C., Aksamit, T. R., Dispenzieri, A. Pulmonary manifestations in patients with POEMS syndrome: a retrospective review of 137 patients. *Chest* 2008;**133**(4):969–74.

15. Lesprit, P., Authier, F. J., Gherardi, R. *et al.* Acute arterial obliteration: a new feature of the POEMS syndrome? *Medicine* 1996;**75**(4):226–32.

16. Dupont, S. A., Dispenzieri, A., Mauermann, M. L., Rabinstein, A. A., Brown, R. D., Jr.. Cerebral infarction in POEMS syndrome: incidence, risk factors, and imaging characteristics. *Neurology* 2009;**73**(16):1308–12.

17. Dispenzieri, A., Kyle, R. A., Lacy, M. Q. *et al.* POEMS syndrome: definitions and long-term outcome. *Blood* 2003;**101** (7):2496–506.

18. Stankowski-Drengler, T., Gertz, M. A., Katzmann, J. A. *et al.* Serum immunoglobulin free light chain measurements and heavy chain isotype usage provide insight into disease biology in patients with POEMS syndrome. *Am. J. Hematol.* 2010;**85**(6):431–4.

19. Ghandi, G. Y., Basu, R., Dispenzieri, A. *et al.* Endocrinopathy in POEMS

syndrome: the Mayo Clinic experience. *Mayo. Clin. Proc.* 2007;**82**(7):836–42.

20. Watanabe, O., Arimura, K., Kitajima, I., Osame, M., Maruyama, I. Greatly raised vascular endothelial growth factor (VEGF) in POEMS syndrome [letter]. *Lancet* 1996;**347** (9002):702.

21. Soubrier, M., Dubost, J. J., Serre, A. F. *et al.* Growth factors in POEMS syndrome: evidence for a marked increase in circulating vascular endothelial growth factor. *Arthritis Rheumatism* 1997;**40**(4):786–7.

22. Hashiguchi, T., Arimura, K., Matsumuro, K. *et al.* Highly concentrated vascular endothelial growth factor in platelets in Crow–Fukase syndrome. *Muscle Nerve* 2000;**23**(7):1051–6.

23. Watanabe, O., Maruyama, I., Arimura, K. *et al.* Overproduction of vascular endothelial growth factor/vascular permeability factor is causative in Crow-Fukase (POEMS) syndrome. *Muscle Nerve* 1998;**21**(11):1390–7.

24. Scarlato, M., Previtali, S. C., Carpo, M. *et al.* Polyneuropathy in POEMS syndrome: role of angiogenic factors in the pathogenesis. *Brain* 2005; **128**(Pt 8):1911–20.

25. Tanaka, O., Ohsawa, T. The POEMS syndrome: report of three cases with radiographic abnormalities. *Radiologe* 1984; **24**(10):472–4.

26. Chong, S. T., Beasley, H. S., Daffner, R. H. POEMS syndrome: radiographic appearance with MRI correlation. *Skeletal Radiol.* 2006;**35**(9):690–5.

27. Sung, J. Y., Kuwabara, S., Ogawara, K., Kanai, K., Hattori, T. Patterns of nerve conduction abnormalities in POEMS syndrome. *Muscle Nerve* 2002; **26**(2):189–93.

28. Saida, K., Kawakami, H., Ohta, M., Iwamura, K. Coagulation and

vascular abnormalities in Crow–Fukase syndrome. *Muscle Nerve* 1997;**20**(4):486–92.

29. Li, J., Zhang, W., Jiao, L. *et al.* Combination of melphalan and dexamethasone for patients with newly diagnosed POEMS syndrome. *Blood* 2011;**117** (24):6445–9.

30. Dispenzieri, A. POEMS syndrome: 2011 update on diagnosis, risk-stratification, and management. *Am. J. Hematol.* 2011;**86**(7):591–601.

31. Samaras, P., Bauer, S., Stenner-Liewen, F. *et al.* Treatment of POEMS syndrome with bevacizumab. *Haematologica* 2007;**92**(10):1438–9.

32. Imai, N., Taguchi, J., Yagi, N. *et al.* Relapse of polyneuropathy, organomegaly, endocrinopathy, M-protein, and skin changes (POEMS) syndrome without increased level of vascular endothelial growth factor following successful autologous peripheral blood stem cell transplantation. *Neuromusc. Disord.* 2009;**19**(5):363–5.

33. Kojima, H., Katsuoka, Y., Katsura, Y. *et al.* Successful treatment of a patient with POEMS syndrome by tandem high-dose chemotherapy with autologous CD34+ purged stem cell rescue. *Int. J. Hematol.* 2006;**84**(2):182–5.

34. Latov, N., Sherman, W. H., Nemni, R. *et al.* Plasma-cell dyscrasia and peripheral neuropathy with a monoclonal antibody to peripheral-nerve myelin. *N. Engl. J. Med.* 1980;**303** (11):618–21.

35. Quarles, R. H., Weiss, M. D. Autoantibodies associated with peripheral neuropathy. *Muscle Nerve* 1999;**22**(7):800–22.

36. Suarez, G. A., Kelly, J. J., Jr. Polyneuropathy associated with monoclonal gammopathy of undetermined significance: further evidence that IgM-MGUS neuropathies are different than

IgG-MGUS. *Neurology* 1993;
43(7):1304–8.

37. Chassande, B., Leger, J. M.,
Younes-Chennoufi, A. B. *et al.*
Peripheral neuropathy associated
with IgM monoclonal
gammopathy: correlations
between M-protein antibody
activity and clinical/
electrophysiological features in
40 cases. *Muscle Nerve* 1998;
21(1):55–62.

38. Nobile-Orazio, E., Meucci, N.,
Baldini, L., Di Troia, A., Scarlato,
G. Long-term prognosis of
neuropathy associated with anti-
MAG IgM M- proteins and its
relationship to immune therapies.
Brain 2000;**123**(Pt 4):710–17.

39. Dyck, P. J., Low, P. A.,
Windebank, A. J. *et al.* Plasma
exchange in polyneuropathy
associated with monoclonal
gammopathy of undetermined
significance. *N. Engl. J. Med.*
1991;**325**(21):1482–6.

40. Dalakas, M. C., Quarles, R. H.,
Farrer, R. G. *et al.* A controlled
study of intravenous
immunoglobulin in
demyelinating neuropathy with
IgM gammopathy. *Ann. Neurol.*
1996;**40**(5):792–5.

41. Mariette, X., Brouet, J. C.,
Chevret, S. *et al.* A randomised
double blind trial versus placebo
does not confirm the benefit of
alpha-interferon in
polyneuropathy associated with
monoclonal IgM [letter].
J. Neurol. Neurosurg. Psychiatry
2000;**69**(2):279–80.

42. Oksenhendler, E., Chevret, S.,
Leger, J. M. *et al.* Plasma exchange
and chlorambucil in
polyneuropathy associated with
monoclonal IgM gammopathy.
IgM-associated Polyneuropathy
Study Group. *J. Neurol.
Neurosurg. Psychiatry* 1995;**59**
(3):243–7.

43. Comi, G., Roveri, L., Swan, A.
et al. A randomised controlled
trial of intravenous

immunoglobulin in IgM
paraprotein associated
demyelinating neuropathy. *J.
Neurol.* 2002;**249**(10):1370–7.

44. Pestronk, A., Florence, J., Miller,
T. *et al.* Treatment of IgM
antibody associated
polyneuropathies using rituximab.
J. Neurol. Neurosurg. Psychiatry
2003;**74**(4):485–9.

45. Dispenzieri, A., Gertz, M. A.,
Witzig, T. E. Cryoglobulinemia
and heavy chain disease. In: Greer,
J. P., editor, *Wintrobe's Clinical
Hematology*. Philadelphia:
Wolters Kluwer Health/Lippincott
Williams & Wilkins; 2009,
pp. 2484–96.

46. Gorevic, P. D., Kassab, H. J., Levo,
Y. *et al.* Mixed cryoglobulinemia:
clinical aspects and long-term
follow-up of 40 patients. *Am.
J. Med.* 1980;**69**(2):287–308.

47. Dispenzieri, A., Gorevic, P. D.
Cryoglobulinemia. *Hematol.
Oncol. Clin. North Am.* 1999;**13**
(6):1315–49.

48. Monti, G., Galli, M., Invernizzi, F.
et al. Cryoglobulinaemias: a
multi-centre study of the early
clinical and laboratory
manifestations of primary and
secondary disease. GISC. Italian
Group for the Study of
Cryoglobulinaemias. *QJM*
1995;**88**(2):115–26.

49. Pascual, M., Perrin, L., Giostra, E.,
Schifferli, J. A. Hepatitis C virus in
patients with cryoglobulinemia
type II. *J. Infect. Dis.* 1990;
162(2):569–70.

50. Ferri, C., Greco, F.,
Longombardo, G. *et al.*
Antibodies to hepatitis C virus in
patients with mixed
cryoglobulinemia. *Arthritis
Rheumatism* 1991;**34**(12):1606–10.

51. Goldman, M., Renversez, J. C.,
Lambert, P. H. Pathological
expression of idiotypic
interactions: immune complexes
and cryoglobulins. *Springer
Seminars Immunopathology*
1983;**6**(1):33–49.

52. Meltzer, M., Franklin, E. C., Elias,
K., McCluskey, R. T., Cooper, N.
Cryoglobulinemia–a clinical and
laboratory study. II.
Cryoglobulins with rheumatoid
factor activity. *Am. J. Med.*
1966;**40**(6):837–56.

53. Mendez, P., Saeian, K.,
Reddy, K. R. *et al.* Hepatitis C,
cryoglobulinemia, and cutaneous
vasculitis associated with unusual
and serious manifestations.
Am. J. Gastroenterol. 2001;
96(8):2489–93.

54. Brouet, J., Clauvel, J., Danon, F.,
Klein, M., Seligmann, M.
Biological and clinical significance
of cryoglobulins. A report of
86 cases. *Am. J. Med.*
1974;**57**:775–88.

55. Donada, C., Crucitti, A.,
Donadon, V. *et al.* Systemic
manifestations and liver disease in
patients with chronic hepatitis
C and type II or III mixed
cryoglobulinaemia. *J. Viral.
Hepat.* 1998;**5**(3):179–85.

56. Montagnino, G. Reappraisal of the
clinical expression of mixed
cryoglobulinemia. *Springer
Seminars Immunopathology*
1988;**10**(1):1–19.

57. Cohen, S. J., Pittelkow, M. R., Su,
W. P. Cutaneous manifestations
of cryoglobulinemia: clinical and
histopathologic study of seventy-
two patients. *J. Am. Acad.
Dermatol.* 1991;**25**(1 Pt 1):21–7.

58. Cavaletti, G., Petruccioli, M. G.,
Crespi, V. *et al.* A clinicopathological and follow up study
of 10 cases of essential type II
cryoglobulinaemic neuropathy.
J. Neurol. Neurosurg. Psychiatry
1990;**53**(10):886–9.

59. Ammendola, A., Sampaolo, S.,
Ambrosone, L. *et al.* Peripheral
neuropathy in hepatitis-related
mixed cryoglobulinemia:
electrophysiologic follow-up
study. *Muscle Nerve* 2005;
31(3):382–5.

60. Cordonnier, D., Vialtel, P.,
Renversez, J. C. *et al.* Renal

241

Chapter

18

Treatment of emergent peripheral neuropathy in plasma cell disorders

Charise Gleason, Melanie Watson and Sagar Lonial

Introduction

Peripheral neuropathy (PN) occurs due to damage, inflammation or dysfunction to the peripheral nervous system, most likely as a result of injury to axons, myelin sheaths or the cell bodies. The extent of impaired function depends on the type of nerves affected – motor, sensory or autonomic. The onset of symptoms is variable and can present gradually or in a more rapid fashion. Symptoms range from temporary numbness, tingling, paresthesias, sensitivity to touch and weakness to more severe symptoms ranging from burning pain, muscle wasting, and to the extent of paralysis [1,2]. Typically, the longest nerves in the extremities are first affected with symmetric length dependent spreading from distal to proximal nerves [3]. The most common clinical manifestation of PN occurs in a "stocking and glove" pattern and the patients may complain of losing hand grip by dropping things or having difficulty picking up small objects. Patients with autonomic symptoms may experience labile blood pressure changes, orthostatic hypotension, irregular heart rates, changes in gastrointestinal motility, swallowing or respiratory problems [2]. PN tends to have a severe impact on quality of life and functional abilities in cancer patients and can impact overall survival or severity of full dose effective therapy [1].

Mechanism of peripheral neuropathy

Peripheral neuropathy is known to be associated with both dysproteinemias and their associated treatments. The damage or degeneration of the peripheral nerves involves sensory, motor, or autonomic nerve fibers. Some degree of PN may be present in up to 54% of newly diagnosed patients with plasma cell dyscrasias

such as monoclonal gammopathy of undetermined significance (MGUS), multiple myeloma (MM), POEMS (polyneuropathy, organomegaly, endocrinopathy, monoclonal gammopathy and skin changes syndrome), Castleman's disease, Waldenstrom's macroglobulinemia and light chain amyloidosis [1,4,5]. Neuropathy can result from nerve compression or interactions between the monoclonal protein and nerve fibers.

The strongest association between dysproteinemias and PN is found with IgM paraproteins. IgM antibodies and light chains bind to myelin-associated glycoprotein (MAG) targeting neural antigens of the myelin sheet, damaging the interface between Schwann cell and axons. Anti-MAG antibodies are found in approximately 70% of patients with neuropathy-associated IgM monoclonal gammopathy [6]. Up to 50% of patients with IgM gammopathies have symptomatic neuropathy and are categorized as IgM MGUS [7]. The presence of high anti-MAG antibodies in patients with IgM monoclonal gammopathies is known to predict the development of clinical neuropathy [8]. Clinically, the patients presenting with high anti-MAG IgM antibodies are older patients that develop paresthesias of the distal lower extremities gradually extending to the proximal lower extremities over a prolonged period of one to two decades [9]. The clinical course begins with gait ataxia, tremors, loss of vibratory and position sense and distal limb weakness progressing to proximal muscle weakness [7]. Electrophysiologic studies have shown a demyelinating process with nerve biopsies demonstrating deposits of IgM paraprotein and complement on nerve myelin and abnormally wide myelin lamellae. The intercalation of anti-MAG between the layers of myelin accounts for the widening of lamellae and demyelination [10].

Myeloma, ed. Stephen A. Schey, Kwee L. Yong, Robert Marcus and Kenneth C. Anderson. Published by Cambridge University Press. © Cambridge University Press 2014.

Therapies such as plasma exchange, steroids, cytotoxic drugs, intravenous immunoglobulin and monoclonal antibodies have been used in an attempt to target the IgM paraprotein in patients with anti-MAG with varying response. While 50% of patients may respond to these agents, the results are short lived and long-term follow up is lacking. Immune therapies may be effective in half of patients but come with considerable side effects and should be limited to patients impaired in their daily life or in a progressive phase of disease [7]. The relationship of neuropathy associated with IgA or IgG have not been described in detail.

Neuropathy is often a manifestation of systemic amyloidosis and most frequently seen in patients with hereditary transthyretin (TTR) amyloidosis [11] and characterized by predominant sensorimotor and autonomic involvement due to endoneurial and polyvisceral extracellular deposition of amyloid [12]. At the time of diagnosis, 17%–20% of patients with AL or primary amyloidosis will have PN, with symptoms often predating the diagnosis [11,13–15]. Small fiber neuropathy is often seen in amyloidosis and may be a result of pro-inflammatory cytokines and vasoactive peptides [1,4,5,16]. PN associated with amyloidosis is usually a painful, progressive, symmetric, distal sensory neuropathy that progresses to motor neuropathy and associated with autonomic dysfunction [8,17,18]. Nerve biopsies have revealed amyloid deposits in vessel walls and connective tissue with axonal degeneration [5] but the pathogenesis remains unclear. The definition of nerve involvement is primarily clinical and can be established with a sural nerve biopsy or evidence of amyloid involvement at an alternate site [19]. Cryoglobulins are also known to be associated with the nerve damage and amyloid deposits in patients with light chain amyloidosis associated PN, but their role in causation is unclear [20]. Among patients with primary amyloidosis and AL amyloidosis, the presence of PN is known to be a poor risk feature. The median survival in primary amyloidosis and AL amyloidosis patients presenting with a prominent neuropathy is 25 months [21]. Autonomic dysfunction from amyloid may range from mild postural hypotension to profound hypotension with bowel and bladder dysfunction [19].

Symptoms of nerve damage

The symptoms of PN are related to the type of affected nerve and may present over a period of days, weeks, or years. Large sensory nerves are enclosed within myelin sheaths that register and transmit vibration, touch and position sense. Sensory nerve damage can cause a more complex range of symptoms including painful parasthesias, dysesthesias, cold sensitivity, numbness, tingling, alteration in proprioception, or changes in reflexes. Small sensory fibers without myelin sheaths transmit pain and temperature. Injury to these fibers can render over-sensitization of the pain receptors and interfere with the ability to feel pain or temperature changes. PN associated with motor nerves that affect the muscles of movement manifest as muscle weakness. Autonomic nervous system associated PN may present as gastrointestinal disturbances such as diarrhea or constipation, sexual dysfunction, urinary retention, orthostatic hypotension, and gastrointestinal motility and swallowing issues [2].

Chemotherapy-induced peripheral neuropathy

Chemotherapy-induced peripheral neuropathy (CIPN) remains a major dose cause of morbidity in the treatment of plasma cell disorders, especially with the proteosome inhibitor bortezomib and the immunomodulatory agent thalidomide. The management of CIPN has largely been supportive [22]. Besides bortezomib and thalidomide, various cytotoxic therapies such as taxanes, platinum compounds, and vinca-alkaloids are associated with CIPN [23, 24]. These cytotoxic agents have played a lesser role in the treatment of plasma cell dyscrasias in the last decade, nevertheless are still used. Primary nerve toxicity with platinum drugs occurs at the dorsal root ganglion (DRG) with small sensory fibers affected most frequently. These nerves have little capacity for regeneration and therefore the majority of the damage is predominantly sensory and irreversible [2]. Treatment options can be limited as they may exacerbate existing PN and further impact overall quality of life. Other factors to consider that can affect CIPN include age, chemotherapy dose, cumulative dosing, therapy duration, co-administration of other neurotoxic agents, and pre-existing conditions such as AL amyloidosis, alcoholism, diabetes, etc. [25].

Immunomodulatory agents
Thalidomide

Thalidomide is an immunomodulatory agent which is part of a class of small molecule anticancer and anti-inflammatory drugs with broad biologic activities

Table 18.1 Dose modifications for bortezomib and thalidomide induced PN per NCI CTCAE v3.0 toxicity criteria

Toxicity grade of PN	Bortezomib	Thalidomide
Grade 1 toxicity (paresthesias, weakness and/or loss of reflexes) without pain or loss of function	Observation	Observation
Grade 1 toxicity with pain or grade 2 toxicity (interfering with function but not with activities of daily living)	Bortezomib should be reduced to 1 mg/m^2	Thalidomide should be reduced to 50% dose or withhold thalidomide therapy until toxicity resolves and reinitiate with 50% dose reduction
Grade 2 toxicity with pain or grade 3 (interfering with activities of daily living)	Withhold bortezomib therapy until toxicity resolves. Reinitiate with reduced dose of bortezomib at 0.7 mg/m^2 and change treatment schedule to once weekly	Withhold thalidomide therapy until toxicity resolves or ≤ grade 1. Thalidomide should be discontinued if neuropathy does not improve to ≤ grade 1.
Grade 4 toxicities (sensory neuropathy which is disabling or motor neuropathy that is life threatening or leads to paralysis).	Bortezomib should be discontinued	Thalidomide should be discontinued

(although the molecular mechanism has largely been undefined) [26]. Thalidomide was first used in the 1950s as a sedative-hypnotic drug and as an anti-emetic. It was withdrawn from the market in 1961 and, even at that time, incidents of neuropathy were reported [27]. The major predictor of developing peripheral neuropathy while on thalidomide was duration of exposure with the rate of development rising dramatically between six and 12 months from 40% to almost 75% [28]. Based on these findings and a systematic review of the data, it is recommended that optimal dosing of thalidomide should be no more than six months [29,30]. Because of the toxicity of thalidomide over extended exposure time, it recommended to avoid daily doses higher than 200 mg [29]. PN remains one of the most relevant side effects reported with thalidomide use.

The mechanisms of action for thalidomide and its anti-myeloma effects are thought to be mediated by multiple immunomodulatory targets as well as angiogenesis inhibition via vascular endothelial growth factor blockade [31]. TNF-α synthesis is inhibited and there is a blockade of NF-κB [32,33]. Owing to the anti-angiogenetic properties of thalidomide, there are direct toxic effects on neurons of the posterior root ganglia through effects of thalidomide on NF-κB [24]. The neurologic complications of thalidomide occur after prolonged exposure with clinical manifestations including bilateral and symmetrical sensory disorders.

Age, sex and prior therapy were not predictive and motor involvement is rare except in extreme cases. Typically patients experience distal paresthesias and hyperasthesias that initially affect the toes and fingers and may extend proximally. Later in the course, proprioception and vibratory sensation may be affected, leading to difficulty ambulating [24]. Thalidomide is most commonly reported to produce length-dependent axonal neuropathy [34]. Sinus bradycardia may occur as a result of autonomic neuropathy in patients receiving thalidomide and can be severe enough to cause syncope [35]. Dose modifications for thalidomide induced PN are included in Table 18.1 and if caught early may improve. Up to 90% of patients with a grade 2 or above neuropathy improved to a lower grade of neuropathy within four months [36]. If treatment is not stopped, PN can progress to permanent nerve damage and could become irreversible. A dose modification schedule is shown in Table 18.1.

Lenalidomide

Lenalidomide is a second generation immunomodulatory drug class and an analog of thalidomide with more potent anti-inflammatory and antiangiogenic activities than thalidomide. It has a more favorable side effect profile than thalidomide with less neurotoxicity reported. In phase 1 and 2 trials in relapsed/refractory patients [37], lenalidomide did not cause significant neuropathy and phase 3 studies confirmed the results. Grade 3–4 neuropathy was reported in less than 5% of patients [38,39]. There are few case reports that lenalidomide is associated with mild to moderated PN most notably in combination with other neurotoxic drug use such as vincristine, thalidomide or bortezomib [40], but in practical clinical settings, lenalidomide induced PN is rare and usually mild.

Pomalidomide

Pomalidomide is a newer immunomodulatory agent currently used in clinical trials with data suggesting it to be the most potent in the class [41]. Data from this phase II trial noted a total of 24 patients (40%) experiencing PN during treatment (grade 1, $n = 18$; grade 2, $n = 5$; grade 3, $n = 1$); and of those 24 patients, 14% had neuropathy at baseline. Among 33 patients with no reported neuropathy at baseline, 30% reported neuropathy during treatment and all grade 1. In lenalidomide refractory patients, Lacy et al. [42] report that a total of nine patients (26%) experienced PN during treatment (grade 1, $n = 6$; grade 2 = 3). There are currently no available data on incidence.

Proteosome inhibitors

Bortezomib

Bortezomib is a first-generation proteosome inhibitor that is a boronic acid derivative that reversibly inhibits the 26S proteosome leading to cell cycle arrest and apoptosis. Management of bortezomib induced PN (BIPN) remains an important clinical issue and the mechanism the neuropathy remains unknown. Proteasome inhibition may result in the accumulation of damaged protein, which may interfere with neuronal function [43]. BIPN typically occurs in the early cycles of therapy after a median of three months, and plateau around cycle 5 of therapy [44, 45]. PN can also occur subacutely as early as cycle 1 of therapy. BIPN was first observed in phase 1 studies [46–48] and as a result effort was made to assess PN in the pivotal phase 2 trials [49,50]. The phase 2 trials included a total 256 patients with 37% of these patients reporting PN, though grade 3 occurred in only 14%. The PN is usually more sensory than motor with pain, paresthesia, burning, numbness, sensory loss and dysesthesia overall most commonly affecting the feet [51]. BIPN was less frequent with a lower dose or weekly schedule of bortezomib [45,50]. Burning sensations may occur

at rest, and are usually confined to the soles of the feet though can be present in fingers and the palmar sides of the hands [20].

While motor impairment is rare, motor neuropathy consisting of mild to severe distal weakness in the lower extremities may occur in approximately 10% of patients with cases of grade 4 motor neurotoxicity [52,53]. Study reports note that PN associated with bortezomib tends to be a cumulative, dose related adverse effect that increases in prevalence through the first five cycles of therapy and most patients experienced resolution of improvement of their neuropathic symptoms with dose modification or completion of therapy [45]. Symptoms of autonomic neuropathy may also complicate bortezomib therapy. Bortezomib has been traditionally dosed IV on a once weekly or twice weekly schedule. Newer phase 3 data comparing IV versus subcutaneous route of administration report significantly lower all grade PN events with acceptable local tolerability at subcutaneous site [54]. Since bortezomib induced neuropathy is dose dependent and often reversible, a regular clinical evaluation of symptoms and performance status and use of an algorithm with treatment modifications is essential. A dose modification schedule is included in Table 18.1.

Carfilzomib

Carfilzomib is a novel proteosome inhibitor of the epoxyketone class that is structurally distinct from bortezomib and associated with a low rate of treatment related PN [55–57]. In phase I and II trials, there were no reports noted of dose-limiting PN in patients with relapsed/refractory myeloma [55–57]. In the PX-171–003 phase II trial of relapsed/refractory myeloma, 77% of patients had grade 1 and 2 PN at baseline and, despite this, fewer than 10% of patients developed treatment emergent PN [58]. In the PX-171–004 phase II in patients with relapsed myeloma, 69% presented with a history of PN and 53% with active PN of grade 1 and 2, yet treatment induced PN was again infrequent with 15.3% in cohort 1 and 17.1% in cohort 2 [59]. Only one patient developed a grade 3 PN and no patients developed grade 4 PN. To date, carfizomib appears substantially less neurotoxic than bortezomib.

Predisposing factors

The possibility of predisposing factors related to CIPN has been explored with mixed results. Genotyping has been used to address the hypothesis that there is a genetic variation associated with the risk of developing PN. Results from the Intergroupe Francophone du Myeloma trials and the HOVAN-65/GMMG-HD4 in patients previously not exposed to bortezomib, identified gene expression profiles in MM associated with bortezomib induced PN as well as vincristine induced PN, and significantly associated single-nucleotide polymorphisms (SNPs) [60]. Genes involved with drug induced apoptosis, mitochondrial dysfunction, and peripheral nervous system development were associated with early-onset bortezomib induced PN and peripheral blood analyses identified SNPs located in genes involved with the development and function of the nervous system, DNA repair and apoptosis [60]. Genes involved in late-onset bortezomib induced PN also included genes involved in the nervous system but significant SNPs were identified in inflammatory genes and DNA repair genes. When comparing vincristine induced PN, a different set of genes was identified, suggesting that both myeloma related factors and genetic factors play a role in the development of bortezomib induced PN [60].

Management of agents in the context of pre-existing PN

For many different reasons, patients may have pre-existing PN that may complicate the decisions about how to approach therapy and which agents to use. This can arise for one of two reasons. First, there may be patients with pre-existing PN as a consequence of non-plasma cell related causes such as diabetes, peripheral vascular disease or other acquired causes for PN. Among these patients, the margin for developing treatment related toxicity is much narrower, hence agents such as bortezomib or thalidomide at standard dose and schedule may not be an optimal or first choice. If one were to use bortezomib, it would be preferable to use the subcutaneous route to minimize treatment emergent PN. Other options could include the use of combination treatments where weekly bortezomib can be administered, or the use of the newer proteasome inhibitors, such as carfilzomib or MLN 9708, which appear to have a lower incidence of PN when used in the standard dose and schedule. The use of low dose thalidomide may have a lower incidence of PN, but this can still be an issue among patients with pre-existing PN, and thus the use of thalidomide may need to be minimized or avoided if possible. Alternatives such as lenalidomide could provide good

efficacy with reduced toxicity. Among patients whose PN is related to the underlying plasma cell disorder, the same caution as above needs to be employed; however, in these cases, PN may actually improve with therapy, and thus while vigilance is clearly important, the net result of using agents with the potential for PN may be less PN as a consequence of reduction in disease burden.

Evaluation

PN severity can be quantified with the National Cancer Institute (NCI) Common Terminology Criteria for Adverse Events (CTCAE). The NCI CTCAE v3.0 defines grades 1–5 using clinical descriptions; each assigned a severity. Grade 1 is mild, grade 2 is moderate, grade 3 is severe, grade 4 is life threatening or disabling, and grade 5 defines death related to the adverse event [61] This tool can be used to assess and grade PN objectively and is used widely in clinical trials. Figure 18.1 encompasses the NCI CTCAE v3.0 version with appropriate dose modifications for bortezomib and thalidomide toxicities. The neurotoxicity assessment tool [62](Figure 18.1) can help healthcare providers assess neurotoxicity, though scores do not correlate with the NCI CTCAE [63]. Cavelitti et al. [64] compared assessment tools and note that scores mix impairment, disability and quality of life measures, which could lead to misinterpretation of results. As a result, there is a general recognition that CIPN is still not properly assessed and better assessment and improvements need to be made. Neurophysiologic tests such as electromyography (EMG), nerve conduction studies (NCS), and quantitative sensory tests (QST) have been used to assess the peripheral nervous system. These tests can be expensive and somewhat invasive, and not readily available to all clinicians or patients [2]. It should also be noted that changes on EMG and NCS can lag behind the onset of neurotoxic symptoms.

Pharmacologic interventions

There are many agents proposed in the treatment of PN caused by antineoplastic agents with very little supportive data. Most of the current therapies in management of PN have been extrapolated from studies of neuropathic pain due to diabetes and post-herpetic neuralgia. There have been no prospective randomized studies to evaluate prophylactic pharmacologic interventions. The first line therapies

FACT/GOG-NTX (Version 4)

Figure 18.1 FACT/GOG-NTX (version 4.0).

Please circle or mark one number per line to indicate your response as it applies to the <u>past 7 days.</u>

	ADDITIONAL CONCERNS	Not at all	A little bit	Some-what	Quite a bit	Very much
NTX 1	I have numbness or tingling in my hands.................	0	1	2	3	4
NTX 2	I have numbness or tingling in my feet......................	0	1	2	3	4
NTX 3	I feel discomfort in my hands....................................	0	1	2	3	4
NTX 4	I feel discomfort in my feet..	0	1	2	3	4
NTX 5	I have joint pain or muscle cramps...........................	0	1	2	3	4
H12	I feel weak all over..	0	1	2	3	4
NTX 6	I have trouble hearing...	0	1	2	3	4
NTX 7	I get a ringing or buzzing in my ears.........................	0	1	2	3	4
NTX 8	I have trouble buttoning buttons.................................	0	1	2	3	4
NTX 9	I have trouble feeling the shape of small objects when they are in my hand...	0	1	2	3	4
And	I have trouble walking...	0	1	2	3	4

include opioids, gabapentin and other gabanergic agents (i.e. pregabalin), topical lidocaine, tramadol, tricyclic antidepressants and serotonin norepinephrine reuptake inhibitors (i.e. duloxetine) [65]. Topical application of capsaicin cream also may be of benefit in selected patients [66]. Opioid analgesics and tramadol are recommended as the mainstay of treatment for neuropathic pain.

A wide variety of supplements are currently recommended to treat the symptoms and side effects of PN. Vitamin E, alpha-lipoic acid, glutathione, B vitamins, folic acid, glutamine and acetyl-L-carnitine have been reportedly effective [1,67]. The use of supplements however, remains largely anecdotal and findings were extrapolated from various trials attempting to reduce neuropathy [1,68]. Vitamin E may help with neuropathy associated with platinum-based chemotherapy and has been studied in three small open-labeled studies randomizing 30–47 cancer patients receiving mostly cisplatin to vitamin E or control. The active arms were associated with lower incidence of CIPN compared to the control arm [69–71]. In a phase 3 [72] trial 108 patients treated with cisplatin were randomly assigned to receive vitamin E supplementation or placebo. The severity of neurotoxicity, measured with a validated neurotoxicity score (Total Neuropathy Score [TNS]),

was significantly lower in patients receiving vitamin E than those receiving placebo (mean TNS 1.4 vs. 4.1; $p < 0.01$).

Richardson *et al.* [73] noted potential benefits from the use of supplements, with lower rates of grade 3 neuropathy. The study suggested Vitamin B12 and folic acid deficiencies need to be monitored and corrected to reduce the incidence of PN. High-dose vitamin C is not recommended as it has been indicated to have an inhibitory effect with bortezomib efficacy [74]. Few studies have documented that large doses of pyridoxine (B6) can cause injury to the sensory neurons, especially in the setting of renal insufficiency and in association with a protein-deficient diet [75,76]. L-carnitine and alpha-lipoic acid have been used in Europe for treatment of diabetic neuropathy and docetaxel induced PN [77]. Alpha-lipoic acid has also been shown to improve diabetic neuropathy [78–80]. There are currently trials evaluating the effects of glutamine and glutathione on reducing neuropathy related to platinum-based therapies [81–84].

Conclusion

Treatment for plasma cell disorders has changed with the emergence of newer available agents, with more on the horizon. The novel agents bortezomib and thalidomide have made a tremendous impact on the outcomes of plasma cell dyscrasias including myeloma and amyloidosis. Even though the newer proteasome inhibitors (carfilzomib) and the newer IMiDs (lenalidomide and pomalidomide) are associated with a lower incidence of PN, current therapeutic strategies for plasma cell disorders involve a wide use of both bortezomib and thalidomide. These drugs have led to improved outcomes, but drug induced PN remains a challenge to healthcare providers and has an impact on overall quality of life. Hence, the tools to accurately identify PN and earlier recognition of PN are needed to prevent unwanted consequences.

A major challenge is to identify the subsets of patients that are more prone to develop PN as a result of these therapies. Better understanding of the mechanisms of neurotoxicity will help with identification of more successful neuroprotective strategies. Current electrophysiological assessment techniques by themselves are insufficient to make the diagnosis. A comprehensive assessment tool incorporating the electrophysiological techniques and clinical evaluation with adequate neurological toxicity questioning will aid in the early identification to make appropriate dose reductions and prevent the debilitating consequences of PN.

References

1. Tariman, J., Love, G. et al. Peripheral neuropathy associated with novel therapies in patients with multiple myeloma: concensus statement of the IMF nurse leadership board. Clin. J. Oncol. Nurs. 2008;12(3):29–36.

2. Stubblefield, M. D. et al. NCCN Task Force Report: Management of neuropathy in cancer. Natl Comp. Cancer Network 2009;7 (Suppl 5):S1–26.

3. Kelly, J. The evaluation of peripheral neuropathy. Part I: clinical and laboratory evidence. Rev. Neurol. Dis. 2004;1:133–40.

4. Ropper, A., Gorson, K. Neuropathies associated with paraproteinemia. N. Engl. J. Med. 1998;338:1601–7.

5. Dispenzieri, A., Kyle R. A. Neurological aspects of multiple myeloma and related disorders. Best practice & research. Clin. Haematol. 2005;18(4):673–88.

6. Kuijf, M. L. et al. Detection of anti-MAG antibodies in polyneuropathy associated with IgM monoclonal gammopathy. Neurology 2009;73(9):688–95.

7. Nobile-Orazio, E. et al. Long-term prognosis of neuropathy associated with anti-mag IgM M-proteins and its relationship to immune therapies. J. Peripheral Nerv. System 2000;5(4):239–40.

8. Silberman, J., Lonial, S. Review of peripheral neuropathy in plasma cell disorders. Hematol. Oncol. 2008;26(2):55–65.

9. Steck, A. J. et al. Peripheral neuropathy associated with monoclonal IgM autoantibody. Annals Neurol. 1987;22(6):764–7.

10. Vital, A. Paraproteinemic neuropathies. Brain Pathology 2001;11(4):399–407.

11. Benson, M. D., Kincaid, J. C. The molecular biology and clinical features of amyloid neuropathy. Muscle Nerve 2007;36(4):411–23.

12. Plante-Bordeneuve, V., Said, G. Transthyretin related familial amyloid polyneuropathy. Curr. Opin. Neurol. 2000;13(5):569–73.

13. Kyle, R., Greipp, P. Amyloidosis (AL): clinical and laboratory features in 229 cases. Mayo Clin. Proc. 1983;58:665–83.

14. Duston, M. A. et al. Peripheral neuropathy as an early marker of AL amyloidosis. Arch. Intern. Med. 1989;149(2):358–60.

15. Rajkumar, S. V., Gertz, M. A., Kyle, R. A. Prognosis of patients with primary systemic amyloidosis who present with dominant neuropathy 11 Supported in part by the Quade Amyloidosis Research Foundation and Program Project Grant No. CA 62242, National Cancer Institute (National Institutes of Health). Am. J. Med. 1998; 104(3):232–7.

16. Argyriou, A. A., Iconomou, G., Kalofonos, H. P. Bortezomib-induced peripheral neuropathy in multiple myeloma: a comprehensive review of the literature. Blood 2008;112(5): 1593–9.

17. Sanchorawala, V. AL (immunoglobulin light-chain) amyloidosis. Myeloma Therapy Pursuing the Plasma Cell, 2008:551–69.

18. Reilly, M. M., Staunton, H. Peripheral nerve amyloidosis. Brain Pathology 1996;6(2): 163–77.

19. Gertz, M. A. et al. Definition of organ involvement and treatment response in immunoglobulin light chain amyloidosis (AL): a consensus opinion from the 10th International Symposium on Amyloid and Amyloidosis. Am. J. Hematol. 2005;79(4):319–28.

20. Sonneveld, P., Jongen, J. L. M. Dealing with neuropathy in plasma-cell dyscrasias. Hematology 2010;2010(1):423–30.

21. Kyle, R. A., Gertz, M. A. Primary systemic amyloidosis: clinical and laboratory features in 474 cases. Semin. Hematol. 1995;32(1): 45–59.

22. Hausheer, F. H. et al. Diagnosis, management, and evaluation of

protein-deficient diet. *J. Appl. Toxicol.* 2004;**24**(6):497–500.

77. Gedlicka, C. *et al.* Effective treatment of oxaliplatin-induced cumulative polyneuropathy with alpha-lipoic acid. *J. Clin. Oncol.* 2002;**20**(15):3359–61.

78. Sima, A. A. F. *et al.* Acetyl-L-carnitine improves pain, nerve regeneration, and vibratory perception in patients with chronic diabetic neuropathy. *Diabetes Care* 2005;**28**(1):89–94.

79. Tang, J. *et al.* Alpha-lipoic acid may improve symptomatic diabetic polyneuropathy. *Neurologist* 2007;**13**(3):164–7.

80. Ziegler, D. Treatment of diabetic neuropathy and neuropathic pain. *Diabetes Care* 2008;**31**(Suppl 2):S255–S261.

81. Smyth, J. F. *et al.* Glutathione reduces the toxicity and improves quality of life of women diagnosed with ovarian cancer treated with cisplatin: Results of a double-blind, randomised trial. *Ann. Oncol.*, 1997;**8**(6):569–73.

82. Cascinu, S. *et al.* Neuroprotective effect of reduced glutathione on cisplatin-based chemotherapy in advanced gastric cancer: a randomized double-blind placebo-controlled trial. *J. Clin. Oncol.*, 1995;**13**(1):26–32.

83. Cascinu, S. *et al.* Neuroprotective effect of reduced glutathione on oxaliplatin-based chemotherapy in advanced colorectal cancer: a randomized, double-blind, placebo-controlled trial. *J. Clin. Oncol.*, 2002;**20**(16):3478–83.

84. Wang, W. -S. *et al.* Oral glutamine is effective for preventing oxaliplatin-induced neuropathy in colorectal cancer patients. *The Oncologist* 2007;**12**(3):312–19.

Chapter

19

Management of renal failure in multiple myeloma

Aneel Paulus, Pooja Advani, Nabeel Aslam and
Asher Alban Chanan-Khan

Introduction

Renal failure is a common complication observed in patients with multiple myeloma (MM) and other plasma cell cancers that is generally associated with an adverse clinical outcome [1]. The optimal management of MM patients with renal disease presents a challenge. As numerous drugs are cleared via the kidneys, renal impairment imposes limitation on anti-myeloma therapeutics through decreased drug clearance and enhanced toxicity [1]. Thus optimal renal function assessment is essential, often involving measurements of glomerular filtration rate (GFR), serum creatinine (sCr) levels, and creatinine clearance (CrCl) rates. However, the exact definition and incidence of "renal failure" varies among investigators and depends on the measurement parameter being used. The Kidney Disease Outcomes Quality Initiative (K/DOQI) of the National Kidney Foundation defines kidney disease as either kidney damage or a decreased GFR of <60 ml/min/1.73 m^2 for ≥ 3 months [2]. Using the KDOQI criteria, we observed that 54% of patients seen at Roswell Park Cancer Institute presented with stage ≥ 3 (<60 ml/min/1.73 m^2) kidney disease at the time of diagnosis [3]. When sCr is used to assess kidney function, a value of ≥ 2 mg/dl specifies impairment and is present in approximately 20% of MM patients [4–7]. Although measurement of sCr is simple and relatively the least cumbersome approach, it varies with age, sex and muscle mass, and is not an absolute reflection of renal function [8]. Patients with MM tend to be elderly with normal or low muscle mass and thus sCr may be lower for a given GFR or CrCl rate. As such, the extent of renal insufficiency is often underestimated in these patients when sCr alone is utilized to assess kidney function [8–13].

A more accurate estimation of kidney function can be determined through GFR calculation; however, it is difficult to directly measure [9]. The most commonly used formulas for calculating GFR are the Modification of Diet in Renal Disease (MDRD) [9] and the Cockcroft–Gault formulas [14]. MDRD tends to overvalue GFR in underweight individuals, while the Cockcroft–Gault formula overestimates GFR in heavier patients. The Cockcroft–Gault formula may be preferable for MM patients with normal to low weight. The International Myeloma Working Group (IMWG) recommends using the MDRD formula for the assessment of renal dysfunction in MM patients [15] with subsequent classification into the five stages of renal impairment according to the KDIGO (Kidney Disease Improving Global Outcomes) classification system (Table 19.1).

The MDRD and Cockcroft–Gault prediction equations have only been validated in patients with chronic kidney disease (CKD); thus alternate criteria must be used to assess renal function in MM patients with acute kidney injury (AKI). The RIFLE (risk, injury, failure, loss and end-stage kidney disease) and AKIN (Acute Kidney Injury Network) criteria have been developed to define and classify the severity of AKI [16,17]. Despite being extensively studied in more than 550 000 patients worldwide [18] these criteria have not been validated in MM patients.

Pathogenesis of renal disease in MM

MM related renal failure has a variable and complex pathology (Figure 19.1). Most commonly, renal damage in MM is due to excess nephrotoxic immunoglobulin (Ig) free light chains (FLCs) filtering into the proximal and distal tubules;

Myeloma, ed. Stephen A. Schey, Kwee L. Yong, Robert Marcus and Kenneth C. Anderson. Published by Cambridge University Press. © Cambridge University Press 2014.

Table 19.1 KDIGO classification of chronic kidney disease

Stage of renal damage	Stage 1	Stage 2	Stage 3	Stage 4	Stage 5
Extent of renal damage	Renal damage with normal or increased GFR	Renal damage with mild decrease of GFR	Renal damage with moderate decrease in GFR	Severe decrease in GFR	End stage renal disease
eGFR (ml/min/1.73m^2)	≥90	60–89	30–59	15–29	<15 or on dialysis
Remaining renal function	≥90%	60%–89%	30%–59%	15%–29%	<15%
Prevalence in USA (95% CI)	3.3%	3.0%	4.3%	0.2%	0.1%

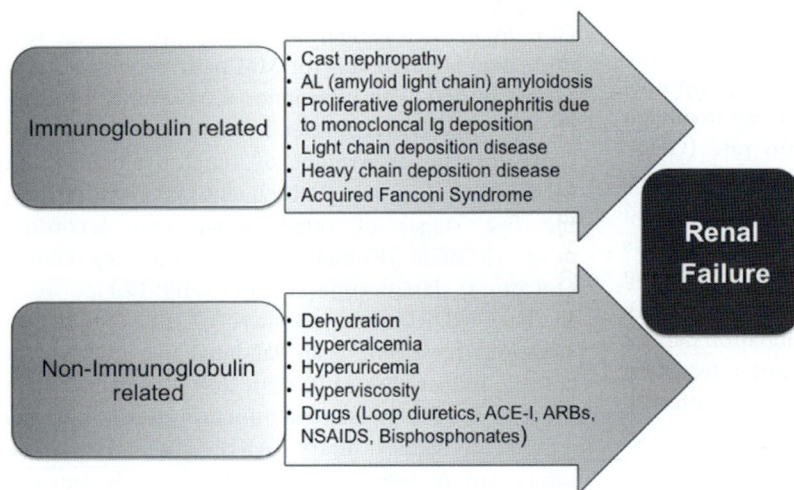

Figure 19.1 Causes of renal disease in multiple myeloma.

relatively sparing the glomeruli. FLC fragments alone may damage the tubules or by forming aggregate casts with secreted intratubular proteins, resulting in obstruction [19]. Other Ig related entities such as amyloidosis, monoclonal Ig deposition diseases, and acquired Fanconi's syndrome also cause renal dysfunction, albeit through different pathogenic mechanisms. These various Ig related renal diseases can rarely present in combination with one another [20]. Non-Ig related causes of renal failure seen in MM include hypercalcemia, volume depletion (reduced renal blood flow), use of nephrotoxic drugs and radiologic contrast dyes, hyperuricemia and hyperviscosity [21].

Cast nephropathy

Cast nephropathy (myeloma kidney) represents the most common diagnosis of renal dysfunction in MM, accounting for 40%–60% of cases [22–24]. Light chains are synthesized as κ (25 kDa) or λ (50 kDa) small molecules and are physiologically filtered across the glomerulus into the proximal tubules. Here, FLCs bind to the multi-ligand receptors, cubilin/megalin and are then endocytosed into the proximal tubular cells via the clathrin dependent endosomal/lysosomal pathway. Subsequently these are degraded within the lysosomes. The overproduction of FLCs in MM results in increased excretion and filtration across

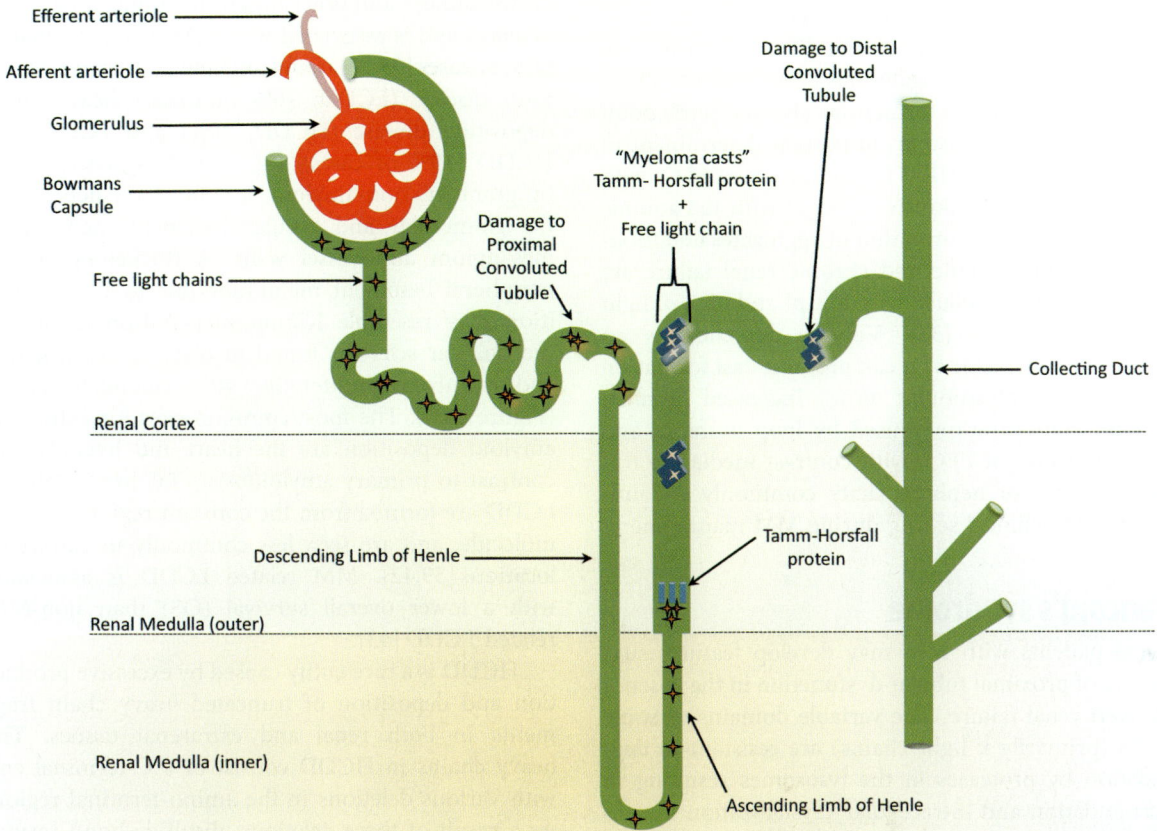

Figure 19.2 Pathogenesis of cast nephropathy in multiple myeloma.

the glomerulus. The latter can overwhelm the lysosomal degradation capacity of proximal tubule cells, resulting in their necrosis and apoptosis [25–28]. When the capacity of the proximal tubule cells to catabolize FLCs is exceeded by their production, FLCs begin to appear in the tubular fluid of the distal nephron where they complex with Tamm–Horsfall proteins (THP) (Figure 19.2). THP, a glycoprotein, is secreted in the thick ascending limb of the loop of Henle and forms the matrix of most urinary casts. The FLCs (via their complementary determining region 3) interact with a 9-amino-acid-binding domain on the THP to form intratubular casts, which result in obstruction of the distal nephron [29]. Volume depletion, acidosis, hypercalcemia and loop diuretics may exacerbate cast formation, thereby encouraging FLC induced renal damage. Addition of

furosemide to rat nephrons previously infused with FLCs demonstrated enhanced cast formation [30]. Increased intraluminal pressure from tubular obstruction contributes to renal dysfunction by decreasing the GFR and interstitial blood flow. Furthermore, endocytosis of FLCs by proximal tubule cells results in NF-κB mediated activation of the proinflammatory cytokines IL-6, IL-8, TNF-α, and MCP-1. In turn, these induce interstitial inflammation and fibrosis [31].

Some patients develop significant renal impairment even in the presence of a small amount of FLCs due to the ability of the light chains to manifest their own unique nephrotoxic effects [30,32]. The ability to form intratubular casts may be determined by certain properties of the FLC. For example, light chains with a greater affinity for THP binding have a higher

257

tendency to produce casts with resulting tubular obstruction. However, in the presence of aggravating factors such as hypovolemia, FLCs with even moderate affinity for THPs may result in cast formation [5]. Likewise, the tendency of the FLC to form high molecular weight aggregates has been shown to influence intratubular cast formation. The isoelectric point (pI) of the FLC is also an important determinant of FLC binding with THP. The interaction of FLCs with a pI above 5.1 (net positive charge) with the anionic THP may promote formation of aggregates and tubular obstruction. Acute and chronic renal failure are reported to be associated with low pI and high pI light chains, respectively [33]. Volume depletion is an important risk factor as it can promote cast formation by slowing intratubular flow. Increased luminal sodium concentration caused by loop diuretics and the interaction of FLCs with contrast media are frequent causes of nephrotoxicity commonly encountered in the clinical setting during MM management.

Fanconi's syndrome

Some patients with MM may develop features suggestive of proximal tubular dysfunction in the absence of overt renal failure. The variable domains of some FLCs (primarily κ light chains) are resistant to degradation by proteases in the lysosomes resulting in accumulation and intracellular crystallization in cells of the proximal tubules [34]. The clinical manifestation is proximal renal tubular acidosis (Fanconi's syndrome). The crystalline inclusions interfere with the function of the membrane transporters resulting in glucosuria, phosphaturia, aminoaciduria, bicarbonaturia, hypophosphatemia and hypouricemia [35].

Amyloidosis

AL (primary) amyloidosis refers to the renal deposition of FLCs in an anti-parallel beta-pleated sheet configuration [36]. This is noted in approximately 30% of patients with MM, and is most commonly affiliated with IgD myeloma [37]. The amyloid deposits are predominantly composed of N-terminal fragments of the λ light chain variable regions [38]. The glomeruli are involved in most cases (80%) causing non-specific proteinuria while amyloid deposition in the renal vessels and tubular-interstitium (10%) results in renal dysfunction without nephrotic syndrome [38].

Monoclonal Ig deposition disease

Monoclonal Ig deposition disease refers to infiltration of the kidneys and other organs by monoclonal paraproteins and is associated with MM in approximately 65% of cases [39]. Variants include light chain deposition disease (LCDD, 70% of cases), heavy chain deposition disease (HCDD, 20%) and LCDD plus HCDD (10% of cases) [40]. LCDD is characterized by granular, non-amyloid, κ-light chain deposits in the glomerular and tubular basement membranes, mesangium and vessel walls. A thickening of the peripheral basement membrane due to FLC deposition may resemble Kimmelstiel–Wilson lesions or the nodular sclerosis found in diabetic nephropathy and membranoproliferative glomerulonephritis [40] (Figure 19.3). The most common sites for extrarenal amyloid deposition are the heart and liver [41]. In contrast to primary amyloidosis, FLC precipitates in LCDD are formed from the constant region of the Ig molecule, and are seen less commonly in extrarenal locations [39,42]. MM related LCDD is associated with a lower overall survival (OS) than non-MM related LCDD [43].

HCDD is a rare entity caused by excessive production and deposition of truncated heavy chain fragments in both renal and extrarenal tissues. The heavy chains in HCDD consist of a C-terminal end with various deletions in the amino-terminal region. As a result of these deletions, disulfide bond formation between light chains and heavy chains do not occur thereby allowing free heavy chain deposition [44]. HCDD is classified according to the type

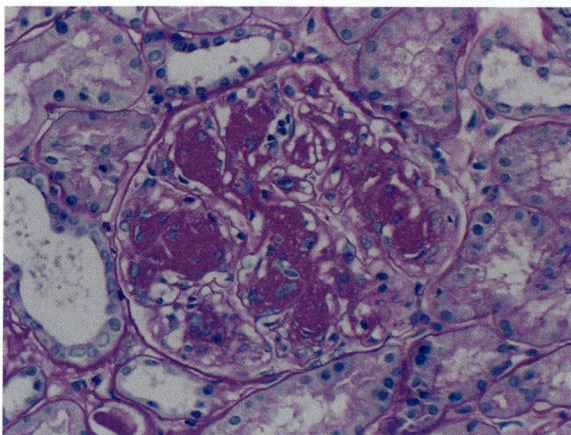

Figure 19.3 Nodular sclerosing glomerulopathy in LCDD. (Courtesy of Dr. Samih H. Nasr.)

of Ig (α-HCD, γ-HCD, and μ-HCD in order of frequency) implicated in deposition and extended follow up shows progressive renal failure in almost all HCDD cases [45].

Diagnosis of renal disease in MM

Asymptomatic proteinurea and an increase in sCr are suggestive of renal disease in MM patients. A measurement of 24 h CrCl, urine protein electrophoresis (UPEP) with immunofixation (IFE), serum protein electrophoresis (SPEP) with IFE and measurement of plasma FLC are recommended for initial assessment of MM type, burden and effect on kidneys (Figures 19.4a, b). A renal biopsy to confirm diagnosis of cast nephropathy, LCCD or amyloidosis should be performed whenever possible as renal histology provides critical information with regard to survival [24]. No specific gross abnormalities are identified in the kidneys of patients with cast nephropathy. Features suggestive of myeloma kidney are typically identified in the tubular-interstitial compartment, whereas the glomeruli and vasculature are usually normal. Typical light microscopy findings include large, irregular, refractile, angulated casts with fracture planes, surrounded by multinucleated giant cells, reflecting cytokine induced inflammatory reaction [46] (Figure 19.5a). These structures are strongly eosinophilic, non-argyrophilic and stain Periodic acid–Schiff stain positive [47,48].

In cases of suspected primary amyloidosis, confirmation of diagnosis of systemic disease is achieved through biopsy of subcutaneous fat, rectal, or renal tissue [42]. Upon tissue examination, amyloid deposits produce an apple green birefringence under polarized light when stained with Congo red dye, and can be found anywhere in the kidney but predominantly in the glomeruli [49] (Figure 19.5b). Renal ultrasound is also beneficial, as it may show kidney enlargement [3].

LCDD and primary amyloidosis share considerable overlap and may both present with heavy proteinurea, hypoalbuminemia, and edema similar to that seen in nephrotic syndromes [42]. Almost all patients with LCDD present with severe renal dysfunction, which manifests as tubulointerstitial fibrosis due to involvement of the tubular basement membrane and Bowman's capsule [50]. FLC deposition may also occur in the glomeruli and the presentation is that of a nephrotic syndrome [40]. In contrast to primary amyloidosis, FLC precipitates in LCDD do not stain with Congo red or thioflavine-T. Also, the light chain seen in primary amyloidosis is of the λ variant in approximately 80% of patients [49], whereas LCDD cases are associated with κFLCs [39]. Diagnosis of LCDD is supported by immunofluorescence and electron microscopy of renal tissues (Figure 19.5c).

Patients with acquired Fanconi's syndrome often present with glycosuria, aminoaciduria, hypophosphatemia

(a)

(b)

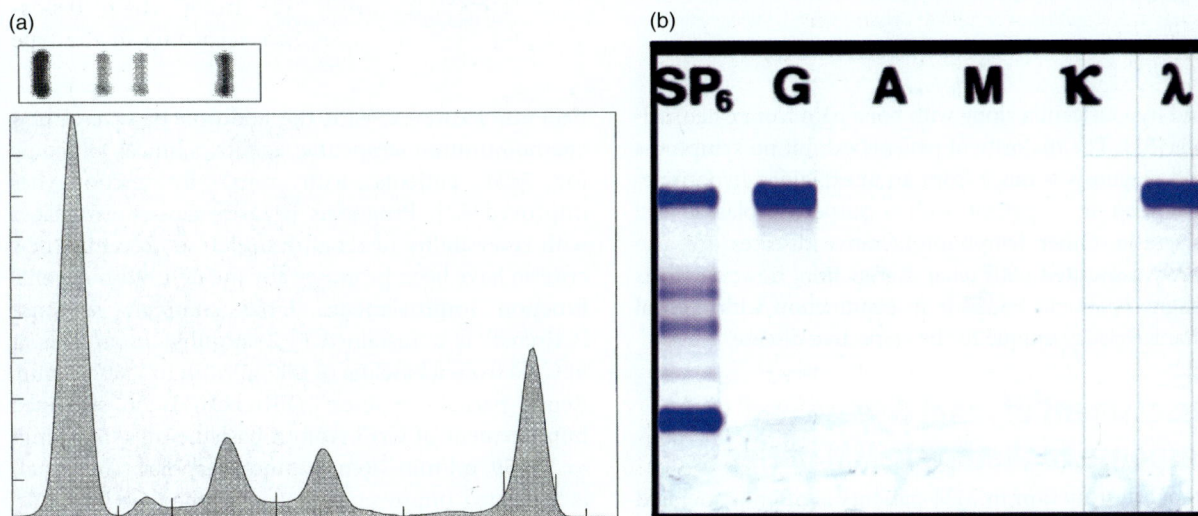

Figure 19.4 (a) Protein electrophoresis showing monoclonal spike in Gamma region (spike on right side). (Courtesy of Dr. Daniel Iancu.) (b) Protein immunofixation electrophoresis showing positivity for immunoglobulin-G with lambda free light chain expression. (Courtesy of Dr. Daniel Iancu.)

259

(a)

(b)

(c)

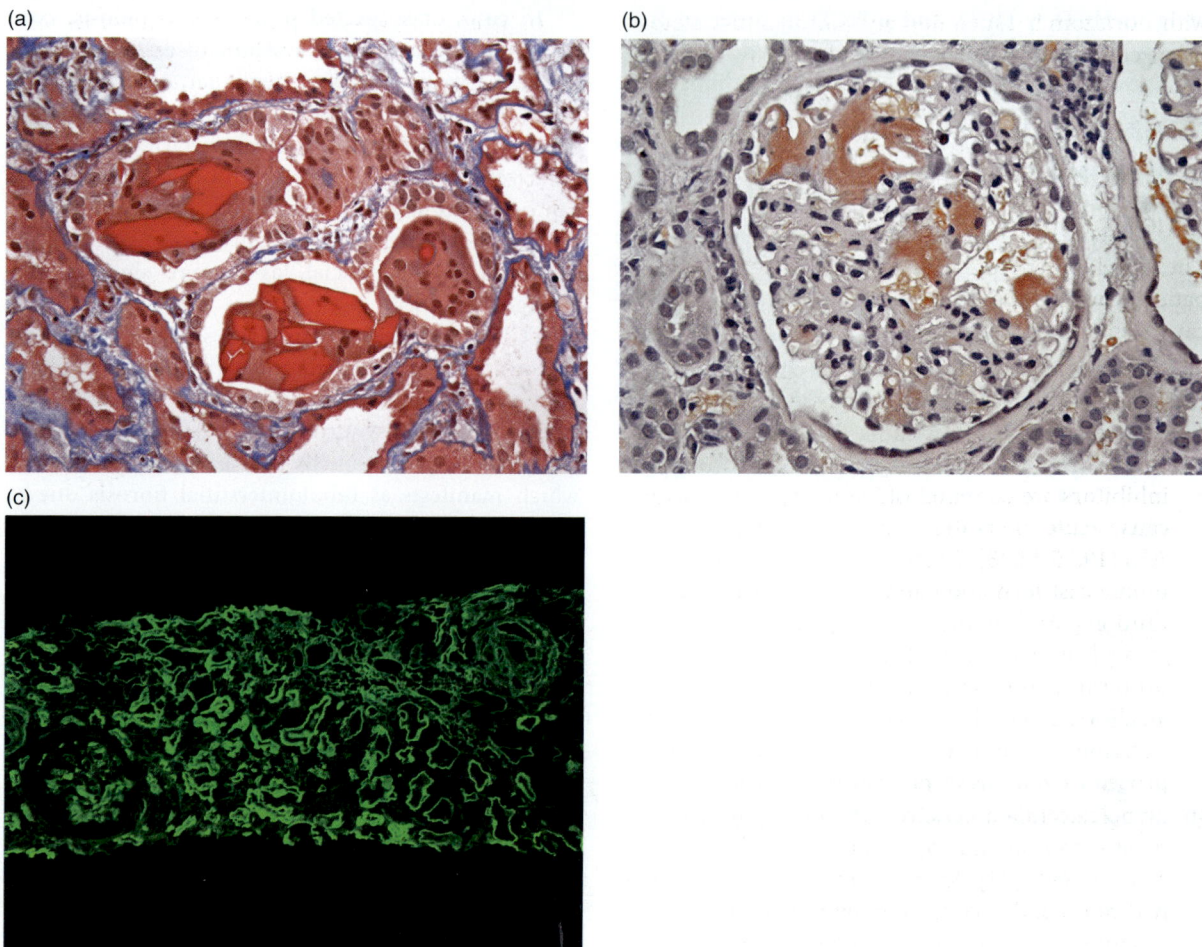

Figure 19.5 (a) Myeloma casts stained red with trichome. (Courtesy of Dr. Samih H. Nasr.) (b) Glomerular amyloid deposits stained with Congo red. (Courtesy of Dr. Samih H. Nasr.) (c) Diffuse linear staining of glomerular and tubular basement membrane for kappa free light chains in LCDD. (Courtesy of Dr. Samih H. Nasr.)

and hypouricemia along with bone pain from osteomalacia [51]. The majority of patients exhibit no symptoms and diagnosis is made from an unexplained hypouricemia seen in a patient with a suspected plasma cell dyscrasia. Other lymphoproliferative diseases are also rarely associated with renal dysfunction; however, their diagnosis should be made in conjunction with clinical characteristics unique to the respective disease.

Assessment of renal disease and response to therapy in MM patients

Renal dysfunction in MM patients is often associated with advanced disease, a higher tumor burden and overall poor survival, with a median survival of <1 year with a worse outcome in dialysis-dependent patients. However, with the addition of several new chemoimmunotherapeutic agents, clinical outcome for MM patients with renal dysfunction has improved [52]. Prognosis is more closely associated with reversibility of renal dysfunction. Recently, new criteria have been proposed for the definition of renal function improvement: Renal complete response (CRrenal) is a sustained (≥ 2 months) improvement of CrCl from a baseline of ≤ 50 ml/min to ≥ 60 ml/min. Renal partial response (PRrenal) is a sustained improvement of CrCl from a baseline of ≤ 15 ml/min to 30–59 ml/min. Renal minor response (MRrenal) is sustained improvement of a baseline CrCl of <15 ml/min to 15–29 ml/min [53,54]. Using these criteria, Roussou *et al.* reported renal response (CRrenal + PRrenal) in 82% and 51% of patients treated primarily with bortezomib containing and immunomodulatory drugs containing regimens, respectively [55].

Management of renal failure in MM patients

Patients with acute kidney injury

The development of acute kidney injury (AKI) in patients with MM is multifactorial, thus specific causes should be first identified.

(a) Nephrotoxic drugs such as non-steroidal anti-inflammatory medications, aminoglycosides, renal-excreted antibiotics, angiotensin-converting enzyme inhibitors and angiotensin II receptor inhibitors are common offending agents that may cause acute interstitial nephritis leading to AKI [19,25,42,48]. Loop diuretics cause renal tubule cast formation and should be used with caution [56]. The first step of managing AKI due to nephrotoxic agents is to remove the offending drug through hydration and urine alkalinization [57]. Intravenous contrast dyes are nephrotoxic and may require prophylactic post-procedure dialysis to prevent renal injury [58].

(b) Hypercalcemia and dehydration are among the most common and correctable causes of AKI in MM patients [21]. Rapid correction with rigorous hydration and specific therapy to decrease calcium levels should be urgently initiated. Bisphosphonates (zoledronic acid and pamidronate) are commonly used but can also cause further renal damage in the setting of AKI [59,60]. Nevertheless, if bisphosphonates are to be used they should be administered when the GFR is >30 ml/min [15]. When administering zoledronic acid in patients with CrCl between 30 and 60 ml/min, dose adjustment is recommended [61]. No adjustments are recommended for pamidronate in patients with CrCl >30 ml/min [62].

    Calcitonin is a feasible alternative to bisphosphonates and effectively lowers serum calcium without renal toxicity [28].

(c) Plasmapheresis has been used to rapidly decrease the offending monoclonal protein levels to improve renal recovery [63–65]. However recent analysis of 104 MM patients treated with plasmapheresis and chemotherapy, failed to demonstrate any improvement in clinical outcome [66], despite previous reports of its potential advantage [57,67]. Pozzi *et al.* reported recovery of renal function with plasma exchange in 61% vs. 27% of the patients without [57]. Leung *et al.* reported two out of nine patients who became dialysis-independent and had a ≥50% reduction in serum FLCs after plasma exchange therapy [67]. If plasmapheresis is used, five to seven sessions over a ten-day period with concomitant anti-myeloma therapy is recommended. The need for additional sessions and response should be determined by quantification of monoclonal proteins within two days after completion of the first course of plasma exchange [3].

Filtration of serum FLC via novel dialyzers

High concentrations of nephrotoxic serum FLCs with subsequent formation of harmful casts are a major cause of acute (and chronic) renal disease in patients with MM [40,68–72]. FLC filtration is contingent upon molecular size and generally monomeric κ chains are filtered rapidly at 40% of the GFR within 2–4 h, whereas dimeric λ chains are cleared within 3–6 h at 20% of the GFR [73]. In patients with end-stage renal disease (ESRD), filtration of FLCs may take up to 2–3 days. The normal reference range for serum FLC is between 0.26 and 1.65. An abnormal ratio reflects one light chain variant being produced in higher amounts than the other, and is indicative of residual myeloma [74].

In MM, serum FLC concentrations may be several thousand times higher than those found in normal individuals, hence their filtration is generally delayed. Efficient removal of serum FLCs, before they enter the renal circulation is critical for preservation of physiologic renal function.

Traditional small pore, "low flux" dialyzer membranes have a molecular cut off of approximately 20 kDa and are not able to filter larger molecules such as FLCs. With the advent of new high cut off dialyzers, serum FLCs can be removed quickly [28,75]. As such, they should be considered early in management of chronic renal insufficiency due to cast nephropathy, as cast obstruction lasting even one month may result in irreversible renal damage [76]. Recently, Hutchison *et al.* tested the efficiency of a novel high flux dialyzer capable of filtering molecules up to

65 kDa in size, in patients with plasma cell dyscrasias who were concomitantly treated with anti-myeloma agents. Two dialyzers were connected in a series for optimal extended filtration of FLCs. Nineteen out of 27 patients with dialysis-dependent, renal biopsy confirmed cast nephropathy met study criteria. Use of extended high cut off hemodialysis and chemotherapy resulted in 13 patients with a decrease in serum FLC concentrations and dialysis-independence within a median of 27 days (range, 13–120 days). An expected limitation of the large pore dialyzer was significant albumin depletion, as the molecular cut off of the membrane was 65 kDa (similar to that of albumin). As such, patients were routinely given 20–40 g of 20% human albumin solution per dialysis treatment [72].

Patients with chronic kidney disease

Standard dialysis

Oliguric MM patients who have not responded to general measures for the restoration of renal function may be managed via renal replacement therapy, which includes long-term hemodialysis, peritoneal dialysis [15,72], and in limited cases renal transplant [77]. Long-term dialysis is a beneficial approach to consider in patients who have progressed to ESRD, but the decision to dialyze should be made with caution. Hemodialysis is more commonly utilized than peritoneal dialysis due to the latter being associated with a higher risk of bacterial peritonitis in MM patients and inefficient FLC removal [77]. Although recent advancements have been made in the management of dialysis-dependent MM patients, the median survival of these patients has been reported as 3.5 years [11]. The most common cause of death related to dialysis-dependent MM is due to malignancy (36.1%); however, cardiovascular (17.2%) and infectious (14.7%) causes should also be considered [77].

Renal transplant

There is limited experience with renal transplantation for the treatment of MM related kidney disease; however, improved survival and prolonged allograft function have been noted in some patients [78–83]. Spontaneous development of MM after renal allograft is rare, but in patients with pre-existing myeloma the post-transplant recurrence rate maybe as high as 67% [80]. Hence, patients with active MM are not

recommended to undergo renal transplant [84] but may be considered for renal allograft if complete remission for a minimum of one year has been demonstrated [3]. Interestingly, a diagnosis of monoclonal gammopathy of unknown significance (MGUS) is not a contraindication to renal transplantation; however, MGUS has been reported to transform into MM post-transplant [84].

Conventional anti-myeloma agents

A number of investigators have reported acceptable response rates (40%–50%) with the use of conventional anti-myeloma agents in MM patients with renal failure [5,56,85,86]. Preferred regimens usually have relied on dexamethasone [56,86] with a renal response rate reported in 73% of patients treated with high-dose steroids [85]. Conventional anti-myeloma agents such as melphalan can be associated with increased toxicities and should therefore be cautiously employed [56,86,87]. Although the use of alkylator and/or anthracycline-based regimens has largely been surpassed by novel agents [88–95], dexamethasone in conjunction with novel agents is a feasible therapeutic option, capable of inducing quick results [85].

Bortezomib

Bortezomib is an FDA approved therapeutic agent for MM patients with renal impairment who may be either dialysis-dependent or -independent. This first-in-class proteasome inhibitor prevents degradation of Iκ-B, resulting in downregulation of the potent transcription factor NF-κB [96,97]. Upregulation of NF-κB in the renal tubular cells of proteinuric patients has been shown to promote inflammation causing interstitial fibrosis [98]. Bortezomib may potentially resolve this inflammatory process through its effect on intratubular NF-κB, thereby reversing renal damage [99]. The pharmacokinetic profile of bortezomib is not affected by renal function status as bortezomib is metabolized through oxidative deboronation by the hepatic cytochrome P-450 enzymes CYP3A4, CYP2C19, and CYP1A2 [100–103]. Bortezomib requires no dose-modification in MM patients with renal impairment, regardless of dialysis status [104].

Numerous clinical studies have demonstrated the efficacy and tolerability of bortezomib in MM patients with varying degrees of renal impairment [54,104–117] (Table 19.2). Jagannath *et al.*

Table 19.2 Activity of bortezomib alone or in combination with other agents in multiple myeloma patients with renal failure

Study	N/disease type	Regimen	Baseline renal impairment	Response (CR + PR)	Changes in renal impairment
VISTA phase 3 study [105]	344 previously untreated MM	VMP	GFR ≤30 ml/min 6%	74% (37% CR)	Renal impairment reversal (baseline CrCl <50 ml/min to CrCl >60 ml/min) seen in 44%, in a median of 2.1 months. Rate of reversal significantly higher in patients aged <75 vs. ≥75 years, and in patients with CrCl >30 vs. ≤30 ml/min
			GFR 31–50 ml/min 27%	67% (29% CR)	
			GFR >50 ml/min 67%	72% (30% CR)	
APEX phase 3 study [106]	313 relapsed MM	Single-agent bortezomib	CrCl <30 ml/min 5%	47%	Not reported
			CrCl 30–50 ml/min 14%	37%	
			CrCl 51–80 ml/min 44%	40%	
			CrCl >80 ml/min 38%	36%	
DOXIL-MMY-3001 phase 3 study [115]	324 relapsed/refractory MM	Bortezomib + pegylated liposomal doxorubicin	CrCl <60 (>30) ml/min 29%	49% (27% CR+VGPR)	Steady, statistically significant, and clinically meaningful improvement from baseline in mean CrCl seen in patients with CrCl <60 ml/min in both arms
			CrCl ≥60 ml/min 71%	47% (29% CR +VGPR)	
	322 relapsed/refractory MM	Single-agent bortezomib	CrCl <60 (>30) ml/min 30%	42% (22% CR +VGPR)	
			CrCl ≥60 ml/min 70%	44% (18% CR +VGPR)	
HOVON-65/GMMG-HD4 phase 3 study [107]	308 previously untreated MM	PAD	SCr >5 mg/dl	After induction: 60% (20% VGPR) After transplant: 60% (40% VGPR)	Not reported
			SCr 2–5 mg/dl	After induction: 58% (26% VGPR) After transplant: 84% (16% CR, 42% CR +VGPR)	
			SCr <2 mg/dl	After induction: 79% (7% CR, 43% CR +VGPR) After transplant: 89% (22% CR, 62% CR +VGPR)	

Table 19.2 (cont.)

Study	N/disease type	Regimen	Baseline renal impairment	Response (CR + PR)	Changes in renal impairment
SUMMIT/CREST phase 2 studies [108]	256 relapsed and/or refractory MM	Bortezomib ± dexamethasone	CrCl < 30 ml/ min 4%	30%[a]	Mean SCr ↓ then stable above normal range
			CrCl 30–50 ml/ min 16%	24%[a]	Not reported
			Cr Cl 51–80 ml/ min 39%	33%[a]	

[a] CR+PR+MR; ARF, acute renal failure; BD, bortezomib, dexamethasone; CrCl, creatinine clearance; CR, complete response; eGFR, estimated GFR; FLC, free light chain; GFR, glomerular filtration rate; MR, minimal response; PAD, bortezomib, doxorubicin, dexamethasone; PR, partial response; SCr, serum creatinine; VGPR, very good PR; VMP, bortezomib, melphalan, prednisone.

initially reported on the performance of bortezomib, in patients with dialysis-independent renal dysfunction, in an analysis of two phase 2 studies (CREST and SUMMIT). A total of 256 patients with relapsed/ refractory MM were treated with bortezomib; a majority of patients also received dexamethasone. Results indicated that renal impairment does not seem to significantly impact bortezomib response rates, discontinuation rate or the toxicity profile [108].

The impact of single-agent bortezomib, versus high-dose dexamethasone has been explored in relapsed/refractory MM patients with varying degrees of renal insufficiency demonstrating superior results [106]. In a subset analysis of 333 patients randomized to the bortezomib arm of the phase 3 APEX study, response rates, time to progression (TTP) and OS were shown to be similar across all renal cohorts. A median time to first response was seen within 0.7–1.6 months, exhibiting the rapid activity of bortezomib irrespective of renal function status. Bortezomib related toxicity was similar across all renal cohorts however patients with moderate to severe renal dysfunction were more likely to discontinue therapy due to adverse events than those with mild or no renal impairment [106]

Renal dysfunction maybe reversed in patients treated with bortezomib-based regimens and has been reported in a number of studies. In a retrospective, multi-center analysis of dialysis-requiring advanced MM patients treated with bortezomib-based therapies, we reported an overall response rate (ORR) of 75% (20/24 patients) and complete response rate of 25%. Dialysis independence was achieved in three patients demonstrating the ability of bortezomib containing regimens to revert kidney damage [118]. In the VISTA trial, Dimopoulos *et al.* assessed 344 treatment naïve MM patients with mild to moderate renal dysfunction, and demonstrated reversal of renal failure (GFR <50 ml/min at baseline to >60 ml/min) in 44% of patients receiving bortezomib. An improved toxicity profile was also observed in patients who achieved reversal of renal impairment versus those who did not [105].

Thalidomide

Thalidomide and its analog lenalidomide are immunomodulating drugs (IMiDs) and are effective treatments for active MM [119]. Thalidomide is primarily metabolized via non-enzymatic hydrolysis but hepatic CYP2C enzymes may also play a crucial role in the pharmacodynamic properties of the drug [120]. As such, the pharmacokinetic profile of thalidomide is not affected by renal disease and shows minimal correlation with creatinine clearance, thus allowing for optimal dosing of the drug [121]. Tosi *et al.* initially demonstrated efficacy of thalidomide +/− dexamethasone in 20 advanced MM patients with renal disease. Recovery of adequate renal function was noted in 12/15 responding patients and a ≥50% reduction of serum creatinine was observed in 45% of the overall cohort of patients. The toxicity profile of thalidomide was not affected by renal impairment and appeared similar to that observed in patients with adequate renal function [122]. Kastritis *et al.* reported feasibility of thalidomide in 15 newly diagnosed patients (total $n = 41$) who received thalidomide and dexamethasone +/− bortezomib. Reversal of renal failure to a maintained sCr level of <1.5 mg/dl

Table 19.3. Activity of thalidomide in multiple myeloma patients with renal failure

Study	N/disease type	Regimen	Baseline renal impairment	Response (CR + PR)	Changes in renal impairment
Single-center prospective study [147]	31 front-line MM	Thalidomide–dexamethasone	CrCl ≤50 ml/min, 7 dialysis dependent	ORR: 74% ≥VGPR: 26%	Renal function improved in 82% vs 37% of patients achieving ≥PR vs. <PR ($p = 0.04$)
Single-center consecutive patient series [148]	29 front-line MM	Thalidomide–dexamethasone ± cyclophosphamide	SCr ≥2 mg/dl	66%	55% of patients showed reversal of renal failure in a median of 0.8 months 45% of patients had a 50% SCr decrease in a median of 1.2 months
Single-center consecutive patient series [85]	41 front-line MM	Thalidomide–dexamethasone, VTD, or BD ($n = 15$) or high-dose dexamethasone-based regimens ($n = 26$)	Median SCr 3.4 mg/dl; 10 patients required dialysis	53% (64% in patients receiving thalidomide or bortezomib, vs. 46%)	Reversal (<1.5 mg/dl) in 73–80% in patients receiving thalidomide or bortezomib, vs. 69% 80% dialysis patients became independent
Single-center consecutive patient series [122]	20 relapsed/refractory MM	Single-agent thalidomide or thalidomide–dexamethasone	SCr > 2 mg/dl	45%/75%*	Recovery (<2 mg/dl) in 60%
Hyperkalemia case studies [123]	8 relapsed or refractory MM	Thalidomide; thalidomide plus dexamethasone; TVAD; CTAD	"Significant renal failure"; 6 dialysis-dependent	2 remission, 2 plateau	Not reported

CrCl, creatinine clearance; CR, complete response; CTAD, cyclophosphamide, thalidomide, doxorubicin, dexamethasone; MR, minimal response; PAD, bortezomib, doxorubicin, dexamethasone; PR, partial response; SCr, serum creatinine; TVAD, thalidomide, vincristine, doxorubicin, dexamethasone; VGPR, very good PR.

was observed in 73% of all patients, within a median time of 1.9 months (range, 0.1–20 months). Overall response to therapy was 53%, including a 64% ORR observed in patients receiving thalidomide/bortezomib. Thalidomide-related toxicity was similar to that observed in patients with normal renal function [85]. It is important to note that severe hyperkalemia has been reported in MM patients with dialysis-dependent renal dysfunction who were receiving thalidomide-based therapy [123]. Data from additional studies in which thalidomide containing regimens were used in the treatment of MM patients with renal failure are presented in Table 19.3.

Lenalidomide

Lenalidomide is a structurally similar yet more potent derivative of thalidomide. It effectively inhibits cell proliferation and is generally associated with less neuropathy, constipation and fatigue, which are frequently seen with thalidomide use [124,125]. Unlike its parent compound, lenalidomide is cleared via the kidneys mainly through glomerular filtration and active tubular secretion [126]. Based on pharmacokinetic studies by Chen et al., lenalidomide dose reduction in patients with renal disease is recommended as follows: dose at 10 mg/day in patients with CrCl of 30–50 ml/min; dose at 15 mg every other day in patients with CrCl of ≤30ml/min who are dialysis independent, and dose at 5 mg once daily in patients who are dialysis dependent [126,127]

Lenalidomide-based regimens are also reported to be effective in MM patients with renal dysfunction; however, there are limited data in this patient population as sCr above 2 mg/dl was an exclusion criterion in the majority of clinical trials [127–133] (Table 19.4). A combined analysis of two studies (MM-009 and MM-010 phase 3 trials), testing lenalidomide plus dexamethasone demonstrated the ORR and quality of response to be similar across all renal subgroups. Patients with mild (CrCl ≥60 ml/min, $n = 243$), moderate (≥30–60 ml/min, $n = 82$) and severe renal dysfunction (<30 ml/min, $n = 16$), achieved ≥VGPR rates of 34%, 26% and 38%, respectively. Except for patients with severe renal disease, TTP, OS and progression-free survival were relatively similar in the remaining renal subgroups and comparable to those patients with normal renal functionality. Lenalidomide toxicity, particularly thrombocytopenia, was more commonly observed in patients with severe renal disease, and required more dose modifications. In patients with moderate to severe renal disease, 72% demonstrated significant improvement in renal function after being treated with lenalidomide plus dexamethasone [127]. Klein et al. further established the efficacy of lenalidomide plus dexamethasone by reporting an ORR of 67%, 60%, and 49% in patients with CrCl of ≥80, ≥50–≤80 and <50 ml/min, respectively [132]. In a small series of dialysis-dependent MM patients treated with lenalidomide plus dexamethasone, improvement of renal function was noted in 57% with one patient becoming dialysis independent [133]. Recovery of physiologic renal function following lenalidomide treatment has been recently reported in a primary bortezomib-refractory MM patient with severe renal disease. Following a 12-month course of a lenalidomide-containing regimen, and subsequent autologous stem cell transplant (ASCT), the patient remained in PRrenal at two years out from initiation of lenalidomide therapy [134].

The addition of novel agents in the therapeutic armamentarium against MM has greatly improved the clinical outcome of MM patients with concomitant renal disease. However, renal impairment continues to carry an adverse prognosis despite use of novel agents. To examine this finding, we retrospectively analyzed the clinical outcome of 175 consecutive MM patients treated at Roswell Park Cancer Institute with IMiDs and/or bortezomib therapy at our institution. Among the patients analyzed, 86% received treatment with either an IMiD ($n = 130$) or bortezomib ($n = 97$) at some point during the course of their disease. Median survival for patients with normal renal function and mild, moderate, and severe renal impairment was 76.1, 55.3, 67.4 and 24.9 months, respectively ($p = 0.21$). Importantly, a decline in renal function was found to be associated with a similar decrease in survival, indicating that patients with renal impairment continue to have a poor prognosis despite availability of novel agents [135].

The role of high-dose chemotherapy with autologous stem cell transplant (ASCT)

In suitably aged patients with good performance status, ASCT may be a viable option for the treatment of MM. In dialysis-dependent MM patients, who received a melphalan (200 mg/m^2) conditioning therapy followed by ASCT, a five-year OS of 36% and a median survival of 41 months was reported by Lee and colleagues. Moreover, 24% of patients evaluable for response in renal function achieved dialysis independence within a median of four months post-ASCT [136]. Stem cell mobilization was not affected by renal function status, and melphalan dosed at 140 mg/m^2 appeared to be equally effective and less toxic compared to a dose of 200 mg/m^2. However, incidence of adverse events was significantly higher in the cohort of patients who received melphalan at 200 mg/m^2, particularly in the dialysis-dependent group. OS was significantly lower in older aged patients who had refractory disease, and a low serum albumin [4,136]. Thus, ASCT for the treatment of MM patients with renal disease remains a feasible therapeutic modality [4,136–143]. Patients who have a higher likelihood of achieving a better clinical outcome (good performance status, young age and chemosensitive disease) may possibly benefit from

Table 19.4   Activity of lenalidomide in multiple myeloma patients with renal failure

Study	N/disease type	Regimen	Baseline renal impairment	Response (CR + PR)	Changes in renal impairment
MM-009/MM-010 phase 3 studies [127]	341 relapsed or refractory MM	Lenalidomide + dexamethasone	CrCl <30 ml/min (severe impairment) 5% CrCl ≥30–<60 ml/min (moderate impairment) 24% CrCl ≥60 ml/min (mild or no impairment) 71%	50% (6% CR, 38% ≥VGPR) 56%(16% CR, 27% ≥VGPR) 64%(16% CR, 34% ≥VGPR)	72% with moderate/severe impairment showed improvement in CrCl by at least one level
Single-center retrospective study [132]	167 relapsed or refractory MM	Lenalidomide + dexamethasone	CrCl <50 ml/min 20% (33 patients) CrCl ≥50–<80 ml/min 24% (40 patients) CrCl ≥80 ml/min 56% (94 patients)	49% (3% CR, 12% ≥VGPR) 60% (10% CR, 30% ≥VGPR) 67% (15% CR, 28% ≥VGPR)	34 patients had improvement in renal function, and 20 had worsening renal function; response rates were higher in patients with stable or improving renal function vs. worsening
Multicenter phase 2 study [131]	75 relapsed/refractory MM	Lenalidomide + dexamethasone	CrCl ≤60 ml/min (28 patients)	69% overall, 73% in patients with renal impairment	Not reported
Single-center analysis from a phase 2 study [128]	72 front-line MM	Lenalidomide + dexamethasone	CrCl ≤40 ml/min 19% (14 patients)	Not reported	21% (3/14) showed increased CrCl
Expanded access program analysis [129]	69 relapsed MM	Lenalidomide ± corticosteroids	Elevated SCr (>1.0 mg/dl in females; >1.5 mg/dl in males), 33% Normal SCr, 67%	61% 54%	SCr decreased in 39%, increased in 26% SCr decreased in 39%, increased in 32%
Multicenter retrospective analysis [133]	15 relapsed MM	Lenalidomide + dexamethasone	Dialysis dependent	60% (29% CR)	One patient became independent of dialysis after achieving PR
Consecutive patient series [130]	50 relapsed/refractory MM	Lenalidomide + dexamethasone	CrCl <50 ml/min 24% (n = 12) CrCl >50 ml/min 76% (n = 38)	60.5% (8% CR, 33% ≥VGPR) 58% (15% CR, 25% ≥VGPR)	25% CR^{renal} 16% MR^{renal} NA

CrCl, creatinine clearance; CR, complete response; GFR, glomerular filtration rate; MR, minimal response; PR, partial response; SCr, serum creatinine; VGPR, very good PR.

this procedure. However, with the advent of novel agents, OS, TTP, and reversal of renal function to physiologic levels is comparable (if not better) to ASCT.

Conclusion

Renal impairment is often a presenting sign of an undiagnosed plasma cell dyscrasia. Thus, prompt restoration and/or preservation of normal renal function are critical in the treatment of MM patients, particularly those with severe kidney impairment. The MDRD and Cockcroft–Gault formulas are helpful in determining renal function status; KDIGO criteria provide a framework for staging of renal disease. Assessment of AKI should be performed using the AKIN and RIFLE criteria.

As etiology of MM related kidney failure is multifactorial, management of the patient is based on rectifying the underlying pathology responsible for kidney damage. Causes of renal failure in MM maybe categorized into Ig related, non-Ig related or, more commonly, a combination of both. When suspected in the confirmed MM patient, investigational studies for diagnosis of renal disease include serum chemistries and SPEP; random and 24-h urine sample measurements of CrCl and UPEP, along with IFE. Renal biopsy remains the gold standard for the accurate pathological diagnosis of renal disease in MM and should be performed if feasible.

MM-associated renal failure is a medical emergency. The duration of kidney dysfunction (AKI versus CKD) is crucial in determining the appropriate treatment modality. Initial management of AKI due to myeloma cast nephropathy includes vigorous volume expansion and alkalinization of urine. Supportive care in conjunction with calcitonin and cautious use of bisphosphonates is recommended for renal dysfunction due to hypercalcemia. Plasmapheresis, for the reduction of monoclonal proteins may potentially benefit select patients when used with chemotherapy and dialysis. For the expedient removal of FLCs, novel dialyzers with large-pore membranes have demonstrated improved efficacy and filtration compared to traditional dialyzers. A randomized prospective trial is currently underway examining the use of high cut off dialyzers in conjunction with bortezomib for the treatment of MM patients with cast nephropathy [144].

The goal of managing patients with CKD is to preserve and, if possible, to restore physiologic renal

potential. In select patients, this may be achieved through ASCT. However, more feasible means are dialysis and anti-myeloma therapies that include conventional chemotherapy based-regimens, and novel chemoimmunotherapy-based regimens. Traditionally, high-dose dexamethasone-based therapies have been the mainstay of MM with renal failure, largely due to their rapid antimyeloma effects. The availability of novel therapeutic agents, particularly bortezomib, which has demonstrated significant activity in decreasing overall tumor burden and reversing renal dysfunction, has changed the treatment paradigm of managing MM with associated kidney disease. As such, the IMWG recommends the combination of bortezomib plus dexamethasone for MM patients with renal disease of any stage. This combination has demonstrated a superior renal response than older regimens such as VAD or dexamethasone alone, which has traditionally been the treatment of choice [55]. Thalidomide and lenalidomide also represent effective therapeutic options; however, due to lack of data from randomized trials, thalidomide should be used with caution in MM patients with renal disease. Similarly, lenalidomide should be administered at the recommended reduced dose. Prospective trials, examining the role of dose-adjusted lenalidomide and newer proteasome inhibitors in patients with varying degrees of renal impairment are currently underway. Efficacy of a second-generation, irreversible proteasome inhibitor, carfilzomib, is being investigated in a number of clinical trials with preliminary data demonstrating its activity and safety in patients with MM [145]. At a meeting of the American Society of Clinical Oncologists, Badros *et al* presented their results from a phase II study in which carfilzomib was administered to 39 relapsed/refractory MM patients with varying degrees of renal impairment [146]. Carfilzomib was dosed at 15 mg/m^2 IV, administered on days 1, 2, 8, 9, 15, and 16 of a 28-day cycle for the first cycle, escalating to 20 mg/m^2 for the second cycle and 27 mg/m^2 for cycle 3. Anemia and thrombocytopenia were the most common grade 3/4 toxicities reported, independent of renal status. These preliminary findings are encouraging and demonstrate that carfilzomib can be used to treat patients with advanced MM with concomitant renal disease without being dose adjusted. Final results from this trial and others are eagerly anticipated, as they will best characterize the role of newer generation antimyeloma agents in the optimal treatment of MM patients with renal impairment.

References

1. Winearls, C. G. Acute myeloma kidney. *Kidney Int.* 1995; **48**(4):1347–61.

2. K/DOQI *clinical practice guidelines for chronic kidney disease: evaluation, classification, and stratification*; 2000 [database on the Internet].

3. Ailawadhi, S., Chanan-Khan, A. Management of Multiple Myeloma Patients with Renal Dysfunction. In: Lonial, S., editor, *Myeloma Therapy: Pursuing the Plasma Cell (Contemporary Hematology)*. Humana Press; 2008, pp. 499–516.

4. Badros, A., Barlogie, B., Siegel, E. *et al.* Results of autologous stem cell transplant in multiple myeloma patients with renal failure. *Br. J. Haematol.* 2001; **114**(4):822–9.

5. Blade, J., Fernandez-Llama, P., Bosch, F. *et al.* Renal failure in multiple myeloma: presenting features and predictors of outcome in 94 patients from a single institution. *Arch. Intern. Med.* 1998;**158**(17):1889–93.

6. Kyle, R. A., Gertz, M. A., Witzig, T. E. *et al.* Review of 1027 patients with newly diagnosed multiple myeloma. *Mayo. Clin. Proc.* 2003;**78**(1):21–33.

7. Sakhuja, V., Jha, V., Varma, S. *et al.* Renal involvement in multiple myeloma: a 10-year study. *Ren. Fail.* 2000;**22**(4):465–77.

8. Manjunath, G., Sarnak, M. J., Levey, A. S. Estimating the glomerular filtration rate. Dos and don'ts for assessing kidney function. *Postgrad. Med.* 2001;**110**(6):55–62; quiz 11.

9. Levey, A. S., Bosch, J. P., Lewis, J. B. *et al.* A more accurate method to estimate glomerular filtration rate from serum creatinine: a new prediction equation. Modification of Diet in Renal Disease Study

Group. *Ann. Intern. Med.* 1999;**130**(6):461–70.

10. Knudsen, L. M., Hippe, E., Hjorth, M., Holmberg, E., Westin, J. Renal function in newly diagnosed multiple myeloma–a demographic study of 1353 patients. The Nordic Myeloma Study Group. *Eur. J. Haematol.* 1994;**53**(4):207–12.

11. Knudsen, L. M., Hjorth, M., Hippe, E. Renal failure in multiple myeloma: reversibility and impact on the prognosis. Nordic Myeloma Study Group. *Eur. J. Haematol.* 2000;**65**(3):175–81.

12. Bostom, A. G., Kronenberg, F., Ritz, E. Predictive performance of renal function equations for patients with chronic kidney disease and normal serum creatinine levels. *J. Am. Soc. Nephrol.* 2002;**13**(8):2140–4.

13. Duncan, L., Heathcote, J., Djurdjev, O., Levin, A. Screening for renal disease using serum creatinine: who are we missing? *Nephrol. Dial. Transplant* 2001; **16**(5):1042–6.

14. Cockcroft, D. W., Gault, M. H. Prediction of creatinine clearance from serum creatinine. *Nephron* 1976;**16**(1):31–41.

15. Dimopoulos, M. A., Terpos, E., Chanan-Khan, A. *et al.* Renal impairment in patients with multiple myeloma: a consensus statement on behalf of the International Myeloma Working Group. *J. Clin. Oncol.* 2010; **28**(33):4976–84.

16. Bellomo, R., Ronco, C., Kellum, J. A., Mehta, R. L., Palevsky, P. Acute renal failure – definition, outcome measures, animal models, fluid therapy and information technology needs: the Second International Consensus Conference of the Acute Dialysis Quality Initiative (ADQI) Group. *Crit. Care* 2004;**8**(4):R204–12.

17. Mehta, R. L., Kellum, J. A., Shah, S. V. *et al.* Acute Kidney Injury Network: report of an initiative to improve outcomes in acute

kidney injury. *Crit. Care* 2007; **11**(2):R31.

18. Srisawat, N., Hoste, E. E., Kellum, J. A. Modern classification of acute kidney injury. *Blood Purif.* 2010;**29**(3):300–7.

19. Alexanian, R., Barlogie, B., Dixon, D. Renal failure in multiple myeloma. Pathogenesis and prognostic implications. *Arch. Intern. Med.* 1990;**150**(8):1693–5.

20. Lorenz, E. C., Sethi, S., Poshusta, T. L. *et al.* Renal failure due to combined cast nephropathy, amyloidosis and light-chain deposition disease. *Nephrol. Dial. Transplant* 2010;**25**(4):1340–3.

21. Blade, J., Rosinol, L. Renal, hematologic and infectious complications in multiple myeloma. *Best Pract. Res. Clin. Haematol.* 2005;**18**(4):635–52.

22. Pasquali, S., Zucchelli, P., Casanova, S. *et al.* Renal histological lesions and clinical syndromes in multiple myeloma. Renal Immunopathology Group. *Clin. Nephrol.* 1987;**27**(5):222–8.

23. Ivanyi, B. Renal complications in multiple myeloma. *Acta. Morphol. Hung.* 1989;**37**(3–4):235–43.

24. Montseny, J. J., Kleinknecht, D., Meyrier, A. *et al.* Long-term outcome according to renal histological lesions in 118 patients with monoclonal gammopathies. *Nephrol. Dial. Transplant* 1998; **13**(6):1438–45.

25. Basnayake, K., Cheung, C. K., Sheaff, M. *et al.* Differential progression of renal scarring and determinants of late renal recovery in sustained dialysis dependent acute kidney injury secondary to myeloma kidney. *J. Clin. Pathol.* 2010;**63**(10):884–7.

26. Batuman, V., Verroust, P. J., Navar, G. L. *et al.* Myeloma light chains are ligands for cubilin (gp280). *Am. J. Physiol.* 1998; **275**(2 Pt 2):F246–54.

27. Klassen, R. B., Allen, P. L., Batuman, V., Crenshaw, K.,

269

Hammond, T. G. Light chains are a ligand for megalin. *J. Appl. Physiol.* 2005;**98**(1):257–63.

28. Wirk, B. Renal failure in multiple myeloma: a medical emergency. *Bone Marrow Transplant* 2011, Feb 21.

29. Huang, Z. Q., Sanders, P. W. Biochemical interaction between Tamm-Horsfall glycoprotein and Ig light chains in the pathogenesis of cast nephropathy. *Lab. Invest.* 1995;**73**(6):810–17.

30. Haynes, R. J., Read, S., Collins, G. P., Darby, S. C., Winearls, C. G. Presentation and survival of patients with severe acute kidney injury and multiple myeloma: a 20-year experience from a single centre. *Nephrol. Dial. Transplant* 2010;**25**(2):419–26.

31. Sengul, S., Zwizinski, C., Simon, E. E. *et al.* Endocytosis of light chains induces cytokines through activation of NF-kappaB in human proximal tubule cells. *Kidney Int.* 2002;**62**(6):1977–88.

32. Kyle, R. A., Gertz, M. A. Primary systemic amyloidosis: clinical and laboratory features in 474 cases. *Semin. Hematol.* 1995;**32**(1): 45–59.

33. Melcion, C., Mougenot, B., Baudouin, B. *et al.* Renal failure in myeloma: relationship with isoelectric point of immunoglobulin light chains. *Clin. Nephrol.* 1984;**22**(3): 138–43.

34. Truong, L. D., Mawad, J., Cagle, P., Mattioli, C. Cytoplasmic crystals in multiple myeloma-associated Fanconi's syndrome. A morphological study including immunoelectron microscopy. *Arch. Pathol. Lab. Med.* 1989; **113**(7):781–5.

35. Orfila, C., Lepert, J. C., Modesto, A., Bernadet, P., Suc, J. M. Fanconi's syndrome, kappa light-chain myeloma, non-amyloid fibrils and cytoplasmic crystals in renal tubular epithelium. *Am. J. Nephrol.* 1991;**11**(4):345–9.

36. Kisilevsky, R., Young, I. D. Pathogenesis of amyloidosis. *Baillieres Clin. Rheumatol.* 1994; **8**(3):613–26.

37. Jancelewicz, Z., Takatsuki, K., Sugai, S., Pruzanski, W.. IgD multiple myeloma. Review of 133 cases. *Arch. Intern. Med.* 1975; **135**(1):87–93.

38. Sanchorawala, V. Light-chain (AL) amyloidosis: diagnosis and treatment. *Clin. J. Am. Soc. Nephrol.* 2006;**1**(6): 1331–41.

39. Pozzi, C., D'Amico, M., Fogazzi, G. B. *et al.* Light chain deposition disease with renal involvement: clinical characteristics and prognostic factors. *Am. J. Kidney Dis.* 2003;**42**(6):1154–63.

40. Lin, J., Markowitz, G. S., Valeri, A. M. *et al.* Renal monoclonal immunoglobulin deposition disease: the disease spectrum. *J. Am. Soc. Nephrol.* 2001; **12**(7):1482–92.

41. Buxbaum, J., Gallo, G. Nonamyloidotic monoclonal immunoglobulin deposition disease. Light-chain, heavy-chain, and light- and heavy-chain deposition diseases. *Hematol. Oncol. Clin. North. Am.* 1999; **13**(6):1235–48.

42. Dimopoulos, M. A., Kastritis, E., Rosinol, L., Blade, J., Ludwig, H. Pathogenesis and treatment of renal failure in multiple myeloma. *Leukemia* 2008;**22**(8):1485–93.

43. Lorenz, E. C., Gertz, M. A., Fervenza, F. C. *et al.* Long-term outcome of autologous stem cell transplantation in light chain deposition disease. *Nephrol. Dial. Transplant* 2008;**23**(6): 2052–7.

44. Goossens, T., Klein, U., Kuppers, R. Frequent occurrence of deletions and duplications during somatic hypermutation: implications for oncogene translocations and heavy chain disease. *Proc. Natl. Acad. Sci. USA* 1998;**95**(5):2463–8.

45. Aucouturier, P., Khamlichi, A. A., Touchard, G. *et al.* Brief report: heavy-chain deposition disease. *N Engl. J. Med.* 1993;**329**(19): 1389–93.

46. Herrera, G., Picken, M. M. Renal diseases associated with plasma cell dyscrasias, amyloidosis, waldenstroms macroglobulinemia, cryoglobulinemic nephropathies. In: Jennette, J. C., Olson, J. L., Schwartz, M. M., Silva, F. G., editors. *Heptinstall's Pathology of the Kidney. 6th edition*, Philadelphia: Lippincott Williams & Wilkins; 2007, p. 861.

47. Sanders, P. W., Herrera, G. A., Kirk, K. A., Old, C. W., Galla, J. H. Spectrum of glomerular and tubulointerstitial renal lesions associated with monotypical immunoglobulin light chain deposition. *Lab. Invest.* 1991; **64**(4):527–37.

48. Pirani, C. L., Valeri, A., D'Agati, V., Appel, G. B. Renal toxicity of nonsteroidal anti-inflammatory drugs. *Contrib. Nephrol.* 1987;**55**:159–75.

49. Obici, L., Perfetti, V., Palladini, G., Moratti, R., Merlini, G. Clinical aspects of systemic amyloid diseases. *Biochim. Biophys. Acta* 2005;**1753**(1):11–22.

50. Buxbaum, J. N., Chuba, J. V., Hellman, G. C., Solomon, A., Gallo, G. R. Monoclonal immunoglobulin deposition disease: light chain and light and heavy chain deposition diseases and their relation to light chain amyloidosis. Clinical features, immunopathology, and molecular analysis. *Ann. Intern. Med.* 1990;**112**(6):455–64.

51. Ma, C. X., Lacy, M. Q., Rompala, J. F. *et al.* Acquired Fanconi syndrome is an indolent disorder in the absence of overt multiple myeloma. *Blood* 2004;**104**(1): 40–2.

52. Dimopoulos, M. A., Terpos, E. Renal insufficiency and failure.

Hematology Am. Soc. Hematol. Educ. Program **2010**;2010:431–6.

53. Ludwig, H., Adam, Z., Hajek, R. *et al.* Recovery of renal impairment by bortezomib-doxorubicin-dexamethasone (BDD) in multiple myeloma (MM) patients with acute renal failure. Results from an ongoing phase II study. *ASH Annual Meeting Abstracts* 2007 November 16;**110**(11):3603.

54. Dimopoulos, M. A., Roussou, M., Gavriatopoulou, M. *et al.* Reversibility of renal impairment in patients with multiple myeloma treated with bortezomib-based regimens: identification of predictive factors. *Clin. Lymphoma Myeloma* 2009; **9**(4):302–6.

55. Roussou, M., Kastritis, E., Christoulas, D. *et al.* Reversibility of renal failure in newly diagnosed patients with multiple myeloma and the role of novel agents. *Leuk. Res.* 2010;**34**(10): 1395–7.

56. Durie, B. G., Kyle, R. A., Belch, A. *et al.* Myeloma management guidelines: a consensus report from the Scientific Advisors of the International Myeloma Foundation. *Hematol. J.* 2003; **4**(6):379–98.

57. Pozzi, C., Pasquali, S., Donini, U. *et al.* Prognostic factors and effectiveness of treatment in acute renal failure due to multiple myeloma: a review of 50 cases. Report of the Italien Renal Immunopathology Group. *Clin. Nephrol.* 1987;**28**(1):1–9.

58. Terpos, E., Cibeira, M. T., Blade, J., Ludwig, H. Management of complications in multiple myeloma. *Semin. Hematol.* 2009;**46**(2):176–89.

59. Markowitz, G. S., Fine, P. L., Stack, J. I. *et al.* Toxic acute tubular necrosis following treatment with zoledronate (Zometa). *Kidney Int.* 2003; **64**(1):281–9.

60. Terpos, E., Sezer, O., Croucher, P. I. *et al.* The use of bisphosphonates in multiple myeloma: recommendations of an expert panel on behalf of the European Myeloma Network. *Ann. Oncol.* 2009;**20**(8):1303–17.

61. Zometa (zoledronic acid): *Prescribing information*: Novartis Pharmaceuticals Corporation; 2007.

62. Aredia (pamidronate): *Prescribing information*: Novartis Pharmaceuticals Corporation; 2007.

63. Feest, T. G., Burge, P. S., Cohen, S. L. Successful treatment of myeloma kidney by diuresis and plasmaphoresis. *Br. Med. J.* 1976;1 (6008):503–4.

64. Misiani, R., Remuzzi, G., Bertani, T. *et al.* Plasmapheresis in the treatment of acute renal failure in multiple myeloma. *Am. J. Med.* 1979;**66**(4):684–8.

65. Locatelli, F., Pozzi, C., Pedrini, L. *et al.* Steroid pulses and plasmapheresis in the treatment of acute renal failure in multiple myeloma. *Proc. Eur. Dial. Transplant Assoc.* 1980;17:690–4.

66. Clark, W. F., Stewart, A. K., Rock, G. A. *et al.* Plasma exchange when myeloma presents as acute renal failure: a randomized, controlled trial. *Ann. Intern. Med.* 2005; **143**(11):777–84.

67. Leung, N., Gertz, M. A., Zeldenrust, S. R. *et al.* Improvement of cast nephropathy with plasma exchange depends on the diagnosis and on reduction of serum free light chains. *Kidney Int.* 2008;**73**(11):1282–8.

68. Sanders, P. W. Pathogenesis and treatment of myeloma kidney. *J. Lab. Clin. Med.* 1994; **124**(4):484–8.

69. Torra, R., Blade, J., Cases, A. *et al.* Patients with multiple myeloma requiring long-term dialysis: presenting features, response to therapy, and outcome in a series

of 20 cases. *Br. J. Haematol.* 1995;**91**(4):854–9.

70. Ying, W. Z., Sanders, P. W. Mapping the binding domain of immunoglobulin light chains for Tamm–Horsfall protein. *Am. J. Pathol.* 2001;**158**(5): 1859–66.

71. Herrera, G. A., Sanders, P. W. Paraproteinemic renal diseases that involve the tubulo-interstitium. *Contrib. Nephrol.* 2007;**153**:105–15.

72. Hutchison, C. A., Bradwell, A. R., Cook, M. *et al.* Treatment of acute renal failure secondary to multiple myeloma with chemotherapy and extended high cut-off hemodialysis. *Clin. J. Am. Soc. Nephrol.* 2009;**4**(4):745–54.

73. Winearls, C. G.. Myeloma kidney. In: Johnson, R., Feehally, J., editors, *Comprehensive Clinical Nephrology*: Mosby; 2003.

74. Katzmann, J. A., Clark, R. J., Abraham, R. S. *et al.* Serum reference intervals and diagnostic ranges for free kappa and free lambda immunoglobulin light chains: relative sensitivity for detection of monoclonal light chains. *Clin. Chem.* 2002; **48**(9):1437–44.

75. Hutchison, C. A., Cockwell, P., Reid, S. *et al.* Efficient removal of immunoglobulin free light chains by hemodialysis for multiple myeloma: in vitro and in vivo studies. *J. Am. Soc. Nephrol.* 2007;**18**(3):886–95.

76. Tanner, G. A., Evan, A. P. Glomerular and proximal tubular morphology after single nephron obstruction. *Kidney Int.* 1989; **36**(6):1050–60.

77. Tsakiris, D. J., Stel, V. S., Finne, P. *et al.* Incidence and outcome of patients starting renal replacement therapy for end-stage renal disease due to multiple myeloma or light-chain deposit disease: an ERA-EDTA Registry study. *Nephrol. Dial. Transplant* 2010;**25**(4):1200–6.

78. Passweg, J., Bock, H. A., Tichelli, A., Thiel, G. 'Transient multiple myeloma' after intense immunosuppression in a renal transplant patient. *Nephrol. Dial. Transplant* 1993;**8**(12):1393–4.

79. Walker, F., Bear, R. A. Renal transplantation in light-chain multiple myeloma. *Am. J. Nephrol.* 1983;**3**(1):34–7.

80. Penn, I. Evaluation of transplant candidates with pre-existing malignancies. *Ann. Transplant* 1997;**2**(4):14–17.

81. Foster, K., Cohen, D. J., D'Agati, V. D., Markowitz, G. S. Primary renal allograft dysfunction. *Am. J. Kidney Dis.* 2004;**44**(2):376–81.

82. Dagher, F., Sammett, D., Abbi, R. *et al.* Renal transplantation in multiple myeloma. Case report and review of the literature. *Transplantation* 1996; **62**(11):1577–80.

83. Humphrey, R. L., Wright, J. R., Zachary, J. B., Sterioff, S., DeFronzo, R. A. Renal transplantation in multiple myeloma. A case report. *Ann. Intern. Med.* 1975;**83**(5):651–3.

84. Kasiske, B. L., Cangro, C. B., Hariharan, S. *et al.* The evaluation of renal transplantation candidates: clinical practice guidelines. *Am. J. Transplant* 2001;1. Suppl **2**:3–95.

85. Kastritis, E., Anagnostopoulos, A., Roussou, M. *et al.* Reversibility of renal failure in newly diagnosed multiple myeloma patients treated with high dose dexamethasone-containing regimens and the impact of novel agents. *Haematologica* 2007;**92**(4): 546–9.

86. Barosi, G., Boccadoro, M., Cavo, M. *et al.* Management of multiple myeloma and related-disorders: guidelines from the Italian Society of Hematology (SIE), Italian Society of Experimental Hematology (SIES) and Italian Group for Bone Marrow Transplantation (GITMO).

Haematologica 2004;**89**(6): 717–41.

87. Carlson, K., Hjorth, M., Knudsen, L. M. Toxicity in standard melphalan-prednisone therapy among myeloma patients with renal failure – a retrospective analysis and recommendations for dose adjustment. *Br. J. Haematol.* 2005;**128**(5):631–5.

88. Dimopoulos, M., Spencer, A., Attal, M. *et al.* Lenalidomide plus dexamethasone for relapsed or refractory multiple myeloma. *N. Engl. J. Med.* 2007;**357**(21): 2123–32.

89. Macro, M., Divine, M., Uzunhan, Y. *et al.* Dexamethasone +thalidomide (Dex/Thal) compared to VAD as a pre-transplant treatment in newly diagnosed multiple myeloma (MM): a randomized trial. *ASH Annual Meeting Abstracts* 2006 November 16;**108**(11):57.

90. Rajkumar, S. V., Rosinol, L., Hussein, M. *et al.* Multicenter, randomized, double-blind, placebo-controlled study of thalidomide plus dexamethasone compared with dexamethasone as initial therapy for newly diagnosed multiple myeloma. *J. Clin. Oncol.* 2008;**26**(13):2171–7.

91. Richardson, P. G., Sonneveld, P., Schuster, M. *et al.* Extended follow-up of a phase 3 trial in relapsed multiple myeloma: final time-to-event results of the APEX trial. *Blood* 2007;**110**(10): 3557–60.

92. Weber, D. M., Chen, C., Niesvizky, R. *et al.* Lenalidomide plus dexamethasone for relapsed multiple myeloma in North America. *N. Engl. J. Med.* 2007;**357**(21):2133–42.

93. Zonder, J. A., Crowley, J., Hussein, M. A. *et al.* Lenalidomide and high-dose dexamethasone compared with dexamethasone as initial therapy for multiple myeloma: a randomized Southwest Oncology Group trial

(S0232). *Blood* 2010;**116**(26): 5838–41.

94. Harousseau, J. L., Attal, M., Avet-Loiseau, H. *et al.* Bortezomib plus dexamethasone is superior to vincristine plus doxorubicin plus dexamethasone as induction treatment prior to autologous stem-cell transplantation in newly diagnosed multiple myeloma: results of the IFM 2005–01 phase III trial. *J. Clin. Oncol.* 2010; **28**(30):4621–9.

95. Sonneveld, P., Schmidt-Wolf, I., van der Holt, B. *et al.* HOVON-65/GMMG-HD4 randomized phase III trial comparing bortezomib, doxorubicin, dexamethasone (PAD) vs VAD followed by high-dose melphalan (HDM) and maintenance with bortezomib or thalidomide in patients with newly diagnosed multiple myeloma (MM). *ASH Annual Meeting Abstracts* 2010 November 19;**116**(21):40.

96. Boccadoro, M., Morgan, G., Cavenagh, J. Preclinical evaluation of the proteasome inhibitor bortezomib in cancer therapy. *Cancer Cell Int.* 2005;**5**(1):18.

97. Chari, A., Mazumder, A., Jagannath, S. Proteasome inhibition and its therapeutic potential in multiple myeloma. *Biologics* 2010;**4**:273–87.

98. Mezzano, S. A., Barria, M., Droguett, M. A. *et al.* Tubular NF-kappaB and AP-1 activation in human proteinuric renal disease. *Kidney Int.* 2001;**60**(4): 1366–77.

99. Ludwig, H., Drach, J., Graf, H., Lang, A., Meran, J. G. Reversal of acute renal failure by bortezomib-based chemotherapy in patients with multiple myeloma. *Haematologica* 2007;**92**(10): 1411–14.

100. Millennium Pharmaceuticals Inc. *VELCADE® (bortezomib) for Injection. Prescribing information.* Cambridge, MA, USA 2009; Issued December 2009, Rev 10.

101. Labutti, J., Parsons, I., Huang, R. et al. Oxidative deboronation of the peptide boronic acid proteasome inhibitor bortezomib: contributions from reactive oxygen species in this novel cytochrome P450 reaction. *Chem. Res. Toxicol.* 2006;**19**(4):539–46.

102. Uttamsingh, V., Lu, C., Miwa, G., Gan, L. S. Relative contributions of the five major human cytochromes P450, 1A2, 2C9, 2C19, 2D6, and 3A4, to the hepatic metabolism of the proteasome inhibitor bortezomib. *Drug Metab. Dispos.* 2005;**33**(11):1723–8.

103. Pekol, T., Daniels, J. S., Labutti, J. et al. Human metabolism of the proteasome inhibitor bortezomib: identification of circulating metabolites. *Drug Metab. Dispos.* 2005;**33**(6):771–7.

104. Mulkerin, D., Remick, S., Takimoto, C. et al. Safety, tolerability, and pharmacology of bortezomib in cancer patients with renal failure requiring dialysis: results from a prospective phase 1 study. *ASH Annual Meeting Abstracts* 2007;**110**(11):3477.

105. Dimopoulos, M. A., Richardson, P. G., Schlag, R. et al. VMP (bortezomib, melphalan, and prednisone) is active and well tolerated in newly diagnosed patients with multiple myeloma with moderately impaired renal function, and results in reversal of renal impairment: cohort analysis of the phase III VISTA study. *J. Clin. Oncol.* 2009;**27**(36):6086–93.

106. San-Miguel, J. F., Richardson, P. G., Sonneveld, P. et al. Efficacy and safety of bortezomib in patients with renal impairment: results from the APEX phase 3 study. *Leukemia* 2008;**22**(4):842–9.

107. Scheid, C., Sonneveld, P., Schmidt-Wolf, I. et al. Influence of renal function on outcome of VAD or bortezomib, doxorubicin, dexamethasone (PAD) induction treatment followed by high-dose melphalan (HDM): a subgroup analysis from the HOVON-65/GMMG-HD4 randomized phase III trial for newly diagnosed multiple myeloma. *ASH Annual Meeting Abstracts* 2010;**116**(21):2396.

108. Jagannath, S., Barlogie, B., Berenson, J. R. et al. Bortezomib in recurrent and/or refractory multiple myeloma. Initial clinical experience in patients with impared renal function. *Cancer* 2005;**103**(6):1195–200.

109. Ludwig, H., Adam, Z., Hajek, R. et al. Light chain-induced acute renal failure can be reversed by bortezomib-doxorubicin-dexamethasone in multiple myeloma: results of a phase II study. *J. Clin. Oncol.* 2010;**28**(30):4635–41.

110. Li, J., Zhou, D. B., Jiao, L. et al. Bortezomib and dexamethasone therapy for newly diagnosed patients with multiple myeloma complicated by renal impairment. *Clin. Lymphoma Myeloma* 2009;**9**(5):394–8.

111. Stefanikova, Z., Roziakova, L. Reversibility of renal failure in multiple myeloma patients treated with bortezomib-based regimens: a single centre experience [abstract]. *Haematologica* 2010;**95**:593.

112. Ailawadhi, S., Mashtare, T. L., Coignet, M. V. et al. Renal dysfunction does not affect clinical response in multiple myeloma (MM) patients treated with bortezomib-based regimens. *ASH Annual Meeting Abstracts* 2007;**110**(11):1477.

113. Malani, A. K., Gupta, V., Rangineni, R. Bortezomib and dexamethasone in previously untreated multiple myeloma associated with renal failure and reversal of renal failure. *Acta Haematol.* 2006;**116**(4):255–8.

114. Basu, S., Cook, M., Hutchison, C. A. et al. High rate of renal recovery in patients with cast nephropathy treated by removal of free light chains using extended hemodialysis: a phase 1/2 clinical trial [abstract]. *Haematologica* 2007;**92**:213.

115. Blade, J., Sonneveld, P., San Miguel, J. F. et al. Pegylated liposomal doxorubicin plus bortezomib in relapsed or refractory multiple myeloma: efficacy and safety in patients with renal function impairment. *Clin. Lymphoma Myeloma.* 2008;**8**(6):352–5.

116. Knauf, W. U., Otremba, B., Overkamp, F., Kornacker, M. Bortezomib in relapsed multiple myeloma: results of a non-interventional study by office-based haematologists. *Onkologie* 2009;**32**(4):175–80.

117. Aggarwal, S., Jauhri, M., Negi, A., Kohli, S., Minhas, S. Frontline management of myeloma with bortezemib and dexamethasone – focus on renal failure – a study from India [abstract]. *Blood* 2010;**116**:5045.

118. Chanan-Khan, A. A., Kaufman, J. L., Mehta, J. et al. Activity and safety of bortezomib in multiple myeloma patients with advanced renal failure: a multicenter retrospective study. *Blood* 2007;**109**(6):2604–6.

119. Kumar, S., Rajkumar, S. V. Thalidomide and lenalidomide in the treatment of multiple myeloma. *Eur. J. Cancer* 2006;**42**(11):1612–22.

120. Li, Y., Hou, J., Jiang, H. et al. Polymorphisms of CYP2C19 gene are associated with the efficacy of thalidomide based regimens in multiple myeloma. *Haematologica* 2007;**92**(9):1246–9.

121. Eriksson, T., Hoglund, P., Turesson, I. et al. Pharmacokinetics of thalidomide in patients with impaired renal function and while on and off

273

dialysis. *J. Pharm. Pharmacol* 2003;**55**(12):1701–6.

122. Tosi, P., Zamagni, E., Cellini, C. *et al*. Thalidomide alone or in combination with dexamethasone in patients with advanced, relapsed or refractory multiple myeloma and renal failure. *Eur. J. Haematol.* 2004;**73**(2):98–103.

123. Harris, E., Behrens, J., Samson, D. *et al*. Use of thalidomide in patients with myeloma and renal failure may be associated with unexplained hyperkalaemia. *Br. J. Haematol.* 2003;**122**(1): 160–1.

124. Bartlett, J. B., Dredge, K., Dalgleish, A. G. The evolution of thalidomide and its IMiD derivatives as anticancer agents. *Nat. Rev. Cancer* 2004;**4**(4): 314–22.

125. Hussein, M. A. Lenalidomide: patient management strategies. *Semin. Hematol.* 2005; **42**(4 Suppl 4):S22–5.

126. Chen, N., Lau, H., Kong, L. *et al*. Pharmacokinetics of lenalidomide in subjects with various degrees of renal impairment and in subjects on hemodialysis. *J. Clin. Pharmacol.* 2007;**47**(12):1466–75.

127. Dimopoulos, M., Alegre, A., Stadtmauer, E. A. *et al*. The efficacy and safety of lenalidomide plus dexamethasone in relapsed and/or refractory multiple myeloma patients with impaired renal function. *Cancer* 2010; **116**(16):3807–14.

128. Niesvizky, R., Naib, T., Christos, P. J. *et al*. Lenalidomide-induced myelosuppression is associated with renal dysfunction: adverse events evaluation of treatment-naive patients undergoing front-line lenalidomide and dexamethasone therapy. *Br. J. Haematol.* 2007;**138**(5):640–3.

129. Reece, D. E., Masih-Khan, E., Chen, C. *et al*. Use of lenalidomide (Revlimid(R) +/– corticosteroids in relapsed/ refractory multiple myeloma

patients with elevated baseline serum creatinine levels. *ASH Annual Meeting Abstracts* 2006;**108**(11):3548.

130. Dimopoulos, M. A., Christoulas, D., Roussou, M. *et al*. Lenalidomide and dexamethasone for the treatment of refractory/ relapsed multiple myeloma: dosing of lenalidomide according to renal function and effect on renal impairment. *Eur. J. Haematol.* 2010; **85**(1):1–5.

131. Quach, H., Fernyhough, L., Henderson, R. *et al*. Lower-dose lenalidomide and dexamethasone reduces toxicity without compromising efficacy in patients with relapsed/refractory myeloma, who are aged >=60 years or have renal impairment: planned interim results of a prospective multicentre phase II trial. *ASH Annual Meeting Abstracts* 2010;**116**(21):1961.

132. Klein, U., Neben, K., Hielscher, T. *et al*. Lenalidomide in combination with dexamethasone: effective regimen in patients with relapsed or refractory multiple myeloma complicated by renal impairment. *Ann. Hematol.* 2011;**90**(4):429–39.

133. de la Rubia, J., Roig, M., Ibanez, A. *et al*. Activity and safety of lenalidomide and dexamethasone in patients with multiple myeloma requiring dialysis: a Spanish multicenter retrospective study. *Eur. J. Haematol.* 2010;**85**(4): 363–5.

134. Ludwig, H., Zojer, N. Renal recovery with lenalidomide in a patient with bortezomib-resistant multiple myeloma. *Nat. Rev. Clin. Oncol.* 2010;**7**(5):289–94.

135. Patel, M., Sher, T., Ailawadhi, S. *et al*. Novel agents overcome the adverse prognosis imparted by compromised renal function in patients with multiple myeloma. *ASH Annual Meeting Abstracts* 2008;**112**(11):2726.

136. Lee, C. K., Zangari, M., Barlogie, B. *et al*. Dialysis-dependent renal failure in patients with myeloma can be reversed by high-dose myeloablative therapy and autotransplant. *Bone Marrow Transplant* 2004;**33**(8):823–8.

137. Ballester, O. F., Tummala, R., Janssen, W. E. *et al*. High-dose chemotherapy and autologous peripheral blood stem cell transplantation in patients with multiple myeloma and renal insufficiency. *Bone Marrow Transplant* 1997;**20**(8):653–6.

138. Royer, B., Arnulf, B., Martinez, F. *et al*. High dose chemotherapy in light chain or light and heavy chain deposition disease. *Kidney Int.* 2004;**65**(2):642–8.

139. Carlson, K. Melphalan 200 mg/m^2 with blood stem cell support as first-line myeloma therapy: impact of glomerular filtration rate on engraftment, transplantation-related toxicity and survival. *Bone Marrow Transplant* 2005;**35**(10):985–90.

140. Raab, M. S., Breitkreutz, I., Hundemer, M. *et al*. The outcome of autologous stem cell transplantation in patients with plasma cell disorders and dialysis-dependent renal failure. *Haematologica* 2006;**91**(11): 1555–8.

141. Bird, J. M., Fuge, R., Sirohi, B. *et al*. The clinical outcome and toxicity of high-dose chemotherapy and autologous stem cell transplantation in patients with myeloma or amyloid and severe renal impairment: a British Society of Blood and Marrow Transplantation study. *Br. J. Haematol.* 2006;**134**(4): 385–90.

142. Hassoun, H., Flombaum, C., D'Agati, V. D. *et al*. High-dose melphalan and auto-SCT in patients with monoclonal Ig deposition disease. *Bone Marrow Transplant* 2008; **42**(6):405–12.

143. Parikh, G. C., Amjad, A. I., Saliba, R. M. *et al.* Autologous hematopoietic stem cell transplantation may reverse renal failure in patients with multiple myeloma. *Biol. Blood Marrow Transplant* 2009;**15**(7):812–16.

144. Hutchinson, C. A., Cook, M., Heyne, N. *et al.* European trial of free light chain removal by extended hemodialysis in cast nephropathy (EuLITE): a randomized controlled trial. *Trials* 2008;**9**:55.

145. Khan, M. L., Stewart, A. K. Carfilzomib: a novel second-generation proteasome inhibitor. *Future Oncology* 2011;7(5): 607–12.

146. Badros, A. Z., Vij, R., Martin, T. *et al.* Phase II study of carfilzomib in patients with relapsed/ refractory multiple myeloma and renal insufficiency. *ASCO Meeting Abstracts* 2010;**28**(15 suppl):8128.

147. Tosi, P., Zamagni, E., Tacchetti, P. *et al.* Thalidomide-dexamethasone as induction therapy before autologous stem cell transplantation in patients with newly diagnosed multiple myeloma and renal insufficiency. *Biol. Blood Marrow Transplant* 2010; **16**(8):1115–21.

148. Seol, Y., Chung, J., Kwon, B. *et al.* Treatment for patients with multiple myeloma complicated by renal failure by thalidomide-based regimens. [abstract]. *J. Clin. Oncol.* 2010;**28**:e13093.

Chapter

20

The management of infection in myeloma

Christopher P. Conlon

Introduction

Myeloma is primarily a disease of older age groups with the median age of diagnosis above 60 years. Although, in the past, the prognosis was poor, this has changed over the past decade with the advent of new therapies and the use of autologous stem cell transplantation. Whereas formerly the infective problems associated with myeloma were the consequence of the disease itself and were often the mode of presentation, now the disease can be viewed as more chronic and infections are more commonly related to either the therapies used or the longer term complications of myeloma itself. Nevertheless, infections still account for the majority of deaths in the first 120 days after diagnosis. This chapter will address the risk factors for infection in myeloma and will outline the more common infective complications and their management, as well as considering what preventive measures can be taken.

Risk factors for infection

Immunodeficiency

The hallmark of myeloma is B cell dysregulation, usually manifested by hypogammaglobulinemia. This leads to an increased risk of bacterial infections, particularly those due to encapsulated organisms such as *Streptococcus pneumoniae* and *Haemophilus influenzae*. Other common bacterial infections that may present early on are *Staphylococcus aureus* and *Eschericia coli* [1]. However, there is ample evidence that the disease also affects cellular immunity with abnormalities of T lymphocytes, dendritic cells and NK cells. Although the cellular defects may be more subtle and do not normally manifest early in myeloma, they undoubtedly contribute to some of the complications of chemotherapy [2].

Disease-related organ damage and co-morbidities

A significant minority of patients with myeloma present with renal impairment either as a result of tubular damage from myeloma proteins or from hypercalcemia. Such renal dysfunction can impair the response to infections, particularly those due to bacteria [3]. Severe bone pain or vertebral collapse are not uncommon and often lead to the use of opiate analgesics. Both pain and the opiates may compromise respiratory effort and increase the risk of respiratory tract infections. Fractures related to myeloma can be associated with an increased risk of osteomyelitis. In addition, the use of bisphosphonates, such as zolendroic acid, in myeloma is associated with a risk of osteonecrosis of the jaw which may, in turn, be complicated by jaw osteomyelitis [4]. More rarely, patients may develop other organ damage from the development of amyloidosis. Finally, because the disease affects older patients, the decline of the immune system with age may be considered another factor increasing the risk of infections. The risk factors for infection in myeloma are shown in Table 20.1.

The complications of myeloma therapy

Many of the new treatments for myeloma are immunosuppressive. The infection risk is compounded by the fact that patients survive longer but are usually immunocompromised during the therapy and for some time afterwards. High-dose steroids, such as dexamethasone, are commonly used in the induction phase of treatment and act to reduce cellular immunity. This increases the risk of infections such as mucosal candidiasis and herpesvirus infections. Bortezomib is now widely used in

Myeloma, ed. Stephen A. Schey, Kwee L. Yong, Robert Marcus and Kenneth C. Anderson. Published by Cambridge University Press. © Cambridge University Press 2014.

Table 20.1 Risk factors for infection in myeloma

Risk factor	Type of infection
Hypogammaglobulinemia	Bacterial pneumonia and bacteremia
Renal impairment	Bacterial infections
Bony lesions	Bacterial osteomyelitis
Bisphosphonates	Jaw osteonecrosis/osteomyelitis
High-dose steroids	Herpes virus infections; fungal disease
Induction chemotherapy	Neutropenic sepsis (bacterial)
Bortezomib	Varicella-zoster
Stem cell transplant	
Early	Neutropenic sepsis; *Clostridium difficile*
Late	Cytomegalovirus; invasive fungal infection

Table 20.2 Variable risk of infection with myeloma over time

Risk period	Type of infection
Diagnosis	Bacterial infections
Induction chemotherapy	Bacterial infections (neutropenia)
	Mucosal fungal infections (mucositis, neutropenia) Herpes virus infections (steroids) Invasive fungal infections (steroids)
Autologous stem cell transplant	
Early	Bacterial infections (neutropenia) Clostridium difficile (antibiotics, steroids) Invasive fungal infections (steroids; neutropenia)
Late	Invasive fungal infections; PCP (low CD4 cells) Cytomegalovirus; VZV
Salvage therapy	VZV (bortezomib) Neutropenic sepsis (lenalidomide, dexamethasone) Invasive fungal infections (low CD4 cells)

induction and has been associated with a greatly increased risk of varicella-zoster virus (VZV) infection [5]. In animal models, this drug affects antigen processing and impairs cytotoxic T-cell function, thus increasing susceptibility to viral infections [6]. Thalidomide and lenalidomide affect T cells but also can be lead to neutropenia, although this is much more marked with lenalidomide. Lenalidomide is associated with an increase in neutropenia but has not, in itself, been associated with a greatly increased infection risk. Clearly autologous stem cell transplantation has marked effects on infection risks. Neutropenic sepsis is a problem early on, while invasive fungal infections and viral infections may present later.

In addition to the effects of therapy on the immune system, some of the complications of treatment can increase the risk of infections in other ways. Thalidomide and lenalidomide are both procoagulant and increase the risk of venous thromboembolism. Infected pulmonary emboli can be a problem and clots involving central venous catheters may increase the risk of line-related bacteremia. The newer drugs, including bortezomib, might lead to peripheral neuropathy which, in turn, may increase the risk of foot and soft tissue infection. Infections may occur at any stage of myeloma and its treatment (Table 20.2)

Bacterial infections and their management

At the time of diagnosis, or when starting induction therapy, infections with common bacteria predominate. The hypogammaglobulinemia of myeloma predisposes to infection with encapsulated bacteria, especially *Streptococcus pneumoniae* (pneumococcus) and *Haemophilus influenzae*. These infections commonly present as pneumonia but may present with sepsis syndrome and bacteraemia [7]. Pneumococcal infection (Figure 20.1) in this setting is best treated with parenteral antibiotics. Generally, beta-lactams, such as benzylpenicillin or amoxicillin in adequate doses are the best treatments. Initially, in a septic patient, broader spectrum antibiotics might be started but the treatment can be narrowed once culture results become available. However, over the past decade, penicillin-resistant pneumococci have emerged in some parts of the world, notably in part of the United States and in southern Europe. If local experience suggests the possibility of penicillin

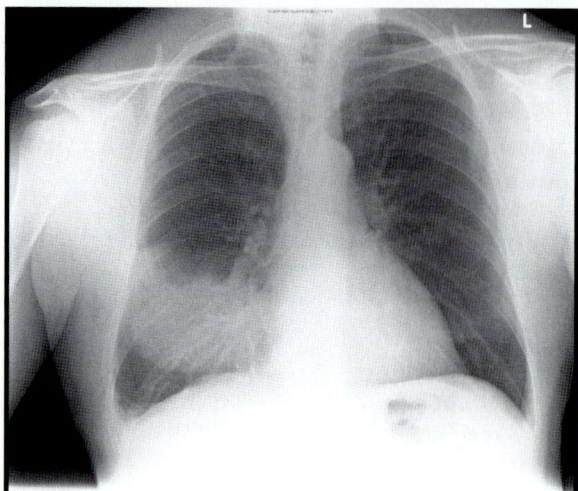

Figure 20.1 Chest X-ray showing consolidation caused by *Streptococcus pneumoniae*.

resistance, clinicians often add a second antibiotic, such as a macrolide or a quinolone, to ensure adequate coverage. In fact, most studies have shown that, even in the presence of penicillin resistance, large doses of a beta lactam antibiotic result in similar outcomes in pneumococcal pneumonia to those seen with other regimens although a recent meta-analysis suggests otherwise [8]. Pneumococcal bacteremia, however, may do better with combination therapy [9]. Infections with *H. influenzae* will usually respond to treatment with co-amoxiclav (amoxicillin with clavulanic acid) or similar agents that will deal with beta-lactamase producing strains. Patients with myeloma also present with infections due to *Staphylococcus aureus*, usually in the form of bacteremia. These infections require parenteral therapy with a beta-lactamase stable antibiotic, such as flucloxacillin. However, if the rate of methicillin-resistant *S. aureus* (MRSA) in the community or hospital is significant, other agents, such as glycopeptides, linezolid or daptomycin, may be more appropriate. It is important to recognize that *S. aureus* is particularly prone to metastatic spread from a focus of infection to other sites in the body. Particular attention should be paid to the possibility of joint involvement or endocarditis in patients presenting with *S. aureus* bacteremia. Other bacteria, such as *E. coli*, will need to be treated according to their identification and antibiotic susceptibility pattern, with appropriate advice from infectious diseases or microbiology specialists. One of the increasing

concerns in Gram-negative infections is the rise in the number of such bacteria producing extended spectrum beta-lactamases (ESBL). The genes encoding these antibiotic-destroying enzymes are becoming more widespread, leading to real problems with resistant Gram-negative organisms both in the community and in hospitals [10]. At present carbapenem antibiotics, such as meropenem, are used in this setting. However, there are now carbapenemase-producing Enterobacteriaceae, for example *Klebsiella* species, that can only be treated by drugs, such as colistin. Tigecycline, a new glycylcycline antibiotic, has also been used in this setting but, at the time of writing, there are concerns about the efficacy and safety of this compound.

The past decade has also seen an alarming increase in the prevalence of infections due to *Clostridium difficile* [11]. Quinolones and third-generation cephalosporins have been identified as risk factors in the development of this infection. The use of proton pump inhibitors, often given with high-dose corticosteroid therapy, is known to increase the risk of *C. difficile* infection and it is likely, though not proven, that steroids themselves may predispose to this problem or lead to more severe disease. Myeloma patients may be particularly prone to *C. difficile*, partly because of the age groups affected, and partly because of the likelihood of being exposed to broad spectrum antibiotics in conjunction with immunodeficiency. There appears to be an increasing prevalence of *C. difficile* infection following stem cell transplantation [12].

Though rarely reported with myeloma, clinicians should be aware of the risk of reactivation of tuberculosis (TB) with the use of powerful immunosuppressive therapy, particularly after stem cell transplantation. Patients from endemic areas, or those who have received TB treatment in the past, are particularly at risk. In addition, sometimes non-tuberculous mycobacteria are implicated in line-related infections. Diagnosis and management of mycobacterial infections are beyond the scope of this chapter but, should they be encountered in patients with myeloma, expert help should be sought.

Neutropenic fever

At some stage, either during induction chemotherapy or following stem cell transplantation, patients usually become neutropenic. Neutropenic episodes may be complicated either by fever, bacteremia or severe sepsis syndrome. Most hospitals and hematology units will have protocols to deal with febrile neutropenia and there may be national guidelines [13]. Not all such episodes of fever will be infective in origin but, because the consequences of bacterial sepsis are so severe, broad spectrum antibiotics are routinely administered. The principles are to give antibiotic therapy to cover a range of Gram-positive and Gram-negative bacteria, with the specific choice of antibiotics governed by local experience of the bacterial isolates from this group of patients. In practice, a broad spectrum, anti-pseudomonal beta-lactam, such as piperacillin-tazobactam, or a carbapenem, such as meropenem, is used that will cover many organisms, including resistant coliforms and *Pseudomonas aeruginosa*. Sometimes a dose of an aminoglycoside, such as gentamicin, is added initially so that rare, resistant organisms are also covered, including MRSA. Antibiotic therapy can then be modified according to the culture results or the response of the patient. Generally, antibiotic therapy is continued until the fever has settled for 48 h, the neutrophil count has recovered and the patient has improved. In patients who are relatively well and in whom the period of neutropenia is expected to be short, it might be possible to treat them as outpatients after initial assessment. In these cases oral antibiotic therapy should cover the typical Gram-positive and Gram-negative organisms [14]. A combination of ciprofloxacin and clindamycin would be appropriate in many settings.

If the fever does not settle within 48–72 h, many clinicians will escalate therapy. This may involve adding a glycopeptide, such as vancomycin, to cover coagulase negative staphylococci or MRSA infections. In practice, the addition of a glycopeptide like this is rarely helpful and does not improve outcomes. Frequently, physicians add an antifungal drug empirically if the fever persists for more than 5–7 days after the start of antibiotics because of the increased risk of invasive fungal infections with prolonged neutropenia. However, such fungal infections are responsible for only a minority of episodes of febrile neutropenia. In recognition of this (and the high cost and potential side effects and drug interactions with antifungal drugs) current efforts are aimed at trying to identify those at risk of invasive fungal infections. Some risk factors for invasive fungal infections are well described, including the prolonged periods of neutropenia, the use of high-dose corticosteroids, graft-versus-host disease and prior CMV infections [15].

Efforts to diagnose fungal infections early, with the view to pre-emptive treatment, have involved the use of PCR or various antigen-detection assays. Although the use of polymerase chain reaction (PCR) to identify invasive *Aspergillus* infections has met with success in some centers, there are no validated commercial assays, false positives are common and such PCRs will only identify one species of fungus. More commonly used are assays to detect galactomannan, an *Aspergillus*-specific polysaccharide but, again, results vary from center to center and there are issues concerning cost and reproducibility. Serial measurements are often undertaken in high risk patients, with a rise in the level triggering the administration of an antifungal drug. False positive reactions can be a problem, particularly in patients receiving piperacillin-tazobactam and one group has found problems with false positive galactomannan assays in the setting of myeloma, especially in those with IgG subtype disease [16].

Fungal infections
Candida infections

The use of corticosteroids, along with chemotherapy agents that cause neutropenia, increases the likelihood of mucosal candida infections. Most of these infections are caused by *Candida albicans* and are easily treatable. Although topical therapy with nystatin or miconazole troches is usually effective, some patients may need systemic therapy with oral fluconazole for severe local infection as the pseudohyphae can penetrate deep into mucosal tissue. Patients with a lot of azole exposure can develop azole-resistant mucosal candidiasis, often with non-albicans species, such as *C. glabrata*. In cases where fluconazole appears less effective, it is important to take samples for culture and sensitivity in order to detect such resistance and to guide therapy.

The main concern in patients undergoing chemotherapy that produces neutropenia or in those receiving autologous stem cell transplants is the development of invasive fungal infections. Colonization of indwelling central lines with candida may lead to candidemia. In addition to causing fever and the potential to cause a sepsis syndrome, metastatic candida infection can occur. Patients with candidemia need to be assessed for this possibility, including an ophthalmic review to look for candida endophthalmitis. If the organism is known to be *Candida albicans* or if the patient is relatively well and stable, high-dose fluconazole (starting at 800 mg daily) can be used. For moderately or severely ill patients or those who have had significant prior exposure to azole antifungals, it is preferable to use an echinocandin, such as caspofungin or micafungin [17]. Therapy can be adjusted according to the state of the patient or when culture and sensitivity results are available. Treatment should continue for at least two weeks after the candida has been cleared from the blood, although metastatic spread of the candida merits more prolonged therapy. Because candida readily adheres to plastic, it is essential to change any central lines or other catheters.

Mold infections

Invasive filamentous fungi, or mold, infections are probably more common and more likely to lead to serious morbidity and death compared to invasive candida infections in the setting of myeloma. The most common infection is that due to *Aspergillus* species [18], [19]. *Aspergillus fumigatus* is the most commonly encountered species but others, such as *A. flavus* or *A. niger*, also occur. Outbreaks of aspergillosis on hematology wards have been associated with hospital building works, probably because such work increases the probability that *Aspergillus* spores will become airborne and inhaled by patients at risk. However, many infections are probably acquired in the community [20]. Because *Aspergillus* conidia are usually inhaled, initial infection usually occurs in the lung. Although the disease may be focal, it can progress and lead to invasive pulmonary aspergillosis (IPA). Early infection may just manifest as a fever, hence the role of empiric antifungals in febrile neutropenia. Patients may also develop symptoms related to lung involvement, such as chest pain if the pleura are involved and, more rarely and later in the course, cough and hemoptysis. One of the hallmarks of aspergillosis in the lung is that it is angio-invasive. As a consequence, disease may spread elsewhere; notably to the brain, leading to focal signs, seizures or reduced Glasgow coma score. Mortality with invasive aspergillosis is high, ranging from 30% to 50% in most studies. Patients with myeloma who receive autologous stem cell transplants are at risk but the risk is several-fold lower than in other patients with hematological malignancy receiving allogeneic transplants.

Clinical signs of IPA, other than fever, are often absent so early use of imaging is recommended. Chest X-ray changes are usually late but chest CT scans are more likely to show abnormalities, such as patchy infiltrates. The classic "halo sign" is relatively unusual but is useful if present. This may progress to the radiological sign of an "air crescent" as the neutrophil count recovers (Figure 20.2). Radiographic abnormalities should prompt an attempt to culture the fungus but, often, co-morbidities or thrombocytopenia may preclude invasive investigations. Because of this,

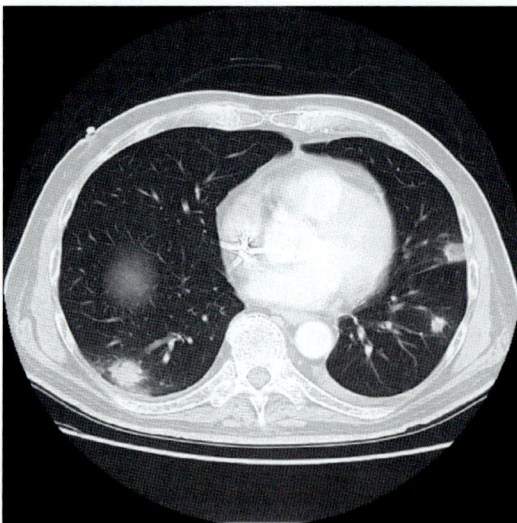
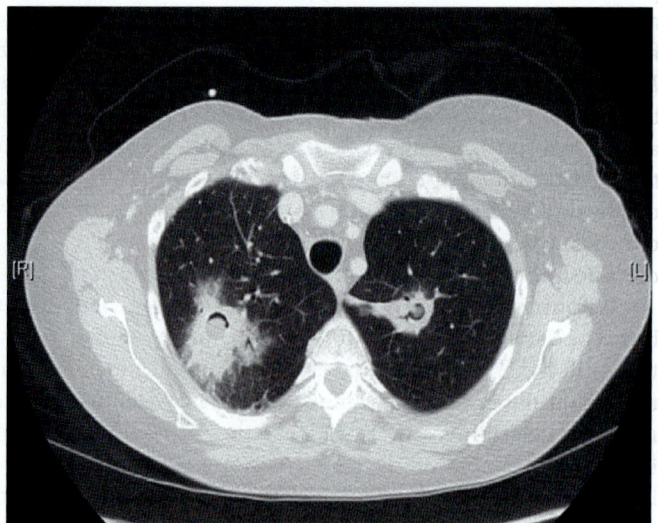

(a)   (b)

Figure 20.2 (a) Chest CT of invasive pulmonary aspergillosis: halo sign. (b) Chest CT of invasive pulmonary aspergillosis: air crescent sign.

indirect diagnostic methods have been used to supplement clinical suspicions. PCR remains a problem, partly because of the high rate of false positives and partly because there are no standard, commercially available assays. Antigen detection using a commercially available ELISA that detects galactomannan, a component of the *Aspergillus* cell wall, has been more successful and is used in many centers. Twice-weekly assays can be used with the addition of chest CT imaging to determine when to start antifungal therapy. Such approaches can reduce costs and toxicity but have not been shown to be superior to using empiric antifungal therapy [21]. There are still problems with the sensitivity and specificity of the assay, and controversy surrounds the cut off level of the assay, but it can probably be considered to have a good negative predictive value.

In addition to aspergillosis, other mold infections that occur in the immunosuppressed hematology patients are *Fusarium* species and mucormycosis. Infection with *Fusarium*, which is also angio-invasive, can mimic aspergillosis with either lung or sinus involvement. *Fusarium* species are more likely to be associated with central line infection. In severe cases, *Fusarium* spreads in the bloodstream and results in skin lesions and abscesses. This mold is much more likely to result in positive blood cultures than other molds. Fungi causing mucormycosis are rarely cultured from blood and are notable for causing locally destructive lesions in the sinuses; rhinocerebral mucormycosis. Skin lesions can also occur and the pulmonary infections are indistinguishable clinically and radiographically from aspergillosis. Mortality from mucormycosis approaches 80%. Importantly, *Fusarium* is usually resistant to amphotericin B and the species causing mucormycosis are usually resistant to azoles, so antifungal therapy needs to be targeted accurately if either type of mold is identified or suspected. There is a suggestion that the incidence of mucomyosis is increasing since the widespread use of azole antifungal prophylaxis [22].

Treatment of invasive mold infections requires broad spectrum systemic antifungal therapy. Clearly the antifungal drug should be chosen appropriately if the fungus has been identified and attempts should be made to determine the antifungal sensitivity of the isolate. More commonly, the diagnosis of fungal infection is probable but not proven and therapy is started in the absence of a microbiological diagnosis. Therefore, treatment is aimed at aspergillosis as the most common infection. The "gold standard" treatment in the past was amphotericin B deoxycholate but, largely because of concerns about renal toxicity, lipid-based formulations of amphotericin B have supplanted this in most centers. These drugs rarely produce more than a 50% success rate in this condition. More recently newer antifungal agents have become available. Extended spectrum third generation azoles, voriconazole, posaconazole and ravuconazole all have good activity against *Aspergillus*. Voriconazole has the advantage of being available intravenously as well as orally and is frequently used as first line therapy for suspected mold infections. The other new group of antifungals is the echinocandins such as caspofungin, micafungin and anidulafungin. These drugs are usually used in salvage therapy for unresponsive disease but, increasingly, some centers use them as first line agents. Both the azoles and the echinocandins are better tolerated than amphotericin B and less nephrotoxic. However, liver function abnormalities do occur, as do rashes. Voriconazole has been associated with odd visual symptoms, including hallucinations, but these usually resolve despite continued use of the drug. Clinical trials have failed to distinguish any of these systemic antifungals from one another for the treatment of invasive mold infections although there is some suggestion that the newer agents may be superior to amphotericin B [23]. Although combinations of antifungal drugs (e.g. azole plus echinocandin) have shown some promise in animal models, the experience in humans is mixed and combination therapy cannot be recommended.

Surgical treatment of mold infections is sometimes appropriate, along with systemic antifungal drugs. Isolated lung lesions due to *Aspergillus* can be resected as can aspergillosis of the sinuses. Mucormycosis in the sinuses usually needs surgery along with amphotericin B treatment and skin lesions should be excised.

Pneumocystis jirovecii

Pneumonia due to *Pneumocystis jirovecii* is a risk for any immunocompromised patient. Human disease was thought to be due to *Pneumocystis carinii* but this is now known to be the species infecting rodents. *Pneumocystis* is also now known to be a fungus from genetic analysis. *Pneumocystis* pneumonia (PCP) generally occurs in the face of T-lymphocyte dysfunction and may be a risk in myeloma, particularly after stem

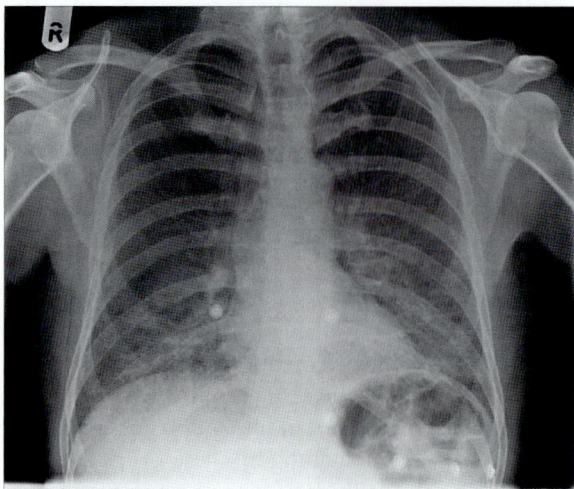

Figure 20.3 Chest X-ray with subtle bilateral changes of *Pneumocystis* pneumonia.

cell transplantation. High-dose steroids or prolonged steroid therapy are also risk factors. PCP usually presents with fever and breathlessness and although many patients present with an acute pneumonic illness, the onset may be insidious [24]. Hypoxia with minimal exertion is typical even though clinical examination of the chest is often normal. The chest radiograph usually shows mid zone bilateral perihilar infiltrates (Figure 20.3) that appear as ground glass shadowing on CT scanning of the lungs. Unilateral disease can occur and, occasionally, the chest X-ray is normal (though the CT is not). Diagnosis is usually by bronchoscopy and broncho-alveolar lavage when the cysts can be identified by cytology or immuno-fluorescence. Induced sputum will yield the diagnosis in some instances but the yield probably relies on the skill and experience of the staff performing the sputum induction. Although PCR has been used to identify *P. jirovecii*, there are no validated commercial assays available.

Treatment of proven or suspected PCP is with high dose co-trimoxazole and oxygen. If myelosuppression is a concern, other treatments include intravenous pentamidine or a combination of clindamycin and primaquine. Although adjunctive corticosteroids have been shown to be effective in the management of PCP in the setting of HIV, there are no data to support their use in PCP in other settings, such as hematological malignancy. Indeed, it is often the use of high-dose steroids that has led to the occurrence of PCP in the latter case. Treatment with co-trimoxazole

should continue for at least two weeks even if clinical resolution is more rapid.

Cryptococcus and dimorphic fungi

Cryptococcus var neoformans is widely distributed in nature whereas *Cryptococcus var gatii* is less so. The former is more likely to cause disease in immuno-compromised patients. In myeloma, the risks are either with prolonged high dose steroid therapy or after stem cell transplantation. Although cryptococci usually enter via the respiratory route and can cause a pneumonic illness, the most common presentation is with meningitis. Cryptococcal meningitis can be quite subtle, with fever and headache but an absence of neck stiffness. Sometimes cranial nerve palsies occur, particularly sixth nerve palsies secondary to raised intracranial pressure. Bloodstream spread can also occur and may result in skin lesions that look a bit like giant molluscum contagiosum lesions. Rarely direct skin inoculation can occur, producing soft tissue infection.

The diagnosis of cryptococcal meningitis is made by lumbar puncture. The cerebrospinal fluid (CSF) pressure is usually elevated and often markedly so. The CSF may appear normal macroscopically but, along with some lymphocytes, is characterized by the presence of the yeast cells. These typically have a large gelatinous capsule which can be demonstrated by India ink staining of the CSF. Detection of crypto-coccal antigen (CRAG) in CSF is helpful and might also be positive in blood or urine. The best treatment for cryptococcal meningitis is a combination of amphotericin B and 5-flucytosine given for at least the first two weeks. Once the patient has improved, CSF cultures have become sterile and the CSF pressure has fallen, follow-on treatment with oral fluconazole (400 mg daily) can be started. Fluconazole should be avoided as first line treatment as it is much less likely to sterilize the CSF compared to amphotericin B and 5-flucytosine [25]. Fluconazole should be continued long term until the patient is no longer immunosuppressed. Rare isolates of *C. neoformans* have been reported with reduced sensitivity to fluconazole so it is important to ensure that antifungal sensitivity testing is performed on the isolates.

Some fungi exist as yeast forms at around 37°C (i.e. human body temperature) and as molds at lower temperatures, such as found in soil. These dimorphic fungi are geographically restricted and none is endemic to Europe. However, they may cause disease in patients who have lived in or visited endemic areas in the past and later become immunosuppressed, so it is important to take a detailed travel history before embarking on myeloma treatment. *Histoplasma capsulatum*, the most common, is found in parts of the Midwest in North America and in parts of Central and South America. *Coccidioides immitis* and *Blastomyces dermatitidis* are restricted to the Western Hemisphere as is *Paracoccidiodes brasiliensis*, although the latter is confined to Latin America. By contrast *Penicillium marneffei* is only found in Southeast Asia. Individuals may harbor these fungi asymptomatically but become ill when immunosuppressed; usually after high-dose corticosteroids or after stem cell transplantation. Disseminated disease is the most common problem in this setting, with frequent lung involvement. Skin and central nervous system involvement can also occur. Diagnosis is by culturing the fungus or demonstrating it in histological sections. Good serological tests exist for *Histoplasma* and *Coccidioides*. Infectious diseases advice should be sought regarding treatment and duration of therapy.

Viral infections

Herpes viruses

The most common viral infections in patients with myeloma are those due to herpes viruses. *Herpes simplex* can be a problem in any patient who is immunocompromised, with outbreaks of cold sores or genital herpes. More commonly in myeloma, infections with *Varicella-zoster virus* (VZV) are the problem. Bortezomib has been associated with a much higher risk of VZV infections compared to other drugs used to treat myeloma. Although VZV infections usually present as dermatomal zoster, there is a higher risk of dissemination in the immunocompromised patient, which can involve the viscera and, rarely, the central nervous system. The diagnosis is usually clinical but can be confirmed by PCR of vesicle fluid. The treatment of choice for VZV infections is aciclovir. This will need to be given intravenously at a dose of 10 mg/kg every 8 h (depending on renal function) to patients unable to take oral therapy or those who are ill. For less severely affected patients, the prodrug valaciclovir can be given orally and will result in blood levels of aciclovir almost as high as those achieved by intravenous therapy.

Cytomegalovirus (CMV) infections are really only a problem in myeloma following stem cell transplantation [26]. Here the T cell dysfunction from conditioning and immunosuppresion increases the risk of CMV reactivation. Reactivation is the most common problem and is most likely in patients who are CMV-seropositive at the outset of treatment but CMV can also be acquired *de novo* [27]. Infection may initially manifest as a fever but can also present with organ-specific symptoms or signs. Apart from fever, pneumonitis, with progressive hypoxia, is probably the most common, and serious, problem but gastrointestinal disease, with diarrhoea (sometimes with blood) occurs, as does hepatitis. Rarely, CMV can cause a pancytopenia or affect the central nervous system. In the rare myeloma patient receiving an allogeneic stem cell transplant, there is also the risk of late CMV disease occurring with graft-versus-host disease. In this setting CMV retinitis is an increasingly recognized problem. Diagnosis of CMV disease as a cause of fever can be made by either PCR for CMV DNA or antigen detection (pp65) in peripheral blood. A rise in the semi-quantitative PCR, or a rising antigen titer, indicate the need for treatment. Organ-specific disease can be diagnosed by the clinical symptoms in conjunction with increasing CMV viremia or by demonstration of the virus in the tissue when biopsied. Tissue diagnosis is preferred, particularly in pneumonitis, as CMV shedding can occur in the absence of disease. Classical CMV inclusions may be seen or the virus may be demonstrated by immunohistology. Treatment of CMV disease relies on intravenous ganciclovir. For disease affecting the gut or the eye, this is probably sufficient. Many practitioners will treat CMV pneumonitis with a combination of ganciclovir and intravenous immunoglobulin (IVIG) or CMV-specific IgG [28]. The evidence base for this is not compelling but the practice is driven by the high mortality associated with lung involvement. Ganciclovir-resistant CMV occurs and needs to be treated either with foscarnet or cidofovir, both of which have more troublesome side effects than ganciclovir. Foscarnet is a particular problem in myeloma because of its renal toxicity and electrolyte disturbance, along with neurological side-effects, but may be necessary to avoid marrow toxicity. Cidofovir can also be nephrotoxic and is marrow-suppressive. The role of the new anti-CMV drug, maribavir, is uncertain at this stage.

More recently in stem cell transplant recipients, disease from reactivation of human herpesvirus

6 (HHV6) has been recognized. Although this might just cause a fever, the most important syndrome is a form of limbic encephalitis with seizures and cognitive impairment [29]. There is no recognized treatment for this complication. Respiratory viruses, such as adenovirus, respiratory syncytial virus (RSV) and metapneumovirus may cause upper and lower respiratory disease but there are no established treatments that have shown to be effective.

Hepatitis viruses

In addition to herpesviruses, hepatitis viruses can also cause problems in immunosuppressed patients. This can either be from reactivation of hepatitis B or hepatitis C in a patient carrying these viruses or as a result of transmission via allogeneic stem cell transplant donors. Hepatitis B may be reactivated by high-dose steroid therapy or following stem cell transplantation. This is usually manifested by a hepatitis flare and, rarely, by fulminant hepatitis. In addition to those already known to be HBsAg positive, patients who are HBsAg negative but hepatitis B core antibody (HBcAb) positive may reactivate [30]. Those who become antigen positive should be treated with an appropriate anti-hepatitis B drug such as lamivudine or entecavir, with appropriate infectious diseases or hepatology advice. There may be a risk of hepatitis C reactivation as well but this is less clear and not reported as a problem in myeloma. It is possible that the presence of hepatitis viruses increases the risk of diseases such as myeloma but the data are far from conclusive.

Protozoan parasites and helminths

Protozoans

Generally, protozoan infections are rare as a complication in myeloma. The most common is *Toxoplasma gondii*. This parasite, usually dormant after asymptomatic infection, can become reactivated in the immunocompromised patient. In myeloma, this is most likely to arise after stem cell transplantation, particularly if the patient has received an allogeneic transplant. Symptomatic infection usually results in encephalitis or cerebral abscesses but pulmonary infection and disseminated disease also occur. Individuals who are seronegative for toxoplasma IgG are unlikely to develop disease and there is some suggestion that seropositive patients are less likely to reactivate if the bone marrow donor is also

seropositive [31]. Diagnosis of disease can be made from tissue biopsy or from documenting a rising antibody titer. More recently PCR of toxoplasma DNA from blood has been used to diagnose disease in immunocompromised patients. Treatment is with combination therapy; either clindamycin plus pyrimethamine, or sulphadiazine plus pyrimethamine. Because of concerns about marrow suppression with these folate antagonists, folinic acid is often given.

The other protozoan parasite that could potentially complicate therapy for myeloma is *Leishmania*. Patients from endemic countries may harbor this parasite and there is a slight risk that reactivation could occur if the individual is immunosuppressed. Symptoms and signs include fever, pancytopenia and hepato-splenomegaly. Treatment is with liposomal amphotericin B but expert advice should be sought.

Helminth infections

The only worm likely to complicate myeloma treatment is *Strongyloides stercoralis* [32]. This is the only important helminth infection in this setting because of the possibility of auto-infection; not a feature of other worm infections in humans. Immunosuppression, such as occurs with stem cell transplantation, can lead to a hyperinfection syndrome with the helminth larvae migrating from the gut widely through tissues. In rare instances, the central nervous system is involved as the larvae penetrate the meninges, carrying Gram-negative bacteria from the gut with them and causing severe bacterial meningitis. Hyperinfection is a serious problem and only occasionally responds to treatment with specific anti-helminth drugs, such as ivermectin. Consideration should be given to screening patients from endemic areas prior to stem cell transplantation, using stool microscopy and serology.

Strategies for preventing infection in myeloma patients

Given the increased risk of infection in patients with myeloma, it is reasonable to consider what preventive measures can be put in place to mitigate the risks. These measures range from general things, such as good line care, through to antimicrobial chemoprophylaxis and vaccination. It might be helpful to assess the various risk factors present in an individual patient before deciding whether, and which, prophylactic measures are required.

Antimicrobial prophylaxis

Perhaps the most useful drug for prophylaxis in myeloma is co-trimoxazole (trimethoprim-sulphamethoxazole), ideally given on a daily basis. The risk of PCP is considerable for patients receiving high dose corticosteroids as part of their treatment and this risk can be reduced by prophylactic co-trimoxazole. This drug has the added benefit of preventing toxoplasmosis and, as a general broad-spectrum antibiotic, may reduce the incidence of bacterial infections, such as *S. pneumoniae*.

The use of other antibiotics in myeloma is controversial. There are some who recommend their use in patients receiving high-dose dexamethasone along with various chemotherapy regimens as this treatment is associated with a high risk of bacterial infection [33]. Such prophylaxis might also be used in high risk patients undergoing re-treatment. One suggestion has been to assess the response to a single dose of G-CSF in patients just before autografting and to focus on those with poor responses as they seem to be more likely to have infective complications [34]. However, there are concerns about selecting more resistant organisms if prophylaxis is used and there is a risk of provoking diarrhoea from *Clostridium difficile* infection of the gut.

Because of the increased incidence of VZV infection when bortezomib is used to treat myeloma, some form of aciclovir prophylaxis should be used. Aciclovir is usually the drug of choice as it is well tolerated and cheap [35]. Aciclovir should also be used prophylactically in other patients if there is a history of recurrent cold sores or genital herpes, or if they are seropositive for VZV. Although not strictly prophylactic, ganciclovir or valganciclovir can be given as pre-emptive treatment if CMV antigenemia is being monitored on a weekly basis and the levels rise [36]. This should be considered in patients who have had a lot of treatment in the past or in those undergoing stem cell transplantation.

Antifungal prophylaxis is most commonly given in the form of oral fluconazole, mainly to reduce the incidence of oro-pharyngeal candidiasis. It is not likely to prevent invasive disease. Third generation antifungals, such as voriconazole, should be used as secondary prophylaxis in patients who have already been diagnosed with invasive aspergillosis in the past and are still undergoing myeloma treatment. Posaconazole is the only drug shown to be effective for primary prophylaxis and, hence, licensed for this indication but this should be reserved for patients at high risk of invasive fungal infection [37]. In high risk patients, such as those undergoing stem cell transplantation, some centers routinely measure galactomannan and initiate systemic antifungal therapy pre-emptively if the galactomannan levels rise rather than use primary prophylaxis.

Immunoglobulin and vaccinations

One study has shown that the administration of intravenous immunoglobulin (IVIG) every four weeks can reduce bacterial infections in patients with myeloma but this was done in patients receiving older, more moderate chemotherapy in the absence of prophylactic antibiotics [38]. However, a more recent meta-analysis has concluded that there is little benefit from IVIG in myeloma [39]. Immunoglobulin therapy is costly and potentially dangerous as it is a human blood product. It is probably best reserved just for patients with severe immunoglobulin deficiency who have already had recurrent bacterial infections.

Vaccination against the common encapsulated bacteria that cause infections in myeloma appears reasonable but there is no good evidence that this is effective. It is unlikely that myeloma patients would form good antibody responses to the vaccines but there are no data on the response, in these patients, to the newer conjugate vaccines. With the increasing use of bortezomib, it could be useful to vaccinate patients who are VZV IgG negative with an inactivated VZV vaccine. A VZV subunit (glycoprotein E) vaccine with adjuvant is currently in clinical trials but there are no efficacy data yet on which to base a decision. Live attenuated VZV vaccine should not be given to non-immune patients with myeloma. Although influenza vaccine is often given to immunocompromised patients, there is no evidence that it is protective in myeloma. It may be more helpful to ensure that the patient's immediate family are immunized and to have a low threshold to starting a neuraminidase inhibitor, such as oseltamivir, during the influenza season if the patient develops a fever.

General measures

As pneumonia is one of the most common infective problems in myeloma, supporting patients in stopping smoking is an important intervention. It is also important to minimize renal injury as renal impairment increases the risk of infection. Attention should be paid to appropriate prevention of venous thrombo-embolism and to monitoring of blood sugar during corticosteroid therapy. Good dental and oral hygiene may reduce the risk of jaw osteonecrosis in those receiving bisphosphonates. It is also important that indwelling central venous catheters are handled carefully with good hand hygiene and strict aseptic measures.

Conclusions

Infections remain a problem in the management of myeloma and, as advances in myeloma treatment continue, it is likely that new infective problems will arise. Although diagnostic tests have improved and clinicians are more alert to the risk of infections, there are increasing problems with drug resistance, particularly in bacterial infections. Fungal infections are likely to become more important with the increasing use of stem cell transplantation and longer survival of this patient group. Newer azoles and echinocandins represent better drugs than have previously been available but have not noticeably increased survival in a significant way. Earlier diagnosis of invasive fungal infection is crucial and there has been some progress with the use of antigen detection and better imaging, but there is still a need to show that this results in better survival.

References

1. Augustson, B. M., Begum, G., Dunn, J. A. *et al.* Early mortality after diagnosis of multiple myeloma: analysis of patients entered onto the United Kingdom Medical Research Council trials between 1980 and 2002–Medical Research Council Adult Leukaemia Working Party. *J. Clin. Oncol.* 2005;**23**(36):9219–26.

2. Schutt, P., Brandhorst, D., Stellberg, W. *et al.* Immune parameters in multiple myeloma patients: influence of treatment and correlation with opportunistic infections. *Leuk. Lymphoma* 2006;**47**(8):1570–82.

3. Engelich, G., Wright, D. G., Hartshorn, K. L. Acquired disorders of phagocyte function complicating medical and surgical illnesses. *Clin. Infect. Dis.* 2001; **33**(12):2040–8.

4. Wimalawansa, S. J. Bisphosphonate-associated osteomyelitis of the jaw: guidelines for practicing clinicians. *Endocr. Pract.* 2008; **14**(9):1150–68.

5. Chanan-Khan, A., Sonneveld, P., Schuster, M. W. *et al.* Analysis of herpes zoster events among bortezomib-treated patients in the phase III APEX study. *J. Clin. Oncol.* 2008;**26**(29):4784–90.

6. Basler, M., Lauer, C., Beck, U., Groettrup, M. The proteasome inhibitor bortezomib enhances the susceptibility to viral infection. *J. Immunol.* 2009;**183**(10): 6145–50.

7. Costa, D. B., Shin, B., Cooper, D. L. Pneumococcemia as the presenting feature of multiple myeloma. *Am. J. Hematol.* 2004;**77**(3):277–81.

8. Tleyjeh, I. M., Tlaygeh, H. M., Hejal, R., Montori, V. M., Baddour, L. M. The impact of penicillin resistance on short-term mortality in hospitalized adults with pneumococcal pneumonia: a systematic review and meta-analysis. *Clin. Infect. Dis.* 2006;**42** (6):788–97.

9. Baddour, L. M., Yu, V. L., Klugman, K. P. *et al.* Combination antibiotic therapy lowers mortality among severely ill patients with pneumococcal bacteremia. *Am. J. Respir. Crit. Care. Med.* 2004;**170**(4):440–4.

10. Arnan, M., Gudiol, C., Calatayud, L. *et al.* Risk factors for, and clinical relevance of, faecal extended-spectrum beta-lactamase producing Escherichia coli (ESBL-EC) carriage in neutropenic patients with haematological malignancies. *Eur. J. Clin. Microbiol. Infect. Dis.* 2011;**30**(3):355–60.

11. Kelly, C. P., LaMont, J. T. Clostridium difficile – more difficult than ever. *N. Engl. J. Med.* 2008;**359**(18):1932–40.

12. Chopra, T., Chandrasekar, P., Salimnia, H. *et al.* Recent epidemiology of Clostridium difficile infection during hematopoietic stem cell transplantation. *Clin. Transplant* 2011;**25**(1):E82–7.

13. Freifeld, A. G., Bow, E. J., Sepkowitz, K. A. *et al.* Clinical practice guideline for the use of antimicrobial agents in neutropenic patients with cancer: 2010 update by the infectious diseases society of America. *Clin. Infect. Dis.* 2011;**52**(4): e56–93.

14. Moores, K. G. Safe and effective outpatient treatment of adults with chemotherapy-induced neutropenic fever. *Am. J. Health. Syst. Pharm.* 2007;**64**(7):717–22.

15. Marr, K. A., Carter, R. A., Boeckh, M., Martin, P., Corey, L. Invasive aspergillosis in allogeneic stem cell transplant recipients: changes in epidemiology and risk factors. *Blood* 2002;**100**(13):4358–66.

16. Mori, Y., Nagasaki, Y., Kamezaki, K. *et al.* High incidence of false-positive Aspergillus galactomannan test in multiple myeloma. *Am. J. Hematol.* 2010;**85**(6):449–51.

17. Pappas, P. G., Kauffman, C. A., Andes, D. et al. Clinical practice guidelines for the management of candidiasis: 2009 update by the Infectious Diseases Society of America. Clin. Infect. Dis. 2009;48 (5):503–35.

18. Lortholary, O., Ascioglu, S., Moreau, P. et al. Invasive aspergillosis as an opportunistic infection in nonallografted patients with multiple myeloma: a European Organization for Research and Treatment of Cancer/ Invasive Fungal Infections Cooperative Group and the Intergroupe Francais du Myelome. Clin. Infect. Dis. 2000;30(1):41–6.

19. Segal, B. H. Aspergillosis. N. Engl. J. Med. 2009;360(18):1870–84.

20. Panackal, A. A., Li, H., Kontoyiannis, D. P. et al. Geoclimatic influences on invasive aspergillosis after hematopoietic stem cell transplantation. Clin. Infect. Dis. 2010;50(12):1588–97.

21. Cordonnier, C., Pautas, C., Maury, S. et al. Empirical versus preemptive antifungal therapy for high-risk, febrile, neutropenic patients: a randomized, controlled trial. Clin. Infect. Dis. 2009;48 (8):1042–51.

22. Sun, H. Y., Singh, N. Mucormycosis: its contemporary face and management strategies. Lancet. Infect. Dis. 2011;11 (4):301–11.

23. Hahn-Ast, C., Glasmacher, A., Muckter, S. et al. Overall survival and fungal infection-related mortality in patients with invasive fungal infection and neutropenia after myelosuppressive chemotherapy in a tertiary care centre from 1995 to 2006. J. Antimicrob. Chemother. 2010;65 (4):761–8.

24. Roblot, F., Le Moal, G., Godet, C. et al. Pneumocystis carinii pneumonia in patients with hematologic malignancies: a descriptive study. J. Infect. 2003;47 (1):19–27.

25. Saag, M. S., Graybill, R. J., Larsen, R. A. et al. Practice guidelines for the management of cryptococcal disease. Infectious Diseases Society of America. Clin. Infect. Dis. 2000;30(4):710–18.

26. Fassas, A. B., Bolanos-Meade, J., Buddharaju, L. N. et al. Cytomegalovirus infection and non-neutropenic fever after autologous stem cell transplantation: high rates of reactivation in patients with multiple myeloma and lymphoma. Br. J. Haematol. 2001;112(1):237–41.

27. Kroger, N., Zabelina, T., Kruger, W. et al. Patient cytomegalovirus seropositivity with or without reactivation is the most important prognostic factor for survival and treatment-related mortality in stem cell transplantation from unrelated donors using pretransplant in vivo T-cell depletion with anti-thymocyte globulin. Br. J. Haematol. 2001;113(4):1060–71.

28. Boeckh, M., Ljungman, P. How we treat cytomegalovirus in hematopoietic cell transplant recipients. Blood 2009;113 (23):5711–19.

29. Zerr, D. M., Fann, J. R., Breiger, D. et al. HHV-6 reactivation and its effect on delirium and cognitive functioning in hematopoietic cell transplantation recipients. Blood 2011;117(19):5243–9.

30. Matsue, K., Aoki, T., Odawara, J. et al. High risk of hepatitis B-virus reactivation after hematopoietic cell transplantation in hepatitis B core antibody-positive patients. Eur. J. Haematol. 2009;83(4):357–64.

31. Derouin, F., Pelloux, H. Prevention of toxoplasmosis in transplant patients. Clin. Microbiol. Infect. 2008;14(12):1089–101.

32. Orlent, H., Crawley, C., Cwynarski, K., Dina, R., Apperley, J. Strongyloidiasis pre and post autologous peripheral blood stem cell transplantation. Bone.

Marrow. Transplant 2003;32(1): 115–17.

33. Cesana, C., Nosari, A. M., Klersy, C. et al. Risk factors for the development of bacterial infections in multiple myeloma treated with two different vincristine-adriamycin-dexamethasone schedules. Haematologica 2003;88(9):1022–8.

34. Straka, C., Sandherr, M., Salwender, H. et al. Testing G-CSF responsiveness predicts the individual susceptibility to infection and consecutive treatment in recipients of high-dose chemotherapy. Blood 2011;117(7):2121–8.

35. Vickrey, E., Allen, S., Mehta, J., Singhal, S. Acyclovir to prevent reactivation of varicella zoster virus (herpes zoster) in multiple myeloma patients receiving bortezomib therapy. Cancer 2009;115(1):229–32.

36. Ayala, E., Greene, J., Sandin, R. et al. Valganciclovir is safe and effective as pre-emptive therapy for CMV infection in allogeneic hematopoietic stem cell transplantation. Bone. Marrow. Transplant 2006;37(9):851–6.

37. Cornely, O. A., Maertens, J., Winston, D. J. et al. Posaconazole vs. fluconazole or itraconazole prophylaxis in patients with neutropenia. N. Engl. J. Med. 2007;356(4):348–59.

38. Chapel, H. M., Lee, M., Hargreaves, R., Pamphilon, D. H., Prentice, A. G. Randomised trial of intravenous immunoglobulin as prophylaxis against infection in plateau-phase multiple myeloma. The UK Group for Immunoglobulin Replacement Therapy in Multiple Myeloma. Lancet 1994;343(8905):1059–63.

39. Raanani, P., Gafter-Gvili, A., Paul, M. et al. Immunoglobulin prophylaxis in chronic lymphocytic leukemia and multiple myeloma: systematic review and meta-analysis. Leuk. Lymphoma 2009;50(5):764–72.

Index